TENTH EDITION

Ross and Wilson

Anatomy
and
Physiology
in Health and Illness

For Elsevier:

Senior Commissioning Editor: Ninette Premdas
Project Development Manager: Mairi McCubbin
Project Manager: Frances Affleck
Senior Designer: Sarah Russell
Illustrations Manager: Bruce Hogarth

TENTH EDITION

Ross and Wilson

Anatomy and Physiology

in Health and Illness

Anne Waugh BSc(Hons) MSc CertEd SRN RNT ILTM

Acting Head, School of Acute and Continuing Care Nursing,
Napier University, Edinburgh, UK

Allison Grant BSc PhD RGN

Lecturer, Department of Biological and Biomedical Sciences,
Glasgow Caledonian University, Glasgow, UK

Illustrations by Graeme Chambers

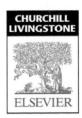

EDINBURGH, LONDON, NEW YORK, OXFORD, PHILADELPHIA, ST LOUIS, SYDNEY, TORONTO 2006

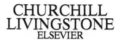

An imprint of Elsevier Limited

Main Edition
First edition 1963
Second edition 1966
Third edition 1968
Fourth edition 1973
Fifth edition 1981
Sixth edition 1987
Seventh edition 1990
Eighth edition 1996
Ninth edition 2001
Tenth edition 2006
  Reprinted 2007, 2008

ISBN: 978-0-443-10101-4

International Student Edition
First published 1991
Eighth edition 1996
Ninth edition 2001
Tenth edition 2006
  Reprinted 2006, 2007 (twice), 2008

ISBN: 978-0-443-10102-1

British Library Cataloguing in Publication Data
A catalogue record for this book is available from the British Library

Library of Congress Cataloging in Publication Data
A catalog record for this book is available from the Library of Congress

Notice
Neither the Publisher nor the Authors assumes any responsibility for any loss or injury and/or damage to persons or property arising out of or related to any use of the material contained in this book. It is the responsibility of the treating practitioner, relying on independent expertise and knowledge of the patient, to determine the best treatment and method of application for the patient.

The Publisher

Working together to grow
libraries in developing countries

www.elsevier.com | www.bookaid.org | www.sabre.org

ELSEVIER   BOOK AID International   Sabre Foundation

ELSEVIER   your source for books, journals and multimedia in the health sciences

www.elsevierhealth.com

The publisher's policy is to use paper manufactured from sustainable forests

Printed in China

Contents

Preface

Ross and Wilson has been a core text for students of anatomy and physiology for over 40 years. This latest edition is aimed at healthcare professionals including nurses, students of nursing, the allied health professions, complementary and alternative medicine, paramedics and ambulance technicians, many of whom have found previous editions invaluable. It retains the straightforward approach to the description of body systems and how they work, and the normal anatomy and physiology is followed by a section that covers common disorders and diseases: pathology.

The human body is described system by system. The reader must, however, remember that physiology is an integrated subject and that, although the systems are considered in separate chapters, they must all function cooperatively to maintain health. The first three chapters provide an overview of the body and describe its main structures.

The later chapters are organised into three further sections, reflecting those areas essential for normal body function: communication; intake of raw materials and elimination of waste; and protection and survival. A new chapter on genetics has been included, reflecting the increasing importance of this branch of science in human affairs; a section outlining the fetal circulation and functions of the placenta has been added; and the musculoskeletal material has been collated and integrated into one new chapter, making it more straightforward for the reader. Much of the material for this edition has been revised and rewritten, and new diagrams included.

Features introduced in the last edition have been retained and revised, including learning outcomes and a list of common prefixes, suffixes and roots, providing examples of common terminology used in the study of anatomy and physiology. Some biological values, extracted from the text, are presented as an Appendix for easy reference. In some cases, slight variations in 'normals' may be found in other texts and used by different medical practitioners.

The material presented in this textbook is supported by the accompanying *Colouring and Workbook*, which gives students the opportunity to test their learning and improve their revision skills.

Edinburgh, 2006

Anne Waugh
Allison Grant

Acknowledgements

The 10th edition of this textbook would not have been possible without the efforts of many people. In preparing this edition, we have continued to build on the foundations established by Kathleen Wilson and we would like to acknowledge her immense contribution to the success of this title.

We are grateful to Graeme Chambers for his patience in the preparation of the new and revised artwork.

We are also grateful to readers of the ninth edition for their feedback and constructive comments, many of which have influenced the current revision.

We are also grateful to the staff of Churchill Livingstone, particularly Mairi McCubbin, Ninette Premdas, Kirsty Guest and Nina Mosgrove, for their support and hospitality.

Thanks are also due to our families, Andy, Michael, Seona and Struan, for their continued patience, support and acceptance of lost evenings and weekends.

Common prefixes, suffixes and roots

Prefix/suffix/root	To do with	Examples in the text
a-/an-	*lack of*	anuria, agranulocyte, asystole, anaemia
-aemia	*of the blood*	anaemia, hypoxaemia, uraemia, hypovolaemia
angio-	*vessel*	angiotensin, haemangioma
anti-	*against*	antidiuretic, anticoagulant, antigen, antimicrobial
-blast	*germ, bud*	reticuloblast, osteoblast
brady-	*slow*	bradycardia
broncho-	*bronchus*	bronchiole, bronchitis, bronchus
card-	*heart*	cardiac, myocardium, tachycardia
chole-	*bile*	cholecystokinin, cholecystitis, cholangitis
cyto-/-cyte	*cell*	erythrocyte, cytosol, cytoplasm, cytotoxic
derm-	*skin*	dermatitis, dermatome, dermis
dys-	*difficult*	dysuria, dyspnoea, dysmenorrhoea, dysplasia
-ema	*swelling*	oedema, emphysema, lymphoedema
endo-	*inner*	endocrine, endocytosis, endothelium
erythro-	*red*	erythrocyte, erythropoietin, erythropoiesis
exo-	*outside*	exocytosis, exophthalmos
extra-	*outside*	extracellular, extrapyramidal
-fferent	*carry*	afferent, efferent
gast-	*stomach*	gastric, gastrin, gastritis, gastrointestinal
-gen-	*origin/production*	gene, genome, genetic, antigen, pathogen, allergen
-globin	*protein*	myoglobin, haemoglobin
haem-	*blood*	haemostasis, haemorrhage, haemolytic
-hydr-	*water*	dehydration, hydrostatic, hydrocephalus
hepat-	*liver*	hepatic, hepatitis, hepatomegaly, hepatocyte
hyper-	*excess/above*	hypertension, hypertrophy, hypercapnia
hypo-	*below/under*	hypoglycaemia, hypotension, hypovolaemia
intra-	*within*	intracellular, intracranial, intraocular
-ism	*condition*	hyperthyroidism, dwarfism, rheumatism
-itis	*inflammation*	appendicitis, hepatitis, cystitis, gastritis
lact-	*milk*	lactation, lactic, lacteal
lymph-	*lymph tissue*	lymphocyte, lymphatic, lymphoedema
lyso-/-lysis	*breaking down*	lysosome, glycolysis, lysozyme
-mega-	*large*	megaloblast, acromegaly, splenomegaly, hepatomegaly
micro-	*small*	microbe, microtubules, microvilli

Prefix/suffix/root	To do with	Examples in the text
myo-	*muscle*	myocardium, myoglobin, myopathy, myosin
neo-	*new*	neoplasm, gluconeogenesis, neonate
nephro-	*kidney*	nephron, nephrotic, nephroblastoma, nephrosis
neuro-	*nerve*	neurone, neuralgia, neuropathy
-oid	*resembling*	myeloid, sesamoid, sigmoid
-oma	*tumour*	carcinoma, melanoma, fibroma
-ophth-	*eye*	xerophthalmia, ophthalmic, exophthalmos
-ory	*referring to*	secretory, sensory, auditory, gustatory
osteo-	*bone*	osteocyte, osteoarthritis, osteoporosis
-path-	*disease*	athogenesis, neuropathy, nephropathy
-plasm	*substance*	cytoplasm, neoplasm
pneumo-	*lung/air*	pneumothorax, pneumonia, pneumotoxic
poly-	*many*	polypeptide, polyuria, polycythaemia
-rrhagia	*excessive flow*	menorrhagia
-rrhoea	*discharge*	dysmenorrhoea, diarrhoea, rhinorrhoea
sub-	*under*	subphrenic, subarachnoid, sublingual
tachy-	*excessively fast*	tachycardia
thrombo-	*clot*	thrombocyte, thrombosis, thrombin, thrombus
-tox-	*poison*	toxin, cytotoxic, hepatotoxic
-uria	*urine*	anuria, polyuria, haematuria, nocturia
vas, vaso-	*vessel*	vasoconstriction, vas deferens, vascular

The body and its constituents

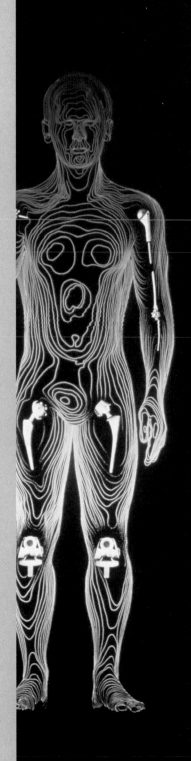

Introduction to the human body

1

The human body is rather like a highly technical and sophisticated machine. It operates as a single entity, but is made up of a number of systems that work interdependently. Each system is associated with a specific, and sometimes related, function that is normally essential for the well-being of the individual. Should one system fail, the consequences are likely to extend to other systems, and may reduce the ability of the body to function normally. Integrated working of the body systems ensures the ability of the individual to survive. The human body is therefore complex in both structure and function, and this book aims to explain the fundamental structures and processes involved.

Anatomy is the study of the structure of the body and the physical relationships involved between body systems. *Physiology* is the study of how the systems of the body work, and the ways in which their integrated cooperation maintains life and health of the individual. *Pathology* is the study of abnormalities and how they affect body functions, often causing illness. Building on the normal anatomy and physiology, relevant illnesses are considered at the end of the later chapters.

Levels of structural complexity

Learning outcome

After studying this section you should be able to:

■ describe the levels of structural complexity within the body.

Within the body are different levels of structural organisation and complexity (Fig. 1.1). The lowest level is chemical. *Atoms* combine to form *molecules*, of which there are a vast range in the body. The structures, properties and functions of important biological molecules are considered in Chapter 2. *Cells* are the smallest independent units of living matter and there are trillions of them within the body. They are too small to be seen with the naked eye, but when magnified using a microscope different types can be distinguished by their size, shape and the dyes they absorb when stained in the laboratory. Each cell type has become *specialised*, and carries out a particular function that contributes to body needs. In complex organisms such as the human body, cells with similar structures and functions are found together, forming *tissues*. The structure and functions of cells and tissues are explored in Chapter 3.

Organs are made up of a number of different types of tissue and have evolved to carry out a specific function.

Systems consist of a number of organs and tissues that together contribute to one or more survival needs of the body. The human body has several systems, which work interdependently carrying out specific functions. All are required for health. The structure and functions of body systems are considered in later chapters.

The internal environment and homeostasis

Learning outcomes

After studying this section you should be able to:

■ define the terms internal environment and homeostasis

■ compare and contrast negative and positive feedback control mechanisms

■ outline the potential consequences of homeostatic imbalance.

The *external environment* surrounds the body and provides the oxygen and nutrients required by all body cells. Waste products of cellular activity are eventually excreted into the external environment. The skin provides a barrier between the dry external environment (the atmosphere) and the aqueous (water-based) environment of most body cells.

The *internal environment* is the water-based medium in which body cells exist. Cells are bathed in fluid called *interstitial* or *tissue fluid*. Oxygen and other substances they require must pass from the internal transport systems through the interstitial fluid to reach them. Similarly, cellular waste products must move through the interstitial fluid to the transport systems to be excreted.

Each cell is surrounded by the *plasma membrane*, which provides a potential barrier to substances entering or leaving. The structure of membranes (p. 30) confers certain properties, in particular *selective permeability* or *semipermeability*. This prevents large molecules moving between the cell and the interstitial fluid (Fig. 1.2). Smaller particles can usually pass through the membrane, some more readily than others, and therefore the chemical composition of the fluid inside is different from that outside the cell.

Homeostasis

The composition of the internal environment is tightly controlled, and this fairly constant state is called

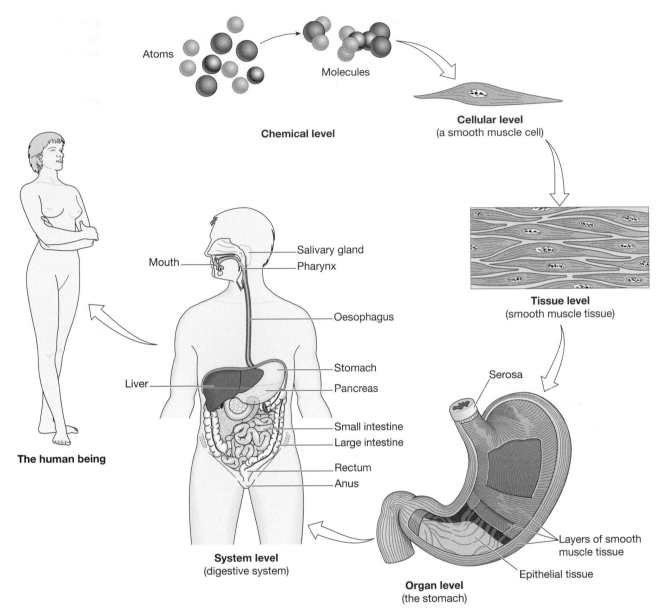

Atoms

Molecules

Chemical level

Cellular level
(a smooth muscle cell)

Tissue level
(smooth muscle tissue)

Mouth
Salivary gland
Pharynx

Oesophagus

Liver
Stomach
Pancreas

Serosa

Small intestine
Large intestine

Rectum
Anus

The human being

Layers of smooth
muscle tissue

Epithelial tissue

System level
(digestive system)

Organ level
(the stomach)

Figure 1.1 The levels of structural complexity.

homeostasis. Literally, this term means 'unchanging', but in practice it describes a dynamic, ever-changing situation kept within narrow limits. When this balance is threatened or lost, there is a serious risk to the well-being of the individual. There are many factors in the internal environment which must be maintained within narrow limits and some of them are listed in Box 1.1.

Homeostasis is maintained by control systems that detect and respond to changes in the internal environment. A control system (Fig. 1.3) has three basic components: detector, control centre and effector. The *control centre* determines the limits within which the variable factor should be maintained. It receives an input from the

detector, or sensor, and integrates the incoming information. When the incoming signal indicates that an adjustment is needed, the control centre responds and its output to the *effector* is changed. This is a dynamic process that allows constant readjustment of many physiological variables.

Negative feedback mechanisms

In systems controlled by negative feedback, the effector response decreases or negates the effect of the original stimulus, maintaining or restoring homeostasis (thus the term negative feedback). Control of body temperature is

5

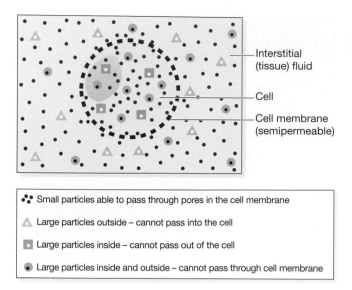

Figure 1.2 legend:

- Small particles able to pass through pores in the cell membrane
- Large particles outside – cannot pass into the cell
- Large particles inside – cannot pass out of the cell
- Large particles inside and outside – cannot pass through cell membrane

Figure 1.2 Diagram of a cell with a semipermeable membrane.

Box 1.1 Examples of physiological variables

Core temperature
Water and electrolyte concentrations
pH (acidity or alkalinity) of body fluids
Blood glucose levels
Blood and tissue oxygen and carbon dioxide levels
Blood pressure

similar to the non-physiological example of a domestic central heating system. The thermostat (temperature detector) is sensitive to changes in room temperature (variable factor). The thermostat is connected to the boiler control unit (control centre), which controls the boiler (effector). The thermostat constantly compares the information from the detector with the preset temperature and, when necessary, adjustments are made to alter the room temperature. When the thermostat detects the room temperature is low, it switches the boiler on. The result is output of heat by the boiler, warming the room. When the preset temperature is reached, the system is reversed. The thermostat detects the higher room temperature and turns the boiler off. Heat production from the boiler stops and the room slowly cools as heat is lost. This series of events is a negative feedback mechanism and it enables continuous self-regulation or control of a variable factor within a narrow range.

Body temperature is a physiological variable controlled by negative feedback (Fig. 1.4). When body tem-

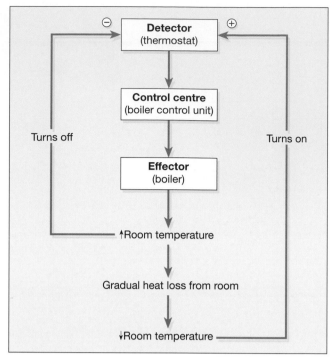

Figure 1.3 Example of a negative feedback mechanism: control of room temperature by a domestic boiler.

perature falls below the preset level, this is detected by specialised temperature sensitive nerve endings. They transmit this information to groups of cells in the hypothalamus of the brain, which form the control centre. The control centre then activates mechanisms that raise body temperature (effectors). These include:

- stimulation of skeletal muscles causing shivering
- narrowing of the blood vessels in the skin reducing the blood flow to, and heat loss from, the peripheries
- behavioural changes, e.g. we put on more clothes or curl up.

When body temperature rises to within the normal range, the temperature sensitive nerve endings no longer stimulate the cells of the control centre and therefore the output of this centre to the effectors ceases.

Most of the homeostatic controls in the body use negative feedback mechanisms to prevent sudden and serious changes in the internal environment. Many more of these are explained in the following chapters.

Positive feedback mechanisms

There are only a few of these *amplifier* or *cascade systems* in the body. In positive feedback mechanisms, the stimulus progressively increases the response, so that as long as the stimulus is continued the response is progressively

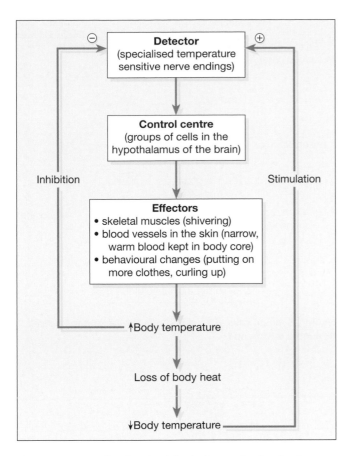

Figure 1.4 Example of a physiological negative feedback mechanism: control of body temperature.

Survival needs of the body

Learning outcomes

After studying this section you should be able to:

■ describe the roles of the body transport systems

■ outline the roles of the nervous and endocrine systems in internal communication

■ outline how raw materials are absorbed by the body

■ state the waste materials eliminated from the body

■ outline activities undertaken by an individual for protection and survival.

By convention, the body systems are described separately in the study of anatomy and physiology, but in reality they are all interdependent. This section provides an introduction to body activities, linking them to survival needs (Table 1.1). The later chapters build on this framework, exploring human structure and functions in health and illness using a systems approach.

amplified. Examples include blood clotting and uterine contractions during labour.

During labour, contractions of the uterus are stimulated by the hormone *oxytocin*. These force the baby's head into the cervix of the uterus, stimulating stretch receptors there. In response to this, more oxytocin is released, further strengthening the contractions and maintaining labour. After the baby is born the stimulus (stretching of the cervix) is no longer present so the release of oxytocin stops (see Fig. 9.5, p. 217).

Homeostatic imbalance

This arises when the fine control of a factor in the internal environment is inadequate and the level of the factor falls outside the normal range. If the control system cannot maintain homeostasis, an abnormal state develops that may threaten health, or even life. Many such situations are explained in later chapters.

Survival need	Body activities
Communication	Transport systems: blood, circulatory system, lymphatic system
	Internal communication: nervous system, endocrine system
	External communication: special senses, verbal and non-verbal communication
Intake of raw materials and elimination of waste	Intake of oxygen
	Diet
	Elimination of waste: carbon dioxide, urine, faeces
Protection and survival	Protection against the external environment: skin
	Resistance and immunity: non-specific and specific defence mechanisms
	Body movement
	Transmission of inherited characteristics
	Reproduction

Table 1.1 **Survival needs and related body activities**

Communication

In this section, transport and communication are considered. Transport systems ensure that all cells have access to the internal and external environments; the blood, the circulatory system and lymphatic system are involved. All communication systems involve receiving, collating and responding to appropriate information.

There are different systems for communicating with the internal and external environments. Internal communication involves mainly the nervous and endocrine systems; these are important in the maintenance of homeostasis and regulation of vital body functions. Communication with the external environment involves the special senses, and verbal and non-verbal activities, and all of these also depend on the nervous system.

Transport systems

Blood

The blood transports substances around the body through a large network of blood vessels. In adults the body contains 5 to 6 litres of blood (see Ch. 4). It consists of two parts – a fluid called *plasma* and *blood cells* suspended in the plasma.

Plasma. This is mainly water with a wide range of substances dissolved or suspended in it. These include:

- nutrients absorbed from the alimentary canal
- oxygen absorbed from the lungs
- chemical substances synthesised by body cells, e.g. hormones
- waste materials produced by all cells to be eliminated from the body by excretion.

Blood cells. There are three distinct groups, classified according to their functions (Fig. 1.5).

Erythrocytes (red blood cells) are concerned with the transport of oxygen and, to a lesser extent, carbon dioxide between the lungs and all body cells.

Leukocytes (white blood cells) are mainly concerned with protection of the body against microbes and other potentially damaging substances that gain entry to the body. There are several types of leukocytes, which carry out their protective functions in different ways. These cells are larger and less numerous than erythrocytes.

Platelets (thrombocytes) are tiny cell fragments that play an essential part in blood clotting.

Circulatory system (Ch. 5)

This consists of a network of blood vessels and the heart (Fig. 1.6).

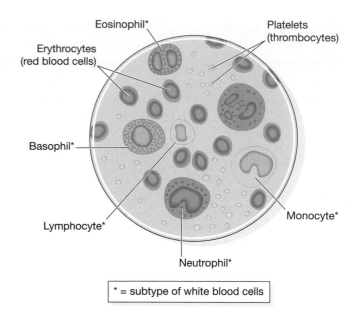

Figure 1.5 **Blood cells after staining in the laboratory viewed through a microscope.**

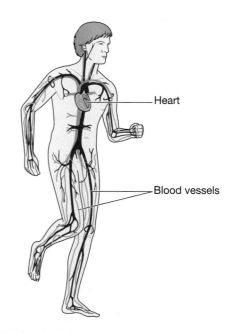

Figure 1.6 **The circulatory system.**

Blood vessels. There are three types:

- *arteries*, which carry blood away from the heart
- *veins*, which return blood to the heart
- *capillaries*, which link the arteries and veins.

Capillaries are tiny blood vessels with very thin walls consisting of only one layer of cells. They are the site of exchange of substances between the blood and body tissues, e.g. nutrients, oxygen and cellular waste products. Blood vessels form a network that transports blood to:

- the lungs (*pulmonary circulation*) where oxygen is absorbed from the air in the lungs and, at the same time, carbon dioxide is excreted from the blood into the air
- cells in all other parts of the body (*general* or *systemic circulation*).

Heart. The heart is a muscular sac. It pumps blood round the body and maintains the blood pressure in the lungs and general circulation.

The heart muscle is not under conscious (voluntary) control. At rest, the heart contracts, or beats, between 65 and 75 times per minute. The rate may be greatly increased during exercise, when the oxygen and nutritional needs of the muscles moving the limbs are increased, and in some emotional states.

The rate at which the heart beats can be counted by taking the *pulse*. The pulse can be felt most easily where a superficial artery can be pressed gently against a bone. The wrist is the site most commonly used for this purpose.

Lymphatic system

The lymphatic system (Ch. 6) consists of a series of *lymph vessels*, which begin as blind-ended tubes in the spaces between the blood capillaries and tissue cells (Fig. 1.7). Structurally they are similar to veins and blood capillaries but the pores in the walls of the lymph capillaries are larger than those of the blood capillaries. *Lymph* is tissue fluid containing large molecules, e.g. proteins, fragments of damaged tissue cells and microbes. It is transported along lymph vessels and returned to the bloodstream.

There are collections of *lymph nodes* situated at various points along the length of the lymph vessels. Lymph is filtered as it passes through the lymph nodes, and microbes and other materials are removed.

The lymphatic system provides the sites for formation and maturation of *lymphocytes*, the white blood cells involved in immunity (Ch. 15).

Internal communication

Communication and the nervous system

The nervous system is a rapid communication system (Ch. 7). The main components are shown in Figure 1.8.

The *central nervous system* consists of:

- the *brain*, situated inside the skull
- the *spinal cord*, which extends from the base of the skull to the lumbar region and is protected from injury by the bones of the spinal column.

The *peripheral nervous system* is a network of nerve fibres, which are:

- *sensory* or *afferent*, providing the brain with 'input' from organs and tissues, or
- *motor* or *efferent*, which convey nerve impulses carrying 'output' from the brain to effector organs: the muscles and glands.

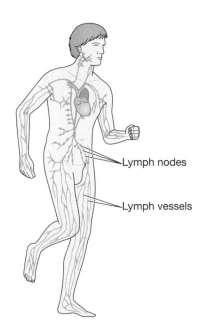

Figure 1.7 The lymphatic system: lymph nodes and vessels.

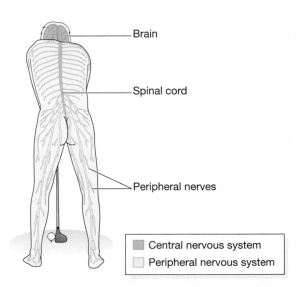

Brain

Spinal cord

Peripheral nerves

☐ Central nervous system
☐ Peripheral nervous system

Figure 1.8 The nervous system.

The *somatic (common) senses* are pain, touch, heat and cold, and they arise following stimulation of specialised sensory receptors at nerve endings found throughout the skin.

There are different receptors in muscles and joints that respond to changes in the position and orientation of the body, maintaining posture and balance. Yet other receptors are activated by stimuli in internal organs and maintain control of vital body functions, e.g. heart rate, respiratory rate and blood pressure. Stimulation of any of these receptors sets up impulses that are conducted to the brain in sensory (afferent) nerves. Communication along nerve fibres (cells) is by electrical impulses that are generated when nerve endings are stimulated.

Communication between nerve cells is also required, since more than one nerve is involved in the chain of events occurring between the initial stimulus and the reaction to it. Nerves communicate with each other by releasing a chemical (the *neurotransmitter*) into tiny gaps between them. The neurotransmitter quickly travels across the gap and either stimulates or inhibits the next nerve cell, thus ensuring the message is transmitted.

Sensory nerves and chemical substances circulating in the blood provide information to appropriate parts of the brain, which collates it and then responds via motor (efferent) nerves to effector organs, often through a negative feedback mechanism (see Fig. 1.3). Some of these activities are understood and perceived, e.g. pain, whereas others take place subconsciously, e.g. changes in blood pressure. Nerve impulses travel at great speed along nerve fibres leading to rapid responses, and adjustments to many body functions therefore occur within a few seconds.

Reflex actions are fast involuntary, and usually protective motor responses to specific stimuli. They include:

- withdrawal of a finger from a very hot surface
- constriction of the pupil in response to bright light
- control of blood pressure.

Communication and the endocrine system
The endocrine system consists of a number of discrete *glands* situated in different parts of the body. They synthesise and secrete chemical messengers called *hormones* that circulate round the body in the blood. Hormones stimulate *target glands* or *tissues*, influencing metabolic and other cellular activities and regulating body growth and maturation. Endocrine glands detect and respond to levels of particular substances in the blood, including specific hormones. Changes in blood hormone levels are usually controlled by negative feedback mechanisms (see Fig. 1.3). The endocrine system provides slower and more precise control of body functions than the nervous system.

Communication with the external environment

Special senses
These senses arise following stimulation of specialised sensory receptor cells located in sensory organs or tissues in the head. The senses and the special organs involved are shown in Box 1.2.

Although these senses are usually considered to be separate and different from each other, one sense is rarely used alone (Fig. 1.9). For example, when the smell of smoke is perceived then other senses such as sight and sound are used to try and locate the source of a fire. Similarly, taste and smell are closely associated in the enjoyment, or otherwise, of food. The brain collates incoming information with information from the memory and initiates a response by setting up electrical impulses in motor (efferent) nerves to effector organs, muscles and glands. Such responses enable the individual to escape from the fire, or to prepare the digestive system for eating.

Verbal communication
Sound is a means of communication that is produced in the larynx as a result of blowing air through the space between the *vocal cords* during expiration. Speech is the manipulation of sound by contraction of the muscles of the throat and cheeks, and movements of the tongue and lower jaw.

> **Box 1.2 The special senses and related sense organs**
>
> Sight – eyes
> Hearing – ears
> Balance – ears
> Smell – nose
> Taste – tongue

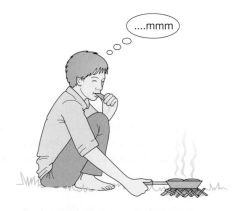

Figure 1.9 Combined use of the special senses: vision, hearing, smell and taste.

Non-verbal communication

Posture and movements are associated with non-verbal communication, e.g. nodding the head and shrugging the shoulders. The skeletal system provides the bony framework of the body (Ch. 16), and movement takes place at joints between bones. Skeletal muscles that move the skeleton attach bones to one another, spanning one or more joints in between. They are stimulated by the part of the nervous system under conscious (voluntary) control. Some non-verbal communication, e.g. changes in facial expression, may not involve the movement of bones.

Intake of raw materials and elimination of waste

This section considers substances taken into and excreted from the body. Oxygen, water and food are taken in, and carbon dioxide, urine and faeces are excreted.

Intake of oxygen

Oxygen gas makes up about 21% of atmospheric air. A continuous supply is essential for human life because it is needed for most chemical activities that take place in the body cells. Oxygen is necessary for the series of chemical reactions that result in the release of energy from nutrients.

The upper respiratory system carries air between the nose and the lungs during breathing (Ch. 10). Air passes through a system of passages consisting of the pharynx (also part of the digestive tract), the larynx (voice box), the trachea, two bronchi (one bronchus to each lung) and a large number of bronchial passages (Fig. 1.10). These end in alveoli, millions of tiny air sacs in each lung. They are surrounded by a network of tiny capillaries and are the sites where vital gas exchange between the lungs and the blood takes place (Fig. 1.11).

Nitrogen, which makes up about 80% of atmospheric air, is breathed in and out, but in this gaseous form it cannot be used by the body. The nitrogen needed by the body is present in protein-containing foods, mainly meat and fish.

Diet

Nutrition is considered in Chapter 11. A balanced diet is important for health and provides *nutrients*, substances that are absorbed, usually following digestion, and promote body function. Nutrients include water, carbohydrates, proteins, fats, vitamins and mineral salts. They are required for:

- maintaining water balance within the body
- energy production, mainly carbohydrates and fats

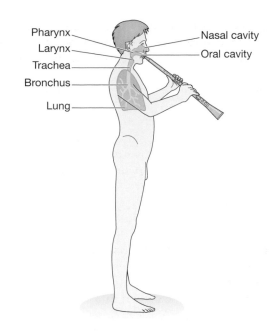

Figure 1.10 The respiratory system.

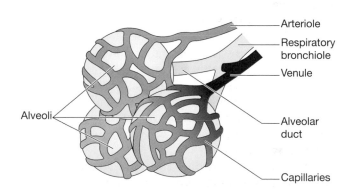

Figure 1.11 Alveoli: the site of gas exchange.

- synthesis of large and complex molecules, using mineral salts, proteins, fats, carbohydrates and vitamins
- cell building, growth and repair, especially proteins.

Digestion

The digestive system has evolved because food is chemically complex and seldom in a form the body cells can use. Its function is to break down, or digest, food so that it can be absorbed into the circulation and then used by body cells. The digestive system consists of the alimentary canal and accessory glands (Fig. 1.12).

Alimentary canal. This is essentially a tube that begins at the mouth and continues through the pharynx,

11

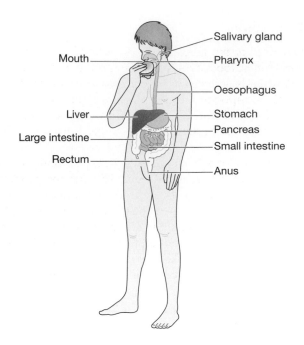

Figure 1.12 **The digestive system.**

oesophagus, stomach, small and large intestines, rectum and anus.

Glands. The accessory organs situated outside the alimentary canal with ducts leading into it are the *salivary glands*, the *pancreas* and the *liver*. There are also many tiny glands situated in the walls of the alimentary canal. Most of these glands synthesise *digestive enzymes* that are involved in the chemical breakdown of food.

Metabolism

This is the sum total of the chemical activity in the body. It consists of two groups of processes:

- *anabolism*, building or synthesising large and complex substances
- *catabolism*, breaking down substances to provide energy and raw materials for anabolism, and substances for excretion as waste.

The sources of energy are mainly the carbohydrates and fats provided by the diet. If these are in short supply, proteins are used.

Elimination of waste

Carbon dioxide

This is a waste product of cellular metabolism. Because it dissolves in body fluids to make an acid solution, it must be excreted in appropriate amounts to maintain pH (acidity or alkalinity) within the normal range. The main route of carbon dioxide excretion is through the lungs.

Urine

This is formed by the kidneys, which are part of the urinary system (Ch. 13). The organs of the urinary system are shown in Figure 1.13. Urine consists of water and waste products mainly of protein breakdown, e.g. urea. Under the influence of hormones from the endocrine system, the kidneys regulate water balance. They also play a role in maintaining blood pH within the normal range. The bladder stores urine until it is excreted during *micturition*.

Faeces

The waste materials from the digestive system are excreted as faeces during *defaecation*. They contain:

- indigestible food residue that remains in the alimentary canal because it cannot be absorbed
- bile from the liver, which contains the waste products from the breakdown of red blood cells
- large numbers of microbes.

Protection and survival

In this section relevant activities are outlined under the following headings: protection against the external environment, resistance and immunity, movement, transmission of inherited characteristics and reproduction.

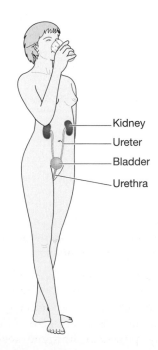

Figure 1.13 **The urinary system.**

Protection against the external environment

On the body surface, the skin (Ch. 14) provides this. It consists of two layers: the epidermis and the dermis.

The epidermis lies superficially and is composed of several layers of cells that grow towards the surface from its deepest layer. The surface layer consists of dead cells that are constantly being rubbed off and replaced from below. The epidermis constitutes the barrier between the moist internal environment and the dry atmosphere of the external environment.

The dermis contains tiny *sweat glands* that have little canals or ducts, leading to the surface. Hairs grow from follicles in the dermis. The layers of the skin form a barrier against invasion by microbes, chemicals and dehydration.

The dermis is rich in sensory nerve endings sensitive to pain, temperature and touch. It is a vast organ that constantly provides the central nervous system with sensory input from the body surfaces. The skin also plays an important role in regulation of body temperature.

Resistance and immunity

The body has many means of self-protection from invaders (Ch. 15). They are divided into two categories: specific and non-specific defence mechanisms.

Non-specific defence mechanisms

These are effective against any invaders. The protection provided by the skin is outlined above. In addition there are other protective features at body surfaces, e.g. *mucus* secreted by mucous membranes traps microbes and other foreign materials on its sticky surface. Some body fluids contain *antimicrobial substances*, e.g. gastric juice contains hydrochloric acid, which kills most ingested microbes. Following successful invasion other non-specific processes may occur, including the *inflammatory response*, which is also involved in tissue healing.

Specific defence mechanisms

The body generates a specific (immune) response against any substance it identifies as foreign. Such substances are called *antigens* and include:

- bacteria and other microbes
- cancer cells or transplanted tissue cells
- pollen from flowers and plants.

Following exposure to an antigen, lifelong immunity against further invasion by the same antigen often develops. Over a lifetime, an individual gradually builds up immunity to millions of antigens. Allergic reactions are abnormally powerful immune responses to an antigen that usually poses no threat to the body.

Movement

Movement of the whole body, or parts of it, is essential for obtaining food, avoiding injury and reproduction.

Most body movement is under conscious (voluntary) control. Exceptions include protective movements that are carried out before the individual is aware of them, e.g. the reflex action of removing the finger from a very hot surface.

The musculoskeletal system includes the bones of the skeleton, *skeletal muscles* and *joints*. The skeleton provides the rigid body framework and movement takes place at joints between two or more bones. Skeletal muscles (Fig. 1.14), under the control of the voluntary nervous system, maintain posture and balance, and move the skeleton. A brief description of the skeleton is given in Chapter 3, and a more detailed account of bones, muscles and joints is presented in Chapter 16.

Transmission of inherited characteristics

Individuals with the most advantageous genetic makeup are most likely to survive, reproduce and pass their genes on to the next generation. This is the basis of natural selection, i.e. 'survival of the fittest'. Chapter 17 explores the processes involved in the transmission of inherited characteristics.

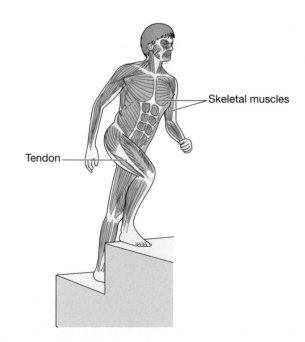

Skeletal muscles

Tendon

Figure 1.14 The skeletal muscles.

Reproduction (Ch. 18)

Successful reproduction is essential in order to ensure the continuation of a species and genetic characteristics from one generation to the next. Fertilisation occurs when a female egg cell or *ovum* fuses with a male sperm cell or *spermatozoon*. Ova are produced by two *ovaries* situated in the female pelvis (Fig. 1.15). Usually only one ovum is released at a time and it travels towards the *uterus* in the *uterine tube*. The spermatozoa are produced in large numbers by the two *testes*, situated in the *scrotum*. From each testis, spermatozoa pass through a duct called the *deferent duct* (vas deferens) to the *urethra*. During sexual intercourse (coitus) the spermatozoa are deposited in the *vagina*.

They then pass upwards through the uterus and fertilise the ovum in the uterine tube. The fertilised ovum (*zygote*) then passes into the uterus, embeds itself in the uterine wall and grows to maturity during pregnancy or *gestation*, in about 40 weeks. The newborn baby is entirely dependent on others for food and protection that was provided by the mother's body before birth.

One ovum is produced about every 28 days during the childbearing years between *puberty* and the *menopause*.

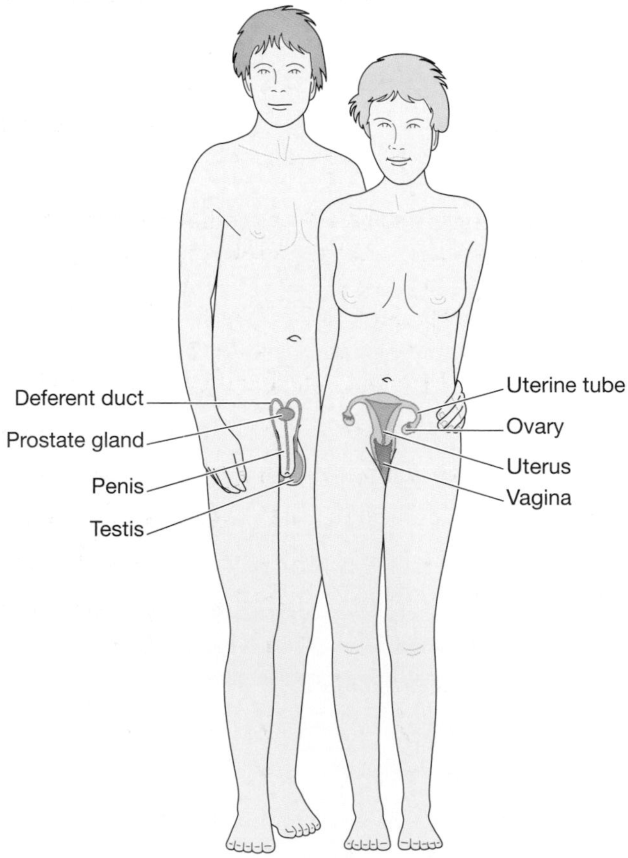

Figure 1.15 The reproductive systems: male and female.

When the ovum is not fertilised it passes out of the uterus accompanied by menstrual bleeding, known as *menstruation*. In females, the *menstrual cycle* consists of phases associated with changes in hormone levels involving the endocrine system. There is no such cycle in the male but hormones, similar to those of the female, are involved in the production and maturation of spermatozoa.

Introduction to the study of illness

Learning outcomes

After studying this section you should be able to:

- list factors that commonly cause disease
- define the terms aetiology, pathogenesis and prognosis
- name some common disease processes that can affect many of the body systems.

In order to understand the specific diseases described in later chapters, knowledge of the relevant anatomy and physiology is necessary, as well as familiarity with the pathological processes outlined below.

Many different illnesses, disorders and diseases are known, which vary from minor, but often very troublesome conditions, to the very serious. The study of abnormalities can be made much easier when a systematic approach is adopted. In order to achieve this in later chapters where specific diseases are explained, the headings shown in Box 1.3 will be used as a guide. Causes (*aetiology*) are outlined first when there are clear links between them and the effects of the abnormality (*pathogenesis*).

Box 1.3 Suggested framework for understanding diseases

Aetiology: cause of the disease

Pathogenesis: the nature of the disease process and its effect on normal body functioning

Complications: other consequences which might arise if the disease progresses

Prognosis: the likely outcome

Aetiology

Diseases are usually caused by one or more of a limited number of factors that may include:

- genetic abnormalities, either inherited or acquired
- infection by microbes or parasites, e.g. viruses, bacteria or worms
- chemicals
- ionising radiation
- physical trauma
- degeneration, e.g. excessive use or ageing.

In some diseases more than one of the aetiological factors listed above is involved, while in others, no specific cause has been identified and these may be described as *essential, idiopathic* or *spontaneous*. Although the precise cause of a disease may not be known, *predisposing (risk) factors* are usually identifiable. *Iatrogenic* conditions are those that result from healthcare interventions.

Pathogenesis

The main processes causing illness or disease are outlined below. Box 1.4 is a glossary of disease-associated terminology.

Inflammation (p. 371) – this is a tissue response to damage by, e.g. trauma, invasion of microbes*. Inflammatory conditions are recognised by the suffix -itis, e.g. appendicitis.

Tumours (p. 51) – these arise when the rate of cell production exceeds that of normal cell death causing a

---

* The term **microbe**, used throughout the text, includes all types of organisms that can only be seen by using a microscope. Specific microbes are named where appropriate.

> **Box 1.4 Glossary of terminology associated with disease**
>
> **Acute**: a disease with sudden onset often requiring urgent treatment (compare with chronic).
> **Acquired**: a disorder which develops any time after birth (compare with congenital).
> **Chronic**: a long-standing disorder which cannot usually be cured (compare with acute).
> **Congenital**: a disorder which one is born with (compare with acquired).
> **Sign**: an abnormality seen or measured by people other than the patient.
> **Symptom**: an abnormality described by the patient.
> **Syndrome**: a collection of signs and symptoms which tend to occur together.

mass to develop. Tumours are recognised by the suffix -oma, e.g. carcinoma.

Abnormal immune mechanisms (p. 379) – these are responses of the normally protective immune system that cause undesirable effects.

Thrombosis, embolism and infarction (p. 115) – these are the effects and consequences of abnormal changes in the blood and/or blood vessel walls.

Degeneration – this is often associated with normal ageing but may also arise prematurely when structures deteriorate causing impaired function.

Metabolic abnormalities – these cause undesirable metabolic effects, e.g. diabetes mellitus, p. 232.

Genetic abnormalities – these may be either inherited (e.g. phenylketonuria, p. 439) or caused by environmental factors such as exposure to ionising radiation (p. 51).

Introduction to the chemistry of life

2

In all the following chapters, the cells, tissues and organs of the body will be studied in more depth. However, on a smaller scale even than the cell, all living matter is made up of chemical building blocks. The basis of anatomy and physiology is therefore a chemical one, and before launching into the study of the subject it is necessary to consider briefly some aspects of chemistry and biochemistry.

Atoms, molecules and compounds

Learning outcomes

After studying this section, you should be able to:

- define the following terms: atomic number, atomic weight, isotope, molecular weight, ion, electrolyte, pH, acid and alkali

- describe the structure of an atom

- discuss the types of bonds that hold molecules together

- outline the concept of molar concentration

- explain the importance of buffers in the regulation of pH.

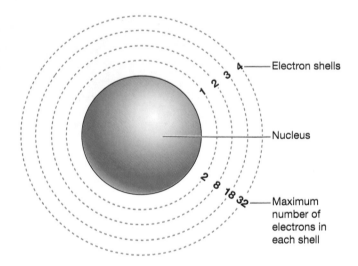

Figure 2.1 **The atom, showing the nucleus and four electron shells.**

Labels: Electron shells; Nucleus; Maximum number of electrons in each shell

Table 2.1 **Characteristics of subatomic particles**

Particle	Mass	Electric charge
Proton	1 unit	1 positive
Neutron	1 unit	neutral
Electron	negligible	1 negative

The *atom* is the smallest unit of an element that can exist as a stable entity. An *element* is a chemical substance whose atoms are all of the same type; e.g. iron contains only iron atoms. *Compounds* contain more than one type of atom; for instance, water is a compound containing both hydrogen and oxygen atoms.

There are 92 naturally occurring elements. The body structures are made up of a great variety of combinations of four of these elements: carbon, hydrogen, oxygen and nitrogen. In addition small amounts of others are present, collectively described as *mineral salts* (p. 276).

Atomic structure

Atoms are mainly empty space, with a tiny central nucleus containing *protons* and *neutrons* surrounded by clouds of tiny orbiting *electrons* (Fig. 2.1). Neutrons carry no electrical charge, but protons are positively charged, and electrons are negatively charged. Because atoms contain equal numbers of protons and electrons, they carry no net charge.

These subatomic particles differ also in terms of their mass. Electrons are so small that their mass is negligible, but the bigger neutrons and protons carry one atomic mass unit each. The physical characteristics of electrons, protons and neutrons are summarised in Table 2.1.

Atomic number and atomic weight

What makes one element different from another is the number of protons in the nuclei of its atoms (Fig. 2.2). For instance, hydrogen has only one proton per nucleus, oxygen has eight and sodium has eleven. The number of protons in the nucleus of an atom is called the *atomic number*; the atomic numbers of hydrogen, oxygen and sodium are therefore 1, 8 and 11 respectively. It therefore follows that each element has its own, unique, atomic number. The *atomic weight* of an element is the sum of the protons and neutrons in the atomic nucleus.

The electrons are shown in Figure 2.1 to be in concentric rings round the nucleus. These shells diagrammatically represent the different energy levels of the electrons in relation to the nucleus, not their physical positions. The first energy level can hold only two electrons and is filled first. The second energy level can hold only eight electrons and is filled next. The third and subsequent energy levels hold increased numbers of electrons, each containing more than the preceding level.

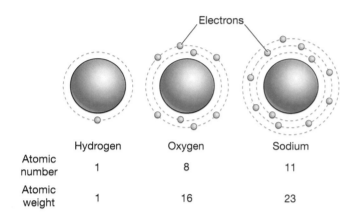

Figure 2.2 The atomic structures of the elements hydrogen, oxygen and sodium.

The *electron configuration* denotes the distribution of the electrons in each element, e.g. sodium is 2 8 1 (Fig. 2.2).

The biochemistry of life depends upon the ability of atoms to react and combine with one another, to produce the wide range of molecules required for biological diversity. The atomic particles important for this are the electrons of the outermost shell. An atom is reactive when it does not have a stable number of electrons in its outer shell, and may donate, receive or share electrons with one or more other atoms to achieve stability. This will be described more fully in the section discussing molecules and compounds.

Isotopes. These are atoms of an element in which there is a *different number of neutrons in the nucleus*. This does not affect the electrical activity of these atoms because neutrons carry no electrical charge, but it does affect their atomic weight. For example, there are three forms of the hydrogen atom. The most common form has one proton in the nucleus and one orbiting electron. Another form (*deuterium*) has one proton and one neutron in the nucleus. A third form (*tritium*) has one proton and two neutrons in the nucleus and one orbiting electron. These three forms of hydrogen are called *isotopes* (Fig. 2.3).

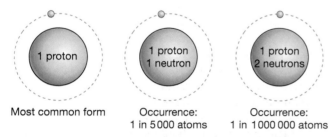

Figure 2.3 The isotopes of hydrogen.

Taking into account the isotopes of hydrogen and the proportions in which they occur, the atomic weight of hydrogen is 1.008, although for many practical purposes it can be taken as 1.

Chlorine has an atomic weight of 35.5, because it exists in two forms; one isotope has an atomic weight of 35 (with 18 neutrons in the nucleus) and the other 37 (with 20 neutrons in the nucleus). Because the proportion of these two forms is not equal, the *average atomic weight* is 35.5.

Molecules and compounds

It was mentioned earlier that the atoms of each element have a specific number of electrons around the nucleus. When the number of electrons in the outer shell of an element is either the maximum number (Fig. 2.1), or a stable proportion of this fraction, the element is described as *inert* or chemically unreactive, i.e. it will not easily combine with other elements to form compounds. These elements are the inert gases – helium, neon, argon, krypton, xenon and radon.

Molecules consist of two or more atoms that are chemically combined. The atoms may be of the same element, e.g. a molecule of atmospheric oxygen (O_2) contains two oxygen atoms. Most molecules, however, contain two or more different elements, e.g. a water molecule (H_2O) consists of two hydrogen atoms and an oxygen atom. As mentioned earlier, when two or more elements combine, the resulting molecule is referred to as a compound.

Compounds that contain the element carbon are classified as *organic*, and all others as *inorganic*. The body contains both.

Covalent and ionic bonds. The vast array of chemical processes on which body functioning is based is completely dependent upon the way atoms come together, bind and break apart. For example, the simple water molecule is a crucial foundation of all life on Earth. If water was a less stable compound, and the atoms came apart easily, human biology could never have evolved. On the other hand, the body is dependent upon the breaking down of various molecules (e.g. sugars, fats) to release energy for cellular activities. When atoms are joined together, they form a chemical bond that is generally one of two types: *covalent* or *ionic*.

Covalent bonds are formed when atoms share their electrons with each other. Most atoms use this type of bond when they come together; it forms a strong and stable link between them. A water molecule is built using covalent bonds. Hydrogen has one electron in its outer shell, but the optimum number for this shell is two. Oxygen has six electrons in its outer shell, but the optimum number for this shell is eight. Therefore, if one oxygen atom and two hydrogen atoms combine, each

19

hydrogen atom will share its electron with the oxygen atom, giving the oxygen atom a total of eight outer electrons and thereby conferring stability. The oxygen atom shares one of its electrons with each of the two hydrogen atoms, so that each hydrogen atom has two electrons in its outer shell, and they too are stable (Fig. 2.4).

Ionic bonds are weaker than covalent bonds and are formed when electrons are transferred from one atom to another. For example, when sodium (Na) combines with chlorine (Cl) to form sodium chloride (NaCl) there is a transfer of the only electron in the outer shell of the sodium atom to the outer shell of the chlorine atom (Fig. 2.5).

This leaves the sodium atom of the compound with eight electrons in its outer (second) shell, and therefore stable. The chlorine atom also has eight electrons in its outer shell, which, although not filling the shell, is a stable number. The two atoms now stick together because they are carrying opposite, mutually attractive, charges. The sodium atom is positively charged because it has given away a negatively charged electron, and the chloride ion is negatively charged because it has accepted sodium's extra electron.

The number of electrons is the only change that occurs in the atoms in this type of reaction. There is no change in the number of protons or neutrons in the atomic nuclei. The chloride atom now has *18 electrons*, each with one negative electrical charge, and *17 protons*, each with one positive charge. The sodium atom has lost one electron, leaving *10 electrons* orbiting round the nucleus containing *11 protons*. When sodium chloride is dissolved in water the two atoms separate. The atoms are charged, because they have traded electrons, so are no longer called atoms, but *ions*. Sodium, with the positive charge, is a *cation*, written Na^+, and chloride is an *anion*, written Cl^-. By convention the number of electrical charges carried by an ion is indicated by the superscript plus or minus signs.

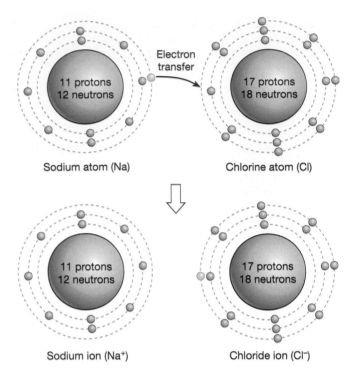

Figure 2.5 **Formation of the ionic compound, sodium chloride.**

Electrolytes

An ionic compound, e.g. sodium chloride, dissolved in water is called an *electrolyte* because it can conduct electricity. Electrolytes are important body constituents because:

- some conduct electricity, essential for muscle and nerve function
- some exert osmotic pressure, keeping body fluids in their own compartments
- some function in acid–base balance, as buffers to resist pH changes in body fluids.

A large number of compounds present in the body are not ionic, and therefore have no electrical properties when dissolved in water, e.g. carbohydrates. Important electrolytes other than sodium and chloride include potassium (K^+), calcium (Ca^{2+}), bicarbonate (HCO_3^-) and phosphate (PO_4^{2-}).

Molecular weight

The molecular weight of a molecule is the sum of the atomic weights of the elements forming its molecules, e.g.:

Water (H_2O)

2 hydrogen atoms	(atomic weight 1)	2
1 oxygen atom	(atomic weight 16)	16
	Molecular weight	= 18

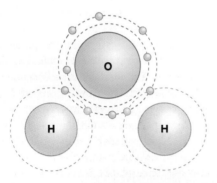

Figure 2.4 **A water molecule, showing the covalent bonds between hydrogen (yellow) and oxygen (green).**

20

Sodium bicarbonate ($NaHCO_3$)

1 sodium atom	(atomic weight 23)	23
1 hydrogen atom	(atomic weight 1)	1
1 carbon atom	(atomic weight 12)	12
3 oxygen atoms	(atomic weight 16)	48
	Molecular weight	= 84

Molecular weight, like atomic weight, is expressed simply as a figure until a scale of measurement of weight is applied.

Molar concentration

This is the term used to express the concentration of substances present in the body fluids.

The mole (mol) is the molecular weight in grams of a substance. One mole of any substance contains 6.023×10^{23} molecules or atoms. For example, 1 mole of sodium bicarbonate (the example above) is 84 grams.

A molar solution is a solution in which 1 mole of a substance is dissolved in 1 litre of solvent. In the human body the solvent is water or fat. A molar solution of sodium bicarbonate is therefore prepared using 84 g of sodium bicarbonate dissolved in 1 litre of solvent.

Molar concentration may be used to measure quantities of electrolytes, non-electrolytes, ions and atoms, e.g. molar solutions of the following substances mean:

1 mole of sodium chloride molecules (NaCl)	= 58.5g per litre
1 mole of sodium ions (Na^+)	= 23g per litre
1 mole of carbon atoms (C)	= 12g per litre
1 mole of atmospheric oxygen (O_2)	= 32g per litre

In physiology this system has the advantage of being a measure of the number of particles (molecules, atoms, ions) of substances present, because molar solutions of different substances contain the same number of particles. It has the advantage over the measure milliequivalents per litre* because it can be used for non-electrolytes, in fact for any substance of known molecular weight.

Many of the chemical substances present in the body are in very low concentrations so it is more convenient to use smaller metric measures, e.g. millimoles per litre (mmol/l) or micromoles per litre (μmol/l) as a biological measure (Table 2.2).

---

*Milliequivalents per litre (mEq/l)

$$\text{Equivalent weight} = \frac{\text{atomic weight}}{\text{number of electrical charges}}$$

Concentration is expressed as:

$$\text{mEq/l} = \frac{\text{mg/l}}{\text{atomic weight}} \times \text{number of electrical charges}$$

Table 2.2 Examples of normal plasma levels

Substance	Amount in moles	Amount in other units
Chloride	97–106 mmol/l	97–106 mEq/l
Sodium	135–143 mmol/l	135–143 mEq/l
Glucose	3.5–5.5 mmol/l	60–100 mg/100 ml
Iron	14–35mmol/l	90–196 mg/100 ml

For substances of unknown molecular weight, e.g. insulin, concentration may be expressed in International Units per millilitre (IU/ml).

Acids, alkalis and pH

The number of hydrogen ions ($[H^+]$) in a solution is a measure of the acidity of the solution. Control of the normal hydrogen ion concentration within the body is an important factor in maintaining a stable internal environment.

An acid substance is one that releases hydrogen ions when in solution. On the other hand, a basic (alkaline) substance accepts hydrogen ions, often with the release of hydroxyl (OH^-) ions. A *salt* releases other anions and cations when dissolved; sodium chloride is therefore a salt because in solution it releases sodium and chloride ions.

The pH scale

A standard scale for the measurement of the hydrogen ion concentration in solution has been developed: the pH scale. The scale measures from 0 to 14, with 7, the midpoint, as neutral; this is the pH of water. Water is a neutral molecule, neither acid nor alkaline, because when the molecule breaks up into its constituent ions, it releases one H^+ and one OH^-, which balance one another. Most body fluids are close to neutral, because strong acids and bases are damaging to living tissues, and body fluids contain *buffers*, themselves weak acids and bases, to keep their pH within narrow ranges.

A pH reading below 7 indicates an *acid solution*, while readings above 7 indicate *alkalinity* (Fig. 2.6). A change of one whole number on the pH scale indicates a tenfold change in $[H^+]$. Therefore, a solution of pH 5 contains ten times as many hydrogen ions as a solution of pH 6.

Litmus paper indicates whether a solution is acid or alkaline by colouring blue for alkaline and red for acid. Other specially treated absorbent papers give an approximate measure of pH by a colour change. When accurate measurements of pH are required, sensitive pH meters are used.

21

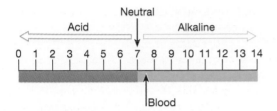

Figure 2.6 The pH scale.

Not all acids ionise completely when dissolved in water. The hydrogen ion concentration is a measure, therefore, of the amount of *dissociated acid* (ionised acid) rather than of the total amount of acid present. Strong acids dissociate more freely than weak acids, e.g. hydrochloric acid dissociates freely into H^+ and Cl^-, while carbonic acid dissociates much less freely into H^+ and HCO_3^-. The number of *free hydrogen ions* in a solution is a *measure of its acidity* rather than an indication of the type of molecule from which the hydrogen ions originated.

Likewise, not all bases dissociate completely. Strong bases dissociate more fully i.e. release more OH^-, than weaker ones.

pH values of the body fluids

Body fluids have pH values that must be maintained within relatively narrow limits for normal cell activity. The pH values are not the same in all parts of the body. The normal range of pH values of certain body fluids are shown in Table 2.3.

The highly acid pH of the gastric juice is maintained by hydrochloric acid secreted by the parietal cells in the walls of the gastric glands. The low pH of the stomach fluids provides the environment best suited to the functioning of the enzyme pepsin that begins the digestion of dietary protein. Saliva has a pH of between 5.4 and 7.5, which is the optimum value for the action of salivary amylase, the enzyme present in saliva which initiates the digestion of carbohydrates. Its action is inhibited when

food containing it reaches the stomach and is mixed with the acidic gastric juice.

Blood has a pH value between 7.35 and 7.45, and outwith this narrow range there is severe disruption of normal physiological and biochemical processes. The metabolic activity of the body cells produces certain acids and alkalis, which alter the pH of the tissue fluid and blood. To maintain the pH within the normal range, there are substances present in blood that act as *buffers*.

Buffers

Optimum pH is maintained by keeping a balance between acids and bases produced by cells. The buffer systems maintain normal body pH by preventing dramatic changes in the pH values of the blood, but can function effectively only if there is some means by which excess acid or alkali can be excreted from the body. The organs most active in this way are the *lungs* and the *kidneys*. The lungs are important regulators of blood pH because they excrete carbon dioxide (CO_2). CO_2 increases $[H^+]$ in body fluids because it combines with water to form carbonic acid, which then dissociates into a bicarbonate ion and a hydrogen ion.

$$CO_2 + H_2O \leftrightarrow H_2CO_3 \leftrightarrow H^+ + HCO_3^-$$

carbon water carbonic hydrogen bicarbonate
dioxide acid ion ion

The lungs help to control blood pH by regulating levels of excreted CO_2. The brain detects the rising $[H^+]$ in the blood and stimulates breathing, causing increased CO_2 loss and a fall in $[H^+]$. Conversely, if the pH becomes too alkaline, the brain can reduce the respiration rate to increase CO_2 levels and increase $[H^+]$, restoring pH towards normal (see Ch. 10).

The kidneys regulate blood pH by increasing or decreasing as required the excretion of hydrogen and bicarbonate ions. If pH falls, hydrogen ion excretion is increased and bicarbonate conserved; the reverse happens if pH rises. In addition, the kidneys generate bicarbonate ions as a by-product of amino acid breakdown in the renal tubules; this process also generates ammonium ions, which are rapidly excreted.

Other buffer systems include body proteins, which absorb excess H^+, and phosphate, which is particularly important in controlling pH inside cells. The buffer and excretory systems of the body together maintain the *acid–base balance* so that the pH range of the blood remains within normal, but narrow, limits.

Acidosis and alkalosis

The buffer systems described above compensate for most pH fluctuations, but these reserves are limited and, in extreme cases, can become exhausted. When the pH falls below 7.35, and all the reserves of alkaline buffers are

Table 2.3 pH values of body fluids	
Body fluid	**pH**
Blood	7.35 to 7.45
Saliva	5.4 to 7.5
Gastric juice	1.5 to 3.5
Bile	6 to 8.5
Urine	4.5 to 8.0

used up, the condition of *acidosis* exists. In the reverse situation, when the pH rises above 7.45, the increased alkali uses up all the acid reserve and the state of *alkalosis* exists.

Acidosis and alkalosis are both damaging to the body, particularly to the central nervous system and the cardiovascular system. In practice, acidotic conditions are commoner than alkalotic ones, because the body tends to produce more acid than alkali. Acidosis may follow respiratory problems, if the lungs are not excreting CO_2 as efficiently as normal, or if the body is producing excess acids (e.g. diabetic ketoacidosis, p. 233) or in kidney disease, if renal H^+ excretion is reduced. Alkalosis may be caused by loss of basic substances through vomiting, diarrhoea, endocrine disorders or diuretic therapy, which stimulates increased renal excretion. Rarely, it may follow increased respiratory effort, such as in an acute anxiety attack where excessive amounts of CO_2 are lost through overbreathing (hyperventilation).

Important biological molecules

Learning outcomes

After studying this section, you should be able to:

■ describe in simple terms the chemical nature of sugars, protein, lipids, nucleotides and enzymes

■ discuss the biological importance of each of these important groups of molecules.

Carbohydrates

The carbohydrates are the sugars. Carbohydrates are composed of carbon, oxygen and hydrogen and the carbon atoms are normally arranged in a ring, with the oxygen and hydrogen atoms linked to them. The structures of glucose, fructose and sucrose are shown in Figure 2.7. When two sugars link up, the reaction occurring expels a molecule of water and the resulting bond is called a *glycosidic linkage*.

Simple sugars, like glucose, can exist as single units, and are referred to as *monosaccharides*. Glucose is the main form in which sugar is used by cells, and blood levels are tightly controlled. Frequently, the monosaccharides are linked together, the resultant molecule ranging from two sugars or *disaccharides*, e.g. sucrose (table sugar), to long chains containing many thousands of monosaccharides. Such complex carbohydrates are called *polysaccharides*, e.g. starch.

Glucose can be broken down (metabolised) in either the presence (*aerobically*) or the absence (*anaerobically*) of oxygen, but the process is much more efficient when O_2 is used. During this process, energy, water and carbon dioxide are released (p. 312). This family of molecules:

- serves as a ready source of energy to fuel cellular activities (p. 312)
- provides a form of energy storage, e.g. glycogen (p. 312)
- forms an integral part of the structure of DNA and RNA (pp. 433, 434)
- can act as receptors on the cell surface, allowing the cell to recognise other molecules and cells.

23

Amino acids and proteins

Amino acids always contain carbon, hydrogen, oxygen and nitrogen, and many in addition carry sulphur. In human biochemistry, 20 amino acids are used as the principal building blocks of protein, although there are others; for instance, there are some amino acids used only in certain proteins, and some are seen only in microbial products. Of the amino acids used in human protein synthesis, there is a basic common structure, including an

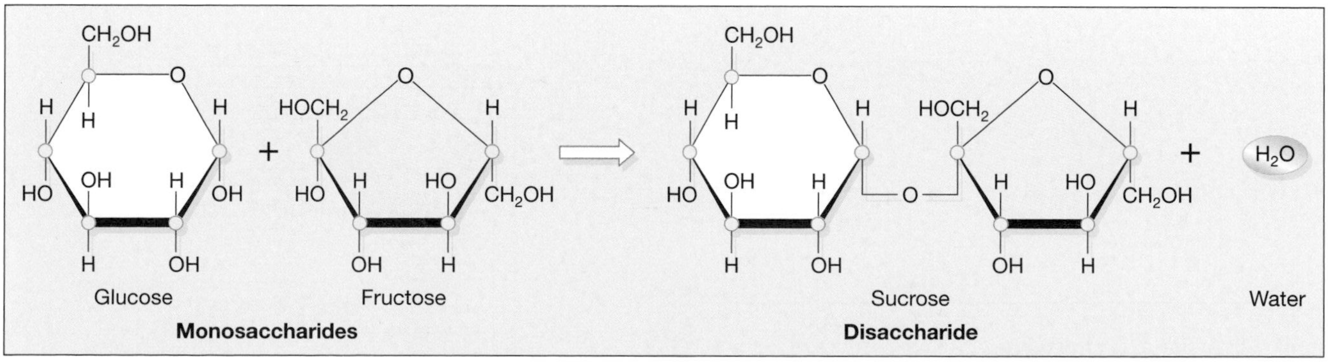

Figure 2.7 The combination of glucose and fructose to make sucrose.

amino group (NH_2), a carboxyl group (COOH) and a hydrogen atom. What makes one amino acid different from the next is a variable side chain. The basic structure and three common amino acids are shown in Figure 2.8. As in formation of glycosidic linkages, when two amino acids join up the reaction expels a molecule of water and the resulting bond is called a *peptide bond*.

Proteins are made from amino acids joined together, and are the main family of molecules from which the human body is built. Protein molecules vary enormously in size, shape, chemical constituents and function. Many important groups of biologically active substances are proteins, e.g.:

- carrier molecules, e.g. haemoglobin (p. 60)
- enzymes (p. 25)
- many hormones, e.g. insulin (p. 222)
- antibodies (p. 375).

Proteins can also be used as an alternative energy source, usually in dietary inadequacy, although the process is much less efficient than when carbohydrates or fats are broken down.

Lipids

Lipids are made up of carbon, hydrogen and oxygen atoms. One group of lipids, the *phospholipids*, forms an integral part of the cell membrane. One notable feature of lipid molecules is that they are strongly hydrophobic (water hating) and therefore lipids do not mix with water. This is important in their function in the cell membrane (p. 30).

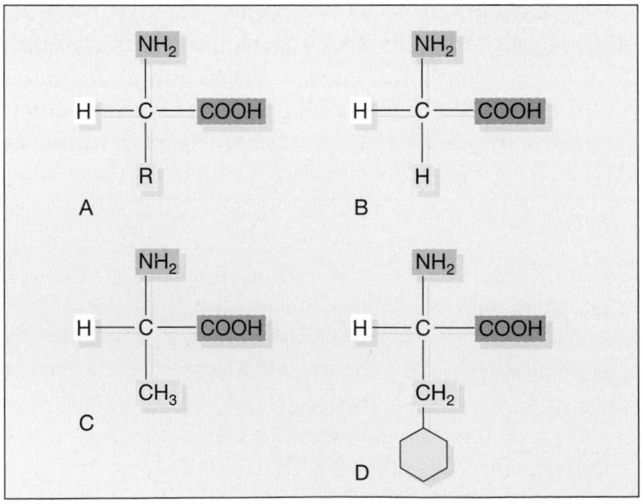

Other types of lipids include certain vitamins (e.g. E and K), an important group of hormones called *steroids*, and the *fats*. A molecule of fat consists of three fatty acids, each linked to a molecule of glycerol (Fig. 2.9). Fats are a source of energy, and provide a convenient form in which to store excess energy intake. When fats are broken down, they release energy, but the process is less efficient than when carbohydrates are used, since it requires more energy for the breakdown reaction to take place. They are used in the body for:

- insulation
- protection of body parts
- energy storage.

Nucleotides

Nucleic acids

These are the largest molecules in the body and are built from components called nucleotides, which consist of three subunits: a sugar, a base and one or more phosphate groups. Nucleic acids are described in more detail in Chapter 17.

Adenosine triphosphate (ATP)

ATP is a nucleotide that contains ribose (the sugar unit), adenine (the base) and three phosphate groups attached to the ribose (Fig. 2.10A). It is sometimes known as the energy currency of the body, which implies that the body has to 'earn' (synthesise) it before it can 'spend' it. Many of the body's huge number of reactions release energy, e.g. the breakdown of sugars in the presence of O_2. The body captures the energy released by these reactions, using it to make ATP from adenosine diphosphate (ADP). When the body needs chemical energy to fuel cellular activities, ATP releases its stored energy, water and a phosphate group through the splitting of a high-energy phosphate bond, and reverts to ADP (Fig. 2.10B).

Figure 2.8 Amino acid structures: A. Common structure, R = variable side chain. **B.** Glycine, the simplest amino acid. **C.** Alanine. **D.** Phenylalanine.

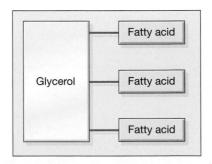

Figure 2.9 Core structure of the fats.

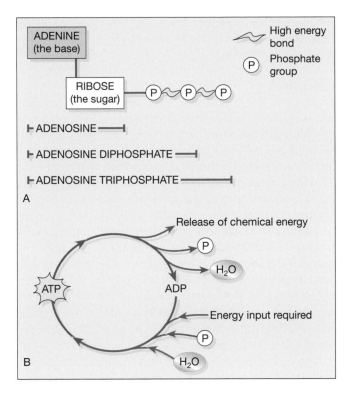

Figure 2.10 **ATP and ADP:** A. Structures. B. Conversion cycle.

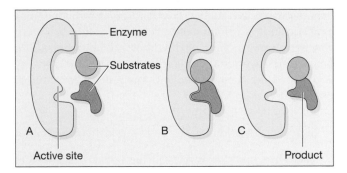

Figure 2.11 **Action of an enzyme:** A. Enzyme and substrates. B. Enzyme–substrate complex. C. Enzyme and product.

The body needs chemical energy to:

- drive synthetic reactions (i.e. building biological molecules)
- fuel movement
- transport substances across membranes.

Enzymes

Many of the body's chemical reactions can be reproduced in a test-tube. Surprisingly, the rate at which the reactions then occur usually plummets to the extent that, for all practical purposes, chemical activity ceases. The cells of the body have developed a solution to this apparent problem – they are equipped with a huge array of enzymes. Enzymes are proteins which act as *catalysts* for biochemical reactions – that is, they speed the reaction up but are not themselves changed by it, and therefore can be used over and over again. Enzymes are very selective and will usually catalyse only one specific reaction. The molecule(s) entering the reaction is called the *substrate* and it binds to a very specific site on the enzyme, called the *active site*. Whilst the substrate(s) is bound to the active site the reaction proceeds, and once it is complete the product(s) of the reaction breaks away from the enzyme and the active site is ready for use again (Fig. 2.11).

Enzyme action is reduced or stopped altogether if conditions are unsuitable. Increased or decreased tem-perature is likely to reduce activity, as is any change in pH. Some enzymes require the presence of a *cofactor*, an ion or small molecule that allows the enzyme to bind its substrate(s). Some vitamins are cofactors in enzyme reactions.

Enzymes can catalyse both synthetic and breakdown reactions, and their names (almost always!) end in ~ase.

Movement of substances within the body

25

Learning outcomes

After studying this section, you should be able to:

- compare and contrast the processes of osmosis and diffusion

- using these concepts, describe how molecules move within and between body compartments.

Within the body, it is essential that substances (e.g. molecules, electrolytes) move around. Nutrients absorbed in the small intestine must travel, or they will never reach the tissues they are destined to nourish. Waste substances must move from the tissues to their exit points from the body. To enter the body from inhaled air, oxygen gas must cross first the alveolar wall and then the wall of the lung capillary to get into the blood. Communication molecules, such as hormones, have to travel from the site of production to their destination. Water itself, the principal constituent of the body, has to move in order to distribute throughout body fluids and keep solutes at appropriate physiological concentrations.

From a physical point of view, substances will always travel from an area of high concentration to one of low concentration, assuming that there is no barrier in the way. Between two such areas, there exists a *concentration gradient* and movement of substances occurs *down* the concentration gradient, or downhill, until concentrations on each side are equal (*equilibrium* is reached). No energy is required for such movement; this process is therefore described as *passive*.

$$\text{high concentration} \xrightarrow{\text{net movement of substance}} \text{low concentration}$$

There are many examples in the body of substances moving *uphill*, i.e. against the concentration gradient; in this case, chemical energy is required, usually in the form of ATP. These processes are described as *active*. Movement of substances across cell membranes by active transport is described on page 33.

Passive movement of substances in the body proceeds usually in one of two main ways – *diffusion* or *osmosis*.

Diffusion

Diffusion refers to the movement of a chemical substance from an area of high concentration to an area of low concentration, and occurs mainly in gases, liquids and solutions. This process enables the transfer of oxygen from the alveoli of the lungs (high concentration) through the alveolar and capillary walls into the blood (low concentration). Sugar molecules heaped at the bottom of a cup of coffee that has not been stirred will, in time, become evenly distributed throughout the liquid by diffusion (Fig. 2.12). The process of diffusion is speeded up if the temperature rises and/or the concentration of the diffusing substance is increased.

Diffusion can also occur across a semipermeable membrane, such as the plasma membrane; in this case, only those molecules able to cross the membrane can diffuse through. For example, the capillary wall is effectively a semipermeable membrane; although water can travel freely in either direction across it, large proteins in the plasma and red blood cells are too big to cross and so remain in the blood.

Osmosis

Osmosis is the movement of water down its concentration gradient across a semipermeable membrane when equilibrium cannot be achieved by diffusion of solute molecules. This is usually because the solute molecules are too large to pass through the pores in the membrane. The force with which this occurs is called the *osmotic pressure*. Water crosses the membrane down its concentration gradient from the side with the lower solute concentration to the side with the greater solute concentration. This dilutes the more concentrated solution, and concentrates the more dilute solution. Osmosis proceeds until equilibrium is reached, at which point the solutions on each side of the membrane are of the same concentration and are said to be *isotonic*. Osmosis can be illustrated using the semipermeable membrane of the red blood cell as an example.

The concentration of water and solutes in the plasma is maintained within a very narrow range because if the plasma water concentration rises, i.e. the plasma becomes more dilute than the intracellular fluid within the red blood cells, then water will move down its concentration gradient across their membranes and into the red blood cells. This may cause the red blood cells to swell and burst. In this situation, the plasma is said to be *hypotonic*. Conversely, if the plasma water concentration falls so that the plasma becomes more concentrated than the intracellular fluid within the red blood cells (the plasma becomes *hypertonic*), water passively moves by osmosis from the blood cells into the plasma and the blood cells shrink (Fig. 2.13).

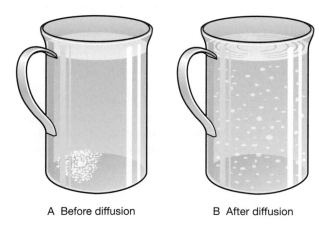

A Before diffusion   B After diffusion

Figure 2.12 The process of diffusion: a spoonful of sugar in a cup of coffee.

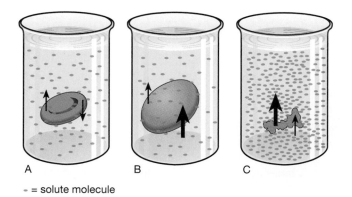

A   B   C

• = solute molecule

Figure 2.13 The process of osmosis. Net water movement when a red blood cell is suspended in solutions of varying concentrations (tonicity): **A.** Isotonic solution. **B.** Hypotonic solution. **C.** Hypertonic solution.

Body fluids

Learning outcomes

After studying this section, you should be able to:

■ define the terms intra- and extracellular fluid

■ using examples, explain why homeostatic control of the composition of these fluids is vital to body function.

The total body water in adults of average build is about 60% of body weight. This proportion is higher in babies and young people and in adults below average weight. It is lower in the elderly and in obesity in all age groups. About 22% of body weight is extracellular water and about 38% is intracellular water (Fig. 2.14).

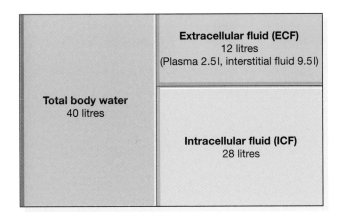

Figure 2.14 **Distribution of body water in a 70 kg person.**

Extracellular fluid

The extracellular fluid (ECF) consists of blood, plasma, lymph, cerebrospinal fluid and fluid in the interstitial spaces of the body. Other extracellular fluids are present in very small amounts; their role is mainly in lubrication, and they include joint (synovial) fluid, pericardial fluid (around the heart) and pleural fluid (around the lungs).

Interstitial or intercellular fluid (tissue fluid) bathes all the cells of the body except the outer layers of skin. It is the medium through which substances pass from blood to the body cells, and from the cells to blood. Every body cell in contact with the ECF is directly dependent upon the composition of that fluid for its well-being. Even slight changes can cause permanent damage, and any change is therefore resisted by the body through one or more of its many control mechanisms. For example, a fall in plasma potassium levels may cause muscle weakness and cardiac arrhythmia, because of increased excitability of muscle and nervous tissue. Rising blood potassium also interferes with cardiac function, and can even cause the heart to stop beating. Potassium levels in the blood are only one of the many parameters under constant, careful adjustment by the homeostatic mechanisms of the body.

Intracellular fluid

The composition of intracellular fluid (ICF) is largely controlled by the cell itself, because there are selective uptake and discharge mechanisms present in the cell membrane. The composition of ICF can therefore be very different from ECF. Thus, sodium levels are nearly ten times higher in the ECF than in the ICF. This concentration difference occurs because, although sodium diffuses into the cell down its concentration gradient, there is a pump in the membrane that selectively pumps it back out again. This concentration gradient is essential for the function of excitable cells (mainly nerve and muscle). Conversely, many substances are found inside the cell in significantly higher amounts than outside, e.g. ATP, protein and potassium.

27

The cells, tissues and organisation of the body

Cells are the smallest functional units of the body. They are grouped together to form *tissues*, each of which has a specialised function, e.g. blood, muscle, bone. Different tissues are grouped together to form *organs*, e.g. heart, stomach, brain. Organs are grouped together to form *systems*, each of which performs a particular function that maintains homeostasis and contributes to the health of the individual (see Fig. 1.1, p. 5). For example, the digestive system is responsible for taking in, digesting and absorbing food and involves a number of organs, including the stomach and intestines. The structure and functions of cells and types of tissue are explored in this chapter.

The terminology used to describe the anatomical relationships of body parts, the skeleton and the cavities within the body are described in the last section of this chapter.

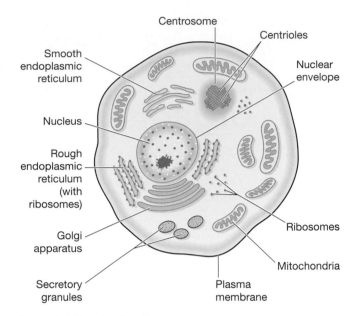

Figure 3.1 **The simple cell.**

The cell: structure and functions

Learning outcomes

After studying this section you should be able to:

■ describe the structure of the plasma membrane

■ explain the functions of the principal organelles

■ outline the process of mitosis

■ compare and contrast active, passive and bulk transport of substances across cell membranes.

The human body develops from a single cell called the *zygote*, which results from the fusion of the ovum (female egg cell) and the spermatozoon (male sex cell). Cell division follows and, as the fetus grows, cells with different structural and functional specialisations develop, all with the same genetic make-up as the zygote. Individual cells are too small to be seen with the naked eye. However, they can be seen when thin slices of tissue are stained in the laboratory and magnified by a microscope.

A cell consists of a *plasma membrane* inside which are a number of *organelles* suspended in a watery fluid called *cytosol* (Fig. 3.1). Organelles, literally 'small organs', have individual and highly specialised functions, and are often enclosed in their own membrane within the cytosol. They include: the *nucleus, mitochondria, ribosomes, endoplasmic reticulum, Golgi apparatus, lysosomes* and the *cytoskeleton*.

Plasma membrane

The plasma membrane (Fig. 3.2) consists of two layers of phospholipids (fatty substances, see p. 24) with protein and sugar molecules embedded in them. Those that extend all the way through the membrane may provide channels that allow the passage of, for example, electrolytes and non-lipid-soluble substances.

The phospholipid molecules have a head, which is electrically charged and *hydrophilic* (meaning 'water

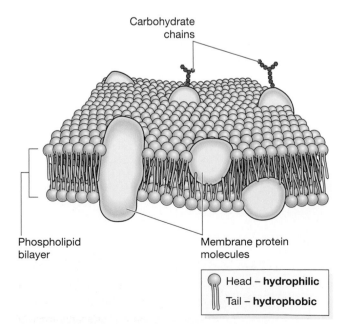

Figure 3.2 **The plasma membrane.**

loving'), and a tail which has no charge and is *hydrophobic* (meaning 'water hating'). The phospholipid bilayer is arranged like a sandwich with the hydrophilic heads aligned on the outer surfaces of the membrane and the hydrophobic tails forming a central water-repelling layer. These differences influence the transfer of substances across the membrane.

The membrane proteins perform several functions:

- branched carbohydrate molecules attached to the outside of some membrane protein molecules give the cell its immunological identity
- they can act as specific receptors (recognition sites) for hormones and other chemical messengers
- some are enzymes (p. 25)
- some are involved in transport across the membrane.

Organelles

Nucleus

Every cell in the body has a nucleus, with the exception of mature erythrocytes (red blood cells). Skeletal muscle and some other cells contain several nuclei. The nucleus is the largest organelle and is contained within the *nuclear envelope*, a membrane similar to the plasma membrane but with tiny pores through which some substances can pass between it and the *cytoplasm*, i.e. the cell contents excluding the nucleus.

The nucleus contains the body's genetic material, which directs all the metabolic activities of the cell. This consists of 46 *chromosomes,* which are made from deoxyribonucleic acid (DNA, p. 433). Except during cell division, the chromosomes resemble a fine network of threads called *chromatin* (see Fig. 3.3).

Mitochondria

Mitochondria are sausage-shaped structures in the cytoplasm, sometimes described as the 'power house' of the cell. They are involved in aerobic respiration, the processes by which chemical energy is made available in the cell. This is in the form of ATP, which releases energy when the cell breaks it down (see Fig. 2.10, p. 25). Synthesis of ATP is most efficient in the final stages of aerobic respiration, a process requiring oxygen (p. 312). The most active cell types have the greatest number of mitochondria, e.g. liver, muscle and spermatozoa.

Ribosomes

These are tiny granules composed of RNA and protein. They synthesise proteins from amino acids, using RNA as the template (see Fig. 17.4, p. 434). When present in free units or in small clusters in the cytoplasm, the ribosomes make proteins for use within the cell. These include the enzymes required for metabolism. Metabolic pathways

consist of a series of steps, each driven by a specific enzyme. Ribosomes are also found on the outer surface of the nuclear envelope and rough endoplasmic reticulum (see below) where they manufacture proteins for export from the cell.

Endoplasmic reticulum (ER)

Endoplasmic reticulum is a series of interconnecting membranous canals in the cytoplasm. There are two types: smooth and rough. Smooth ER synthesises lipids and steroid hormones, and is also associated with the detoxification of some drugs. Rough ER is studded with ribosomes. These are the site of synthesis of proteins that are 'exported' from cells, i.e. enzymes and hormones that are extruded from the parent cell to be used by cells elsewhere.

Golgi apparatus

The Golgi apparatus consists of stacks of closely folded flattened membranous sacs. It is present in all cells but is larger in those that synthesise and export proteins. The proteins move from the endoplasmic reticulum to the Golgi apparatus where they are 'packaged' into membrane-bound vesicles called *secretory granules*. The vesicles are stored and, when needed, move to the plasma membrane, through which the proteins are exported.

Lysosomes

Lysosomes are one type of secretory vesicle formed by the Golgi apparatus. They contain a variety of enzymes involved in breaking down fragments of organelles and large molecules (e.g. RNA, DNA, carbohydrates, proteins) inside the cell into smaller particles that are either recycled, or extruded from the cell as waste material.

Lysosomes in white blood cells contain enzymes that digest foreign material such as microbes.

Cytoskeleton

This consists of tiny strands of protein.

Microfilaments. These are the smallest fibres. They provide structural support, maintain the characteristic shape of the cell and permit contraction e.g. in muscle cells.

Microtubules. These are larger contractile protein fibres that are involved in movement of:

- organelles within the cell
- chromosomes during cell division
- cell extensions (see p. 32).

Centrosome. This directs organisation of microtubules within the cell. It consists of a pair of *centrioles* (small clusters of microtubules) and plays an important role during cell division.

31

Cell extensions. These project from the plasma membrane and their main components are microtubules, which allow movement. They include:

- cilia – small hair-like projections lying along the free border of some cells. They beat in unison moving substances along the surface, e.g. mucus upwards in the respiratory tract (see Fig. 10.12, p. 245)
- flagella – single, long whip-like projections that move cells, e.g. tails of spermatozoa (see Fig. 18.14, p. 453).

Cell division

Most body cells divide by *mitosis*, a process that results in two new genetically identical daughter cells. Formation of *gametes* (sex cells), i.e. ova and spermatozoa, takes place by *meiosis* (see p. 436) and the four daughter cells are genetically different from the parent cell and each other.

The period between cell division is known as *interphase*. Towards the end of interphase, the chromatin replicates and becomes tightly coiled forming double chromosomes, called *chromatids*, in preparation for cell division. In human cells there are 46 chromosomes. The two chromatids of each chromosome are joined at the *centromere*.

Mitosis (Fig. 3.3)

This is a continuous process involving four distinct stages seen by light microscopy.

Prophase. During this stage the chromatids become visible within the nucleus, and the *mitotic apparatus* appears. This consists of two *centrioles* separated by the *mitotic spindle*, which is formed from microtubules. The centrioles migrate, one to each end of the cell, and the nuclear envelope disappears.

Metaphase. The chromatids align on the centre of the spindle, attached by their centromeres.

Anaphase. The centromeres separate, and one of each pair of sister chromatids migrates to each pole (end) of the spindle as the microtubules that form the mitotic spindle contract.

Telophase. The mitotic apparatus disappears, the chromosomes uncoil and the nuclear envelope reforms.

Following telophase, the cytoplasm and plasma membrane divide in half forming two identical daughter cells. The organelles of the daughter cells are incomplete at the end of cell division but they develop as the cell matures during interphase.

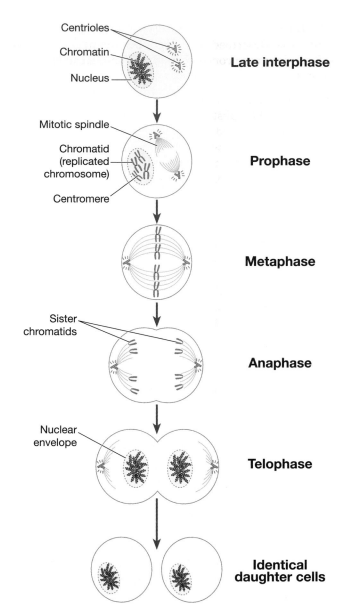

Figure 3.3 **The stages of mitosis.**

The frequency with which cell division occurs varies with different types of cell (p. 40).

Transport of substances across cell membranes

Passive transport

This occurs when substances can cross the semipermeable plasma and organelle membranes and move down the concentration gradient (downhill) without using energy.

Diffusion

This was described on page 26. Small substances diffuse down the concentration gradient, crossing membranes by:

- dissolving in the lipid part of the membrane, e.g. lipid-soluble substances such as oxygen, carbon dioxide, fatty acids, steroids
- passing through water-filled channels, or pores in the membrane, e.g. small water-soluble substances including sodium, potassium, calcium.

Facilitated diffusion

This passive process is used by some substances that are unable to diffuse through the semipermeable membrane unaided, e.g. glucose, amino acids. Specialised protein carrier molecules in the membrane have specific sites that attract and bind substances to be transferred, like a lock and key mechanism. The carrier then changes its shape and deposits the substance on the other side of the membrane (Fig. 3.4). The carrier sites are specific and can be used by only one substance. As there are a finite number of carriers, there is a limit to the amount of a substance which can be transported at any time. This is known as the *transport maximum*.

Osmosis

Osmosis is passive movement of water down its concentration gradient towards equilibrium across a semipermeable membrane and is explained on page 26.

Active transport

This is the transport of substances up their concentration gradient (uphill), i.e. from a lower to a higher concentration. Chemical energy in the form of ATP (p. 24) drives specialised protein carrier molecules that transport substances across the membrane in either direction (see Fig. 3.4). The carrier sites are specific and can be used by only one substance; therefore the rate at which a substance is transferred depends on the number of sites available.

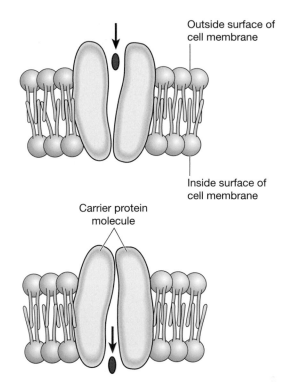

Figure 3.4 **Specialised protein carrier molecules involved in facilitated diffusion and active transport.**

The sodium–potassium pump

This active transport mechanism maintains homeostasis of the electrolytes sodium (Na^+) and potassium (K^+). It may use up to 30% of cellular ATP requirements.

The principal cations are K^+ intracellularly and Na^+ extracellularly. These ions tend to diffuse down their concentration gradients, K^+ outwards and Na^+ into the cell. In order to maintain their concentration gradients, excess Na^+ is constantly pumped out across the cell membrane in exchange for K^+.

Bulk transport (Fig. 3.5)

Transfer of particles too large to cross cell membranes occurs by *pinocytosis* or *phagocytosis*. These particles are

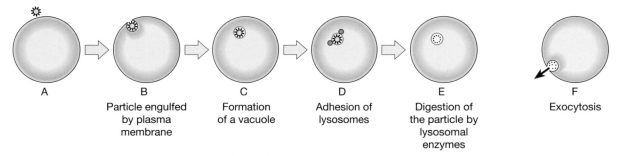

Figure 3.5 **Bulk transport across plasma membranes: A–E.** Phagocytosis. **F.** Exocytosis.

engulfed by extensions of the cytoplasm, which enclose them forming a membrane-bound vacuole. When the vacuole is small, pinocytosis occurs. In phagocytosis larger particles (e.g. cell fragments, foreign materials, microbes) are taken into the cell. Lysosomes then adhere to the vacuole membrane, releasing enzymes which digest the contents.

Extrusion of waste material by the reverse process through the plasma membrane is called *exocytosis*. Secretory granules formed by the Golgi apparatus usually leave the cell in this way, as do any indigestible residues of phagocytosis.

Tissues

Learning outcomes

After studying this section you should be able to:

- describe the structure and functions of epithelial, connective and muscle tissue
- outline the structure and functions of membranes
- compare and contrast the structure and functions of exocrine and endocrine glands.

The tissues of the body consist of large numbers of cells and they are classified according to the size, shape and functions of these cells. There are four main types of tissue. They are:

- epithelial tissue or epithelium
- connective tissue
- muscle tissue
- nervous tissue.

Each has subdivisions.

Epithelial tissue

This group of tissues is found covering the body and lining cavities, hollow organs and tubes. It is also found in glands. The structure of epithelium is closely related to its functions, which include:

- protection of underlying structures from, for example, dehydration, chemical and mechanical damage
- secretion
- absorption.

The cells are very closely packed and the intercellular substance, called the *matrix*, is minimal. The cells usually lie on a *basement membrane*, which is an inert connective tissue made by the epithelial cells themselves.

Epithelial tissue may be:

- *simple*: a single layer of cells
- *stratified*: several layers of cells.

Simple epithelium

Simple epithelium consists of a single layer of identical cells and is divided into four types. It is usually found on absorptive or secretory surfaces, where the single layer enhances these processes, and not usually on surfaces subject to stress. The types are named according to the shape of the cells, which differs according to their functions. The more active the tissue, the taller the cells.

Squamous (pavement) epithelium

This is composed of a single layer of flattened cells (Fig. 3.6). The cells fit closely together like flat stones, forming a thin and very smooth membrane.

Diffusion takes place freely through this thin, smooth lining of the following structures:

- heart
- blood vessels
- lymph vessels
- alveoli of the lungs.

where it is also known as endothelium

Cuboidal (cubical) epithelium

This consists of cube-shaped cells fitting closely together lying on a basement membrane (Fig. 3.7). It forms the kidney tubules and is found in some glands. Cuboidal epithelium is actively involved in secretion, absorption and excretion.

Columnar epithelium

This is formed by a single layer of cells, rectangular in shape, on a basement membrane (Fig. 3.8). It is found lining the organs of the alimentary tract and consists of a mixture of cells; some absorb the products of digestion and others secrete *mucus*. Mucus is a thick sticky substance secreted by specialised columnar cells called *goblet cells* (see Fig. 3.23, p. 41).

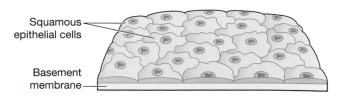

Squamous epithelial cells

Basement membrane

Figure 3.6 Squamous epithelium.

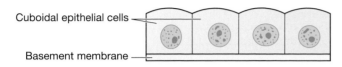

Figure 3.7 Cuboidal epithelium.

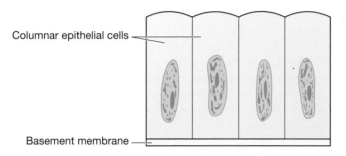

Figure 3.8 Columnar epithelium.

Ciliated epithelium (Fig. 3.9)

Cilia are microscopic, hair-like processes on the free surface of columnar epithelial cells lining certain passageways, e.g. uterine tubes and airways, where their wave-like motion propels materials one-way. In the uterine tubes the cilia propel ova towards the uterus and in the respiratory passages they propel mucus towards the throat.

Stratified epithelia

Stratified epithelia consist of several layers of cells of various shapes. The superficial layers grow up from below. Basement membranes are usually absent. The main function of stratified epithelium is to protect underlying structures from mechanical wear and tear. There are two main types: stratified squamous and transitional.

Stratified squamous epithelium (Fig. 3.10)

This is composed of a number of layers of cells of different shapes representing newly formed and mature cells. In the deepest layers the cells are mainly columnar and, as they grow towards the surface, they become flattened and are then shed.

Non-keratinised stratified epithelium. This is found on wet surfaces subjected to wear and tear but are protected from drying, e.g. the conjunctiva of the eyes, the lining of the mouth, the pharynx, the oesophagus and the vagina.

Keratinised stratified epithelium. This is found on dry surfaces subjected to wear and tear, i.e. skin, hair and nails. The surface layer consists of dead epithelial cells that contain the protein keratin. This forms a tough, relatively waterproof protective layer that prevents drying of the live cells underneath. The surface layer of skin is rubbed off and is replaced from below (see Ch. 14).

Transitional epithelium (Fig. 3.11)

This is composed of several layers of pear-shaped cells. It is found lining the urinary bladder and allows for stretching as the bladder fills.

Connective tissue

Connective tissue is the most abundant tissue in the body. The connective tissue cells are more widely separated from each other than in epithelial tissues, and inter-cellular substance (matrix) is present in considerably larger amounts. There are usually fibres present in the matrix, which may be of a semisolid jelly-like consistency or dense and rigid, depending upon the position and function of the tissue. Most types of connective tissue

35

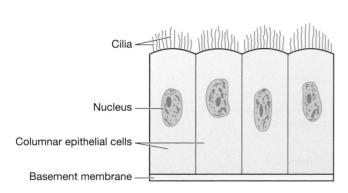

Figure 3.9 Ciliated columnar epithelium.

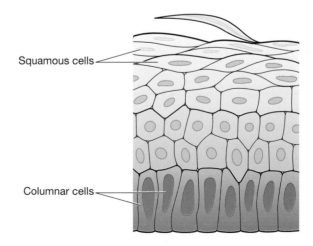

Figure 3.10 Stratified epithelium.

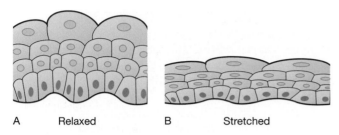

A   Relaxed   B   Stretched

Figure 3.11 Transitional epithelium: A. Relaxed. B. Stretched.

have a good blood supply. Major functions of connective tissue are:

- binding and structural support
- protection
- transport
- insulation.

Cells of connective tissue

Connective tissue, excluding blood (see Ch. 4), is found in all organs supporting the specialised tissue. The different types of cell involved include: fibroblasts, fat cells, macrophages, leukocytes and mast cells.

Fibroblasts. Fibroblasts are large flat cells with irregular processes. They produce *collagen* and *elastic fibres* and a matrix of extracellular material. Very fine collagen fibres, sometimes called *reticulin fibres*, are found in very active tissue, such as the liver and lymphoid tissue. Fibroblasts are particularly active in tissue repair (wound healing) where they may bind together the cut surfaces of wounds or form *granulation tissue* following tissue destruction (see p. 363). The collagen fibres formed during healing shrink as they grow old, sometimes interfering with the functions of the organ involved and with adjacent structures.

Fat cells. Also known as *adipocytes*, these cells occur singly or in groups in many types of connective tissue and are especially abundant in adipose tissue. They vary in size and shape according to the amount of fat they contain.

Macrophages. These are irregular-shaped cells with granules in the cytoplasm. Some are fixed, i.e. attached to connective tissue fibres, and others are motile. They are an important part of the body's defence mechanisms because they are actively phagocytic, engulfing and digesting cell debris, bacteria and other foreign bodies. Their activities are typical of those of the macrophage/monocyte defence system, e.g. monocytes in blood, phagocytes in the alveoli of the lungs, Kupffer cells in liver sinusoids, fibroblasts in lymph nodes and spleen, and microglial cells in the brain.

Leukocytes. White blood cells (p. 63) are normally found in small numbers in healthy connective tissue but neutrophils migrate in significant numbers during infection when they play an important part in tissue defence.

Plasma cells. These develop from B-lymphocytes, a type of white blood cell (see p. 375). They synthesise and secrete specific defensive *antibodies* into the blood and tissues (see Ch. 15).

Mast cells. These cells are similar to basophil leukocytes (see p. 65). They are found in loose connective tissue and under the fibrous capsule of some organs, e.g. liver and spleen, and in considerable numbers round blood vessels. They produce granules containing *heparin*, *histamine* and other substances, which are released when the cells are damaged by disease or injury. Histamine is involved in local and general inflammatory reactions, it stimulates the secretion of gastric juice and is associated with the development of allergies and hypersensitivity states (see p. 380). Heparin prevents coagulation of blood, which may aid the passage of protective substances from blood to affected tissues.

Loose (areolar) connective tissue (Fig. 3.12)

This is the most generalised type of connective tissue. The matrix is semisolid with many fibroblasts and some fat cells, mast cells and macrophages widely separated by elastic and collagen fibres. It is found in almost every part of the body providing elasticity and tensile strength. It connects and supports other tissues, for example:

- under the skin
- between muscles
- supporting blood vessels and nerves
- in the alimentary canal
- in glands supporting secretory cells.

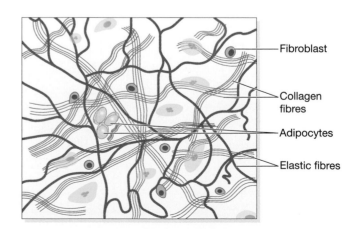

Fibroblast

Collagen fibres

Adipocytes

Elastic fibres

Figure 3.12 Loose (areolar) connective tissue.

Adipose tissue (Fig. 3.13)

Adipose tissue consists of fat cells (adipocytes), containing large fat globules, in a matrix of areolar tissue. There are two types: white and brown.

White adipose tissue. This makes up 20 to 25% of body weight in well-nourished adults. The amount of adipose tissue in an individual is determined by the balance between energy intake and expenditure. It is found supporting the kidneys and the eyes, between muscle fibres and under the skin, where it acts as a thermal insulator and energy store.

Brown adipose tissue. This is present in the newborn. It has a more extensive capillary network than white adipose tissue. When brown tissue is metabolised, it produces less energy and considerably more heat than other fat, contributing to the maintenance of body temperature. In some adults it is present in small amounts.

Dense connective tissue

This contains more fibres and fewer cells than loose connective tissue.

Fibrous tissue (Fig. 3.14)

This tissue is made up mainly of closely packed bundles of collagen fibres with very little matrix. Fibrocytes (old and inactive fibroblasts) are few in number and are found lying in rows between the bundles of fibres. Fibrous tissue is found:

- forming *ligaments*, which bind bones together
- as an outer protective covering for bone, called *periosteum*
- as an outer protective covering of some organs, e.g. the kidneys, lymph nodes and the brain

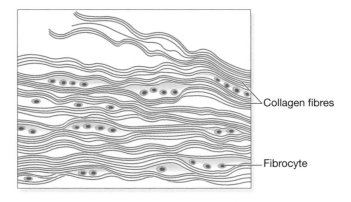

Figure 3.14 Fibrous tissue.

- forming muscle sheaths, called *muscle fascia* (see Fig. 16.52, p. 415), which extend beyond the muscle to become the *tendon* that attaches the muscle to bone.

Elastic tissue (Fig. 3.15)

Elastic tissue is capable of considerable extension and recoil. There are few cells and the matrix consists mainly of masses of elastic fibres secreted by fibroblasts. It is found in organs where stretching or alteration of shape is required, e.g. in large blood vessel walls, the trachea and bronchi, and the lungs.

Blood

This is a fluid connective tissue that is described in detail in Chapter 4.

Lymphoid tissue (Fig. 3.16)

This tissue, also known as reticular tissue, has a semisolid matrix with fine branching reticulin fibres. It contains reticular cells and white blood cells (*monocytes* and

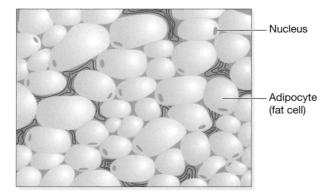

Figure 3.13 Adipose tissue.

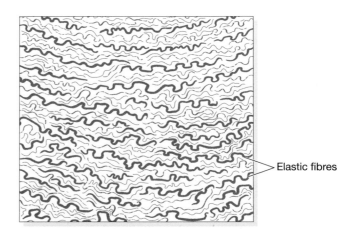

Figure 3.15 Elastic tissue.

37

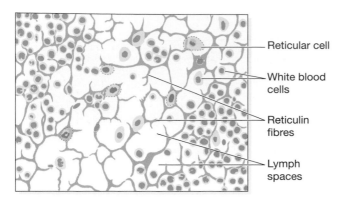

Figure 3.16 Lymphoid tissue.

lymphocytes). Lymphoid tissue is found in lymph nodes and all organs of the lymphatic system (see Fig. 6.1, p. 132).

Cartilage

Cartilage is firmer than other connective tissues; the cells are called *chondrocytes* and are less numerous. They are embedded in matrix reinforced by collagen and elastic fibres. There are three types: hyaline cartilage, fibrocartilage and elastic fibrocartilage.

Hyaline cartilage (Fig. 3.17)

Hyaline cartilage is a smooth bluish-white tissue. The chondrocytes are in small groups within cell nests and the matrix is solid and smooth. Hyaline cartilage provides flexibility, support and smooth surfaces for movement at joints. It is found:

- on the ends of long bones that form joints
- forming the costal cartilages, which attach the ribs to the sternum
- forming part of the larynx, trachea and bronchi.

Fibrocartilage (Fig. 3.18)

This consists of dense masses of white collagen fibres in a matrix similar to that of hyaline cartilage with the cells widely dispersed. It is a tough, slightly flexible, supporting tissue found:

- as pads between the bodies of the vertebrae, the *intervertebral discs*
- between the articulating surfaces of the bones of the knee joint, called *semilunar cartilages*
- on the rim of the bony sockets of the hip and shoulder joints, deepening the cavities without restricting movement
- as *ligaments* joining bones.

Elastic fibrocartilage (Fig. 3.19)

This flexible tissue consists of yellow elastic fibres lying in a solid matrix. The chondrocytes lie between the fibres. It provides support and maintains shape of, e.g. the pinna or lobe of the ear, the epiglottis and part of the tunica media of blood vessel walls.

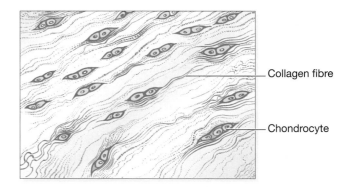

Figure 3.18 Fibrocartilage.

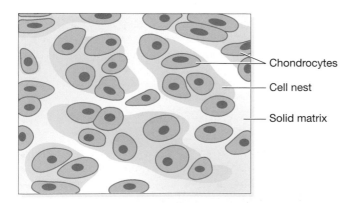

Figure 3.17 Hyaline cartilage.

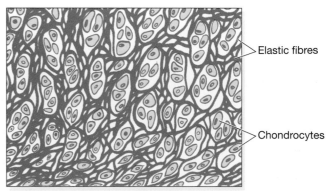

Figure 3.19 Elastic fibrocartilage.

Bone

Bone cells (osteocytes) are surrounded by a matrix of collagen fibres strengthened by inorganic salts, especially calcium and phosphate. This provides bones with their characteristic strength and rigidity. Bone also has considerable capacity for growth in the first two decades of life, and for regeneration throughout life. Two types of bone can be identified by the naked eye:

- *compact bone* – solid or dense appearance
- *spongy* or *cancellous bone* – 'spongy' or fine honeycomb appearance.

These are described in detail in Chapter 16.

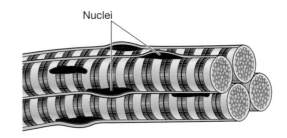

Figure 3.20 **Skeletal muscle fibres.**

Muscle tissue

Muscle tissue is able to contract and relax, providing movement within the body and of the body itself. Muscle contraction requires an adequate blood supply to provide sufficient oxygen, calcium and nutrients and to remove waste products. There are three types of specialised contractile cells, also known as *fibres*: skeletal muscle, smooth muscle and cardiac muscle.

Skeletal muscle tissue (Fig. 3.20)

This type is described as skeletal because it forms those muscles that move the bones [of the skeleton], *striated* because striations (stripes) can be seen on microscopic examination and *voluntary* as it is under conscious control. In reality, movements can be finely coordinated, e.g. writing, but may also be controlled subconsciously. For example, maintaining an upright posture does not normally require thought unless a new locomotor skill is being learned, e.g. skating or cycling, and the diaphragm maintains breathing while asleep.

Fibres are cylindrical, contain several nuclei and can be up to 35 cm long. Skeletal muscle contraction is stimulated by motor nerve impulses originating in the brain or spinal cord and ending at the neuromuscular junction (see p. 416). The properties and functions of skeletal muscle are explained in detail in Chapter 16.

Smooth (visceral) muscle tissue (Fig. 3.21)

Smooth muscle may also be described as *non-striated* or *involuntary*. It does not have striations and is not under conscious control. Smooth muscle has the intrinsic ability to contract and relax. Additionally, autonomic nerve impulses, some hormones and local metabolites stimulate contraction. A degree of muscle tone is always present, meaning that smooth muscle is completely relaxed for only short periods. Contraction of smooth

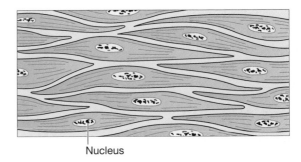

Figure 3.21 **Smooth muscle fibres.**

39

muscle is slower and more sustained than skeletal muscle. It is found in the walls of hollow organs:

- regulating the diameter of blood vessels and parts of the respiratory tract
- propelling contents of the ureters, ducts of glands and alimentary tract
- expelling contents of the urinary bladder and uterus.

When examined under a microscope, the cells are seen to be spindle shaped with only one central nucleus. Bundles of fibres form sheets of muscle, such as those found in the walls of the above structures.

Cardiac muscle tissue (Fig. 3.22)

This type of muscle tissue is found only in the heart wall. It is not under conscious control but, when viewed under a microscope, cross-stripes (striations) characteristic of skeletal muscle can be seen. Each fibre (cell) has a nucleus and one or more branches. The ends of the cells and their branches are in very close contact with the ends and branches of adjacent cells. Microscopically these 'joints',

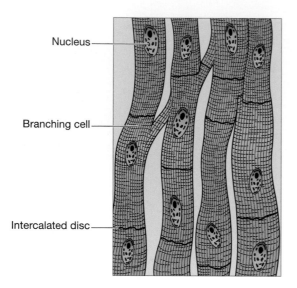

Nucleus

Branching cell

Intercalated disc

Figure 3.22 Cardiac muscle fibres.

or *intercalated discs*, can be seen as lines that are thicker and darker than the ordinary cross-stripes. This arrangement gives cardiac muscle the appearance of a sheet of muscle rather than a very large number of individual fibres. The end-to-end continuity of cardiac muscle cells has significance in relation to the way the heart contracts. A wave of contraction spreads from cell to cell across the intercalated discs, which means that cells do not need to be stimulated individually.

The heart has an intrinsic pacemaker system, which means that it beats in a coordinated manner without external nerve stimulation, although the rate at which it beats is influenced by autonomic nerve impulses, some hormones, local metabolites and other substances (see Ch. 5).

Nervous tissue

Two types of tissue are found in the nervous system:

- excitable cells – these are called *neurones* and they initiate, receive, conduct and transmit information
- non-excitable cells – also known as *glial cells*, these support the neurones.

These are described in detail in Chapter 7.

Tissue regeneration

When tissue regeneration occurs it is essential that some of the original cells are available to replicate by mitosis. The extent to which regeneration is possible depends on the normal rate of turnover of particular types of cell. Those with a rapid turnover regenerate most effectively. There are three types.

Labile cells are those in which replication is normally a continuous process. They include epithelial cells of e.g. skin, mucous membrane, secretory glands, ducts, uterine lining, cells in the bone marrow and spleen, and lymphoid tissue.

Stable cells retain the ability to replicate but do so infrequently. They include liver, kidney and pancreatic cells, fibroblasts, smooth muscle cells, and osteoblasts and osteoclasts in bone.

Permanent cells are unable to replicate after normal growth is complete. They include nerve cells (neurones) and skeletal and cardiac muscle.

Membranes

Epithelial membranes

These membranes are sheets of epithelial tissue and supporting connective tissue that cover or line many internal structures or cavities. The main ones are mucous membrane, serous membrane and the skin (cutaneous membrane, see Ch. 14)

Mucous membrane

This is the moist lining of the alimentary tract, respiratory tract and genitourinary tracts and is sometimes referred to as the *mucosa*. The membrane surface consists of epithelial cells, some of which produce a secretion called *mucus*, a slimy tenacious fluid. As it accumulates the cells become distended and finally burst, discharging the mucus onto the free surface. As the cells fill up with mucus they have the appearance of a goblet or flask and are known as *goblet cells* (Fig. 3.23). Organs lined by mucous membrane have a moist slippery surface. Mucus protects the lining membrane from drying, and mechanical and chemical injury. In the respiratory tract it traps inhaled foreign particles, preventing them from entering the alveoli of the lungs.

Serous membrane

Serous membranes, or *serosa*, secrete serous watery fluid. They consist of a double layer of loose areolar connective tissue lined by simple squamous epithelium. The *parietal* layer lines a cavity and the *visceral* layer surrounds organs (the viscera) within the cavity. The two layers are

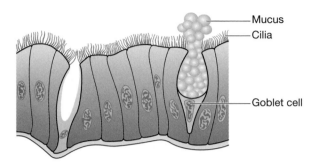

Figure 3.23 Ciliated columnar epithelium with goblet cells.

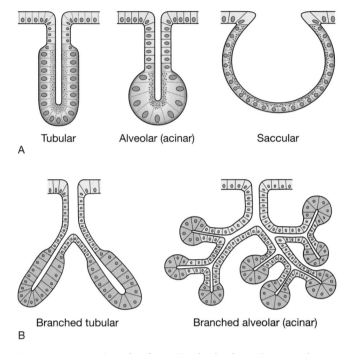

Figure 3.24 Exocrine glands: A. Simple glands. **B.** Compound (branching) glands.

separated by *serous fluid* secreted by the epithelium. There are three sites where serous membranes are found:

- the *pleura* lining the thoracic cavity and surrounding the lungs (p. 246)
- the *pericardium* lining the pericardial cavity and surrounding the heart (p. 81)
- the *peritoneum* lining the abdominal cavity and surrounding abdominal organs (p. 284).

The serous fluid between the visceral and parietal layers enables an organ to glide freely within the cavity without being damaged by friction between it and adjacent organs. For example, the heart changes its shape and size during each beat and friction damage is prevented by the arrangement of pericardium and its serous fluid.

Synovial membrane

This membrane lines the cavities of moveable joints and surrounds tendons that could be injured by rubbing against bones, e.g. over the wrist joint. It is not an epithelial membrane, but instead consists of areolar connective tissue and elastic fibres.

Synovial membrane secretes clear, sticky, oily *synovial fluid*, which lubricates and nourishes the joints (see Ch. 16).

Glands

Glands are groups of epithelial cells that produce specialised secretions. Glands that discharge their secretion onto the epithelial surface of hollow organs, either directly or through a *duct*, are called *exocrine glands*. Secretions of exocrine glands include mucus, saliva, digestive juices and earwax. Exocrine glands vary considerably in size, shape and complexity as shown in Figure 3.24. Other glands discharge their secretions into blood and lymph. These are called *endocrine glands* (ductless glands) and their secretions are *hormones* (see Ch. 9).

41

Organisation of the body

Learning outcomes

After studying this section you should be able to:

- define common anatomical terms
- identify the principal bones of the axial skeleton and the appendicular skeleton
- state the boundaries of the four body cavities
- list the contents of the body cavities.

This part of the chapter provides an overview of anatomical terms and the names and positions of bones. A more detailed account of the bones, muscles and joints is given in Chapter 16.

Anatomical terms

The anatomical position. This is the position assumed in all anatomical descriptions to ensure accuracy and consistency. The body is in the upright position with the head facing forward, the arms at the sides with the palms of the hands facing forward and the feet together.

Median plane. When the body, in the anatomical position, is divided *longitudinally* through the midline into right and left halves it has been divided in the median plane.

Directional terms. These paired terms are used to describe the location of body parts in relation to others, and are explained in Table 3.1.

Regional terms. These are used to describe parts of the body (Fig. 3.25).

The skeleton

The skeleton (Fig. 3.26) is the bony framework of the body. It forms the cavities and fossae (depressions or hollows) that protect some structures, forms the joints and gives attachment to muscles. A detailed description of the bones is given in Chapter 16. Table 16.1 (p. 388) lists the terminology related to the skeleton.

The skeleton is described in two parts: *axial* and *appendicular* (the appendages attached to the axial skeleton).

Axial skeleton

The axial skeleton (axis of the body) consists of the skull, vertebral column, sternum (or breast bone) and the ribs.

Skull

The skull is described in two parts, the *cranium*, which contains the brain, and the *face*. It consists of a number of bones, which develop separately but fuse together as they mature. The only movable bone is the mandible or lower jaw. The names and positions of the individual bones of the skull can be seen in Figure 3.27.

Functions of the skull
The various parts of the skull have specific and different functions (see p. 395) and are, in summary:

- protection of delicate structures including the brain, eyes and inner ears
- maintaining patency of the nasal passages enabling breathing
- eating – the teeth are embedded in the mandible and maxilla; and movement of the mandible, the only movable skull bone, allows chewing.

Vertebral column

This consists of 24 movable bones (vertebrae) plus the sacrum and coccyx. The bodies of the bones are separated

Table 3.1 Paired directional terms used in anatomy

Directional term	Meaning
Medial	Structure is nearer to the midline. *The heart is medial to the humerus*
Lateral	Structure is further from the midline or at the side of the body. *The humerus is lateral to the heart*
Proximal	Nearer to a point of attachment of a limb, or origin of a body part. *The femur is proximal to the fibula*
Distal	Further from a point of attachment of a limb, or origin of a body part. *The fibula is distal to the femur*
Anterior or ventral	Part of the body being described is nearer the front of the body. *The sternum is anterior to the vertebrae*
Posterior or dorsal	Part of the body being described is nearer the back of the body. *The vertebrae are posterior to the sternum*
Superior	Structure nearer the head. *The skull is superior to the scapulae*
Inferior	Structure further from the head. *The scapulae are inferior to the skull*

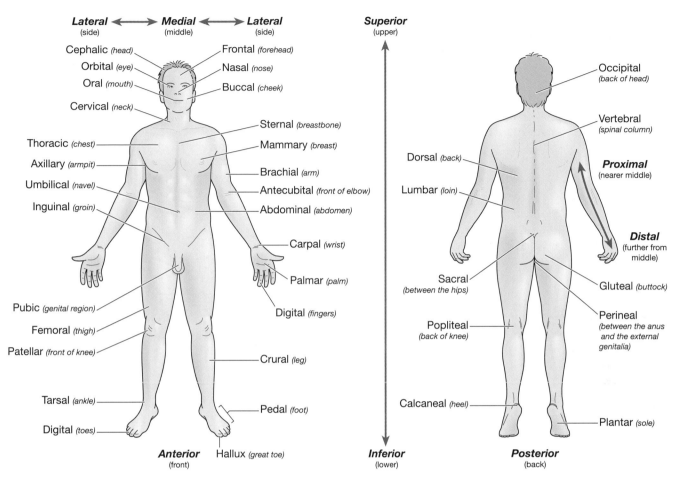

Figure 3.25 Regional and directional terms

from each other by *intervertebral discs*, consisting of cartilage. The vertebral column is described in five parts and the bones of each part are numbered from above downwards (Fig. 3.28):

- 7 cervical
- 12 thoracic
- 5 lumbar
- 1 sacrum (5 fused bones)
- 1 coccyx (4 fused bones).

The first cervical vertebra, called the *atlas*, forms a joint (*articulates*) with the skull. Thereafter each vertebra forms a joint with the vertebrae immediately above and below. More movement is possible in the cervical and lumbar regions than in the thoracic region.

The *sacrum* consists of five vertebrae fused into one bone that articulates with the fifth lumbar vertebra above, the coccyx below and an innominate (pelvic or hip) bone at each side.

The *coccyx* consists of the four terminal vertebrae fused into a small triangular bone that articulates with the sacrum above.

Functions of the vertebral column

The vertebral column has several important functions:

- It protects the spinal cord. In each vertebra is a hole, the *vertebral foramen,* and collectively the foramina form a canal in which the spinal cord lies.
- Adjacent vertebrae form openings (intervertebral foramina), which protect the spinal nerves as they pass from the spinal cord (see Fig. 16.24, p. 398).
- In the thoracic region the ribs articulate with the vertebrae forming joints allowing movement of the ribcage during respiration.

Thoracic cage

The thoracic cage is formed by:

- 12 thoracic vertebrae
- 12 pairs of ribs
- 1 sternum or breast bone.

The arrangement of the bones is shown in Figure 3.29.

43

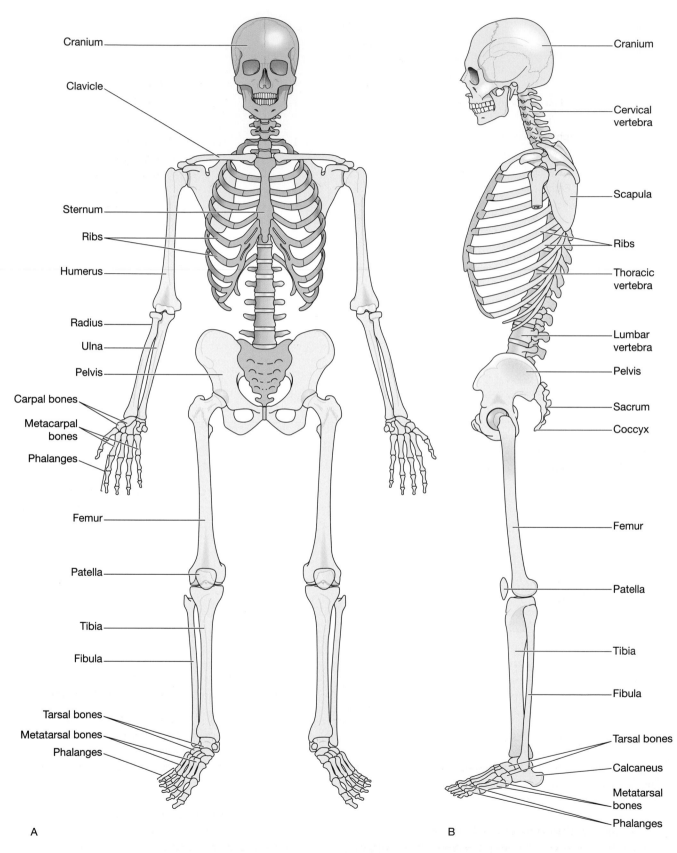

Cranium

Clavicle

Sternum

Ribs

Humerus

Radius

Ulna

Pelvis

Carpal bones

Metacarpal bones

Phalanges

Femur

Patella

Tibia

Fibula

Tarsal bones

Metatarsal bones

Phalanges

Cranium

Cervical vertebra

Scapula

Ribs

Thoracic vertebra

Lumbar vertebra

Pelvis

Sacrum

Coccyx

Femur

Patella

Tibia

Fibula

Tarsal bones

Calcaneus

Metatarsal bones

Phalanges

A

B

44

Figure 3.26 The skeleton: A. Anterior view: axial skeleton – gold, appendicular skeleton – brown. **B.** Lateral view.

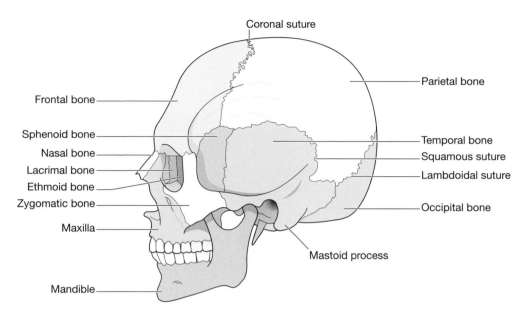

Coronal suture

Parietal bone

Frontal bone

Sphenoid bone

Temporal bone

Nasal bone

Squamous suture

Lacrimal bone

Lambdoidal suture

Ethmoid bone

Zygomatic bone

Occipital bone

Maxilla

Mandible

Mastoid process

Figure 3.27 The skull: bones of the cranium and face.

Functions of the thoracic cage

The functions of the thoracic cage are:

- It protects the thoracic organs including the heart, lungs and large blood vessels.
- It forms joints between the upper limbs and the axial skeleton. The upper part of the sternum, the *manubrium*, articulates with the clavicles forming the only joints between the upper limbs and the axial skeleton.
- It gives attachment to the muscles of respiration:
  - *intercostal muscles* occupy the spaces between the ribs and when they contract the ribs move upwards and outwards, increasing the capacity of the thoracic cage, and inspiration (breathing in) occurs
  - the *diaphragm* is a dome-shaped muscle which separates the thoracic and abdominal cavities. It is attached to the bones of the thorax and when it contracts it assists with inspiration.
- It enables breathing to take place.

Appendicular skeleton

The appendicular skeleton consists of the shoulder girdles and upper limbs, and the pelvic girdle and lower limbs (Fig. 3.26).

The shoulder girdles and upper limbs. Each shoulder girdle consists of a clavicle and a scapula. Each upper limb comprises:

- 1 humerus
- 1 radius
- 1 ulna
- 8 carpal bones
- 5 metacarpal bones
- 14 phalanges.

The pelvic girdle and lower limbs. The bones of the pelvic girdle are the two innominate bones and the sacrum. Each lower limb consists of:

- 1 femur
- 1 tibia
- 1 fibula
- 1 patella
- 7 tarsal bones
- 5 metatarsal bones
- 14 phalanges.

Functions of the appendicular skeleton

The appendicular skeleton has two main functions.

- *Voluntary movement.* The bones, muscles and joints of the limbs are involved in movement of the skeleton. This ranges from very fine finger movements needed for writing to the coordinated movement of all the limbs associated with running and jumping.
- *Protection of delicate structures.* Blood vessels and nerves lie along the length of bones of the limbs and are protected from injury by the associated muscles and skin. These structures are most vulnerable where

45

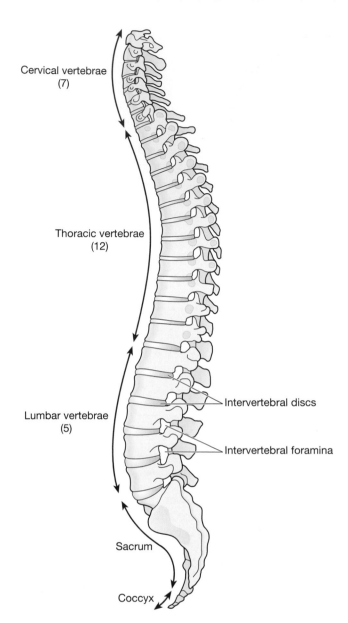

Cervical vertebrae
(7)

Thoracic vertebrae
(12)

Lumbar vertebrae
(5)

Intervertebral discs

Intervertebral foramina

Sacrum

Coccyx

Figure 3.28 The vertebral column – lateral view.

they cross joints and where bones can be felt immediately below the skin.

Cavities of the body

The organs that make up the systems of the body are contained in four cavities: cranial, thoracic, abdominal and pelvic.

Cranial cavity

The cranial cavity contains the brain, and its boundaries are formed by the bones of the skull (Fig. 3.30):

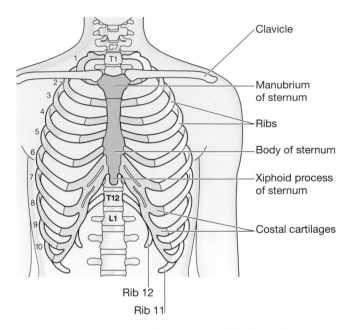

Clavicle

Manubrium
of sternum

Ribs

Body of sternum

Xiphoid process
of sternum

Costal cartilages

Rib 12

Rib 11

Figure 3.29 The structures forming the walls of the thoracic cage.

Anteriorly – 1 frontal bone
Laterally – 2 temporal bones
Posteriorly – 1 occipital bone
Superiorly – 2 parietal bones
Inferiorly – 1 sphenoid and 1 ethmoid bone and parts of the frontal, temporal and occipital bones.

Thoracic cavity

This cavity is situated in the upper part of the trunk. Its boundaries are formed by a bony framework and supporting muscles (Fig. 3.31):

Anteriorly – the sternum and costal cartilages of the ribs
Laterally – 12 pairs of ribs and the intercostal muscles
Posteriorly – the thoracic vertebrae
Superiorly – the structures forming the root of the neck
Inferiorly – the diaphragm, a dome-shaped muscle.

Contents

The main organs and structures contained in the thoracic cavity are (Fig. 3.32):

- the trachea, 2 bronchi, 2 lungs
- the heart, aorta, superior and inferior vena cava, numerous other blood vessels
- the oesophagus
- lymph vessels and lymph nodes
- nerves.

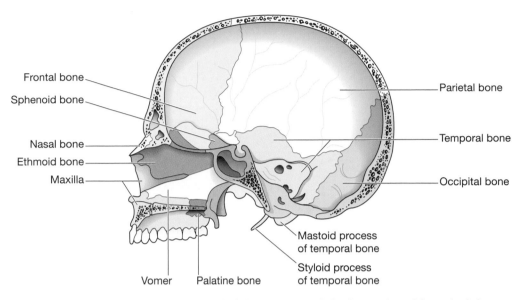

Figure 3.30 Bones forming the right half of the cranium and the face – viewed from the left.

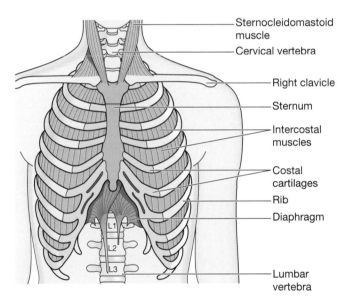

Figure 3.31 Structures forming the walls of the thoracic cavity and associated structures.

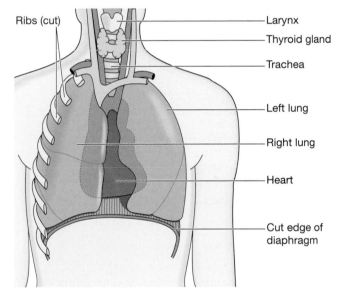

Figure 3.32 Some of the main structures in the thoracic cavity and the root of the neck.

The *mediastinum* is the name given to the space between the lungs including the structures found there, such as the heart, oesophagus and blood vessels.

Abdominal cavity

This is the largest cavity in the body and is oval in shape (Figs 3.33 and 3.34). It is situated in the main part of the trunk and its boundaries are:

Superiorly – the diaphragm, which separates it from the thoracic cavity

Anteriorly – the muscles forming the anterior abdominal wall

Posteriorly – the lumbar vertebrae and muscles forming the posterior abdominal wall

Laterally – the lower ribs and parts of the muscles of the abdominal wall

Inferiorly – it is continuous with the pelvic cavity.

By convention, the abdominal cavity is divided into the nine regions shown in Figure 3.35. This facilitates the description of the positions of the organs and structures it contains.

47

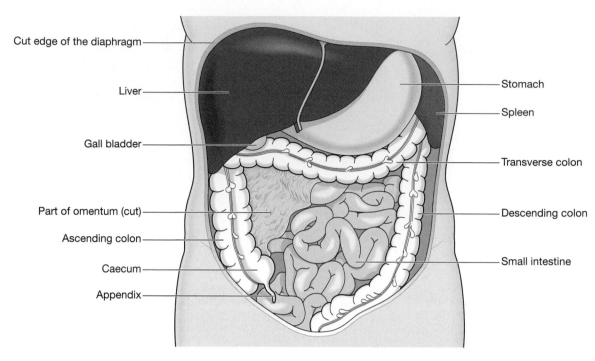

Figure 3.33 Organs occupying the anterior part of the abdominal cavity and the diaphragm (cut).

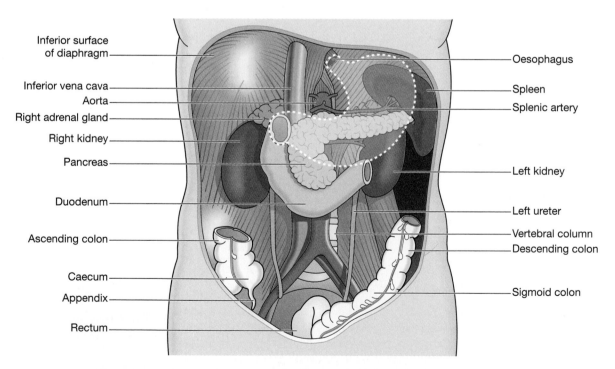

Figure 3.34 Organs occupying the posterior part of the abdominal and pelvic cavities. The broken line shows the position of the stomach.

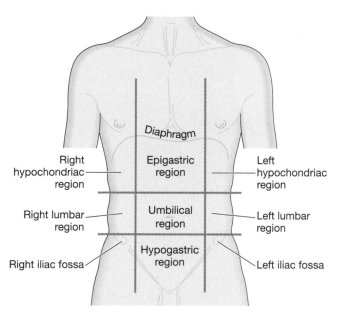

Figure 3.35 Regions of the abdominal cavity.

Contents

Most of the abdominal cavity is occupied by the organs and glands of the digestive system (Figs 3.33 and 3.34). These are:

- the stomach, small intestine and most of the large intestine
- the liver, gall bladder, bile ducts and pancreas.

Other structures include:

- the spleen
- 2 kidneys and the upper part of the ureters
- 2 adrenal (suprarenal) glands
- numerous blood vessels, lymph vessels, nerves
- lymph nodes.

Pelvic cavity

The pelvic cavity is roughly funnel shaped and extends from the lower end of the abdominal cavity (Figs 3.36 and 3.37). The boundaries are:

Superiorly – it is continuous with the abdominal cavity
Anteriorly – the pubic bones
Posteriorly – the sacrum and coccyx
Laterally – the innominate bones
Inferiorly – the muscles of the pelvic floor.

Contents

The pelvic cavity contains the following structures:

- sigmoid colon, rectum and anus
- some loops of the small intestine
- urinary bladder, lower parts of the ureters and the urethra
- in the female, the organs of the reproductive system: the uterus, uterine tubes, ovaries and vagina (Fig. 3.36)

49

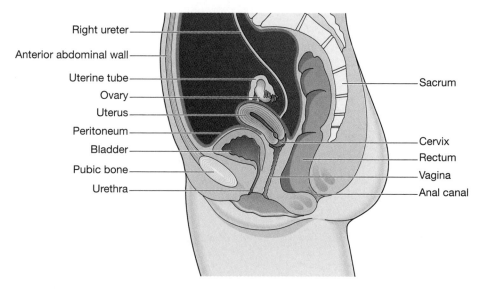

Figure 3.36 Female reproductive organs and other structures in the pelvic cavity.

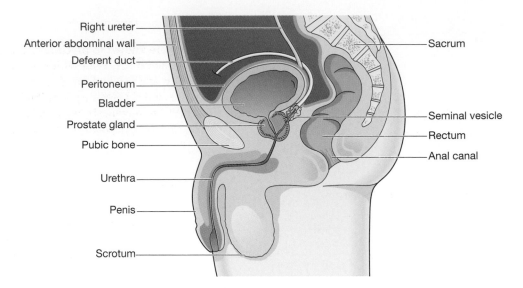

Right ureter
Anterior abdominal wall
Deferent duct
Peritoneum
Bladder
Prostate gland
Pubic bone
Urethra
Penis
Scrotum

Sacrum
Seminal vesicle
Rectum
Anal canal

Figure 3.37 The pelvic cavity and reproductive structures in the male.

- in the male, some of the organs of the reproductive system: the prostate gland, seminal vesicles, spermatic cords, deferent ducts (vas deferens), ejaculatory ducts and the urethra (common to the reproductive and urinary systems) (Fig. 3.37).

Disorders of cells and tissues

Learning outcomes

After studying this section you should be able to:

■ outline the common causes of tumours

■ explain the terms 'well differentiated' and 'poorly differentiated'

■ outline causes of death in malignant disease

■ compare and contrast the effects of benign and malignant tumours.

Neoplasms or tumours

A tumour or *neoplasm* (literally meaning 'new growth') is a mass of tissue that grows faster than normal in an uncoordinated manner, and continues to grow after the initial stimulus has ceased.

Tumours are classified as benign or malignant although a clear distinction is not always possible (see Table 3.2). Benign tumours only rarely change their character and become malignant. Tumours may be classified according to their tissue of origin. For example, an *adenoma* is a benign tumour of glandular tissue whereas an *adenocarcinoma* is a malignant tumour of glandular or secretory epithelial tissue. Malignant tumours are often named according to the tissue they arise from, for example a *carcinoma* originates in epithelial tissue whereas a *sarcoma* arises from connective tissue.

Table 3.2 Differences between benign and malignant tumours

Benign	Malignant
Slow growth	Rapid growth
Cells well differentiated (resemble tissue of origin)	Cells poorly differentiated (may not resemble tissue of origin)
Usually encapsulated	Not encapsulated
No distant spread (metastases)	Spreads (metastasises): – by local infiltration – via lymph – via blood – via body cavities
Recurrence is rare	Recurrence is common

Causes of neoplasms

Some factors are known to precipitate the changes found in tumour cells but the reasons for the uncontrolled cell multiplication are not known. The process of change is *carcinogenesis* and the agents precipitating the change are *carcinogens*. Carcinogenesis may be of genetic and/or environmental origin and a clear-cut distinction is not always possible.

Carcinogens

Environmental agents known to cause malignant changes in cells do so by irreversibly damaging a cell's DNA. It is impossible to specify a maximum 'safe dose' of a carcinogen. A small dose may initiate change but this may not be enough to cause malignancy unless there are repeated doses within a limited period of time that have a cumulative effect. In addition, there are widely varying latent periods between exposure and evidence of malignancy. There may also be other unknown factors. Environmental carcinogens include chemicals, irradiations and oncogenic viruses.

Chemical carcinogens

Some chemicals are carcinogens when absorbed; others are modified after absorption and become carcinogenic. Examples include:

● aniline dyes, which predispose to bladder cancer (p. 354)
● asbestos, which is associated with malignant pleural tumours (mesothelioma, p. 265)
● cigarette smoke, which is the main risk factor for lung cancer (p. 264).

Radiation carcinogens

Exposure to ionising radiation including X-rays, radioactive isotopes, environmental radiation and ultraviolet rays in sunlight may cause malignant changes in some cells and kill others. The cells are affected during mitosis so those normally undergoing continuous controlled division are most susceptible. These labile tissues include skin, mucous membrane, bone marrow, lymphoid tissue and gametes in the ovaries and testes.

Oncogenic viruses

Some viruses are known to cause malignant changes in animals and there are indications of similar involvement in humans. Viruses enter cells and incorporate their DNA or RNA into the host cell's genetic material, which causes mutation. The mutant cells may be malignant. Examples include hepatitis B virus, which can cause liver cancer (p. 332) and human papilloma virus, which is associated with cervical cancer (p. 458).

51

Host factors

Individual characteristics can influence susceptibility to tumours. These include race, diet, age and inherited factors. Tumours of individual tissues and organs are described in the appropriate chapters.

Growth of tumours

Normally cells divide in an orderly manner. Neoplastic cells have escaped from the normal controls and they multiply in a disorderly manner forming a tumour. Blood vessels grow with the proliferating cells, but in some malignant tumours the blood supply does not keep pace with growth and *ischaemia* (lack of blood supply) leads to tumour cell death, called *necrosis*. If the tumour is near the surface, this may result in skin ulceration and infection. In deeper tissues there is fibrosis; e.g. retraction of the nipple in breast cancer is due to the shrinkage of fibrous tissue in a necrotic tumour. The mechanisms controlling the lifespan of tumour cells are poorly understood.

Cell differentiation

Differentiation of cells into specialised cell types with particular structural and functional characteristics occurs at an early stage in fetal development; e.g. epithelial cells develop different characteristics from lymphocytes. Later, when cell replacement occurs, daughter cells have the same appearance, functions and genetic make-up as the parent cell. In benign tumours the cells from which they originate are easily recognised; i.e. tumour cells are *well differentiated*. Tumours with well-differentiated cells are usually benign but some may be malignant. Malignant tumours grow beyond their normal boundaries and show varying levels of differentiation:

- *mild dysplasia* – the tumour cells retain most of their normal features and their parent cells can usually be identified
- *anaplasia* – the tumour cells have lost most of their normal features and their parent cells cannot be identified.

Encapsulation and spread of tumours

Most benign tumours are contained within a fibrous capsule derived partly from the surrounding tissues and partly from the tumour. They neither infiltrate local tissues nor spread to other parts of the body, even when they are not encapsulated.

Malignant tumours are not encapsulated. They spread locally by infiltration, and tumour fragments may spread to other parts of the body in blood or lymph. Some spreading cells may be phagocytosed but others lodge in tissues away from the primary site and grow into *secondary tumours* (metastases). Metastases are often multiple and Table 3.3 shows common sites of primary tumours and their metastases.

Local spread

Benign tumours enlarge and may cause pressure damage to local structures but they do not spread to other parts of the body.

Benign or malignant tumours may:

- damage nerves, causing pain and loss of nerve control of other tissues and organs supplied by the damaged nerves
- compress adjacent structures causing e.g. ischaemia (lack of blood), necrosis (death of tissue), blockage of ducts, organ dysfunction or displacement, or pain due to pressure on nerves.

Additionally *malignant tumours* grow into and infiltrate surrounding tissues and they may erode blood and lymph vessel walls, causing spread of tumour cells to other parts of the body.

Body cavities spread

This occurs when a tumour penetrates the wall of a cavity. The peritoneal cavity is most frequently involved. If, for example, a malignant tumour in an abdominal organ penetrates the visceral peritoneum, tumour cells may metastasise to folds of peritoneum or any abdominal or pelvic organ. Where there is less scope for the movement of fragments within a cavity the tumour tends to bind layers of tissue together, e.g. a pleural tumour binds the visceral and parietal layers together, limiting expansion of the lung.

Table 3.3 Common sites of primary tumours and their metastases

Primary tumour	Metastatic tumours
Bronchi	Adrenal glands, brain
Alimentary tract	Abdominal and pelvic structures, especially liver
Prostate gland	Pelvic bones, vertebrae
Thyroid gland	Pelvic bones, vertebrae
Breast	Vertebrae, brain, bone
Many organs	Lungs

Lymphatic spread

This occurs when malignant tumours grow into lymph vessels. Groups of tumour cells break off and are carried to lymph nodes where they lodge and may grow into secondary tumours. There may be further spread through the lymphatic system, and to blood because lymph drains into the subclavian veins.

Blood spread

This occurs when a malignant tumour erodes the walls of a blood vessel. A *thrombus* (blood clot) may form at the site and *emboli* consisting of fragments of tumour and blood clot enter the bloodstream. These emboli block small blood vessels, causing *infarcts* (areas of dead tissue) and development of metastatic tumours. Phagocytosis of tumour cells in the emboli is unlikely to occur because these are protected by the blood clot. Single tumour cells can also lodge in the capillaries of other body organs. Division and subsequent growth of secondary tumours, or *metastases*, may then occur. The sites of blood-spread metastases depend on the location of the original tumour and the anatomy of the circulatory system. The most common sites of these metastases are bone, the lungs, the brain and the liver.

Effects of tumours

Pressure effects

Both benign and malignant tumours may compress and damage adjacent structures, especially if in a confined space. The effects depend on the site of the tumour but are most marked in areas where there is little space for expansion, e.g. inside the skull, under the periosteum of bones, in bony sinuses and respiratory passages. Compression of adjacent structures may cause ischaemia, necrosis, blockage of ducts, organ dysfunction or displacement, pain due to invasion of nerves or pressure on nerves.

Hormonal effects

Tumours of endocrine glands may secrete hormones, producing the effects of hypersecretion. The extent of cell dysplasia is an important factor. Well-differentiated benign tumours are more likely to secrete hormones than are markedly dysplastic malignant tumours. High levels of hormones are found in the bloodstream as secretion occurs in the absence of the normal stimulus and homeostatic control mechanism. Some malignant tumours produce uncharacteristic hormones, e.g. some lung tumours produce insulin. Endocrine glands may be destroyed by invading tumours, causing hormone deficiency.

Cachexia

This is the severe weight loss accompanied by progressive weakness, loss of appetite, wasting and anaemia that is usually associated with advanced metastatic cancer. The severity is usually indicative of the stage of development of the disease. The causes are not clear.

Causes of death in malignant disease

Infection

Acute infection is a common cause of death when superimposed on advanced malignancy. Predisposition to infection is increased by prolonged bedrest, and by depression of the immune system by cytotoxic drugs and irradiation by X-rays or radioactive isotopes used in treatment. The most commonly occurring infections are pneumonia, septicaemia, peritonitis and pyelonephritis.

Organ failure

A tumour may destroy so much tissue that an organ cannot function. Severe damage to vital organs, such as lungs, brain, liver and kidneys, are common causes of death.

Carcinomatosis

When there is widespread metastatic disease associated with cachexia, severe physiological and biochemical disruption follows causing death.

Haemorrhage

This may occur when a tumour grows into and ruptures the wall of a vein or artery. The most common sites are the gastrointestinal tract, brain, lungs and the peritoneal cavity.

Communication

The blood

4

Blood is a connective tissue. It provides one of the means of communication between the cells of different parts of the body and the external environment, e.g. it carries:

- oxygen from the lungs to the tissues, and carbon dioxide from the tissues to the lungs for excretion
- nutrients from the alimentary tract to the tissues, and cell wastes to the excretory organs, principally the kidneys
- hormones secreted by endocrine glands to their target glands and tissues
- heat produced in active tissues to other less active tissues
- protective substances, e.g. antibodies, to areas of infection
- clotting factors that coagulate blood, minimising bleeding from ruptured blood vessels.

Blood makes up about 7% of body weight (about 5.6 litres in a 70 kg man). This proportion is less in women and considerably greater in children, gradually decreasing until the adult level is reached.

Blood in the blood vessels is always in motion because of the pumping action of the heart. The continual flow maintains a fairly constant environment for the body cells.

Blood volume and the concentration of its many constituents are kept within narrow limits by homeostatic mechanisms.

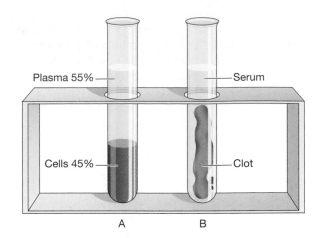

Figure 4.1 **A.** The proportions of blood cells and plasma in whole blood separated by gravity. **B.** A blood clot in serum.

Plasma

The constituents of plasma are water (90 to 92%) and dissolved substances, including:

- plasma proteins
- inorganic salts
- nutrients, principally from digested foods
- waste materials
- hormones
- gases.

Plasma proteins

Plasma proteins, which make up about 7% of plasma, are normally retained within the blood, because they are too big to escape through the capillary pores into the tissues. They are largely responsible for creating the osmotic pressure of blood (normally 25 mmHg or 3.3 kPa), which keeps plasma fluid within the circulation. If plasma protein levels fall, because of either reduced production or loss from the blood vessels, osmotic pressure is also reduced, and fluid moves into the tissues (oedema) and body cavities.

Plasma viscosity (thickness) is due to plasma proteins, mainly albumin and fibrinogen. Viscosity is used as a measure of the body's response to some diseases.

Albumins. These are formed in the liver. They are the most abundant plasma proteins and their main function is to maintain normal plasma osmotic pressure. Albumins also act as carrier molecules for lipids and steroid hormones.

Globulins. Most are formed in the liver and the remainder in lymphoid tissue. Their main functions are:

Composition of blood

Learning outcomes

After studying this section, you should be able to:

- describe the chemical composition of plasma

- discuss the structure, function and formation of red blood cells, including the systems used in medicine to classify the different types

- discuss the functions and formation of the different types of white blood cell

- outline the role of platelets in blood clotting.

Blood is composed of a straw-coloured transparent fluid, *plasma*, in which different types of cells are suspended. Plasma constitutes about 55% and cells about 45% of blood volume (Fig. 4.1A).

- as *antibodies* (immunoglobulins), which are complex proteins produced by lymphocytes that play an important part in immunity. They bind to, and neutralise, foreign materials (antigens) such as micro-organisms (see also p. 376).
- transportation of some hormones and mineral salts; e.g. thyroglobulin carries the hormone thyroxine and transferrin carries the mineral iron
- inhibition of some proteolytic enzymes, e.g. α_2 macroglobulin inhibits trypsin activity.

Clotting factors. These are substances essential for coagulation of blood (p. 66). *Serum* is plasma from which clotting factors have been removed (Fig. 4.1B).

Fibrinogen. This is synthesised in the liver and is essential for blood coagulation.

Inorganic (mineral) salts

These are involved in a wide variety of activities, including muscle contraction, transmission of nerve impulses, formation of secretions and maintenance of acid–base balance. In health the blood is slightly alkaline. Alkalinity and acidity are expressed in terms of pH, which is a measure of hydrogen ion concentration, or $[H^+]$ (p. 21 and Fig. 2.6). The pH of blood is maintained between 7.35 and 7.45 by an ongoing complicated series of chemical activities, involving buffering systems.

Nutrients

In the alimentary tract, food is broken down into small molecules, e.g. monosaccharides, amino acids, fatty acids and glycerol, and are absorbed. Together with mineral salts they are required by all body cells to provide energy, heat, materials for repair and replacement, and for the synthesis of other blood components and body secretions.

Waste products

Urea, creatinine and uric acid are the waste products of protein metabolism. They are formed in the liver and conveyed in blood to the kidneys for excretion.

Hormones (see Ch. 9)

These are substances synthesised by endocrine glands. Hormones pass directly from the endocrine cells into the blood, which transports them to their target tissues and organs elsewhere in the body, where they influence cellular activity.

Gases

Oxygen, carbon dioxide and nitrogen are transported round the body dissolved in plasma. Oxygen and carbon dioxide are also transported in combination with haemoglobin in red blood cells (p. 60). Most oxygen is carried in combination with haemoglobin and most carbon dioxide as bicarbonate ions dissolved in plasma. Atmospheric nitrogen enters the body in the same way as other gases and is present in plasma but it has no physiological function.

Cellular content of blood

There are three types of blood cells (see Fig. 1.5, p. 8).

- erythrocytes (red cells)
- platelets (thrombocytes)
- leukocytes (white cells).

All blood cells originate from *pluripotent stem cells* and go through several developmental stages before entering the blood. Different types of blood cells follow separate lines of development. The process of blood cell formation is called *haemopoiesis* (Fig. 4.2) and takes place within red bone marrow. For the first few years of life, red marrow occupies the entire bone capacity and, over the next 20 years, is gradually replaced by fatty yellow marrow that has no haemopoietic function. In adults, haemopoiesis in the skeleton is confined to flat bones, irregular bones and the ends (*epiphyses*) of long bones, the main sites being the sternum, ribs, pelvis and skull. In addition, some lymphocytes (white blood cells) are produced in lymphoid tissue.

Erythrocytes (red blood cells)

Red blood cells are biconcave discs; they have no nucleus, and their diameter is about 7 micrometres (Fig. 4.3). Their main function is in gas transport, mainly of oxygen, but they also carry some carbon dioxide. Their characteristic shape is suited to their purpose; the biconcavity increases their surface area for gas exchange, and the thinness of the central portion allows fast entry and exit of gases. The cells are flexible so they can squeeze through narrow capillaries, and contain no intracellular organelles, leaving more room for haemoglobin, the large pigmented protein responsible for gas transport.

Measurements of red cell numbers, volume and haemoglobin content are routine and useful assessments made in clinical practice (Table 4.1). The symbols in brackets are the abbreviations commonly used in laboratory reports.

Life span and function of erythrocytes

Erythrocytes are produced in red bone marrow, which is present in the ends of long bones and in flat and irregular

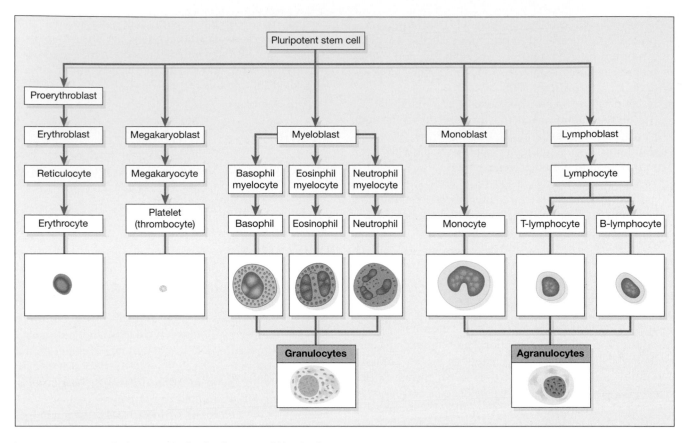

Figure 4.2 **Haemopoiesis:** stages in the development of blood cells.

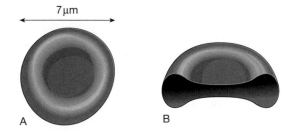

Figure 4.3 **The red blood cell.**

bones. They pass through several stages of development before entering the blood. Their life span in the circulation is about 120 days.

The process of development of red blood cells from pluripotent stem cells takes about 7 days and is called *erythropoiesis* (Fig. 4.2). The immature cells are released into the bloodstream as reticulocytes, and then mature into erythrocytes over a day or two within the circulation. During this time, they lose their nucleus and therefore become incapable of division (Fig. 4.4).

Both vitamin B_{12} and folic acid are required for red blood cell synthesis. They are absorbed in the intestines, although vitamin B_{12} must be bound to intrinsic factor (p. 295) to allow absorption to take place. Both vitamins are present in dairy products, meat and green vegetables. The liver usually contains substantial stores of vitamin B_{12}, several years' worth, but signs of folic acid deficiency appear within a few months.

Oxygen transport

Haemoglobin is a large, complex protein containing a globular protein (globin) and a pigmented iron-containing complex called haem. Each haemoglobin molecule contains four globin chains and four haem units, each with one atom of iron (Fig. 4.5). As each atom of iron can combine with an oxygen molecule, this means that a single haemoglobin molecule can carry up to four molecules of oxygen. An average red blood cell carries about 280 million haemoglobin molecules, giving each cell a theoretical oxygen-carrying capacity of over a billion oxygen molecules!

When all four oxygen-binding sites on a haemoglobin molecule are full, it is described as *saturated*. Haemo-

Table 4.1 Erythrocytes – normal values

Measure	Normal values
Erythrocyte count – number of erythrocytes per litre, or cubic millilitre, (mm³) of blood	Male: $4.5 \times 10^{12}/l$ to $6.5 \times 10^{12}/l$ ($4.5–6.5$ million/mm³) Female: $3.8 \times 10^{12}/l$ to $5.8 \times 10^{12}/l$ ($3.8–5.8$ million/mm³)
Packed cell volume (PCV, haematocrit) – the volume of red cells in 1 l or mm³ of blood	0.40–0.55 l/l
Mean cell volume (MCV) – the volume of an average cell, measured in femtolitres (1 fl = 10^{-15} litre)	80–96 fl
Haemoglobin – the weight of haemoglobin in whole blood, measured in grams/100 ml blood	Male: 13–18 g/100 ml Female: 11.5–16.5 g/100 ml
Mean cell haemoglobin (MCH) – the average amount of haemoglobin per cell, measured in picograms (1 pg = 10^{-12} gram)	27–32 pg/cell
Mean cell haemoglobin concentration (MCHC) – the weight of haemoglobin in 100 ml of red cells	30–35 g/100 ml of red cells

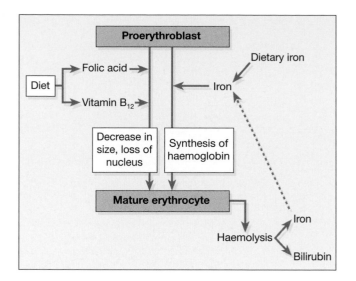

Figure 4.4 Maturation of the erythrocyte.

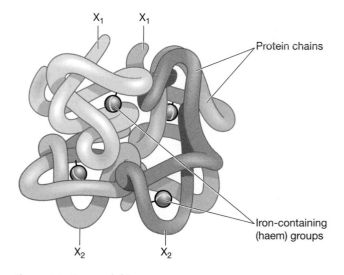

Figure 4.5 Haemoglobin

globin binds reversibly to oxygen to form oxyhaemoglobin, according to the equation:

Haemoglobin + oxygen ↔ oxyhaemoglobin
(Hb)   (O₂)   (HbO)

As the oxygen content of blood increases, its colour changes too. Blood rich in oxygen is bright red because of the high levels of oxyhaemoglobin it contains, compared with blood with lower oxygen levels, which is dark bluish in colour because it is not saturated.

The association of oxygen with haemoglobin is a loose one, so that oxyhaemoglobin releases its oxygen readily, especially under certain conditions.

Low pH. Metabolically active tissues, e.g. exercising muscle, release acid waste products, and so the local pH falls. Under these conditions, oxyhaemoglobin readily breaks down, giving up additional oxygen for tissue use.

Low oxygen levels (hypoxia). When oxygen levels are low, oxyhaemoglobin breaks down, releasing oxygen; e.g. in the body tissues, which constantly consume oxygen keeping levels low. On the other hand, when oxygen levels are high, as they are in the lungs, oxyhaemoglobin formation is favoured.

Temperature. Actively metabolising tissues, which have higher than normal oxygen needs, are warmer than less active ones, which drives the equation above to the left, increasing oxygen dissociation, and ensures that very active tissues receive a higher oxygen supply than less active ones. In the lungs, where the alveoli are exposed to inspired air, the temperature is lower, favouring oxyhaemoglobin formation.

Control of erythropoiesis

The number of red cells remains fairly constant, which means that the bone marrow produces erythrocytes at the rate at which they are destroyed. This is due to a homeostatic negative feedback mechanism (Fig. 4.6).

61

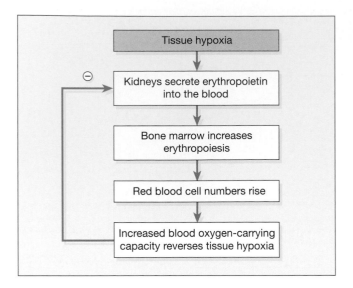

Figure 4.6 Control of erythropoiesis: the role of erythropoietin.

The primary stimulus to increased erythropoiesis is *hypoxia*, i.e. deficient oxygen supply to body cells. This occurs when:

- the oxygen-carrying power of blood is reduced by e.g. haemorrhage or excessive erythrocyte breakdown (*haemolysis*) due to disease
- the oxygen tension in the air is reduced, as at high altitudes.

Hypoxia increases erythrocyte formation by stimulating the production of the hormone *erythropoietin*, mainly by the kidneys. Erythropoietin stimulates an increase in the production of proerythroblasts and the release of increased numbers of reticulocytes into the blood. These changes increase the oxygen-carrying capacity of the blood and reverse tissue hypoxia, the original stimulus. When the tissue hypoxia is overcome, erythropoietin production declines (Fig. 4.6). When erythropoietin levels are low, red cell formation does not take place even in the presence of hypoxia, and *anaemia* (the inability of the blood to carry adequate oxygen for body needs) develops. Erythropoietin regulates normal red cell replacement, i.e. in the absence of hypoxia.

Destruction of erythrocytes

The life span of erythrocytes is about 120 days and their breakdown, or *haemolysis*, is carried out by *phagocytic reticuloendothelial cells*. These cells are found in many tissues but the main sites of haemolysis are the spleen, bone marrow and liver. As erythrocytes age, changes in their cell membranes make them more susceptible to haemolysis. Iron released by haemolysis is retained in

the body and reused in the bone marrow to form new haemoglobin molecules (Fig. 4.4). *Biliverdin* is formed from the haem part of the haemoglobin. It is almost completely reduced to the yellow pigment *bilirubin*, before being bound to plasma globulin and transported to the liver (see Fig. 12.38, p. 308). In the liver it is changed from a fat-soluble to a water-soluble form to be excreted as a constituent of bile.

Blood groups

Individuals have different types of antigen on the surfaces of their red blood cells. These antigens, which are inherited, determine the individual's *blood group*. In addition, individuals make antibodies to these antigens, but not to their own type of antigen, since if they did the antigens and antibodies would react, causing a *transfusion reaction*, which can be fatal. These antibodies circulate in the bloodstream and the ability to make them, like the antigens, is genetically determined and not associated with acquired immunity.

If individuals are transfused with blood of the same group, i.e. possessing the same antigens on the surface of the cells, their immune system will not recognise them as foreign and will not reject them. However, if they are given blood from an individual of a different blood type, i.e. with a different type of antigen on the red cells, their immune system will mount an attack upon them and destroy the transfused cells. This is the basis of the transfusion reaction; the two blood types, the donor and the recipient, are *incompatible*.

There are many different collections of red cell surface antigens, but the most important are the ABO and the Rhesus systems.

The ABO system

About 55% of the population has either A-type antigens (blood group A), B-type antigens (blood group B) or both (blood group AB) on their red cell surface. The remaining 45% have neither A nor B type antigens (blood group O). The corresponding antibodies are called anti-A and anti-B. Blood group A individuals cannot make anti-A (and therefore do not have these antibodies in their plasma), since otherwise a reaction to their own cells would occur; they do, however, make anti-B. Blood group B individuals, for the same reasons, make only anti-A. Blood group AB make neither, and blood group O make both anti-A and anti-B (Fig. 4.7).

Because blood group AB people make neither anti-A nor anti-B antibodies, they are known as *universal recipients*: transfusion of either type A or type B blood into these individuals is likely to be safe, since there are no antibodies to react with them. Conversely, group O

Blood group	Antigen + antibody(ies) present		As donor, is	As recipient, is
A	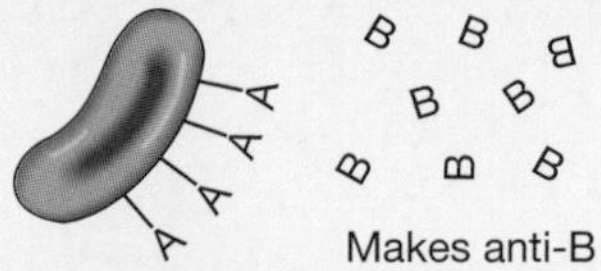 Antigen A	Makes anti-B	Compatible with: A and AB Incompatible with: B and O, because both make anti-A antibodies that will react with A antigens	Compatible with: A and O Incompatible with: B and AB, because type A makes anti-B antibodies that will react with B antigens
B	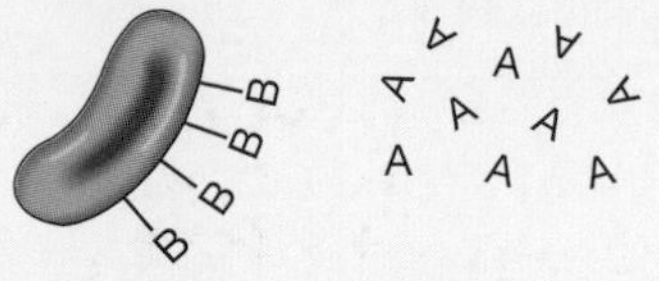 Antigen B	Makes anti-A	Compatible with: B and AB Incompatible with: A and O, because both make anti-B antibodies that will react with B antigens	Compatible with: B and O Incompatible with: A and AB, because type B makes anti-A antibodies that will react with A antigens
AB	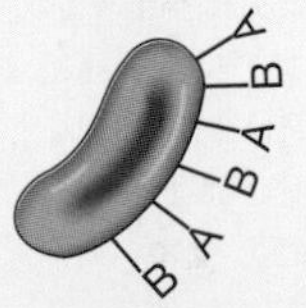 Antigens A and B	Makes neither anti-A nor anti-B	Compatible with: AB only Incompatible with: A, B and O, because all three make antibodies that will react with AB antigens	Compatible with all groups **UNIVERSAL RECIPIENT** AB makes no antibodies and therefore will not react with any type of donated blood
O	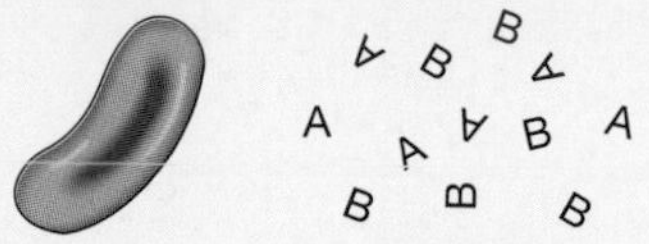 Neither A nor B antigen	Makes both anti-A and anti-B	Compatible with all groups **UNIVERSAL DONOR** O red cells have no antigens, and will therefore not stimulate anti-A or anti-B antibodies	Compatible with: O only Incompatible with: A, AB and B, because type O makes anti-A and anti-B antibodies

Figure 4.7 The ABO system of blood grouping: antigens, antibodies and compatibility.

people have neither A nor B antigens on their red cell membranes, and their blood may be safely transfused into A, B, AB or O types; group O is known as the *universal donor*. The terms *universal donor* and *universal recipient* are misleading, however, since they imply that the ABO system is the only one that needs to be considered. In practice, although the ABO systems may be compatible, other antigen systems on donor/recipient cells may be incompatible, and cause a transfusion reaction (p. 71). For this reason, prior to transfusion, cross-matching is still required to ensure that there is no reaction between donor and recipient bloods.

The Rhesus system

The red blood cell membrane antigen important here is the Rhesus (Rh) antigen, or Rhesus factor. About 85% of people have this antigen; they are Rhesus positive (Rh⁺) and do not therefore make anti-Rhesus antibodies. The remaining 15% have no Rhesus antigen (they are Rhesus negative, or Rh⁻). Rh⁻ individuals are capable of making anti-Rhesus antibodies, but are stimulated to do so only in certain circumstances, e.g. in pregnancy (p. 70), or as the result of an incompatible blood transfusion.

Leukocytes (white blood cells)

These cells have an important function in defending the body against microbes and other foreign materials. Leukocytes are the largest blood cells and they account for about 1% of the blood volume. They contain nuclei and some have granules in their cytoplasm. There are two main types (Table 4.2):

- granulocytes (polymorphonuclear leukocytes)
  – neutrophils, eosinophils and basophils
- agranulocytes
  – monocytes and lymphocytes.

Granulocytes (polymorphonuclear leukocytes)

During their formation, *granulopoiesis*, they follow a common line of development through *myeloblast* to *myelocyte* before differentiating into the three types (Figs 4.2 and 4.8). All granulocytes have multilobed nuclei in their cytoplasm. Their names represent the dyes they take up when stained in the laboratory. Eosinophils take up the red acid dye, eosin; basophils take up alkaline methylene

Table 4.2 Normal leukocyte counts in adult blood

	Number x 10^9/l	Percentage of total
Granulocytes		
Neutrophils	2.5 to 7.5	40 to 75
Eosinophils	0.04 to 0.44	1 to 6
Basophils	0.015 to 0.1	< 1
Agranulocytes		
Monocytes	0.2 to 0.8	2 to 10
Lymphocytes	1.5 to 3.5	20 to 50
Total	5 to 9	100

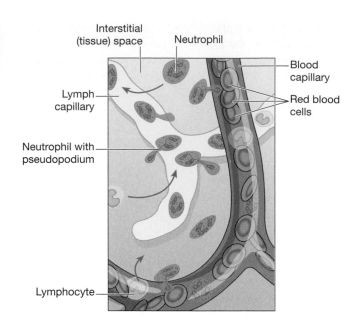

Figure 4.9 Diapedesis of leukocytes.

blue; and neutrophils are purple because they take up both dyes.

Neutrophils

Their main function is to protect against any foreign material entering the body, mainly microbes, and to remove waste materials, e.g. cell debris. They are attracted in large numbers to any area of infection by chemical substances, released by damaged cells, called *chemotaxins*. Neutrophils are highly mobile, and squeeze through the capillary walls in the affected area by *diapedesis* (Fig. 4.9). Thereafter they engulf and kill the microbes by *phagocytosis* (Fig. 4.10). Their nuclei are characteristically complex, with up to six lobes, and their granules are *lysosomes* containing enzymes to digest engulfed material. Pus that may form in an infected area consists of dead tissue cells, dead and live microbes, and phagocytes killed by microbes.

There is a physiological increase in circulating neutrophils following strenuous exercise and in the later stages of normal pregnancy. Numbers are also increased in:

- microbial infection
- extensive tissue damage, e.g. inflammation, myocardial infarction, burns, crush injuries
- metabolic disorders, e.g. diabetic ketoacidosis, acute gout
- leukaemia

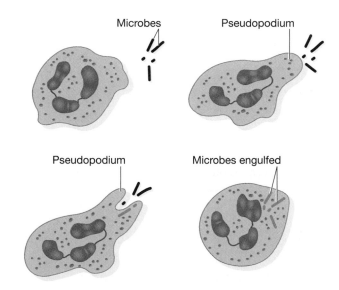

Figure 4.10 Phagocytic action of neutrophils.

- heavy smoking
- use of oral contraceptives.

Eosinophils

Eosinophils, although capable of phagocytosis, are less active in this than neutrophils; their specialised role appears to be in the elimination of parasites, such as worms, which are too big to be phagocytosed. They are equipped with certain toxic chemicals, stored in their granules, which they release when the eosinophil binds an infecting organism.

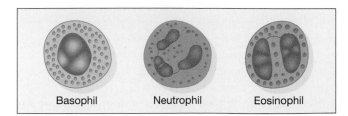

Figure 4.8 The granulocytes (granular leukocytes).

Eosinophils are often found at sites of allergic inflammation, such as the asthmatic airway and skin allergies. There, they promote tissue inflammation by releasing their array of toxic chemicals, but they may also dampen down the inflammatory process through the release of other chemicals, such as an enzyme that breaks down histamine (p. 372).

Basophils

Basophils, which are closely associated with allergic reactions, contain cytoplasmic granules packed with *heparin* (an anticoagulant), *histamine* (an inflammatory agent) and other substances that promote inflammation. Usually the stimulus that causes basophils to release the contents of their granules is an *allergen* (an antigen that causes allergy) of some type. This binds to antibody-type receptors on the basophil membrane. A cell type very similar to basophils, except that it is found in the tissues, not in the circulation, is the *mast cell*. Mast cells release their granule contents within seconds of binding an allergen, which accounts for the rapid onset of allergic symptoms following exposure to, for example, pollen in hay fever (p. 379).

Agranulocytes

The types of leukocyte with a large nucleus and no granules in their cytoplasm are *monocytes* and *lymphocytes* and they make up 25% to 50% of all leukocytes (Figs 4.2 and 4.11).

Monocytes

These are large mononuclear cells that originate in red bone marrow. Some circulate in the blood and are actively motile and phagocytic while others migrate into the tissues where they develop into *macrophages*. Both types of cell produce *interleukin 1*, which:

- acts on the hypothalamus, causing the rise in body temperature associated with microbial infections
- stimulates the production of some globulins by the liver
- enhances the production of activated T-lymphocytes.

Macrophages have important functions in inflammation (p. 371) and immunity.

Lymphocyte   Monocyte

Figure 4.11 The agranulocytes.

The monocyte–macrophage system. This is sometimes called the *reticuloendothelial system*, and consists of the body's complement of monocytes and macrophages. Some macrophages are mobile, whereas others are fixed. Collections of fixed macrophages include:

- *histiocytes* in connective tissues
- *synovial cells* in joints
- *Langerhans cells* in the skin
- *microglia* in the brain
- *Kupffer cells* in the liver
- *alveolar macrophages* in the lungs
- *sinus-lining macrophages* (reticular cells) in the spleen, lymph nodes and thymus gland
- *mesangial cells* in the glomerulus of nephrons in the kidney
- *osteoclasts* in bone.

Macrophages have a diverse range of protective functions. They are actively phagocytic and if they encounter large amounts of foreign or waste material, they tend to multiply at the site and 'wall off' the area, isolating the material, e.g. pockets of tubercular infection in the lungs. They synthesise and release an array of biologically active chemicals, called *cytokines*, including interleukin 1 mentioned earlier. They also have a central role linking the non-specific and specific (immune) systems of body defence (Ch. 15), and produce factors important in inflammation and repair.

Their numbers are increased in microbial infections, collagen diseases and some non-infective bowel conditions.

Lymphocytes

Lymphocytes are smaller than monocytes and have large nuclei. They circulate in the blood and are present in great numbers in lymphatic tissue such as lymph nodes and the spleen. Lymphocytes develop from pluripotent stem cells in red bone marrow and from precursors in lymphoid tissue, then travel in the blood to lymphoid tissue elsewhere in the body where they are *activated*, i.e. they become immunocompetent which means they are able to respond to *antigens* (foreign material). Examples of antigens include:

- cells regarded by lymphocytes as abnormal, e.g. cells that have been invaded by viruses, cancer cells, tissue transplant cells
- pollen from flowers and plants
- fungi
- bacteria
- some large molecule drugs, e.g. penicillin, aspirin.

Although all lymphocytes originate from one type of stem cell, when they are activated in lymphatic tissue, two distinct types of lymphocyte are produced –

65

T-lymphocytes and *B-lymphocytes*. The specific functions of these two cell types are discussed in Chapter 15.

Platelets (thrombocytes)

These are very small non-nucleated discs, 2 to 4 μm in diameter, derived from the cytoplasm of megakaryocytes in red bone marrow (Fig. 4.2). They contain a variety of substances that promote blood clotting, which causes *haemostasis* (cessation of bleeding).

The normal blood platelet count is between $200 \times 10^9/l$ and $350 \times 10^9/l$ (200 000 to 350 000/mm³). The control of platelet production is not yet entirely clear but one stimulus is a fall in platelet count. The kidneys release a substance called *thrombopoietin*, which stimulates platelet synthesis; other cytokines may also be involved.

The lifespan of platelets is between 8 and 11 days and those not used in haemostasis are destroyed by macrophages, mainly in the spleen. About a third of platelets are stored within the spleen rather than in the circulation; this is an emergency store that can be released as required to control excessive bleeding.

Haemostasis

When a blood vessel is damaged, loss of blood is stopped and healing occurs in a series of overlapping processes, in which platelets play a vital part.

1. Vasoconstriction. When platelets come into contact with a damaged blood vessel, their surface becomes sticky and they adhere to the damaged wall. They then release *serotonin* (5-hydroxytryptamine), which constricts (narrows) the vessel, reducing blood flow through it. Other chemicals that cause vasoconstriction, e.g. thromboxanes, are released by the damaged vessel itself.

2. Platelet plug formation. The adherent platelets clump to each other and release other substances, including *adenosine diphosphate* (ADP), which attract more platelets to the site. Passing platelets stick to those already at the damaged vessel and they too release their chemicals. This is a positive feedback system by which many platelets rapidly arrive at the site of vascular damage and quickly form a temporary seal – the *platelet plug*.

3. Coagulation (blood clotting). This is a complex process that also involves a positive feedback system and only a few stages are included here. The factors involved are listed in Table 4.3. Their numbers represent the order in which they were discovered and not the order of participation in the clotting process. Blood clotting results in formation of an insoluble thread-like mesh of *fibrin*,

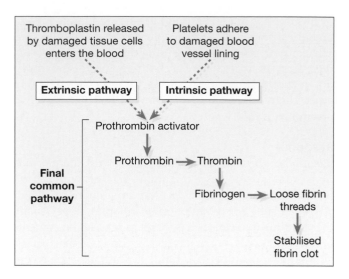

Figure 4.12 Stages of blood clotting (coagulation).

which traps blood cells and is much stronger than the rapidly formed platelet plug. In the final stages of this process *prothrombin activator* acts on the plasma protein *prothrombin* converting it to thrombin.

Thrombin then acts on another plasma protein *fibrinogen* and converts it to fibrin (Fig. 4.12).

Prothrombin activator can be formed by two processes which often occur together: the extrinsic and intrinsic pathways (Fig. 4.12). The *extrinsic pathway* occurs rapidly (within seconds) when there is tissue damage outside the circulation. Damaged tissue releases a complex of chemicals called *thromboplastin* or tissue factor, which initiates coagulation. The *intrinsic pathway* is slower (3–6 minutes) and is confined to the circulation. It is triggered by damage to a blood vessel lining (endothelium) and the effects of platelets adhering to it. After a time the clot

Table 4.3 **Blood clotting factors**	
I	Fibrinogen
II	Prothrombin
III	Tissue factor (thromboplastin)
IV	Calcium (Ca^{2+})
V	Labile factor, proaccelerin, Ac-globulin
VII	Stable factor, proconvertin
VIII	Antihaemophilic globulin (AHG), antihaemophilic Factor A
IX	Christmas factor, plasma thromboplastin component (PTA), antihaemophilic factor B
X	Stuart Prower factor
XI	Plasma thromboplastin antecedent (PTA), antihaemophilic factor C
XII	Hageman factor
XIII	Fibrin stabilising factor

(There is no Factor VI)
Vitamin K is essential for synthesis of Factors II, VII, IX and X.

shrinks because the platelets contract, squeezing out *serum*, a clear sticky fluid that consists of plasma from which clotting factors have been removed. Clot shrinkage pulls the edges of the damaged vessel together, reducing blood loss and closing off the hole in the vessel wall.

4. Fibrinolysis. After the clot has formed the process of removing it and healing the damaged blood vessel begins. The breakdown of the clot, or fibrinolysis, is the first stage. An inactive substance called *plasminogen* is present in the clot and is converted to the enzyme *plasmin* by activators released from the damaged endothelial cells. Plasmin initiates the breakdown of fibrin to soluble products that are treated as waste material and removed by phagocytosis. As the clot is removed, the healing process restores the integrity of the blood vessel wall.

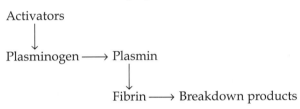

Control of coagulation

The process of blood clotting relies heavily on several self-perpetuating processes – that is, once started, a positive feedback mechanism promotes their continuation. For example, thrombin is a powerful stimulator of its own production. The body therefore possesses several mechanisms to control and limit the coagulation cascade; otherwise once started the clotting process would spread throughout the circulatory system, far beyond requirements. The main controls are:

- the perfect smoothness of normal blood vessel lining means that platelets do not adhere to it
- the binding of thrombin to a special thrombin receptor on the cells lining blood vessels; once bound, thrombin is inactivated
- the presence of natural anticoagulants, e.g. heparin, in the blood, which inactivate clotting factors.

Erythrocyte disorders

Learning outcomes

After studying this section, you should be able to:

■ define the term anaemia

■ compare and contrast the causes and effects of iron deficiency, megaloblastic, aplastic, hypoplastic and haemolytic anaemias

■ explain why polycythaemia occurs.

Anaemias

In anaemia there is not enough haemoglobin available to carry sufficient oxygen from the lungs to supply the needs of the tissues. It occurs when the rate of production of mature cells entering the blood from the red bone marrow does not keep pace with the rate of haemolysis. The classification of anaemia is based on the cause:

- impaired erythrocyte production
  - iron deficiency
  - megaloblastic anaemias
  - hypoplastic anaemia
- increased erythrocyte loss
  - haemolytic anaemias
  - normocytic anaemia.

Red cells may appear abnormal when examined microscopically. Characteristic changes are listed in Table 4.4. Signs and symptoms of anaemia relate to the inability of the blood to supply body cells with enough oxygen, and may represent adaptive measures. Examples include:

- tachycardia; the heart rate increases to improve blood supply and speed circulation

- palpitations (an awareness of the heartbeat), or angina pectoris (p. 123); these are caused by the increased effort of the overworked heart muscle
- breathlessness on exertion; when oxygen requirements increase, respiratory rate and effort rise in an effort to meet the greater demand.

Iron deficiency anaemia

This is the most common form of anaemia in many parts of the world. The normal daily requirement of iron intake in men is about 1 to 2 mg, derived from meat and highly coloured vegetables. The normal daily requirement in women is 3 mg because of blood loss during menstruation and to meet the needs of the growing fetus during pregnancy. Children, during their period of rapid growth, require more than adults.

The amount of haemoglobin in each cell is regarded as below normal when the MCH is less than 27 pg/cell (Table 4.1). The anaemia is regarded as severe when the haemoglobin level is below 9 g/dl blood. It is caused by deficiency of iron in the bone marrow and may be due to dietary deficiency, excessively high requirements or malabsorption.

In this type of anaemia erythrocytes are microcytic and hypochromic because their haemoglobin content is low.

Normal requirements, deficient intake

Because of the relative inefficiency of iron absorption, deficiency occurs frequently, even in individuals whose requirements are normal. The likelihood of deficiency increases if the daily diet is restricted in some way, as in poorly planned vegetarian diets, or in weight-reducing diets where the range of foods eaten is small. Babies dependent on milk may also suffer mild iron deficiency anaemia if weaning on to a mixed diet is delayed much past the first year, since the liver carries only a few months' store and milk is a poor source of iron.

Table 4.4 Terms used to describe red blood cell characteristics

Term	Definition	Example
Normocytic	Cells normal sized	Acute haemorrhage
Microcytic	Cells smaller than normal	Iron deficiency
Macrocytic	Cells bigger than normal	Vitamin B_{12} or folic acid deficiency
Hypochromic	Cells paler than normal	Iron deficiency anaemia
Haemolytic	Rate of cell destruction raised	Autoimmune disease
		Sickle cell anaemia

High requirements, normal or deficient intake

This type of anaemia occurs in pregnancy, when iron requirements are increased both for fetal growth and to support the additional load on the mother's cardiovascular system. It may also occur as a result of chronic blood loss, the causes of which include peptic ulcers, heavy menstrual bleeding (menorrhagia), haemorrhoids or gastrointestinal carcinoma.

Malabsorption

Iron absorption is usually increased following haemorrhage, but may be reduced in abnormalities of the stomach, duodenum or jejunum. Because iron absorption is dependent on an acid environment in the stomach, an increase in gastric pH may reduce it; this may follow removal of part of the stomach, or in pernicious anaemia (see below), where the acid-releasing (parietal) cells of the stomach are destroyed. Loss of surface area for absorption in the intestine e.g. after surgical removal, can also cause deficiency.

Megaloblastic anaemias

Maturation of erythrocytes is impaired when deficiency of vitamin B_{12} and/or folic acid occurs (Fig. 4.4) and abnormally large erythrocytes (megaloblasts) are found in the blood. During normal erythropoiesis (Fig. 4.2) several cell divisions occur and the daughter cells at each stage are smaller than the parent cell because there is not much time for cell enlargement between divisions. When deficiency of vitamin B_{12} and/or folic acid occurs, the rate of DNA and RNA synthesis is reduced, delaying cell division. The cells can therefore grow larger than normal between divisions. Circulating cells are immature, larger than normal and some are nucleated (MCV > 94 fl). The haemoglobin content of each cell is normal or raised. The cells are fragile and their life span is reduced to between 40 and 50 days. Depressed production and early lysis cause anaemia.

Vitamin B_{12} deficiency anaemia

Pernicious anaemia

This is the most common form of vitamin B_{12} deficiency anaemia. It occurs more often in females than males, usually between 45 and 65 years of age. It is an autoimmune disease in which autoantibodies destroy intrinsic factor (IF) and parietal cells in the stomach (p. 295).

Dietary deficiency of vitamin B_{12}

This is rare, except in true vegans, i.e. when no animal products are included in the diet. The store of vitamin B_{12} is such that deficiency takes several years to appear.

Other causes of vitamin B_{12} deficiency

These include the following.

- *Gastrectomy* – this leaves fewer cells available to produce IF after partial resection of the stomach.
- *Chronic gastritis, malignant disease and ionising radiation* – these damage the gastric mucosa including the parietal cells that produce IF.
- *Malabsorption* – if the terminal ileum is removed or inflamed, e.g. in Crohn's disease, the vitamin cannot be absorbed.

Complications of vitamin B_{12} deficiency anaemia

These may appear before the signs of anaemia. Because vitamin B_{12} is used in myelin production, deficiency leads to irreversible neurological damage, commonly in the spinal cord (p. 185). Mucosal abnormalities, such as glossitis (inflammation of the tongue) are also common, although they are reversible.

Folic acid deficiency anaemia

Deficiency in the bone marrow causes a form of megaloblastic anaemia identical to that seen in vitamin B_{12} deficiency, but not associated with neurological damage. It may be due to:

- dietary deficiency, e.g. in infants if there is delay in establishing a mixed diet, in alcoholism, in anorexia and in pregnancy when the requirement is raised
- malabsorption from the jejunum caused by e.g. coeliac disease, tropical sprue or anticonvulsant drugs
- interference with folate metabolism by e.g. cytotoxic and anticonvulsant drugs.

Hypoplastic and aplastic anaemias

Hypoplastic and aplastic anaemias are due to varying degrees of bone marrow failure. Bone marrow function is reduced in hypoplastic anaemia, and absent in aplastic anaemia. Since the bone marrow produces leukocytes and platelets as well as erythrocytes, *leukopenia* (low white cell count) and *thrombocytopenia* (low platelet count) are likely to accompany diminished red cell numbers. When all three cell types are low, the condition is called *pancytopenia*, and is accompanied by anaemia, diminished immunity and a tendency to bleed. The condition is often idiopathic, but the known causes include:

- drugs, e.g. cytotoxic drugs, some anti-inflammatory and anticonvulsant drugs, some sulphonamides and antibiotics
- ionising radiation
- some chemicals, e.g. benzene and its derivatives

- viral disease, including hepatitis
- invasion of bone marrow by, e.g., malignant disease, leukaemia or fibrosis.

Haemolytic anaemias

These occur when red cells are destroyed while in circulation or are removed prematurely from the circulation because the cells are abnormal or the spleen is overactive.

Congenital haemolytic anaemias

In these diseases, genetic abnormality leads to the synthesis of abnormal haemoglobin and increased red cell membrane friability, reducing their oxygen-carrying capacity and life span. The most common forms are sickle cell anaemia and thalassaemia.

Sickle cell anaemia

The abnormal haemoglobin molecules become misshapen when deoxygenated, making the erythrocytes sickle shaped. If the cells contain a high proportion of abnormal molecules, sickling is permanent. The life span of cells is reduced by early haemolysis, which causes anaemia. Sickle cells do not move smoothly through the small blood vessels. This tends to increase the viscosity of the blood, reducing the rate of blood flow and leading to intravascular clotting, ischaemia and infarction.

Blacks are more affected than other races. Some affected individuals have a degree of immunity to malaria because the life span of the sickled cells is less than the time needed for the malaria parasite to mature inside the cells.

Complications. Pregnancy, infection and dehydration predispose to the development of 'sickle crises' due to intravascular clotting and ischaemia, causing severe pain in long bones, chest or the abdomen. The formation of gallstones (*cholelithiasis*) and inflammation of the gall bladder (*cholecystitis*) also occur (p. 333).

Thalassaemia

There is reduced globin synthesis with resultant reduced haemoglobin production and increased friability of the cell membrane, leading to early haemolysis. Severe cases may cause death in infants or young children. This inherited condition is most common in Mediterranean countries.

Haemolytic disease of the newborn

In this disorder, the mother's immune system makes antibodies to the baby's red blood cells, causing haemoly-

sis and phagocytosis of fetal erythrocytes. The antigen system involved is usually (but not always) the Rhesus (Rh) antigen.

A Rh⁻ mother carries no Rh antigen on her red blood cells, but she has the capacity to produce anti-Rh antibodies. If she conceives a child fathered by a Rh⁺ man, and the baby inherits the Rh antigen from him, the baby may also be Rh⁺, i.e. different from the mother. During pregnancy, the placenta protects the baby from the mother's immune system, but at delivery a few fetal red blood cells may enter the maternal circulation. Because

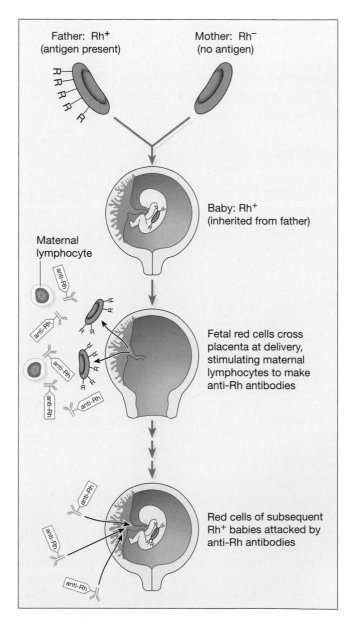

Figure 4.13 The immunity of haemolytic disease of the newborn.

they carry an antigen (the Rh antigen) foreign to the mother, her immune system will be stimulated to produce neutralising antibodies to it. The red cells of second and subsequent Rh⁺ babies are attacked by these maternal antibodies, which can cross the placenta and enter the fetal circulation (Fig. 4.13). In the most severe cases, the baby dies in the womb from profound anaemia. In less serious circumstances, the baby is born with some degree of anaemia, which is corrected with blood transfusions.

The disease is much less common than it used to be, because it was discovered that if a Rh⁻ mother is given an injection of anti-Rh antibodies within 72 hours of the delivery of a Rh⁺ baby, her immune system does not make its own anti-Rh antibodies to the fetal red cells. Subsequent pregnancies are therefore not affected. The anti-Rh antibodies given to the mother bind to, and neutralise, any fetal red cells present in her circulation before her immune system becomes sensitised to them.

Acquired haemolytic anaemias

In this context, 'acquired' means haemolytic anaemia in which no familial or racial factors have been identified. There are several causes.

Chemical agents
These substances cause early or excessive haemolysis, e.g.:

- some drugs, especially when taken long term in large doses, e.g. sulphonamides
- chemicals encountered in the general or work environment, e.g. lead, arsenic compounds
- toxins produced by microbes, e.g. *Streptococcus pyogenes*, *Clostridium perfringens*.

Autoimmunity
In this disease, individuals make antibodies to their own red cell antigens, causing haemolysis. It may be acute or chronic and primary or secondary to other diseases, e.g. carcinoma, viral infection or other autoimmune diseases.

Blood transfusion reactions
Individuals do not normally produce antibodies to their own red blood cell antigens; if they did, the antigens and antibodies would react, causing clumping and lysis of the erythrocytes (see Fig. 4.7). However, if individuals receive a transfusion of blood carrying antigens different from their own, their immune system will recognise them as foreign, make antibodies to them and destroy them (transfusion reaction). This adverse reaction between the blood of incompatible recipients and donors leads to

haemolysis within the cardiovascular system. The breakdown products of haemolysis lodge in and block the filtering mechanism of the nephron, impairing kidney function. Other principal signs of a transfusion reaction include fever, chills, lumbar pain and shock.

Other causes of haemolytic anaemia
These include:

- parasitic diseases, e.g. malaria
- ionising radiation, e.g. X-rays, radioactive isotopes
- destruction of blood trapped in tissues in e.g. severe burns, crush injuries
- physical damage to cells by e.g. artificial heart valves, kidney dialysis machines.

Normocytic normochromic anaemia

In this type the cells are normal but the numbers are reduced, and the proportion of reticulocytes in the blood may be increased as the body tries to restore erythrocyte numbers to normal. This occurs:

- in many chronic conditions, e.g. in chronic inflammation
- following severe haemorrhage
- in haemolytic disease.

Polycythaemia

There is an abnormally large number of erythrocytes in the blood. This increases blood viscosity, slows the rate of flow and increases the risk of intravascular clotting, ischaemia and infarction.

Relative increase in erythrocyte count
This occurs when the erythrocyte count is normal but the blood volume is reduced by fluid loss, e.g. excessive serum exudate from extensive burns.

True increase in erythrocyte count
Physiological. Prolonged hypoxia stimulates erythropoiesis and the number of cells released into the normal volume of blood is increased. This occurs in people living at high altitudes where the oxygen tension in the air is low and the partial pressure of oxygen in the alveoli of the lungs is correspondingly low. Each cell carries less oxygen so more cells are needed to meet the body's oxygen needs.

Pathological. The reason for this increase in circulating red cells, sometimes to twice the normal number, is not

71

known. It may be secondary to other factors that cause hypoxia of the red bone marrow, e.g. cigarette smoking, pulmonary disease, bone marrow cancer.

Leukocyte disorders

Learning outcomes

After studying this section, you should be able to:

- define the terms leukopenia and leukocytosis

- review the physiological importance of abnormally increased and decreased leukocyte numbers in the blood

- discuss the main forms of leukaemia, including the causes, signs and symptoms of the disease.

Leukopenia

In this condition, the total blood leukocyte count is less than $4 \times 10^9/l$ (4000/mm^3).

Granulocytopenia (neutropenia)

This is a general term used to indicate an abnormal reduction in the numbers of circulating granulocytes (polymorphonuclear leukocytes), commonly called neutropenia because 40 to 75% of granulocytes are neutrophils. A reduction in the number of circulating granulocytes occurs when production does not keep pace with the normal removal of cells or when the life span of the cells is reduced. Extreme shortage or the absence of granulocytes is called *agranulocytosis*. A temporary reduction occurs in response to inflammation but the numbers are usually quickly restored. Inadequate granulopoiesis may be caused by:

- drugs, e.g. cytotoxic drugs, phenothiazines, some sulphonamides and antibiotics
- irradiation damage to granulocyte precursors in the bone marrow by e.g. X-rays, radioactive isotopes
- diseases of red bone marrow, e.g. leukaemias, some anaemias
- severe microbial infections.

In conditions where the spleen is enlarged, excessive numbers of granulocytes are trapped, reducing the number in circulation. Neutropenia predisposes to severe infections that can lead to septicaemia and death.

Septicaemia is the presence of significant numbers of active pathogens in the blood. The pathogens are commonly *commensals*, i.e. microbes that are normally present in the body but do not usually cause infection, such as those in the bowel.

Leukocytosis

An increase in the number of circulating leukocytes occurs as a normal protective reaction in a variety of pathological conditions, especially in response to infections. When the infection subsides the leukocyte count returns to normal.

Pathological leukocytosis exists when a blood leukocyte count of more than $11 \times 10^9/l$ (11 000/mm^3) is sustained and is not consistent with the normal protective function. One or more of the different types of cell is involved.

Leukaemia

Leukaemia is a malignant proliferation of white blood cell precursors by the bone marrow. It results in the uncontrolled increase in the production of leukocytes and/or their precursors. As the tumour cells enter the blood the total leukocyte count is usually raised but in some cases it may be normal or even low. The proliferation of immature leukaemic blast cells crowds out other blood cells formed in bone marrow, causing anaemia, thrombocytopenia and leukopenia (pancytopenia). Because the leukocytes are immature when released, immunity is reduced and the risk of infection high.

Causes of leukaemia

Some causes of leukaemia are known but many cases cannot be accounted for. Some people may have a genetic predisposition that is triggered by environmental factors, including viral infection. Other known causes include:

Ionising radiation. Radiation such as that produced by X-rays and radioactive isotopes causes malignant changes in the precursors of white blood cells. The DNA of the cells may be damaged and some cells die while others reproduce at an abnormally rapid rate. Leukaemia may develop at any time after irradiation, even 20 or more years later.

Chemicals. Some chemicals encountered in the general or work environment alter the DNA of the white cell precursors in the bone marrow. These include benzene and its derivatives, asbestos, cytotoxic drugs, chloramphenicol.

Genetic factors. Identical twins of leukaemia sufferers have a much higher risk than normal of developing the disease, suggesting involvement of genetic factors.

Types of leukaemia

Leukaemias are usually classified according to the type of cell involved, the maturity of the cells and the rate at which the disease develops (see Fig. 4.2, p. 60).

Acute leukaemias

These types usually have a sudden onset and affect the poorly differentiated and immature 'blast' cells (Fig. 4.2). They are aggressive tumours that reach a climax within a few weeks or months. The rapid progress of bone marrow invasion impairs its function and culminates in anaemia, haemorrhage and susceptibility to infection. The mucous membranes of the mouth and upper gastrointestinal tract are most commonly affected.

Leukocytosis is usually present in acute leukaemia. The bone marrow is packed with large numbers of immature and abnormal cells.

Acute myeloblastic leukaemia (AML) involves proliferation of myeloblasts (Fig. 4.2), and is most common in adults between the ages of 25 and 60, risk gradually increasing with age. The disease can often be cured, or long-term remission achieved. *Acute lymphoblastic leukaemia* (ALL) is seen mainly in children, who have a better prognosis than adults, with up to 70% achieving cure. The cell responsible here is a primitive B-lymphocyte.

Chronic leukaemias

These conditions are less aggressive than the acute forms and the leukocytes are more differentiated, i.e. at the 'cyte' stage (Fig. 4.2).

Leukocytosis is a feature of chronic leukaemia, with crowding of the bone marrow with immature and abnormal leukocytes, although this varies depending upon the form of the disease.

Chronic myeloid leukaemia (CML) occurs at all ages and, although its onset is gradual, in most patients it eventually transforms into a rapidly progressive stage similar to AML (sometimes ALL) and proves fatal. Death usually occurs within five years. *Chronic lymphocytic leukaemia* (CLL) involves proliferation of B-lymphocytes, and is usually less aggressive than CML. It is most often seen in

the elderly; disease progression is usually slow, and survival times can be as long as 25 years.

Haemorrhagic diseases

Learning outcomes

After studying this section, you should be able to:

- indicate the main causes and effects of thrombocytopenia

- outline how vitamin K deficiency relates to clotting disorders

- explain the term disseminated intravascular coagulation, including its principal causes

- describe the physiological deficiencies present in the haemophilias.

Thrombocytopenia

This is defined as a blood platelet count below $150 \times 10^9/l$ ($150\ 000/mm^3$) but spontaneous capillary bleeding does not usually occur unless the count falls below $30 \times 10^9/l$ ($30\ 000/mm^3$). It may be due to a reduced rate of platelet production or increased rate of destruction.

Reduced platelet production

This is usually due to bone marrow deficiencies, and therefore production of erythrocytes and leukocytes is also reduced, giving rise to pancytopenia. It is often due to:

- platelets being crowded out of the bone marrow in bone marrow diseases, e.g. leukaemias, pernicious anaemia, malignant tumours
- ionising radiation, e.g. X-rays or radioactive isotopes, which damage the rapidly dividing precursor cells in the bone marrow
- drugs that can damage bone marrow, e.g. cytotoxic drugs, chloramphenicol, chlorpromazine, sulphonamides.

Increased platelet destruction

A reduced platelet count occurs when production of new cells does not keep pace with destruction of damaged and worn out cells. This occurs in disseminated intravascular coagulation (see below) and autoimmune thrombocytopenic purpura.

Autoimmune thrombocytopenic purpura. This condition, which usually affects children and young adults,

73

may be triggered by a viral infection such as measles. Antiplatelet antibodies are formed that coat platelets, leading to platelet destruction and their removal from the circulation. A significant feature of this disease is the presence of *purpura*, which are haemorrhages into the skin ranging in size from pinpoints to large blotches. The severity of the disease varies from mild bleeding into the skin to severe haemorrhage. When the platelet count is very low there may be severe bruising, haematuria, gastrointestinal or intracranial haemorrhages.

Vitamin K deficiency

Vitamin K is required by the liver for the synthesis of many clotting factors and therefore deficiency predisposes to abnormal clotting (p. 66).

Haemorrhagic disease of the newborn
Spontaneous haemorrhage from the umbilical cord and intestinal mucosa occurs in babies when the stored vitamin K obtained from the mother before birth has been used up and the intestinal bacteria needed for its synthesis in the infant's bowel are not yet established. This is most likely to occur when the baby is premature.

Deficiency in adults
Vitamin K is fat soluble and bile salts are required in the colon for its absorption. Deficiency may occur when there is liver disease, prolonged obstruction to the biliary tract or in any other disease where fat absorption is impaired, e.g. coeliac disease. Dietary deficiency is rare because a sufficient supply of vitamin K is usually synthesised in the intestine by bacterial action. However, it may occur during treatment with drugs that sterilise the bowel.

Disseminated intravascular coagulation (DIC)

In DIC, the coagulation system is activated within blood vessels, leading to formation of intravascular clots and deposition of fibrin in the tissues. Because of this consumption of clotting factors and platelets, there is a consequent tendency to haemorrhage. DIC is a common complication of a number of other disorders, including:

- severe shock, especially when due to microbial infection

- septicaemia, when endotoxins are released by Gram-negative bacteria
- severe trauma
- premature separation of placenta when amniotic fluid enters maternal blood
- acute pancreatitis when digestive enzymes are released into the blood
- malignant tumours with widely dispersed metastases.

Congenital disorders

The haemophilias
The haemophilias are a group of inherited clotting disorders, carried by genes present on the X-chromosome (i.e. inheritance is sex linked, p. 438). The faulty genes code for abnormal clotting factors (Factor VIII and Christmas factor), and if inherited by a male child always leads to expression of the disease. Women inheriting one copy are *carriers*, but, provided their second X chromosome bears a copy of the normal gene, their blood clotting is normal. It is possible, but unusual, for a woman to inherit two copies of the abnormal gene and have haemophilia.

Those who have haemophilia experience repeated episodes of severe and prolonged bleeding at any site, with little evidence of trauma. Recurrent bleeding into joints is common, causing severe pain and, in the long term, cartilage is damaged. The disease ranges in severity from mild forms, where the defective factor has partial activity, to extreme forms where bleeding can take days or weeks to control.

The two main forms of haemophilia differ only in the clotting factor involved; the clinical picture in both is identical.

- Haemophilia A. In this disease, factor VIII is abnormal and is less biologically active.
- Haemophilia B (Christmas disease). This is less common and factor IX is deficient, resulting in deficiency of thromboplastin (clotting factor III).

von Willebrand's disease
In this disease, a deficiency in the von Willebrand factor causes low levels of factor VIII. As the inheritance is not sex linked, haemorrhages due to impaired clotting occur equally in males and females.

The cardiovascular system

5

The cardiovascular system is divided for descriptive purposes into two main parts.

- The *circulatory system,* consisting of the *heart,* which acts as a pump, and the *blood vessels* through which the *blood* circulates
- The *lymphatic system,* consisting of *lymph nodes* and *lymph vessels,* through which colourless *lymph* flows (see Ch. 6).

The two systems communicate with one another and are intimately associated.

The heart pumps blood into two anatomically separate systems of blood vessels (Fig. 5.1).

- the pulmonary circulation
- the systemic circulation.

The right side of the heart pumps blood to the lungs (the pulmonary circulation) where gas exchange occurs; i.e. CO_2 leaves the blood and enters the lungs, and O_2 leaves the lungs and enters the blood. The left side of the heart pumps blood into the systemic circulation, which supplies the rest of the body. Here, tissue wastes are passed into the blood for excretion, and body cells extract nutrients and O_2.

The circulatory system ensures a continuous flow of blood to all body cells, and its function is subject to continual physiological adjustments in order to maintain an adequate blood supply. Should the supply of oxygen and nutrients to body cells become inadequate, tissue damage occurs and cell death may follow.

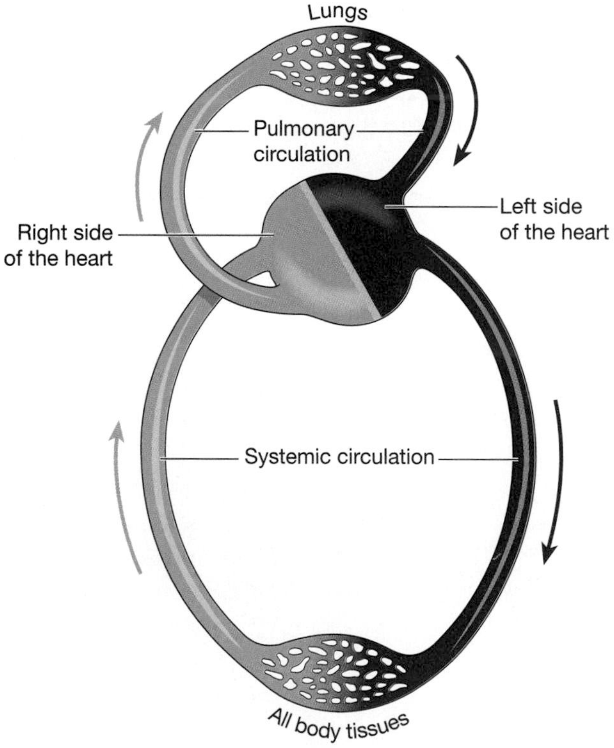

Blood vessels

Learning outcomes

After studying this section, you should be able to:

- describe the structures and functions of arteries, veins and capillaries
- explain the relationship between the different types of blood vessel
- indicate the main factors controlling blood vessel diameter
- explain the mechanisms by which exchange of nutrients, gases and wastes occurs between the blood and the tissues.

The heart pumps blood into vessels that vary in structure, size and function, and there are several types: arteries, arterioles, capillaries, venules and veins (Fig. 5.2).

Arteries and arterioles

These are the blood vessels that transport blood away from the heart. They vary considerably in size and their walls consist of three layers of tissue (Fig. 5.3):

- *tunica adventitia* or outer layer of fibrous tissue
- *tunica media* or middle layer of smooth muscle and elastic tissue
- *tunica intima* or inner lining of squamous epithelium called *endothelium.*

76

Figure 5.1 The relationship between the pulmonary and the systemic circulations.

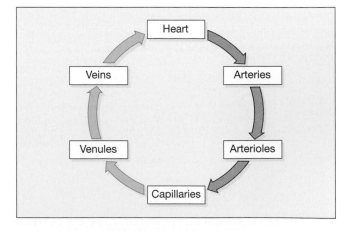

Figure 5.2 The relationship between the heart and the different types of blood vessel.

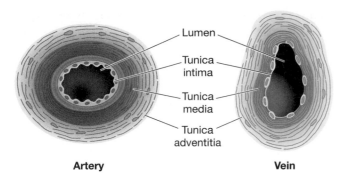

Figure 5.3 Structures of an artery and a vein.

The amount of muscular and elastic tissue varies in the arteries depending upon their size and function. In the large arteries, sometimes called elastic arteries, the tunica media consists of more elastic tissue and less smooth muscle. This allows the vessel wall to stretch, absorbing the pressure wave generated by the heart as it beats. These proportions gradually change as the arteries branch many times and become smaller until in the *arterioles* (the smallest arteries) the tunica media consists almost entirely of smooth muscle. This enables their diameter to be precisely controlled, which regulates the pressure within them. Systemic blood pressure is mainly determined by the resistance these tiny arteries offer to blood flow, and for this reason they are called *resistance vessels*.

Arteries have thicker walls than veins and this enables them to withstand the high pressure of arterial blood.

Anastomoses and end-arteries

Anastomoses are arteries that form a link between main arteries supplying an area, e.g. the arterial supply to the palms of the hand (p. 100) and soles of the feet, the brain, the joints and, to a limited extent, the heart muscle. If one artery supplying the area is occluded, anastomotic arteries provide a *collateral circulation*. This is most likely to provide an adequate blood supply when the occlusion occurs gradually, giving the anastomotic arteries time to dilate.

End-arteries are the arteries with no anastomoses or those beyond the most distal anastomosis, e.g. the branches from the circulus arteriosus (circle of Willis) in the brain or the central artery to the retina of the eye. When an end-artery is occluded the tissues it supplies die because there is no alternative blood supply.

Veins and venules

Veins are blood vessels that return blood at low pressure to the heart. The walls of the veins are thinner than those of arteries but have the same three layers of tissue

(Fig. 5.3). They are thinner because there is less muscle and elastic tissue in the tunica media, because veins carry blood at a lower pressure than arteries. When cut, the veins collapse while the thicker-walled arteries remain open.

When an artery is cut blood spurts at high pressure while a slower, steady flow of blood escapes from a vein.

Some veins possess *valves*, which prevent backflow of blood, ensuring that it flows towards the heart (Fig. 5.4). They are formed by a fold of tunica intima and strengthened by connective tissue. The cusps are *semilunar* in shape with the concavity towards the heart. Valves are abundant in the veins of the limbs, especially the lower limbs where blood must travel a considerable distance against gravity when the individual is standing. They are absent in very small and very large veins in the thorax and abdomen. Valves are assisted in maintaining one-way flow by skeletal muscles surrounding the veins (p. 88).

The smallest veins are called *venules*.

Veins are called *capacitance vessels* because they are distensible, and therefore have the capacity to hold a large proportion of the body's blood. At any one time, about two-thirds of the body's blood is in the venous system. This allows the vascular system to absorb (to an extent) sudden changes in blood volume, such as in haemorrhage; the veins can recoil, helping to prevent a sudden fall in blood pressure.

Capillaries and sinusoids

The smallest arterioles break up into a number of minute vessels called *capillaries*. Capillary walls consist of a single layer of endothelial cells sitting on a very thin basement membrane, through which water and other small-molecule substances can pass. Blood cells and large-

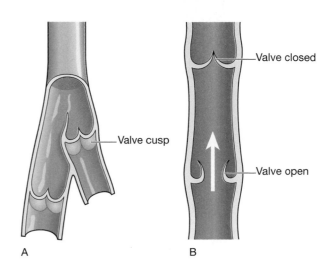

A   B

Figure 5.4 Interior of a vein: A. The valves and cusps. **B.** The direction of blood flow through a valve.

77

molecule substances such as plasma proteins do not normally pass through capillary walls. The capillaries form a vast network of tiny vessels that link the smallest arterioles to the smallest venules. Their diameter is approximately that of an erythrocyte (7 μm). The capillary bed is the site of exchange of substances between the blood and the tissue fluid, which bathes the body cells.

Entry to capillary beds is guarded by rings of smooth muscle (*precapillary sphincters*) that direct blood flow. Hypoxia (low levels of oxygen in the tissues), or high levels of tissue wastes, indicating high levels of activity, dilate the sphincters and increase blood flow through the affected beds.

Sinusoids are wider than capillaries and have extremely thin walls separating blood from the neighbouring cells. In some there are distinct spaces between the endothelial cells. Among the endothelial cells there may be many phagocytic macrophages, e.g. Kupffer cells in the liver. Sinusoids are found in bone marrow, endocrine glands, spleen and liver. Because of their larger lumen, the blood pressure in sinusoids is lower than in capillaries, and blood flow is slower.

Blood supply

The outer layers of tissue of thick-walled blood vessels receive their blood supply via a network of blood vessels called the *vasa vasorum*. Vessels with thin walls and the endothelium of the others receive oxygen and nutrients by diffusion from the blood passing through them.

Control of blood vessel diameter

All blood vessels except capillaries have smooth muscle fibres in the tunica media which are supplied by nerves of the *autonomic nervous system*. These nerves arise from the *vasomotor centre* in the *medulla oblongata* and they change the diameter of the lumen of blood vessels, controlling the volume of blood they contain. Medium-sized and small arteries have more muscle than elastic tissue in their walls. In large arteries, such as the aorta, the middle layer is almost entirely elastic tissue. This means that small arteries and arterioles respond to nerve stimulation whereas the diameter of large arteries varies according to the amount of blood they contain.

Vasodilatation and vasoconstriction

Sympathetic nerves supply the smooth muscle of the tunica media of blood vessels. There is no parasympathetic nerve supply to most blood vessels and therefore the diameter of the vessel lumen and the tone of the smooth muscle is determined by the degree of sympa-

thetic nerve stimulation. There is a baseline (resting) level of nervous activity supplying the smooth muscle in the vessel walls, which can then be increased or decreased as required (Fig. 5.5). Decreased nerve stimulation relaxes the smooth muscle, thinning the vessel wall and enlarging the lumen. This process is called *vasodilatation* and results in increased blood flow under less resistance. Conversely, when nervous activity is increased the smooth muscle of the tunica media contracts and thickens; this process is called *vasoconstriction*.

Resistance to flow of fluids along a tube is determined by three factors: the diameter of the tube; the length of the tube; and the viscosity of the fluid involved. The most important factor determining how easily the blood flows through blood vessels is the first of these variables, that is, the diameter of the resistance vessels (the peripheral resistance). Control of systemic blood pressure is further discussed on p. 89. The degree of vasodilatation/vasoconstriction is important in determining peripheral resistance and systemic blood pressure (p. 89).

The length of the vessels and viscosity of blood could also contribute but in health these are constant and are therefore not significant determinants of changes in blood flow.

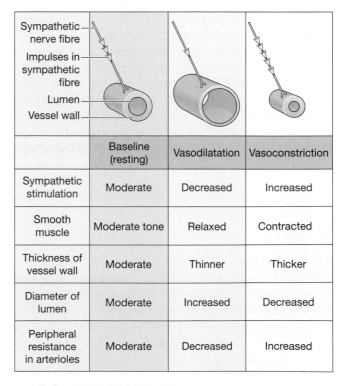

	Baseline (resting)	Vasodilatation	Vasoconstriction
Sympathetic stimulation	Moderate	Decreased	Increased
Smooth muscle	Moderate tone	Relaxed	Contracted
Thickness of vessel wall	Moderate	Thinner	Thicker
Diameter of lumen	Moderate	Increased	Decreased
Peripheral resistance in arterioles	Moderate	Decreased	Increased

Figure 5.5 The relationship between sympathetic stimulation and blood vessel diameter.

Autoregulation

The accumulation of metabolites in local tissues also influences the degree of dilatation of arterioles and capillaries. This mechanism ensures that local blood flow is increased or decreased in response to tissue need. For example in:

- exercise; e.g. lactic acid accumulation in muscle or a rise in tissue temperature causes vasodilatation
- excess CO_2, or tissue hypoxia, both of which signify increased tissue metabolism and which cause local vasodilatation to improve blood supply
- release of vasodilators, such as *nitric oxide* (NO), which increase blood flow through capillary beds. Nitric oxide is very short lived in the tissues, but is thought to have key functions in controlling regional blood flow, reducing clotting and also in body defences.
- tissue damage; e.g. in inflammation, mediators such as histamine, prostaglandins and bradykinin lead to vasodilatation (p. 372)
- situations where the circulation to vital organs, such as the brain and heart, is threatened.

Capillary exchange

Exchange of gases

Internal respiration (Fig. 5.6) is the exchange of gases between capillary blood and local body cells.

Oxygen is carried from the lungs to the tissues in combination with haemoglobin as *oxyhaemoglobin*. Exchange in the tissues takes place between blood at the arterial end of the capillaries and the tissue fluid and then between the tissue fluid and the cells. Oxygen diffuses down its concentration gradient, from the oxygen-rich arterial blood, into the tissues, where oxygen levels are lower because of constant tissue consumption.

Oxyhaemoglobin is an unstable compound and breaks up (dissociates) easily to liberate oxygen. Factors that increase dissociation are discussed on p. 61.

Carbon dioxide is one of the waste products of cell metabolism and, towards the venous end of the capillary, it diffuses into the blood down the concentration gradient. Blood transports carbon dioxide to the lungs for excretion by three different mechanisms:

- dissolved in the water of the blood plasma – 7%
- in chemical combination with sodium in the form of sodium bicarbonate – 70%
- remainder in combination with haemoglobin – 23%.

Exchange of other substances

The nutrients required by the cells of the body are transported round the body in the blood plasma. In passing from the blood to the cells, the nutrients pass through the semipermeable capillary walls into the tissue fluid bathing the cells, then through the cell membrane into the cell (Fig. 5.7). The mechanism of the transfer of water and other substances from the blood capillaries depends mainly upon diffusion and osmosis.

Diffusion (p. 26)

The capillary walls consist of a single layer of epithelial cells that constitutes a semipermeable membrane, which allows substances with small molecules to pass through into tissue fluid, and retains large molecules in the blood. Diffusible substances include dissolved oxygen and carbon dioxide, glucose, amino acids, fatty acids, glycerol, vitamins, mineral salts and water.

79

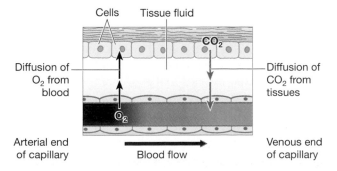

Figure 5.6 The exchange of gases in internal respiration.

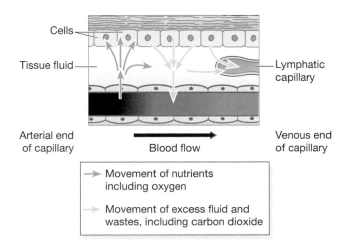

Figure 5.7 Diffusion of nutrients and waste products between capillaries and cells.

Osmosis (p. 26)

Osmotic pressure across a semipermeable membrane draws water from a dilute to a more concentrated solution in an attempt to establish a state of equilibrium. The force of the osmotic pressure depends on the number of non-diffusible particles in the solutions separated by the membrane. The main substances responsible for the osmotic pressure between blood and tissue fluid are the plasma proteins, especially albumin.

Capillary fluid dynamics

The two main forces determining overall fluid movement across the capillary wall are the *hydrostatic pressure* (blood pressure), which tends to push fluid out of the bloodstream, and the *osmotic pressure* of the blood, which tends to pull it back in, and is due mainly to the presence of plasma proteins (Fig. 5.8).

At the arterial end, the hydrostatic pressure is about 5 kPa (35 mmHg), and the opposing osmotic pressure of the blood is only 3 kPa (25 mmHg). The overall force at the arterial end of the capillary therefore drives fluid out of the capillary and into the tissue. This net loss of fluid from the bloodstream must be reclaimed in some way.

At the venous end of the capillary, the situation is reversed. Blood flow is slower than at the arterial end because the hydrostatic pressure drops along the capillary to only 2 kPa (15 mmHg). The osmotic pressure remains unchanged at 3 kPa (25 mmHg) and, because this now exceeds hydrostatic pressure, fluid moves back into the capillary.

This transfer of substances, including water, to the tissue spaces is a dynamic process. As blood flows slowly through the large network of capillaries from the arterial to the venous end, there is constant change. Not all the

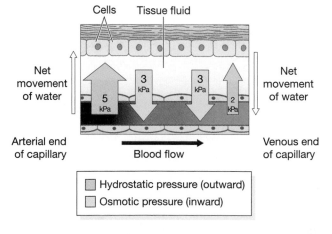

Figure 5.8 Effect of capillary pressures on water movement between capillaries and cells.

water and cell waste products return to the blood capillaries. Of the 24 litres or so of fluid that moves out of the blood across capillary walls every day, only about 21 litres returns to the bloodstream at the venous end of the capillary bed. The excess is drained away from the tissue spaces in the minute lymph capillaries which originate as blind-end tubes with walls similar to, but more permeable than, those of the blood capillaries (Fig. 5.7). Extra tissue fluid and some cell waste materials enter the lymph capillaries and are eventually returned to the bloodstream (Ch. 6).

Heart

Learning outcomes

After studying this section, you should be able to:

- describe the structure of the heart and its position within the thorax

- trace the circulation of the blood through the heart and the blood vessels of the body

- outline the conducting system of the heart

- relate the electrical activity of the cardiac conduction system to the cardiac cycle

- describe the main factors determining heart rate and cardiac output.

The heart is a roughly cone-shaped hollow muscular organ. It is about 10 cm long and is about the size of the owner's fist. It weighs about 225 g in women and is heavier in men (about 310 g).

Position

The heart lies in the thoracic cavity (Fig. 5.9) in the mediastinum (the space between the lungs). It lies obliquely, a little more to the left than the right, and presents a *base* above, and an *apex* below. The apex is about 9 cm to the left of the midline at the level of the 5th intercostal space, i.e. a little below the nipple and slightly nearer the midline. The base extends to the level of the 2nd rib.

Organs associated with the heart (Fig. 5.10)

Inferiorly – the apex rests on the central tendon of the diaphragm

Superiorly – the great blood vessels, i.e. the aorta, superior vena cava, pulmonary artery and pulmonary veins

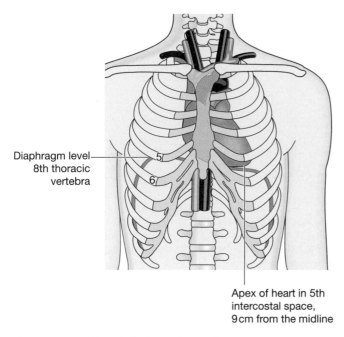

Diaphragm level 8th thoracic vertebra

5

6

Apex of heart in 5th intercostal space, 9 cm from the midline

Figure 5.9 Position of the heart in the thorax.

Posteriorly – the oesophagus, trachea, left and right bronchus, descending aorta, inferior vena cava and thoracic vertebrae
Laterally – the lungs – the left lung overlaps the left side of the heart
Anteriorly – the sternum, ribs and intercostal muscles.

Structure

The heart is composed of three layers of tissue (Fig. 5.11): pericardium, myocardium and endocardium.

Pericardium

The pericardium is made up of two sacs. The outer sac consists of fibrous tissue and the inner of a continuous double layer of serous membrane.

The outer fibrous sac is continuous with the tunica adventitia of the great blood vessels above and is adherent to the diaphragm below. Its inelastic, fibrous nature prevents overdistension of the heart.

The outer layer of the serous membrane, the *parietal pericardium*, lines the fibrous sac. The inner layer, the *visceral pericardium*, or epicardium, which is continuous with the parietal pericardium, is adherent to the heart muscle. A similar arrangement of a double membrane forming a closed space is seen also with the pleura, the membrane enclosing the lungs (see Fig. 10.15, p. 247).

The serous membrane consists of flattened epithelial cells. It secretes serous fluid into the space between the visceral and parietal layers, which allows smooth movement between them when the heart beats. The space between the parietal and visceral pericardium is only a *potential space*. In health the two layers are in close association, with only the thin film of serous fluid between them.

81

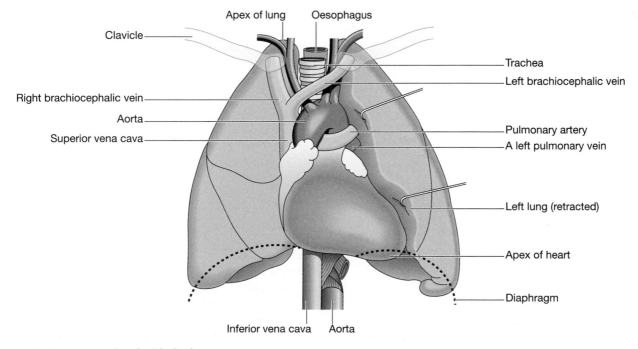

Apex of lung   Oesophagus

Clavicle

Trachea
Left brachiocephalic vein

Right brachiocephalic vein

Aorta

Superior vena cava

Pulmonary artery
A left pulmonary vein

Left lung (retracted)

Apex of heart

Diaphragm

Inferior vena cava   Aorta

Figure 5.10 Organs associated with the heart.

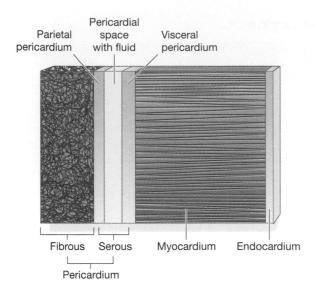

Parietal pericardium — Pericardial space with fluid — Visceral pericardium

Fibrous — Serous — Myocardium — Endocardium

Pericardium

Figure 5.11 Layers of the heart wall.

Myocardium

The myocardium is composed of specialised cardiac muscle found only in the heart (Fig. 5.12). It is not under voluntary control but, like skeletal muscle, cross-stripes are seen on microscopic examination. Each fibre (cell) has a nucleus and one or more branches. The ends of the cells and their branches are in very close contact with the ends and branches of adjacent cells. Microscopically these 'joints', or *intercalated discs*, can be seen as thicker, darker lines than the ordinary cross-stripes. This arrangement gives cardiac muscle the appearance of being a sheet of muscle rather than a very large number of individual

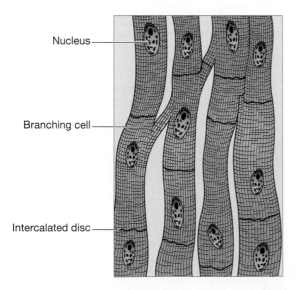

Nucleus

Branching cell

Intercalated disc

Figure 5.12 Cardiac muscle fibres.

cells. Because of the end-to-end continuity of the fibres, each one does not need to have a separate nerve supply. When an impulse is initiated it spreads from cell to cell via the branches and intercalated discs over the whole 'sheet' of muscle, causing contraction. The 'sheet' arrangement of the myocardium enables the atria and ventricles to contract in a coordinated and efficient manner.

The myocardium is thickest at the apex and thins out towards the base (Fig. 5.13). This reflects the amount of work each chamber contributes to the pumping of blood. It is thickest in the left ventricle, which has the greatest workload.

The atria and the ventricles are separated by a ring of fibrous tissue, which does not conduct electrical impulses. Consequently, when a wave of electrical activity passes over the atrial muscle, it can only spread to the ventricles through the conducting system that bridges the fibrous ring from atria to ventricles (p. 85).

Endocardium

This lines the chambers and valves of the heart. It is a thin, smooth, glistening membrane that permits smooth flow of blood inside the heart. It consists of flattened epithelial cells, and it is continuous with the endothelium lining the blood vessels.

Interior of the heart

The heart is divided into a right and left side by the *septum* (Fig. 5.13), a partition consisting of myocardium covered by endocardium. After birth, blood cannot cross the septum from one side to the other. Each side is divided by an *atrioventricular valve* into an upper chamber, the *atrium*, and a lower chamber, the *ventricle*. The atrioventricular valves are formed by double folds of endocardium strengthened by a little fibrous tissue. The *right atrioventricular valve* (tricuspid valve) has three flaps or *cusps* and the *left atrioventricular valve* (mitral valve) has two cusps. Flow of blood in the heart is one way; blood enters the heart via the atria and passes into the ventricles below.

The valves between the atria and ventricles open and close passively according to changes in pressure in the chambers. They open when the pressure in the atria is greater than that in the ventricles. During *ventricular systole* (contraction) the pressure in the ventricles rises above that in the atria and the valves snap shut, preventing backward flow of blood. The valves are prevented from opening upwards into the atria by tendinous cords, called *chordae tendineae*, which extend from the inferior surface of the cusps to little projections of myocardium into the ventricles, covered with endothelium, called *papillary muscles* (Fig. 5.14).

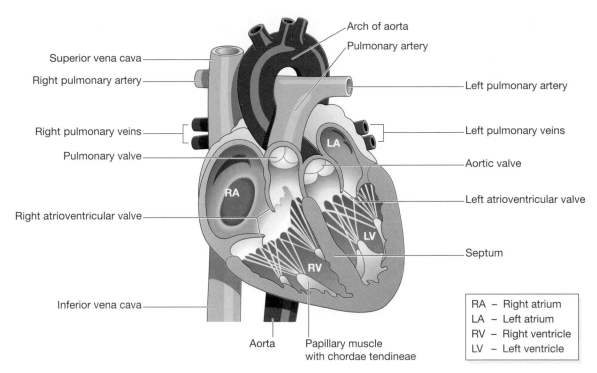

Figure 5.13 **Interior of the heart.**

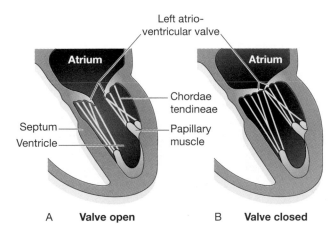

A **Valve open**   B **Valve closed**

Figure 5.14 **The left atrioventricular valve:** A. valve open.
B. valve closed.

Flow of blood through the heart (Fig. 5.15)

The two largest veins of the body, the *superior* and *inferior venae cavae*, empty their contents into the right atrium. This blood passes via the right atrioventricular valve into the right ventricle, and from there it is pumped into the *pulmonary artery* or *trunk* (the only artery in the body which carries deoxygenated blood). The opening of the pulmonary artery is guarded by the *pulmonary valve*, formed by three *semilunar cusps*. This valve prevents the backflow of blood into the right ventricle when the

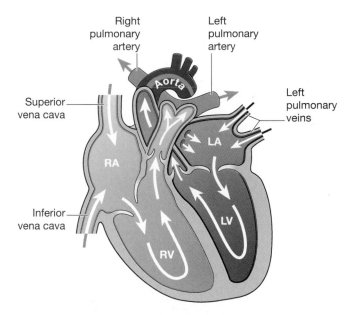

Figure 5.15 **Direction of blood flow through the heart.**

ventricular muscle relaxes. After leaving the heart the pulmonary artery divides into *left* and *right pulmonary arteries*, which carry the venous blood to the lungs where exchange of gases takes place: carbon dioxide is excreted and oxygen is absorbed.

Two *pulmonary veins* from each lung carry *oxygenated blood* back to the *left atrium*. Blood then passes through the left atrioventricular valve into the left ventricle, and from there it is pumped into the aorta, the first artery of the general circulation. The opening of the aorta is guarded by the *aortic valve*, formed by three *semilunar cusps* (Fig. 5.16).

From this sequence of events it can be seen that the blood passes from the right to the left side of the heart via the lungs, or pulmonary circulation (Fig. 5.17). However, it should be noted that both atria contract at the same time and this is followed by the simultaneous contraction of both ventricles.

The muscle layer of the walls of the atria is thinner than that of the ventricles (Fig. 5.13). This is consistent with the amount of work they do. The atria, usually assisted by gravity, propel the blood only through the atrioventricular valves into the ventricles, whereas the ventricles actively pump the blood to the lungs and round the whole body.

The pulmonary trunk leaves the heart from the upper part of the right ventricle, and the aorta leaves from the upper part of the left ventricle.

Blood supply to the heart

Arterial supply (Fig. 5.18). The heart is supplied with arterial blood by the *right and left coronary arteries,* which branch from the aorta immediately distal to the aortic valve (Figs 5.16 and 5.18). The coronary arteries receive about 5% of the blood pumped from the heart, although the heart comprises a small proportion of body weight. This large blood supply, especially to the left ventricle, highlights the importance of the heart to body function. The coronary arteries traverse the heart, eventually forming a vast network of capillaries.

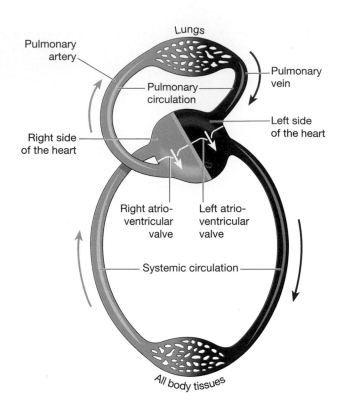

Figure 5.17 Circulation of blood through the heart and the pulmonary and systemic circulations.

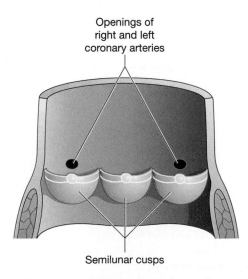

Figure 5.16 The aorta cut open to show the semilunar cusps of the aortic valve.

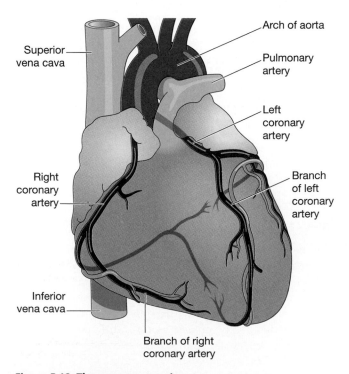

Figure 5.18 The coronary arteries.

Venous drainage. Most of the venous blood is collected into several small veins that join to form the *coronary sinus,* which opens into the right atrium. The remainder passes directly into the heart chambers through little venous channels.

Conducting system of the heart

The heart has an intrinsic system (Fig. 5.19) whereby the cardiac muscle is automatically stimulated to contract without the need for external stimulation. This property is called *autorhythmicity.* However, the intrinsic system can be stimulated or depressed by nerve impulses initiated in the brain and by circulating chemicals, including hormones.

Small groups of specialised neuromuscular cells in the myocardium initiate and conduct impulses, causing coordinated and synchronised contraction of the heart muscle.

Sinoatrial node (SA node)

This small mass of specialised cells lies in the wall of the right atrium near the opening of the superior vena cava. The SA node is the '*pacemaker*' of the heart because it normally initiates impulses more rapidly than other groups of neuromuscular cells. Firing of the SA node causes atrial contraction.

Atrioventricular node (AV node)

This small mass of neuromuscular tissue is situated in the wall of the atrial septum near the atrioventricular valves. Normally, the AV node conducts impulses that arrive via the atria and that originated from the SA node. There is a delay here; the electrical signal takes 0.1 of a second to pass through into the ventricles. This allows the atria to finish contracting before the ventricles start.

The AV node also has a *secondary pacemaker* function and takes over this role if there is a problem with the SA node itself, or with the transmission of impulses from the atria. Its intrinsic firing rate, however, is slower than that set by the SA node.

Atrioventricular bundle (AV bundle or bundle of His)

This is a mass of specialised fibres that originate from the AV node. The AV bundle crosses the fibrous ring that separates atria and ventricles then, at the upper end of the ventricular septum, it divides into *right and left bundle branches*. Within the ventricular myocardium the branches break up into fine fibres, called the *Purkinje fibres*. The AV bundle, bundle branches and Purkinje fibres convey electrical impulses from the AV node to the apex of the myocardium where the wave of ventricular contraction begins, then sweeps upwards and outwards, pumping blood into the pulmonary artery and the aorta.

Nerve supply to the heart

In addition to the intrinsic impulses generated within the conducting system described above, the heart is influenced by autonomic nerves originating in the *cardiovascular centre* in the *medulla oblongata* which reach it through the autonomic nervous system. These consist of *parasympathetic* and *sympathetic nerves* and their actions are antagonistic.

The *vagus nerves* (parasympathetic) supply mainly the SA and AV nodes and atrial muscle. Parasympathetic stimulation reduces the rate at which impulses are produced, decreasing the rate and force of the heartbeat.

The *sympathetic nerves* supply the SA and AV nodes and the myocardium of atria and ventricles. Sympathetic stimulation *increases* the rate and force of the heartbeat.

Factors affecting heart rate

The most important ones are summarized in Box 5.1, and explained in more detail on p. 88.

85

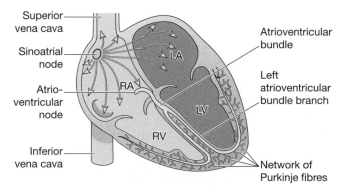

Figure 5.19 The conducting system of the heart.

Labels: Superior vena cava; Sinoatrial node; Atrioventricular node; Inferior vena cava; LA; RA; LV; RV; Atrioventricular bundle; Left atrioventricular bundle branch; Network of Purkinje fibres.

Box 5.1 The main factors affecting heart rate

- Gender
- Autonomic (sympathetic and parasympathetic) nerve activity
- Age
- Circulating hormones, e.g. adrenaline, thyroxine
- Activity and exercise
- Temperature
- The baroreceptor reflex
- Emotional states

The cardiac cycle

The function of the heart is to maintain a constant circulation of blood throughout the body. The heart acts as a pump and its action consists of a series of events known as the *cardiac cycle* (Fig. 5.20).

During each heartbeat, or cardiac cycle, the heart contracts and then relaxes. The period of contraction is called *systole* and that of relaxation, *diastole*.

Stages of the cardiac cycle

The normal number of cardiac cycles per minute ranges from 60 to 80. Taking 74 as an example each cycle lasts about *0.8 of a second* and consists of:

- *atrial systole* – contraction of the atria
- *ventricular systole*– contraction of the ventricles
- *complete cardiac diastole* – relaxation of the atria and ventricles.

It does not matter at which stage of the cardiac cycle a description starts. For convenience the period when the atria are filling has been chosen.

The superior vena cava and the inferior vena cava transport deoxygenated blood into the right atrium *at the same time* as the four pulmonary veins bring oxygenated blood into the left atrium. The atrioventricular valves are open and blood flows passively through to the ventricles. The SA node triggers a wave of contraction that spreads over the myocardium of both atria, emptying the atria and completing ventricular filling (atrial systole 0.1 s). When the electrical impulse reaches the AV node it is slowed down, delaying atrioventricular transmission. This delay means that the mechanical result of atrial stimulation, atrial contraction, lags behind the electrical activity by a fraction of a second. This allows the atria to finish emptying into the ventricles before the ventricles begin to contract. After this brief delay, the AV node triggers its own electrical impulse, which quickly spreads to the ventricular muscle via the AV bundle, the bundle branches and Purkinje fibres. This results in a wave of contraction which sweeps upwards from the apex of the heart and across the walls of both ventricles pumping the blood into the pulmonary artery and the aorta (ventricular systole 0.3 s). The high pressure generated during ventricular contraction is greater than that in the aorta and forces the atrioventricular valves to close, preventing backflow of blood into the atria.

After contraction of the ventricles there is *complete cardiac diastole*, a period of *0.4 seconds*, when atria and ventricles are relaxed. During this time the myocardium recovers in preparation for the next heartbeat, and the atria refill in preparation for the next cycle.

The valves of the heart and of the great vessels open and close according to the pressure within the chambers of the heart. The AV valves are open while the ventricular muscle is relaxed during atrial filling and systole. When the ventricles contract there is a gradual increase in the pressure in these chambers, and when it rises above atrial pressure the atrioventricular valves close. When the ventricular pressure rises above that in the pulmonary artery and in the aorta, the pulmonary and aortic valves open and blood flows into these vessels. When the ventricles relax and the pressure within them falls, the reverse process occurs. First the pulmonary and aortic valves close, then the atrioventricular valves open and the cycle begins again. This sequence of opening and closing valves ensures that the blood flows in only one direction (Fig. 5.21). This figure also shows how the walls of the aorta and other elastic arteries stretch and recoil in response to blood pumped into them.

Heart sounds

The individual is not usually conscious of his heartbeat, but if the ear, or the diaphragm of a stethoscope, is placed on the chest wall a little below the left nipple and slightly nearer the midline the heartbeat can be heard.

There are four heart sounds, each corresponding to a particular event in the cardiac cycle. The first two are most easily distinguished, and sound through the stethoscope like "lub dup". The first sound, *'lub'*, is fairly loud and is due to the closure of the atrioventricular valves. This corresponds with the start of ventricular systole. The second sound, *'dup'*, is softer and is due to the closure of the aortic and pulmonary valves. This corresponds with atrial systole.

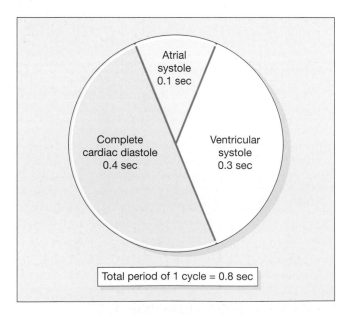

Figure 5.20 The stages of the cardiac cycle.

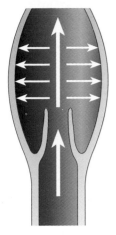 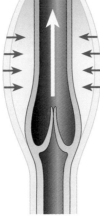

Aortic valve open	Aortic valve closed
Ventricular systole	**Ventricular diastole**

Figure 5.21 The elasticity of the wall of the aorta.

Electrical changes in the heart

As the body fluids and tissues are good conductors of electricity, the electrical activity within the heart can be detected by attaching electrodes to the surface of the body. The pattern of electrical activity may be displayed on an oscilloscope screen or traced on paper. The apparatus used is an *electrocardiograph* and the tracing is an *electrocardiogram* (ECG).

The normal ECG tracing shows five waves which, by convention, have been named P, Q, R, S and T (Fig. 5.22).

The P wave arises when the impulse from the SA node sweeps over the atria.

The QRS complex represents the very rapid spread of the impulse from the AV node through the AV bundle and the Purkinje fibres and the electrical activity of the ventricular muscle.

The T wave represents the relaxation of the ventricular muscle.

The ECG described above originates from the SA node and is known as *sinus rhythm*. The rate of sinus rhythm is 60 to 100 beats per minute. A faster heart rate is called *tachycardia* and a slower heart rate, *bradycardia*.

By examining the pattern of waves and the time interval between cycles and parts of cycles, information about the state of the myocardium and the cardiac conduction system is obtained.

Myocardial energy sources

As mentioned above, the heart receives an excellent blood supply, out of proportion to its size, ensuring a good supply of oxygen and nutrients. Normal energy production in the heart comes from aerobic breakdown of fats and sugars.

Cardiac output

The cardiac output is the amount of blood ejected from the heart. The amount expelled by each contraction of the ventricles is the *stroke volume*. Cardiac output is expressed in litres per minute (l/min) and is calculated by multiplying the stroke volume by the heart rate (measured in beats per minute):

Cardiac output = Stroke volume × Heart rate.

In a healthy adult at rest, the stroke volume is approximately 70 ml and if the heart rate is 72 per minute, the cardiac output is 5 l/minute. This can be greatly increased to meet the demands of exercise to around 25 l/minute, and in athletes up to 35 l/minute. This increase during exercise is called the *cardiac reserve*.

When increased blood supply is needed to meet increased tissue requirements of oxygen and nutrients, heart rate and/or stroke volume can be increased (see Box 5.2).

Stroke volume

The stroke volume is determined by the volume of blood in the ventricles immediately before they contract, i.e. the ventricular end-diastolic volume (VEDV), sometimes called *preload*. In turn, preload depends on the amount of blood returning to the heart through the superior and inferior venae cavae (the *venous return*). Increased VEDV leads to stronger myocardial contraction, and more blood is expelled. In turn the stroke volume and cardiac output rise. This capacity to increase the stroke volume with increasing VEDV is finite, and when the limit is reached, i.e. the cardiac output cannot match the venous return, the cardiac output decreases and the heart begins to fail

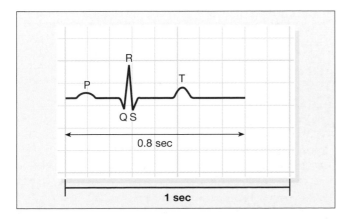

Figure 5.22 Electrocardiogram of one cardiac cycle.

(p. 122). Other factors that increase myocardial contraction include:

- increased sympathetic nerve activity to the heart
- hormones, e.g. adrenaline (epinephrine), noradrenaline (norepinephrine), thyroxine.

Arterial blood pressure. This affects the stroke volume as it creates resistance to blood being pumped from the ventricles into the great arteries. This resistance (sometimes called *afterload*) is determined by the distensibility, or *elasticity*, of the large arteries and the *peripheral resistance* of arterioles.

Blood volume. This is normally kept constant by the kidneys, and if deficient the stroke volume, cardiac output and venous return decrease.

Venous return

Venous return is the major determinant of cardiac output and, normally, the heart pumps out all blood returned to it. The force of contraction of the left ventricle ejecting blood into the aorta is not sufficient to return the blood through the veins and back to the heart. Other factors are involved.

The position of the body. Gravity assists the venous return from the head and neck when standing or sitting and offers less resistance to venous return from the lower parts of the body when an individual is lying flat.

Muscular contraction. Backflow of blood in veins of the limbs, especially when standing, is prevented by valves. The contraction of skeletal muscles surrounding the deep veins compresses them, pushing blood towards the heart (Fig. 5.23). In the lower limbs, this is called the *skeletal muscle pump*.

The respiratory pump. During inspiration, the expansion of the chest creates a negative pressure within the thorax, assisting flow of blood towards the heart. In addition, when the diaphragm descends during inspiration, the increased intra-abdominal pressure pushes blood towards the heart.

Heart rate

The heart rate determines cardiac output. If heart rate rises, cardiac output increases, and if it falls, cardiac output falls too. The main factors determining heart rate are outlined below.

Autonomic nervous system. The intrinsic rate at which the heart beats is a balance between sympathetic and

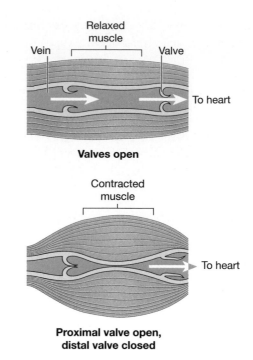

Valves open

Proximal valve open, distal valve closed

Figure 5.23 **The skeletal muscle pump.**

parasympathetic activity and this is the most important factor in determining heart rate.

Circulating chemicals. The hormones adrenaline (epinephrine) and noradrenaline (norepinephrine), secreted by the adrenal medulla, have the same effect as sympathetic stimulation, i.e. they increase the heart rate. Other hormones, including thyroxine, increase heart rate by their metabolic effect. Hypoxia and elevated carbon dioxide levels stimulate heart rate. Electrolyte imbalances may affect it; e.g. hypercalcaemia depresses cardiac function and leads to bradycardia (slow heart rate). Some drugs, such as β-receptor antagonists (e.g. atenolol) used in hypertension, can also cause bradycardia.

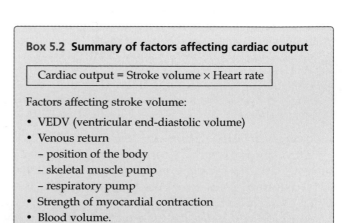

Box 5.2 Summary of factors affecting cardiac output

Cardiac output = Stroke volume × Heart rate

Factors affecting stroke volume:

- VEDV (ventricular end-diastolic volume)
- Venous return
  - position of the body
  - skeletal muscle pump
  - respiratory pump
- Strength of myocardial contraction
- Blood volume.

Position. When the person is upright, the heart rate is usually faster than when lying down.

Exercise. Active muscles need more blood than resting muscles and this is achieved by an increased heart rate and selective vasodilatation.

Emotional states. During excitement, fear or anxiety the heart rate is increased. Other effects mediated by the sympathetic nervous system may be present (see Fig. 7.42, p. 171).

Gender. The heart rate is faster in women than men.

Age. In babies and small children the heart rate is more rapid than in older children and adults.

Temperature. The heart rate rises and falls with body temperature.

Baroreceptor reflex. See p. 90.

A summary of the factors that alter CO is shown in Box 5.2.

Blood pressure

Learning outcomes

After studying this section, you should be able to:

- define the term blood pressure
- describe the main control mechanisms for regulation of blood pressure.

Blood pressure is the force or pressure that the blood exerts on the walls of the blood vessels. Keeping blood pressure within normal limits is very important. If it becomes too high, blood vessels can be damaged, causing clots or bleeding from sites of blood vessel rupture. If it falls too low, then blood flow through tissue beds may be inadequate. This is particularly dangerous for such essential organs as the heart, brain or kidneys.

The systemic arterial blood pressure, usually called simply arterial blood pressure, is the result of the discharge of blood from the left ventricle into the already full aorta.

When the left ventricle contracts and pushes blood into the aorta, the pressure produced within the arterial system is called the *systolic blood pressure*. In adults it is about 120 mmHg or 16 kPa.

When *complete cardiac diastole* occurs and the heart is resting following the ejection of blood, the pressure

within the arteries is much lower and is called *diastolic blood pressure*. In an adult this is about 80 mmHg or 11 kPa. The difference between systolic and diastolic blood pressures is the *pulse pressure*.

Blood pressure varies according to the time of day, the posture, gender and age of the individual. During bedrest at night the blood pressure tends to be lower. It increases with age and is usually higher in women than in men.

Arterial blood pressure is measured with a *sphygmomanometer* and is usually expressed with the systolic pressure written above the diastolic pressure:

$$BP = \frac{120}{80} \text{ mmHg} \quad \text{or} \quad BP = \frac{16}{11} \text{ kPa}$$

The elasticity of the artery walls. There is a considerable amount of elastic tissue in the arterial walls, especially in large arteries. Therefore, when the left ventricle ejects blood into the already full aorta, the aorta expands to accommodate it, and then recoils because of the elastic tissue in the wall. This pushes the blood forwards, into the systemic circulation. This distension and recoil occurs throughout the arterial system. During cardiac diastole the elastic recoil of the arteries maintains the diastolic pressure (Fig. 5.21).

Systemic arterial blood pressure maintains the essential flow of blood into and out of the organs of the body. Blood pressure is determined by *cardiac output* and *peripheral resistance*. Change in either of these parameters tends to alter systemic blood pressure, although the body's compensatory mechanisms usually adjust for any significant change.

$$\text{Blood pressure} = \frac{\text{Cardiac}}{\text{output}} \times \frac{\text{Peripheral}}{\text{resistance}}$$

Cardiac output

The cardiac output is determined by the stroke volume and the heart rate. Factors that affect the heart rate and stroke volume are described above, and they may increase or decrease cardiac output and, in turn, blood pressure. An increase in cardiac output raises both the systolic and diastolic pressure. An increase in stroke volume increases systolic pressure more than it does diastolic pressure.

Peripheral or arteriolar resistance

Arterioles are the smallest arteries and they have a tunica media composed almost entirely of smooth muscle, which responds to nerve and chemical stimulation. Constriction and dilatation of the arterioles are the main determinants of peripheral resistance (p. 77).

Vasoconstriction causes blood pressure to rise and vasodilatation causes it to fall.

When elastic tissue in the tunica media is replaced by inelastic fibrous tissue as part of the ageing process, blood pressure rises.

Dilatation and constriction of arterioles occurs selectively around the body, resulting in changes in the blood flow through organs according to their needs. The highest priorities are the blood supply to the brain and the heart muscle, and in an emergency, supplies to other parts of the body are reduced in order to ensure an adequate supply to these organs. Generally, changes in the amount of blood flowing to any organ depend on how active it is. A very active organ needs more oxygen and nutrients than a resting organ and it produces more waste materials for excretion.

Control of blood pressure (BP)

Blood pressure is controlled in two ways:

- short-term control, on a moment-to-moment basis, which mainly involves the baroreceptor reflex, discussed below, and also chemoreceptors and circulating hormones
- long-term control, which involves regulation of blood volume by the kidneys and the renin–angiotensin–aldosterone system (p. 221).

Short-term blood pressure regulation

The cardiovascular centre (CVC) is a collection of interconnected neurones in the medulla and pons of the brainstem. The CVC receives, integrates and coordinates inputs from:

- baroreceptors (pressure receptors)
- chemoreceptors
- higher centres in the brain.

The CVC sends autonomic nerves (both sympathetic and parasympathetic) to the heart and blood vessels. It controls BP by slowing down or speeding up the heart rate and by dilating or constricting blood vessels. Activity in these fibres is essential for control of blood pressure (Fig. 5.24). The two divisions of the autonomic nervous system, the sympathetic and the parasympathetic divisions, are described more fully in Chapter 7. Their actions relating to the heart and blood vessels are summarised in Table 5.1.

Baroreceptors

These are nerve endings sensitive to pressure changes (stretch) within the vessel, situated in the arch of the aorta and in the carotid sinuses (Fig. 5.25) and are the body's

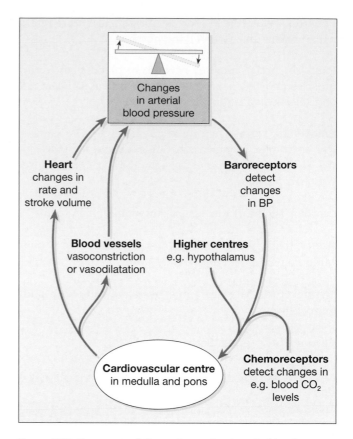

Figure 5.24 Summary of the main mechanisms in blood pressure control.

Table 5.1 The effects of the autonomic nervous system on the heart and blood vessels

	Sympathetic stimulation	Parasympathetic stimulation
Heart	↑rate ↑strength of contraction	↓rate ↓strength of contraction
Blood vessels	Most constrict, but arteries supplying skeletal muscle and brain dilate	There is little parasympathetic supply to most blood vessels

principal moment-to-moment regulatory mechanism for controlling blood pressure. A rise in blood pressure in these arteries stimulates the baroreceptors, increasing their input to the CVC. The CVC responds by increasing parasympathetic nerve activity to the heart; this slows the heart down. At the same time, sympathetic stimulation to the blood vessels is inhibited, causing vasodilatation. The net result is a fall in systemic blood pressure. Conversely, if pressure within the aortic arch and carotid sinuses falls,

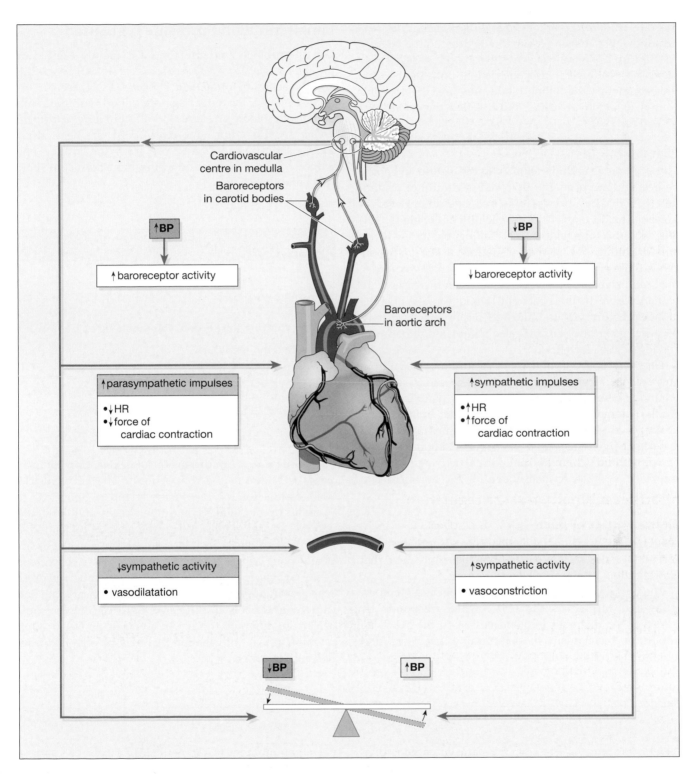

Figure 5.25 The baroreceptor reflex.

91

the rate of baroreceptor discharge also falls. The CVC responds by increasing sympathetic drive to the heart to speed it up. Sympathetic activity in blood vessels is also increased, leading to vasoconstriction. Both these measures counteract the falling blood pressure. Baroreceptor control of blood pressure is also called the *baroreceptor reflex* (Fig. 5.25).

Chemoreceptors

These are nerve endings situated in the carotid and aortic bodies, and are primarily involved in control of respiration (p. 256). They are sensitive to changes in the levels of carbon dioxide, oxygen and the acidity of the blood (pH) (Fig. 5.26). Rising blood CO_2, falling blood O_2 levels and/or falling pH all indicate failing tissue perfusion. When these changes are detected by the chemoreceptors, they send signals to the CVC, which then increases sympathetic drive to the heart and blood vessels, pushing blood pressure up to improve tissue blood supply. Because respiratory effort is also stimulated, blood oxygen levels rise as well.

Chemoreceptor input to the CVC influences its output only when severe disruption of respiratory function occurs or when arterial BP falls to less than 80 mmHg. Similar chemoreceptors are found on the brain surface in the medulla oblongata, and they measure carbon dioxide/oxygen levels and pH of the surrounding cerebrospinal fluid. Changes from normal activate responses similar to those described above for the aortic/carotid receptors.

Higher centres in the brain

Input to the CVC from the higher centres is influenced by emotional states such as fear, anxiety, pain and anger that may stimulate changes in blood pressure.

The hypothalamus in the brain controls body temperature and influences the CVC, which responds by adjusting the diameter of blood vessels in the skin – an important mechanism in determining heat loss and retention (p. 361).

Long-term blood pressure regulation

Long-term blood pressure control is mainly exerted by the *renin–angiotensin–aldosterone system* (RAAS, see p. 221) and the action of *antidiuretic hormone* (ADH, see p. 216). Both of these systems regulate blood volume, thus influencing blood pressure. In addition, *atrial natriuretic peptide* (ANP), a hormone released by the heart itself, causes sodium and water loss from the kidney and reduces blood pressure, opposing the activities of both ADH and the RAAS.

Pulse

Learning outcomes

After studying this section, you should be able to:

- define the term pulse
- list the main sites on the body surface where the pulse is detected
- describe the main factors affecting the pulse.

The pulse is a wave of distension and elongation felt in an artery wall due to the contraction of the left ventricle. Each contraction of the ventricle forces about 60 to 80 millilitres of blood through the already full aorta and into the arterial system. When the aorta is distended, a wave passes along the walls of the arteries and can be felt at any point where a superficial artery can be pressed gently against a bone (Fig. 5.27). The number of pulse beats per minute normally represents the heart rate and varies considerably in different people and in the same person at different times. An average of 60 to 80 is common at rest. Information that may be obtained from the pulse includes:

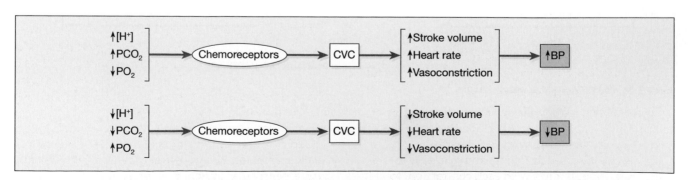

Figure 5.26 The relationship between stimulation of chemoreceptors and arterial blood pressure.

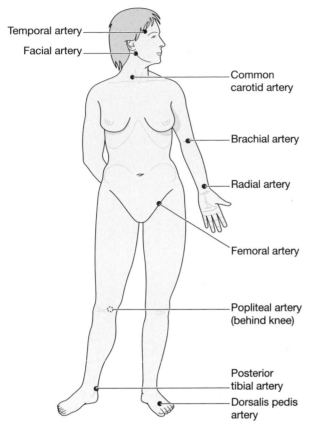

Temporal artery
Facial artery
Common carotid artery
Brachial artery
Radial artery
Femoral artery
Popliteal artery (behind knee)
Posterior tibial artery
Dorsalis pedis artery

Figure 5.27 The main pulse points.

- *the rate* at which the heart is beating
- *the regularity* of the heartbeat – the intervals between beats should be equal
- *the volume or strength* of the beat – it should be possible to compress the artery with moderate pressure, stopping the flow of blood; the compressibility of the blood vessel gives some indication of the blood pressure and the state of the blood vessel wall
- *the tension* – the artery wall should feel soft and pliant under the fingers.

Factors affecting the pulse

In health, the pulse rate and the heart rate are identical. Factors influencing heart rate are summarised on page 85. In certain circumstances, the pulse may be less than the heart rate. This may occur, for example, if:

- the arteries supplying the peripheral tissues are narrowed or blocked and the blood therefore is not pumped through them with each heartbeat
- the heart is diseased or failing, and is unable to generate enough force, with each contraction, to circulate blood to the peripheral arteries.

Circulation of the blood

Learning outcomes

After studying this section, you should be able to:

- describe the circulation of the blood through the lungs, naming the main vessels involved
- list the arteries supplying blood to all major body structures
- describe the venous drainage involved in returning blood to the heart from the body
- describe the arrangement of blood vessels relating to the portal circulation.

Although circulation of blood round the body is continuous (Fig. 5.17) it is convenient to describe it in two parts:

- pulmonary circulation
- systemic or general circulation.

Pulmonary circulation

This is the circulation of blood from the right ventricle of the heart to the lungs and back to the left atrium. In the lungs, carbon dioxide is excreted and oxygen is absorbed.

The pulmonary artery or trunk, carrying *deoxygenated blood*, leaves the upper part of the right ventricle of the heart. It passes upwards and divides into left and right pulmonary arteries at the level of the 5th thoracic vertebra.

The left pulmonary artery runs to the root of the left lung where it divides into two branches, one passing into each lobe.

The right pulmonary artery passes to the root of the right lung and divides into two branches. The larger branch carries blood to the middle and lower lobes, and the smaller branch to the upper lobe.

Within the lung these arteries divide and subdivide into smaller arteries, arterioles and capillaries. The exchange of gases takes place between capillary blood and air in the alveoli of the lungs (p. 255). In each lung the capillaries containing oxygenated blood join up and eventually form two pulmonary veins.

Two pulmonary veins leave each lung, returning oxygenated blood to the left atrium of the heart. During atrial systole this blood is pumped into the left ventricle, and during ventricular systole it is forced into the aorta, the first artery of the general circulation.

93

Systemic or general circulation

The blood pumped out from the left ventricle is carried by the branches of the *aorta* around the body and returns to the right atrium of the heart by the *superior* and *inferior venae cavae*. Figure 5.31 shows the general positions of the aorta and the main arteries of the limbs. Figure 5.32 provides an overview of the venae cavae and the veins of the limbs.

The circulation of blood to the different parts of the body will be described in the order in which their arteries branch off the aorta.

Aorta

The aorta (Fig. 5.28) begins at the upper part of the left ventricle and, after passing upwards for a short way, it arches backwards and to the left. It then descends behind the heart through the thoracic cavity a little to the left of the thoracic vertebrae. At the level of the 12th thoracic vertebra it passes behind the diaphragm then downwards in the abdominal cavity to the level of the 4th lumbar vertebra, where it divides into the *right* and *left common iliac arteries*.

Throughout its length the aorta gives off numerous branches. Some of the branches are *paired*, i.e. there is a right and left branch of the same name, for instance, the right and left renal arteries supplying the kidneys, and some are single or *unpaired*, e.g. the coeliac artery.

The aorta will be described here according to its location:

- thoracic aorta (see below)
- abdominal aorta (p. 102).

Thoracic aorta

This part of the aorta is above the diaphragm and is described in three parts:

- ascending aorta
- arch of the aorta
- descending aorta in the thorax (p. 101).

Ascending aorta

This is the short section of the aorta that rises from the heart. It is about 5 cm long and lies behind the sternum.

The right and left coronary arteries are its only branches and they arise from the aorta just above the level of the

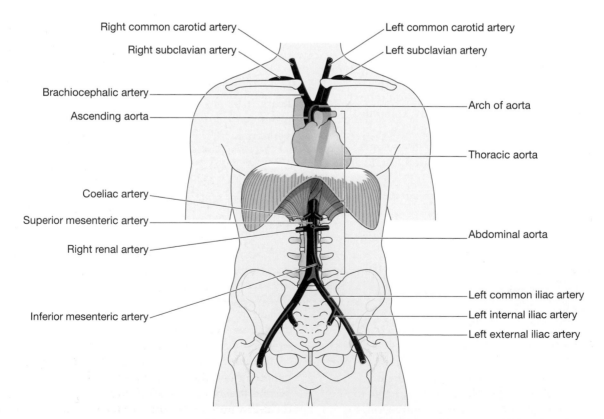

Figure 5.28 The aorta and its main branches.

aortic valve (Fig. 5.16). These important arteries supply the myocardium.

Arch of the aorta

The arch of the aorta is a continuation of the ascending aorta. It begins behind the manubrium of the sternum and runs upwards, backwards and to the left in front of the trachea. It then passes downwards to the left of the trachea and is continuous with the descending aorta.

Three branches are given off from its upper aspect (Fig. 5.29):

- brachiocephalic artery or trunk
- left common carotid artery
- left subclavian artery.

The brachiocephalic artery is about 4 to 5 cm long and passes obliquely upwards, backwards and to the right. At the level of the sternoclavicular joint it divides into the *right common carotid artery* and the *right subclavian artery.*

Circulation of blood to the head and neck

Arterial supply

The paired arteries supplying the head and neck are the *common carotid arteries* and the *vertebral arteries* (Fig. 5.30).

Carotid arteries. The *right common carotid artery* is a branch of the brachiocephalic artery. The *left common carotid artery* arises directly from the arch of the aorta. They pass upwards on either side of the neck and have the same distribution on each side. The common carotid arteries are embedded in fascia, called the *carotid sheath.*

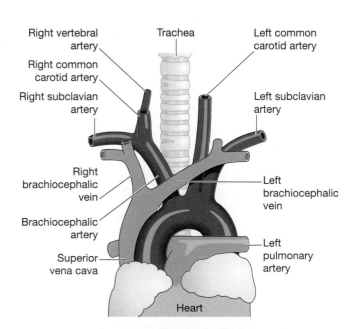

Figure 5.29 The arch of the aorta and its branches.

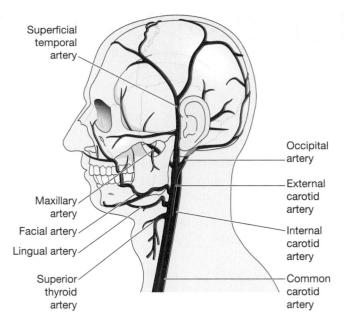

Figure 5.30 Main arteries of the left side of the head and neck.

At the level of the upper border of the thyroid cartilage each divides into an *internal carotid artery* and an *external carotid artery.*

The carotid sinuses are slight dilatations at the point of division (bifurcation) of the common carotid arteries into their internal and external branches. The walls of the sinuses are thin and contain numerous nerve endings of the glossopharyngeal nerves. These nerve endings, or *baroreceptors*, are stimulated by changes in blood pressure in the carotid sinuses. The resultant nerve impulses initiate reflex adjustments of blood pressure through the vasomotor centre in the medulla oblongata (p. 90).

The carotid bodies are two small groups of specialised cells, called *chemoreceptors*, one lying in close association with each common carotid artery at its bifurcation. They are supplied by the glossopharyngeal nerves and their cells are stimulated by changes in the carbon dioxide and oxygen content of blood. The resultant nerve impulses initiate reflex adjustments of respiration through the respiratory centre in the medulla oblongata.

External carotid artery (Fig. 5.30). This artery supplies the superficial tissues of the head and neck, via a number of branches.

- The *superior thyroid artery* supplies the thyroid gland and adjacent muscles.
- The *lingual artery* supplies the tongue, the lining membrane of the mouth, the structures in the floor of the mouth, the tonsil and the epiglottis.
- The *facial artery* passes outwards over the mandible just in front of the angle of the jaw and supplies the muscles of facial expression and structures in the

95

mouth. The pulse can be felt where the artery crosses the jaw bone.

- The *occipital artery* supplies the posterior part of the scalp.
- The *temporal artery* passes upwards over the zygomatic process in front of the ear and supplies the frontal, temporal and parietal parts of the scalp. The pulse can be felt in front of the upper part of the ear.
- The *maxillary artery* supplies the muscles of mastication and a branch of this artery, the *middle meningeal artery*, runs deeply to supply structures in the interior of the skull.

The internal carotid artery. This is a major contributor to the circulus arteriosus (circle of Willis) (Fig. 5.33), which supplies the greater part of the brain. It also has branches that supply the eyes, forehead and nose. It ascends to the base of the skull and passes through the carotid foramen in the temporal bone.

Circulus arteriosus (circle of Willis). The greater part of the brain is supplied with arterial blood by an arrangement of arteries called the *circulus arteriosus* or the *circle of Willis* (Fig. 5.33). Four large arteries contribute to its formation: the two *internal carotid arteries* and the two *vertebral arteries* (Fig. 5.34). The vertebral arteries arise from the subclavian arteries, pass upwards through the foramina in the transverse processes of the cervical vertebrae, enter the skull through the foramen magnum, then join to form the *basilar artery*. The arrangement in the circulus arteriosus is such that the brain as a whole receives an adequate blood supply when a contributing artery is damaged and during extreme movements of the head and neck.

Anteriorly, the two *anterior cerebral arteries* arise from the internal carotid arteries and are joined by the *anterior communicating artery*.

Posteriorly, the two *vertebral arteries* join to form the *basilar artery*. After travelling for a short distance the basilar artery divides to form two *posterior cerebral arteries*, each of which is joined to the corresponding internal carotid artery by a *posterior communicating artery*, completing the circle. The circulus arteriosus is therefore formed by:

- 2 anterior cerebral arteries
- 2 internal carotid arteries
- 1 anterior communicating artery
- 2 posterior communicating arteries
- 2 posterior cerebral arteries
- 1 basilar artery.

From this circle, the *anterior cerebral arteries* pass forward to supply the anterior part of the brain, the *middle cerebral arteries* pass laterally to supply the sides of the brain, and the *posterior cerebral arteries* supply the posterior part of the brain.

Branches of the basilar artery supply parts of the brain stem.

Venous return from the head and neck

The venous blood from the head and neck is returned by *deep* and *superficial* veins.

Superficial veins with the same names as the branches of the external carotid artery return venous blood from the superficial structures of the face and scalp and unite to form the external jugular vein (Fig. 5.35).

The *external jugular vein* begins in the neck at the level of the angle of the jaw. It passes downwards in front of the sternocleidomastoid muscle, then behind the clavicle before entering the *subclavian vein*.

The venous blood from the deep areas of the brain is collected into channels called the *dural venous sinuses*.

The dural venous sinuses of the brain (Figs 5.36 and 5.37) are formed by layers of dura mater lined with endothelium. The dura mater is the outer protective covering of the brain (p. 148). The main venous sinuses are listed below.

- The *superior sagittal sinus* carries the venous blood from the superior part of the brain. It begins in the frontal region and passes directly backwards in the midline of the skull to the occipital region where it turns to the right side and continues as the *right transverse sinus*.
- The *inferior sagittal sinus* lies deep within the brain and passes backwards to form the *straight sinus*.
- The *straight sinus* runs backwards and downwards to become the *left transverse sinus*.
- The *transverse sinuses* begin in the occipital region. They run forward and medially in a curved groove of the skull, to become continuous with the *sigmoid sinuses*.
- The *sigmoid sinuses* are a continuation of the transverse sinuses. Each curves downwards and medially and lies in a groove in the mastoid process of the temporal bone. Anteriorly only a thin plate of bone separates the sinus from the air cells in the mastoid process of the temporal bone. Inferiorly it continues as the internal jugular vein.

The *internal jugular veins* begin at the jugular foramina in the middle cranial fossa and each is the continuation of a sigmoid sinus. They run downwards in the neck behind the sternocleidomastoid muscles. Behind the clavicle they unite with the *subclavian veins*, carrying blood from the upper limbs, to form the *brachiocephalic veins*.

The *brachiocephalic veins* are situated one on each side in the root of the neck. Each is formed by the union of

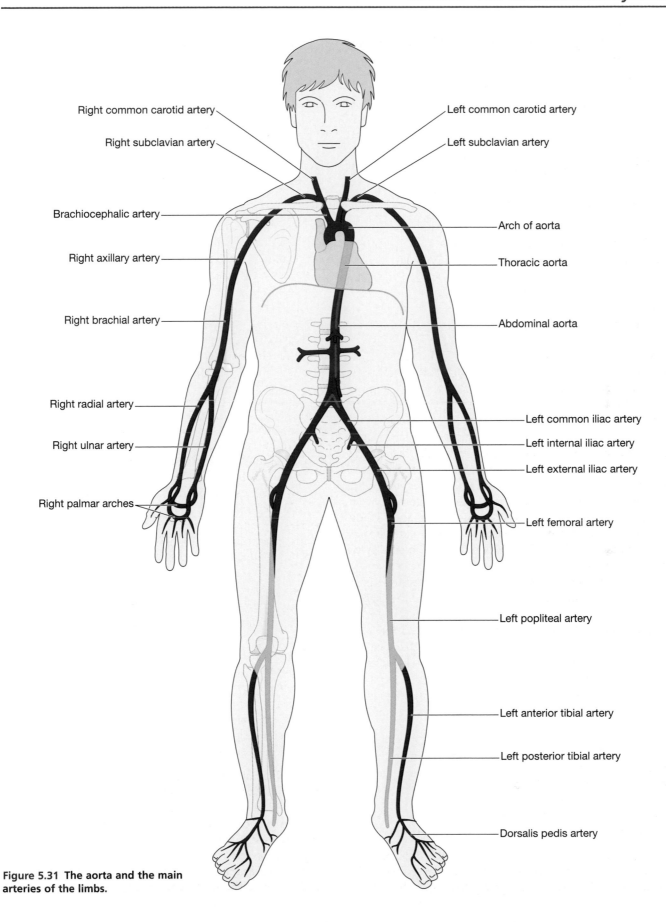

Right common carotid artery

Right subclavian artery

Brachiocephalic artery

Right axillary artery

Right brachial artery

Right radial artery

Right ulnar artery

Right palmar arches

Left common carotid artery

Left subclavian artery

Arch of aorta

Thoracic aorta

Abdominal aorta

Left common iliac artery

Left internal iliac artery

Left external iliac artery

Left femoral artery

Left popliteal artery

Left anterior tibial artery

Left posterior tibial artery

Dorsalis pedis artery

Figure 5.31 The aorta and the main arteries of the limbs.

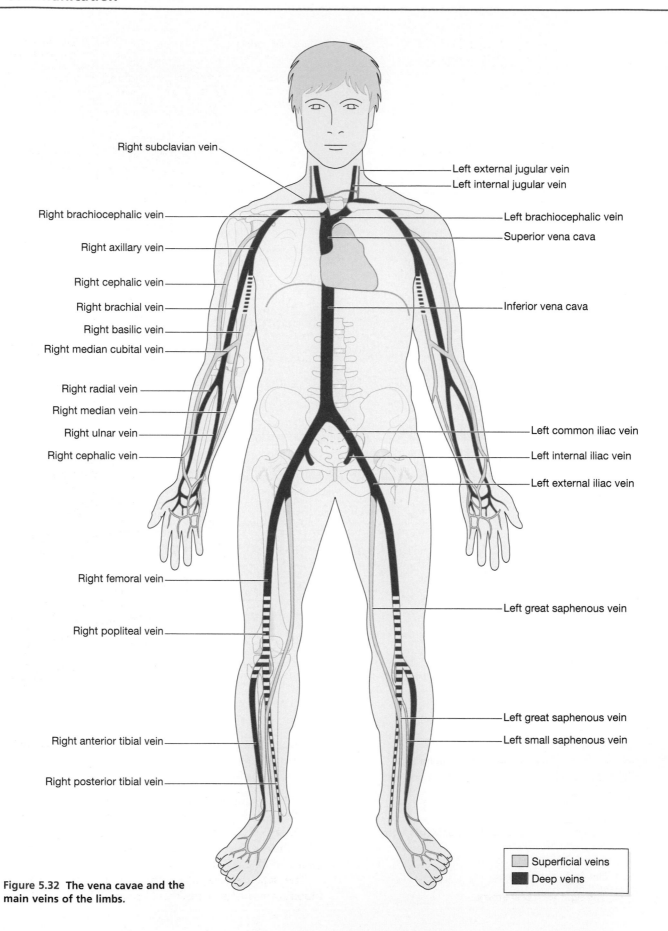

Right subclavian vein

Left external jugular vein

Left internal jugular vein

Right brachiocephalic vein

Left brachiocephalic vein

Superior vena cava

Right axillary vein

Right cephalic vein

Right brachial vein

Inferior vena cava

Right basilic vein

Right median cubital vein

Right radial vein

Right median vein

Right ulnar vein

Left common iliac vein

Left internal iliac vein

Right cephalic vein

Left external iliac vein

Right femoral vein

Left great saphenous vein

Right popliteal vein

Left great saphenous vein

Left small saphenous vein

Right anterior tibial vein

Right posterior tibial vein

Superficial veins

Deep veins

Figure 5.32 The vena cavae and the main veins of the limbs.

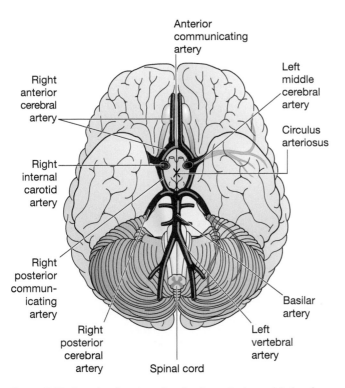

Figure 5.33 Arteries forming the circulus arteriosus (circle of Willis) and its main branches to the brain.

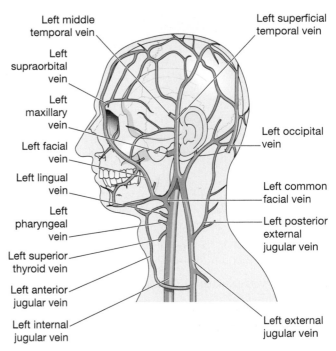

Figure 5.35 Veins of the left side of the head and neck.

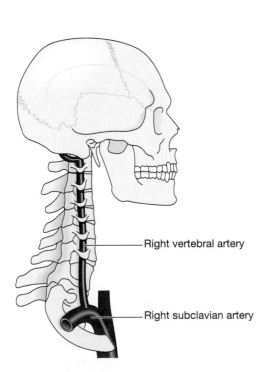

Figure 5.34 The right vertebral artery.

99

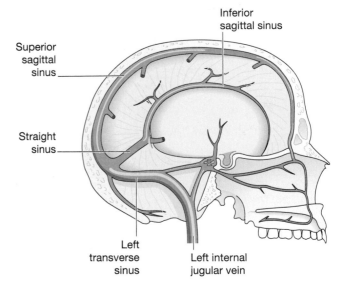

Figure 5.36 Venous sinuses of the brain viewed from the right.

the internal jugular and the subclavian veins. The left brachiocephalic vein is longer than the right and passes obliquely behind the manubrium of the sternum, where it joins the right brachiocephalic vein to form the *superior vena cava* (Fig. 5.38).

The *superior vena cava*, which drains all the venous blood from the head, neck and upper limbs, is about 7 cm

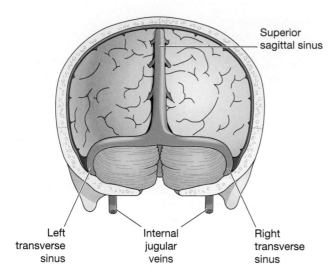

Figure 5.37 **Venous sinuses of the brain viewed from above.**

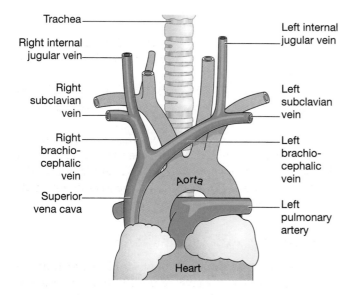

Figure 5.38 **The superior vena cava and the veins that form it.**

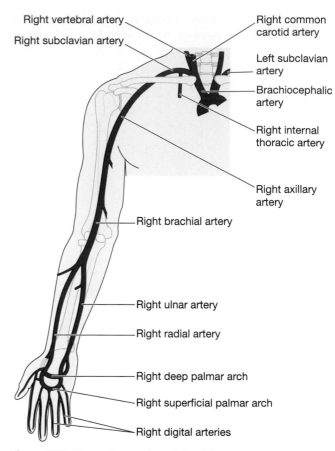

Figure 5.39 **The main arteries of the right arm.**

long. It passes downwards along the right border of the sternum and ends in the right atrium of the heart.

Circulation of blood to the upper limb

Arterial supply

The subclavian arteries. The right subclavian artery arises from the brachiocephalic artery; the left branches from the arch of the aorta. They are slightly arched and pass behind the clavicles and over the first ribs before entering the axillae, where they continue as the *axillary arteries* (Fig. 5.39).

Before entering the axilla, each subclavian artery gives off two branches: the *vertebral artery*, which passes upwards to supply the brain, and the *internal thoracic artery*, which supplies the breast and a number of structures in the thoracic cavity.

The *axillary artery* is a continuation of the subclavian artery and lies in the axilla. The first part lies deeply; then it runs more superficially to become the *brachial artery*.

The *brachial artery* is a continuation of the axillary artery. It runs down the medial aspect of the upper arm, passes to the front of the elbow and extends to about 1 cm below the joint, where it divides into the *radial* and *ulnar arteries*.

The *radial artery* passes down the radial or lateral side of the forearm to the wrist. Just above the wrist it lies superficially and can be felt in front of the radius, as the radial pulse. The artery then passes between the first and second metacarpal bones and enters the palm of the hand.

The *ulnar artery* runs downwards on the ulnar or medial aspect of the forearm to cross the wrist and pass into the hand.

There are anastomoses between the radial and ulnar arteries, called the *deep* and *superficial palmar arches*, from which *palmar metacarpal* and *palmar digital arteries* arise to supply the structures in the hand and fingers.

Venous return from the upper limb

The veins of the upper limb are divided into two groups: deep and superficial veins (Fig. 5.40).

The *deep veins* follow the course of the arteries and have the same names:

- palmar metacarpal veins
- deep palmar venous arch
- ulnar and radial veins
- brachial vein
- axillary vein
- subclavian vein.

The *superficial veins* begin in the hand and consist of the following:

- cephalic vein
- basilic vein
- median vein
- median cubital vein.

The *cephalic vein* begins at the back of the hand where it collects blood from a complex of superficial veins, many of which can be easily seen. It then winds round the radial side to the anterior aspect of the forearm. In front of the elbow it gives off a large branch, the *median cubital vein*, which slants upwards and medially to join the *basilic vein*. After crossing the elbow joint the cephalic vein passes up the lateral aspect of the arm and in front of the shoulder joint to end in the axillary vein. Throughout its length it receives blood from the superficial tissues on the lateral aspects of the hand, forearm and arm.

The *basilic vein* begins at the back of the hand on the ulnar aspect. It ascends on the medial side of the forearm and upper arm then joins the axillary vein. It receives blood from the medial aspect of the hand, forearm and arm. There are many small veins which link the cephalic and basilic veins.

The *median vein* is a small vein that is not always present. It begins at the palmar surface of the hand, ascends on the front of the forearm and ends in the basilic vein or the median cubital vein.

The *brachiocephalic vein* is formed when the subclavian and internal jugular veins unite. There is one on each side.

The *superior vena cava* is formed when the two brachiocephalic veins unite. It drains all the venous blood from the head, neck and upper limbs and terminates in the right atrium. It is about 7 cm long and passes downwards along the right border of the sternum.

Descending aorta in the thorax

This part of the aorta is continuous with the arch of the aorta and begins at the level of the 4th thoracic vertebra. It extends downwards on the anterior surface of the bodies of the thoracic vertebrae (Fig. 5.41) to the level of the 12th thoracic vertebra, where it passes behind the diaphragm to become the abdominal aorta.

The descending aorta in the thorax gives off many *paired branches* which supply the walls of the thoracic cavity and the organs within the cavity, including the:

- *bronchial arteries* that supply the bronchi and their branches, connective tissue in the lungs and the lymph nodes at the root of the lungs
- *oesophageal arteries*, supplying the oesophagus
- *intercostal arteries* that run along the inferior border of the ribs and supply the intercostal muscles, some muscles of the thorax, the ribs, the skin and its underlying connective tissues.

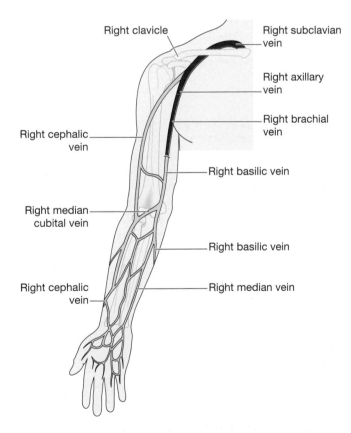

Right clavicle
Right subclavian vein
Right axillary vein
Right brachial vein
Right cephalic vein
Right basilic vein
Right median cubital vein
Right basilic vein
Right cephalic vein
Right median vein

Figure 5.40 The main veins of the right arm. Dark blue indicates deep veins.

101

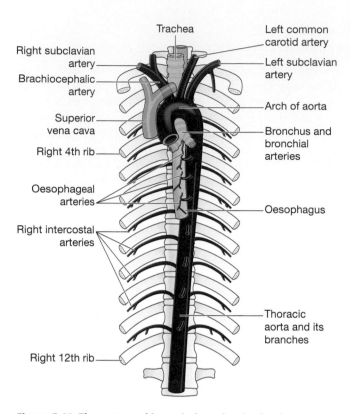

Figure 5.41 **The aorta and its main branches in the thorax.**

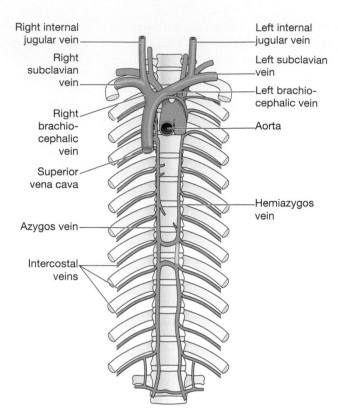

Figure 5.42 **The superior vena cava and the main veins of the thorax.**

Venous return from the thoracic cavity

Most of the venous blood from the organs in the thoracic cavity is drained into the *azygos vein* and the *hemiazygos vein* (Fig. 5.42). Some of the main veins that join them are the *bronchial, oesophageal* and *intercostal veins*. The azygos vein joins the superior vena cava and the hemiazygos vein joins the left brachiocephalic vein. At the distal end of the oesophagus, some oesophageal veins join the azygos vein, and others the left gastric vein. A venous plexus is formed by anastomoses between the veins joining the azygos vein and those joining the left gastric veins, linking the general and portal circulations (see Fig. 12.47, p. 318).

Abdominal aorta

The abdominal aorta is a continuation of the thoracic aorta. The name changes when the aorta enters the abdominal cavity by passing behind the diaphragm at the level of the 12th thoracic vertebra. It descends in front of the bodies of the vertebrae to the level of the 4th lumbar vertebra, where it divides into the *right* and *left common iliac arteries* (Fig. 5.43).

When a branch of the abdominal aorta supplies an organ it is only named here and is described in more detail in association with the organ. However, illustrations showing the distribution of blood from the coeliac, superior and inferior mesenteric arteries are presented here (Figs 5.44 and 5.45).

Many branches arise from the abdominal aorta, some of which are paired and some unpaired.

Paired branches

- *Inferior phrenic arteries* supply the diaphragm.
- *Renal arteries* supply the kidneys and give off branches, the suprarenal arteries, to supply the adrenal glands.
- *Testicular arteries* supply the testes in the male.
- *Ovarian arteries* supply the ovaries in the female.

The testicular and ovarian arteries are much longer than the other paired branches, because these organs

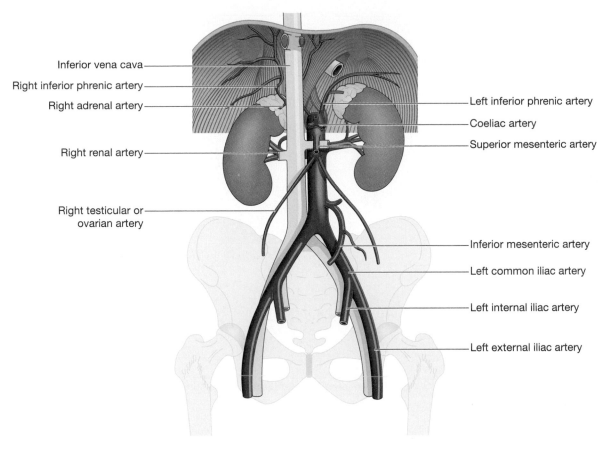

Figure 5.43 The abdominal aorta and its branches.

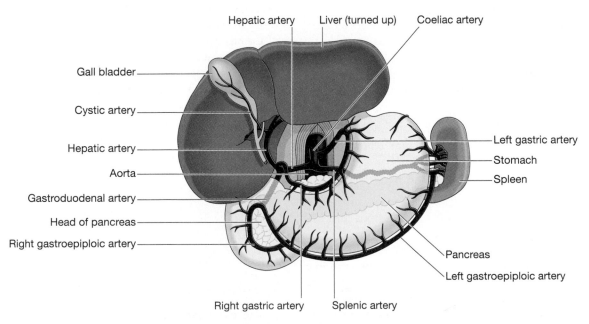

Figure 5.44 The coeliac artery and its branches, and the inferior phrenic arteries.

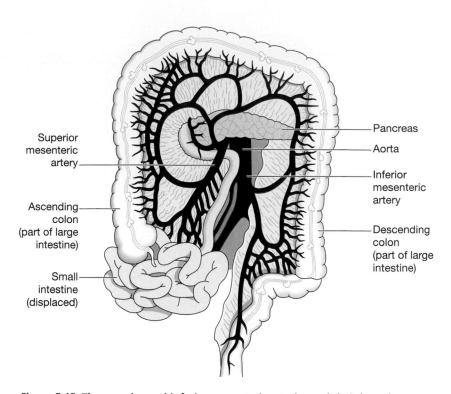

Superior
mesenteric
artery

Ascending
colon
(part of large
intestine)

Small
intestine
(displaced)

Pancreas

Aorta

Inferior
mesenteric
artery

Descending
colon
(part of large
intestine)

Figure 5.45 The superior and inferior mesenteric arteries and their branches.

begin their development in the region of the kidneys. As they grow, they descend into the scrotum and the pelvis respectively, and are accompanied by their blood vessels.

Unpaired branches

The *coeliac artery* (Fig. 5.43) is a short thick artery about 1.25 cm long. It arises immediately below the diaphragm and divides into three branches:

- the *left gastric artery* supplies the stomach
- the *splenic artery* supplies the pancreas and the spleen
- the *hepatic artery* supplies the liver, gall bladder and parts of the stomach, duodenum and pancreas.

The *superior mesenteric artery* (Fig. 5.43) branches from the aorta between the coeliac artery and the renal arteries. It supplies the whole of the small intestine and the proximal half of the large intestine.

The *inferior mesenteric artery* (Fig. 5.43) arises from the aorta about 4 cm above its division into the common iliac arteries. It supplies the distal half of the large intestine and part of the rectum.

Venous return from the abdominal organs

The *inferior vena cava* is formed when the *right* and *left common iliac veins* join at the level of the body of the 5th lumbar vertebra. This is the largest vein in the body, and it carries blood from all parts of the body below the diaphragm to the right atrium of the heart. It passes through the central tendon of the diaphragm at the level of the 8th thoracic vertebra.

Paired testicular, ovarian, renal and adrenal veins join the inferior vena cava.

Blood from the remaining organs in the abdominal cavity passes through the liver via the *portal circulation* before entering the inferior vena cava (Fig. 5.44).

Portal circulation

In all the parts of the circulation described so far, venous blood passes from the tissues to the heart by the most direct route through only one capillary bed. In the portal circulation, venous blood passes from the capillary beds of the abdominal part of the digestive system, the spleen and pancreas to the liver. It then passes through a second capillary bed, the hepatic sinusoids, in the liver before entering the general circulation via the inferior vena cava. In this way, blood with a high concentration of nutrients, absorbed from the stomach and intestines, goes to the liver first. In the liver certain modifications take place, including the regulation of blood nutrient levels.

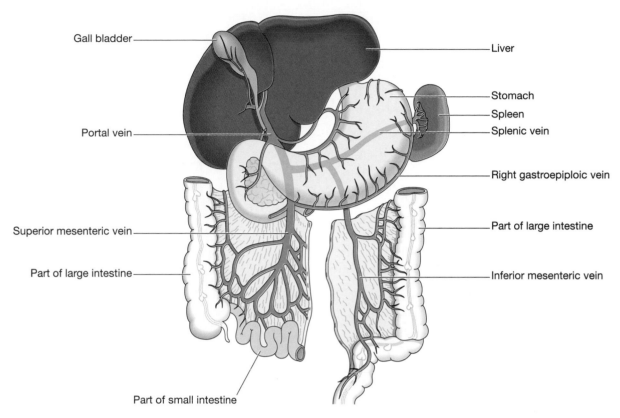

Figure 5.46 Venous drainage from the abdominal organs, and the formation of the portal vein.

105

Portal vein

This is formed by the union of several veins (Figs 5.46 and 5.47), each of which drains blood from the area supplied by the corresponding artery:

- The *splenic vein* drains blood from the spleen, the pancreas and part of the stomach.
- The *inferior mesenteric vein* returns the venous blood from the rectum, pelvic and descending colon of the large intestine. It joins the splenic vein.
- The *superior mesenteric vein* returns venous blood from the small intestine and the proximal parts of the large intestine, i.e. the caecum, ascending and transverse colon. It unites with the *splenic vein* to form the *portal vein*.
- The *gastric veins* drain blood from the stomach and the distal end of the oesophagus, then join the portal vein.
- The *cystic vein*, which drains venous blood from the gall bladder, joins the portal vein.

Hepatic veins

These are very short veins that leave the posterior surface of the liver and, almost immediately, enter the inferior vena cava.

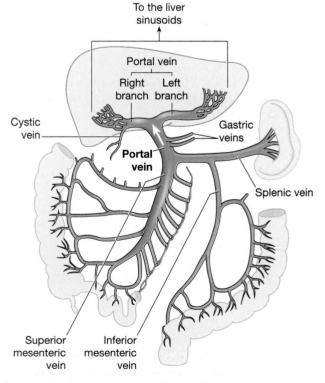

Figure 5.47 The portal vein – origin and termination.

Circulation to the pelvis and lower limb

Arterial supply

Common iliac arteries. The right and left common iliac arteries are formed when the abdominal aorta divides at the level of the 4th lumbar vertebra (Fig. 5.31). In front of the sacroiliac joint each divides into the internal and the external iliac arteries.

The *internal iliac artery* runs medially to supply the organs within the pelvic cavity. In the female, one of the largest branches is the *uterine artery,* which provides the main arterial blood supply to the reproductive organs.

The *external iliac artery* runs obliquely downwards and passes behind the inguinal ligament into the thigh where it becomes the *femoral artery.*

The *femoral artery* (Fig. 5.48) begins at the midpoint of the inguinal ligament and extends downwards in front of the thigh; then it turns medially and eventually passes round the medial aspect of the femur to enter the popliteal space where it becomes the *popliteal artery.* It supplies blood to the structures of the thigh and some superficial pelvic and inguinal structures.

The *popliteal artery* (Fig. 5.49) passes through the popliteal fossa behind the knee, where the pulse can be

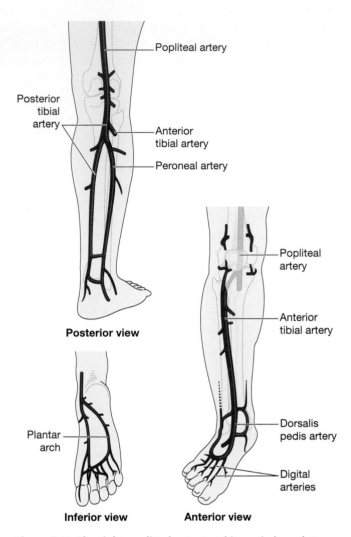

Posterior view

Inferior view   **Anterior view**

Figure 5.49 The right popliteal artery and its main branches.

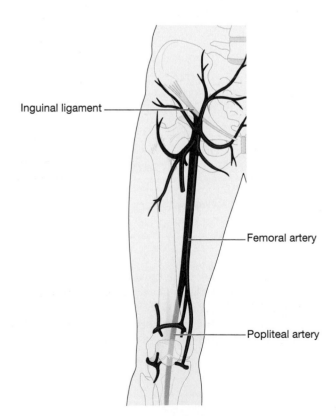

Figure 5.48 The femoral artery and its main branches.

felt. It supplies the structures in this area, including the knee joint. At the lower border of the popliteal fossa it divides into the anterior and posterior tibial arteries.

The *anterior tibial artery* (Fig. 5.49) passes forwards between the tibia and fibula and supplies the structures in the front of the leg. It lies on the tibia, runs in front of the ankle joint and continues over the dorsum (top) of the foot as the *dorsalis pedis artery.*

The *dorsalis pedis artery* is a continuation of the anterior tibial artery and passes over the dorsum of the foot, where the pulse can be felt, supplying arterial blood to the structures in this area. It ends by passing between the first and second metatarsal bones into the sole of the foot where it contributes to the formation of the plantar arch.

The *posterior tibial artery* (Fig. 5.49) runs downwards and medially on the back of the leg. Near its origin it gives off a large branch called the *peroneal artery*, which supplies the lateral aspect of the leg. In the lower part it becomes superficial and passes medial to the ankle joint to reach the sole of the foot, where it continues as the *plantar artery*.

The *plantar artery* supplies the structures in the sole of the foot. This artery, its branches and the dorsalis pedis artery form the *plantar arch* from which the digital branches arise to supply the toes.

Venous return

There are both deep and superficial veins in the lower limb (Fig. 5.30). Blood entering the superficial veins passes to the deep veins through *communicating veins*. Movement of blood towards the heart is partly dependent on contraction of skeletal muscles. Backward flow is prevented by a large number of valves. Superficial veins receive less support from surrounding tissues than deep veins.

Deep veins. The deep veins accompany the arteries and their branches and have the same names. They are the:

- *femoral vein*, which ascends in the thigh to the level of the inguinal ligament, where it becomes the external iliac vein
- *external iliac vein*, the continuation of the femoral vein where it enters the pelvis lying close to the femoral artery. It passes along the brim of the pelvis, and at the level of the sacroiliac joint it is joined by the *internal iliac vein* to form the *common iliac vein*
- *internal iliac vein*, which receives tributaries from several veins draining the organs of the pelvic cavity
- *two common iliac veins*, which begin at the level of the sacroiliac joints. They ascend obliquely and end a little to the right of the body of the 5th lumbar vertebra by uniting to form the *inferior vena cava*.

Superficial veins (Fig. 5.50). The two main superficial veins draining blood from the lower limbs are the small and the great saphenous veins.

The *small saphenous vein* begins behind the ankle joint where many small veins which drain the dorsum of the foot join together. It ascends superficially along the back of the leg and in the popliteal space it joins the *popliteal vein* – a deep vein.

The *great saphenous vein* is the longest vein in the body. It begins at the medial half of the dorsum of the foot and

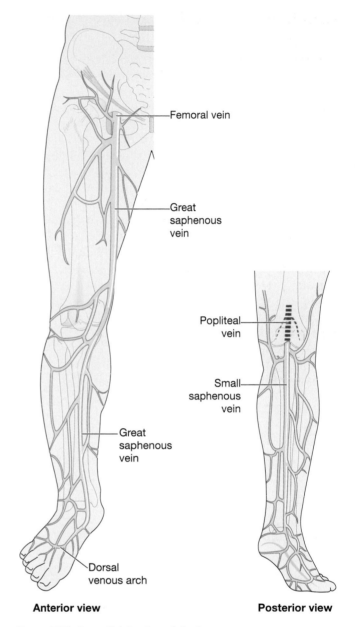

Figure 5.50 Superficial veins of the leg.

107

runs upwards, crossing the medial aspect of the tibia and up the inner side of the thigh. Just below the inguinal ligament it joins the *femoral vein*.

Many *communicating veins* join the superficial veins, and the superficial and deep veins of the lower limb.

Summary of the main blood vessels

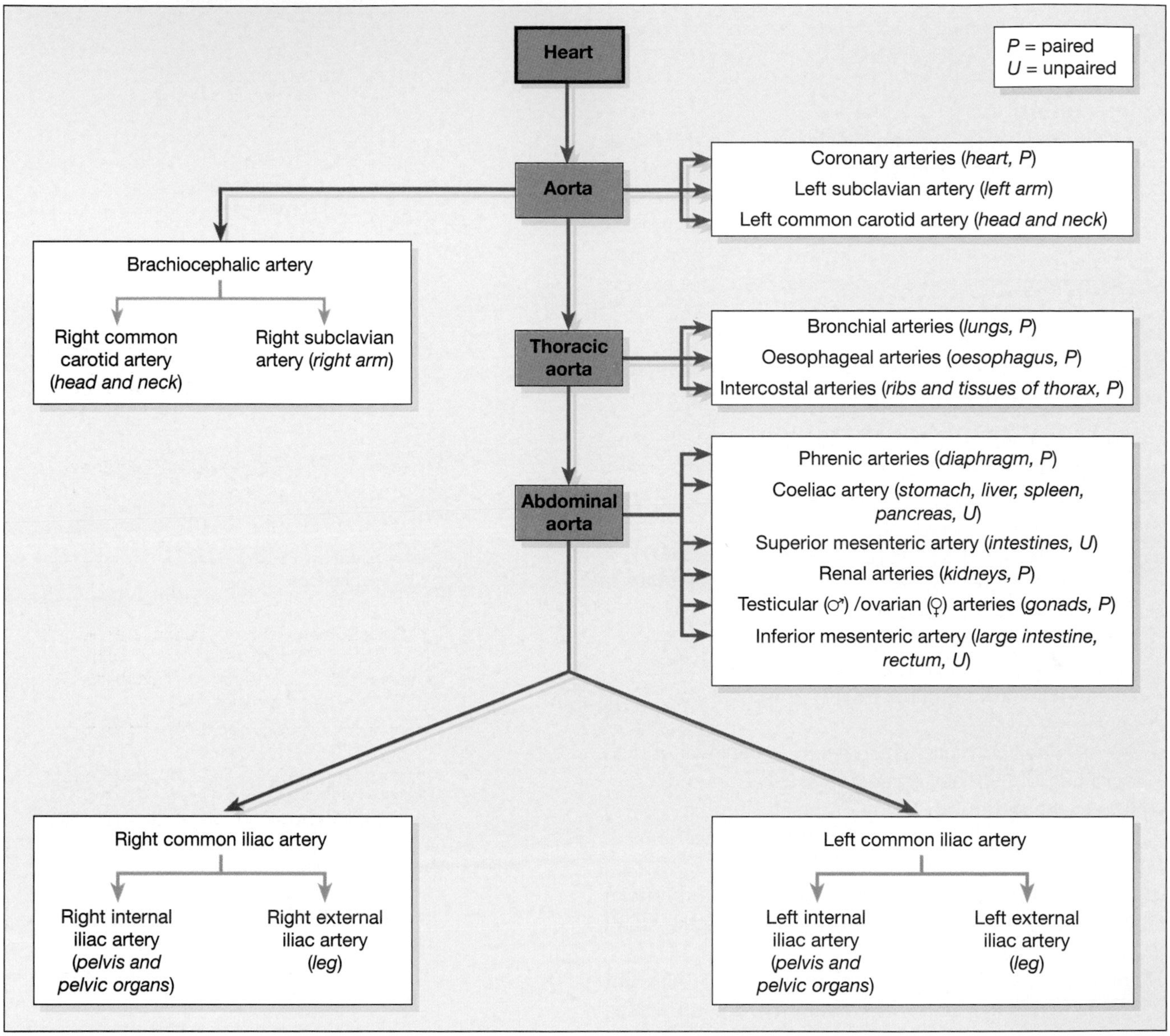

Figure 5.51 A. The aorta and main arteries of the body.

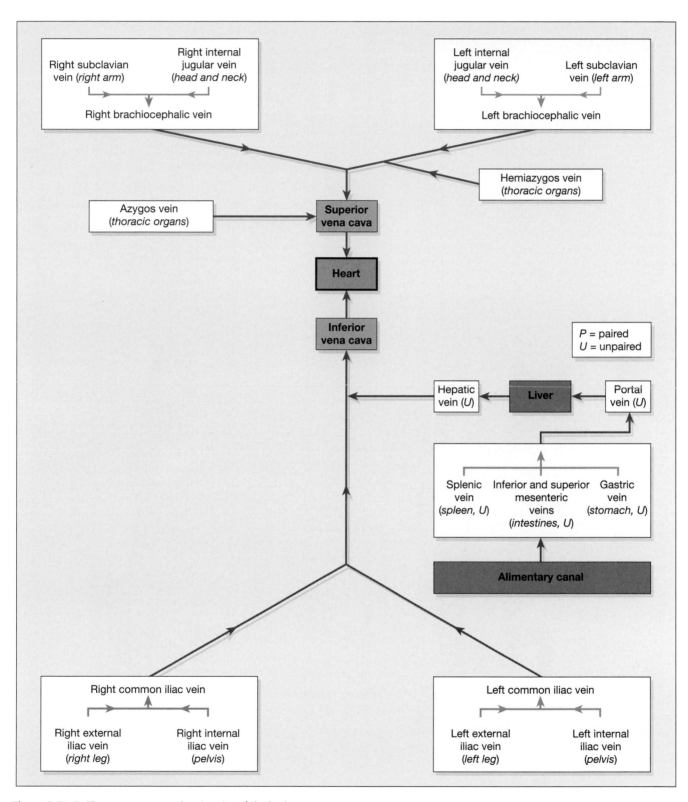

Figure 5.51 B. The venae cavae and main veins of the body.

Fetal circulation

Learning outcomes

- Describe the fetal circulation
- Outline the functions of the placenta
- Compare blood flow through the heart, lungs and liver before and shortly after birth.

Features of the fetal circulation

During pregnancy, the fetus develops its own blood supply to provide its tissues with oxygen and nutrients and to remove carbon dioxide and other wastes. This is known as the *fetal circulation* (Fig. 5.52). Because the lungs, gastrointestinal system and kidneys do not begin to function till after birth, certain unique modifications are present in the fetal circulation to divert blood flow to meet pre-natal requirements:

- 2 *umbilical arteries*, which are extensions of the internal iliac arteries, carry deoxygenated fetal blood to the placenta

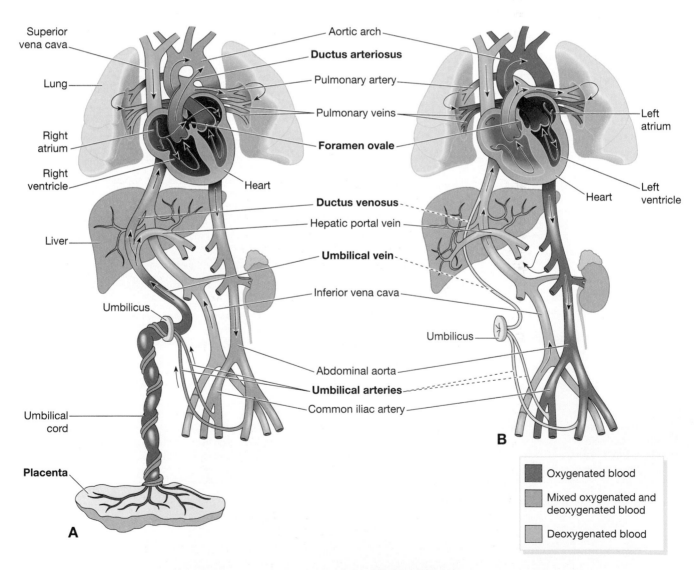

Figure 5.52 A. Fetal circulation before birth. B. Changes to the fetal circulation at birth.

- the *placenta* is attached to the uterine wall and enables exchange of substances between the fetus and the mother
- the *umbilical vein* carries oxygenated blood back to the fetus
- the *ductus venosus* is a continuation of the umbilical vein that returns blood directly into the inferior vena cava, and most blood therefore bypasses the non-functional liver
- the *foramen ovale* forms a valve-like opening (see Fig. 5.64) allowing blood to flow between the right and left atria, so that most blood bypasses the non-functional fetal lungs
- the *ductus arteriosus*, a small vessel that connects the pulmonary artery to the descending thoracic aorta, diverts more blood into the systemic circulation, meaning that very little blood passes through the fetal lungs.

The *umbilical cord* extends from the placenta to the fetus. It is about 50 cm long and consists mainly of the two umbilical arteries and the umbilical vein, and enters the fetus at the *umbilicus*.

Placenta

This is a temporary structure that provides an interface between the mother and fetus, and allows exchange of substances between their circulatory systems. It develops from the surface of the fertilized ovum embedded into the maternal uterine endometrium (Fig. 5.53). It is expelled from the uterus during the final stage of labour soon after birth, when it is no longer needed.

Structure

The mature placenta is pancake-shaped, weighs around 500 g, has a diameter of 20 cm and is about 2.5 cm thick, although wide individual variations occur. The fetal side of the placenta is attached to the uterine wall and consists of an extensive network of fetal capillaries bathed in maternal blood. Whilst the fetal capillaries are in very close proximity to the maternal blood supply, the two circulations are completely separate.

Functions

The fetal circulation allows exchange to take place, mainly by diffusion.

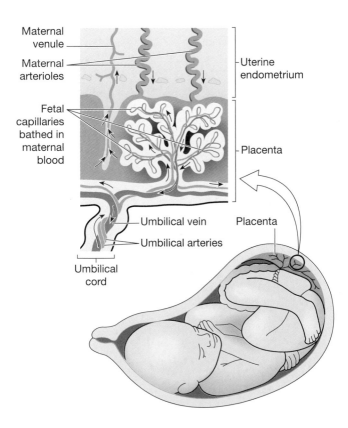

Figure 5.53 Structure of the placenta.

Exchange of nutrients and wastes. Substances involved include:

- oxygen and nutrients from the mother, needed for fetal growth and development
- fetal carbon dioxide and other wastes, for excretion by the mother.

Protection of the fetus. Temporary passive immunity (p. 378) lasting for a few months is provided by *maternal antibodies* that cross the placenta before birth.

Indirect exchange between the fetal and maternal circulations provides a 'barrier' to potentially harmful substances, including microbes and drugs, although some may cross into the fetus, causing abnormal development. They include:

- alcohol
- some infectious microbes, e.g. the virus that causes German measles (rubella)
- other substances and some drugs, which are then known as *teratogens*.

Maintenance of pregnancy. The placenta has an essential endocrine function because it secretes the hormones that maintain pregnancy.

Human chorionic gonadotrophin (hCG). This hormone is secreted in early pregnancy, peaking at around 8 or 9 weeks and thereafter in smaller amounts. hCG stimulates the *corpus luteum* (Ch. 18) to continue secreting progesterone and oestrogen which prevent menstruation and maintain the uterine endometrium, sustaining pregnancy in the early weeks (see Fig. 18.9).

Progesterone and oestrogen. As pregnancy progresses, the placenta takes over secretion of these hormones from the corpus luteum, which degenerates after about 12 weeks. From 12 weeks until delivery, the placenta secretes increasing levels of oestrogen and progesterone. These hormones are essential for maintenance of pregnancy.

Changes at birth (Fig. 5.52B)

When the baby takes its first breath the lungs inflate for the first time, increasing pulmonary blood flow. Blood returning from the lungs increases the pressure in the left atrium, closing the flap over the foramen ovale and preventing blood flow between the atria. Blood entering the right atrium is therefore diverted into the right ventricle and into the pulmonary circulation through the pulmonary veins. As the pulmonary circulation is established (see Fig. 5.1), blood oxygen levels increase, causing constriction and closure of the ductus arteriosus. If these adaptations do not take place after birth, they become evident as congenital abnormalities (see Figs 5.63 and 5.64). When the placental circulation ceases soon after birth, the umbilical vein, ductus venosus and umbilical arteries collapse, as they are no longer required.

Shock

Learning outcomes

After studying this section, you should be able to:

- define the term shock

- describe the main physiological changes that occur during shock

- explain the underlying pathophysiology of the main causes of shock.

Shock occurs when the metabolic needs of cells are not being met because of inadequate blood flow. In effect, there is a reduction in circulating blood volume, in blood pressure and in cardiac output. This causes tissue hypoxia, an inadequate supply of nutrients and the accumulation of waste products. A number of different types of shock are described.

Hypovolaemic shock

This occurs when the blood volume is reduced by 15 to 25%. Cardiac output may fall because of low blood volume and hence low venous return, as a result of different situations.

- severe haemorrhage – whole blood is lost
- extensive burns – serum is lost
- severe vomiting and diarrhoea – water and electrolytes are lost.

Cardiogenic shock

This occurs in acute heart disease when the damaged heart muscle cannot maintain an adequate cardiac output, e.g. in myocardial infarction.

Septic shock (bacteraemic, endotoxic)

This is caused by severe infections in which bacterial toxins are released into the circulation. These toxins trigger a massive inflammatory and immune response, and many powerful mediators are released. Because the response is not controlled, it can cause multiple organ dysfunction, including hypotension because of widespread vasodilatation, depression of myocardial contractility, poor tissue perfusion and tissue death (necrosis).

Neurogenic shock (vasovagal attack, fainting)

The causes include sudden acute pain, severe emotional experience, spinal anaesthesia and spinal cord damage. Excessive parasympathetic activity or decreased sympathetic activity reduces the heart rate, and in turn, the cardiac output. Extensive vasodilatation causes sudden hypotension. These changes effectively reduce the blood supply to the brain, causing fainting. The period of unconsciousness is usually short.

Anaphylactic shock

Anaphylaxis is a severe allergic response that may be triggered in sensitive individuals by substances like penicillin, peanuts or latex rubber. Vasodilatation, provoked by systemic release of mediators, e.g. histamine and bradykinin, causes venous pooling and hypotension. Severe bronchoconstriction leads to respiratory difficulty and hypoxia. Onset is usually sudden, and in severe cases can cause death in a matter of minutes if untreated.

Physiological changes during shock

In the short term, these are associated with physiological attempts to restore an adequate blood circulation – *compensated shock* (Fig. 5.54). If the state of shock persists, the longer-term changes may be irreversible.

Compensatory shock

As the blood pressure falls, a number of reflexes are stimulated and hormone secretions increased in an attempt to restore it. These raise blood pressure by increasing peripheral resistance, blood volume and cardiac output.

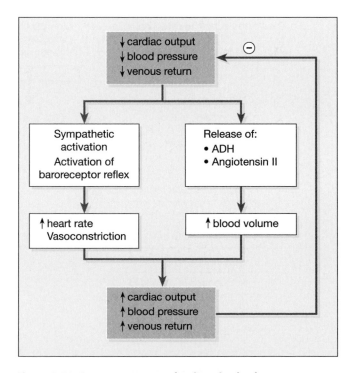

Figure 5.54 Compensatory mechanisms in shock.

Increased sympathetic stimulation increases heart rate and cardiac output, and also causes vasoconstriction, all of which increase blood pressure. Low blood volume and increased osmolarity of the blood cause secretion of ADH (p. 216) and activation of the renin–angiotensin aldosterone system (p. 221). Consequent release of aldosterone reduces water and sodium excretion and promotes vasoconstriction. The veins also constrict, helping to reduce venous pooling and support venous return.

If these compensatory mechanisms, plus any medical interventions available, are sufficient, then perfusion of the heart and brain can be maintained, and the patient's condition may be stabilised.

Uncompensated shock

If the insult is more severe, shock becomes a self-perpetuating sequence of deteriorating cardiovascular function – *uncompensated shock* (Fig. 5.55). Hypoxia causes cellular metabolism to switch to anaerobic pathways (p. 313), resulting in accumulation of lactic acid and progressive acidosis, which damages capillaries. The capillaries then become more permeable, leaking fluid from the vascular system into the tissues, further lowering blood pressure and tissue perfusion. Also, the accumulation of waste products causes vasodilation, making it harder for control mechanisms to support blood pressure. Organs, including the heart, are deprived of oxygen and may start to fail.

Eventually, the cardiovascular system reaches the stage when, although its compensatory mechanisms are running at maximum, it is unable to supply the brain's requirements. As the brain, including the cardiovascular and respiratory centres in the brainstem, becomes starved of oxygen and nutrients, it begins to fail and there is loss of central control of the body's compensatory mechanisms. Circulatory collapse follows. Finally, degenerating cardiovascular function leads to irreversible and progressive brainstem damage, and death follows.

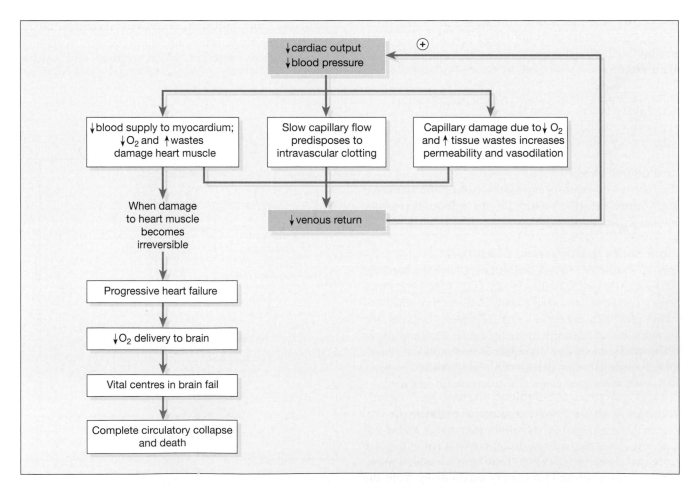

Figure 5.55 Uncompensated shock

Thrombosis and embolism

Learning outcomes

After studying this section, you should be able to:

- define the terms thrombosis, embolism and infarction

- explain, in general terms, the effects of the above on the body

- describe the main causes of venous thrombosis.

Embolus

This is a mass of any material carried in the blood. It is usually a fragment of a *thrombus* (an intravascular blood clot) from elsewhere in the vascular system, but other materials include:

- fragments of atheromatous plaques (p. 117)
- fragments of vegetations from heart valves, e.g. infective endocarditis (p. 124)
- tumour fragments, which may cause metastases
- amniotic fluid, during childbirth
- fat, from bone fractures
- air, from puncture of a blood vessel by a broken rib or during a clinical procedure
- nitrogen bubbles in decompression sickness (the 'bends')
- pus from an abscess.

Thrombus formation

The risk of a thrombus developing within a blood vessel is increased by any condition that slows blood flow, damages the smooth intimal lining of blood vessels or increases blood coagulability.

Blood flow is slowed. This may happen in immobility, e.g. prolonged sitting or in bedrest, or if a blood vessel is compressed by an adjacent structure such as a tumour, or if blood pressure is low for a prolonged period, as in shock.

Damage to the intimal lining of blood vessels. This may be caused by atherosclerosis or trauma.

Increased blood coagulability. Factors here include oestrogen (either naturally produced or taken in oral contraceptive drugs), dehydration, pregnancy and childbirth, the presence of an intravenous cannula, some malignant diseases and some disorders of blood clotting.

Emboli originating in an *artery* travel away from the heart until they reach an artery too narrow to let them pass, and lodge there, partly or completely blocking blood supply to distal tissues. Emboli originating in *veins* travel towards the heart, and from there travel to the lungs in the pulmonary artery. They then lodge in the first branch too narrow to let it pass. Lung tissue supplied by the blocked vessel becomes ischaemic and dies (pulmonary embolism). There may be multiple small emboli or one or more large ones. Massive pulmonary embolism blocks a main pulmonary artery and usually causes sudden collapse and death.

Infarction

This is the term given to tissue death because of interrupted blood supply. The consequences of interrupting tissue blood supply depend on the size of the artery blocked and the function of the tissues affected. *Ischaemia* means tissue damage because of reduced blood supply (Fig. 5.56).

Embolism

Embolism occurs when a travelling embolus, whatever its nature, lodges in and obstructs a blood vessel. The most serious consequences include pulmonary embolism, or blockage of a coronary artery (myocardial infarction, p. 124) or a cerebral artery (cerebral infarction, p. 180).

115

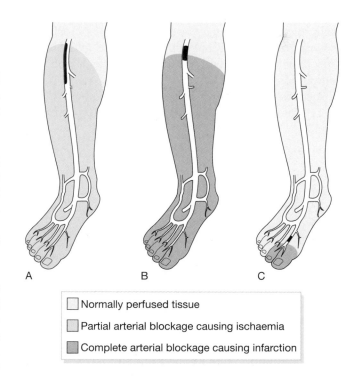

A   B   C

☐ Normally perfused tissue

☐ Partial arterial blockage causing ischaemia

☐ Complete arterial blockage causing infarction

Figure 5.56 Ischaemia and infarction.

Blood vessel pathology

Learning outcomes

After studying this section, you should be able to:

- discuss the main causes, effects and complications of arterial disease, including atheroma, arteriosclerosis and aneurysm

- discuss the underlying abnormality in varicose veins

- list the predisposing factors and the common sites of occurrence of varicose veins

- describe the main tumours that affect blood vessels.

Box 5.3 Predisposing factors in atherosclerosis

(Modifiable factors are shown in purple.)
- Heredity – family history
- Obesity
- Gender – males are more susceptible than females, until after the female menopause
- Diet – high in refined carbohydrates and/or saturated fats and cholesterol
- Increasing age
- Smoking cigarettes
- Diabetes mellitus
- Excessive emotional stress
- Hypertension
- Sedentary lifestyle
- Hyperlipidaemia
- Excessive alcohol consumption

Atheroma

Pathological changes

Atheromatous plaques are patchy changes that develop in the tunica intima of large and medium-sized arteries. They consist of accumulations of cholesterol and other lipid compounds, excess smooth muscle and fat-filled monocytes (foam cells). The plaque is covered with a fibrous cap. As plaques grow they spread along the artery wall forming swellings that protrude into the lumen. Eventually the whole thickness of the wall and long sections of the vessel may be affected (Fig. 5.57). Plaques may rupture, exposing subintimal materials to the blood. This may cause thrombosis and vasospasm and will compromise blood flow.

Arteries most commonly involved are those in the heart, brain, kidneys, small intestine and lower limbs.

Causes of atheroma

The origin of atheromatous plaques is uncertain. *Fatty streaks* present in artery walls of infants are usually absorbed but their incomplete absorption may be the origin of atheromatous plaques in later life.

Atherosclerosis (the presence of plaques) is considered to be a disease of older people because it is usually in these age groups that clinical signs appear. Plaques, however, start to form in childhood in developed countries.

The incidence of atheroma is widespread in developed countries. Why atheromatous plaques develop is not clearly understood, but the predisposing factors appear to exert their effects over a long period. This may mean that the development of atheroma can be delayed or even arrested by a change in lifestyle (Box 5.3).

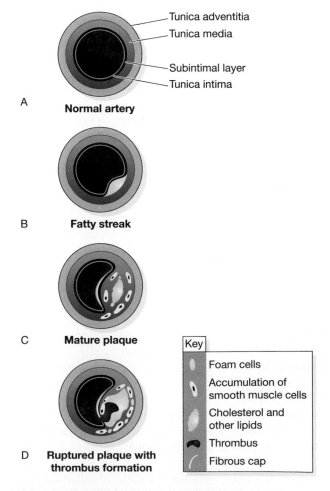

A   **Normal artery**

— Tunica adventitia
— Tunica media
— Subintimal layer
— Tunica intima

B   **Fatty streak**

C   **Mature plaque**

D   **Ruptured plaque with thrombus formation**

Key	
	Foam cells
	Accumulation of smooth muscle cells
	Cholesterol and other lipids
	Thrombus
	Fibrous cap

Figure 5.57 Stages in the formation of an atheromatous plaque.

Effects of atheroma

Atheromatous plaques may cause partial or complete obstruction of an artery. The blockage may be complicated by clot formation. The consequences of this depend on the site and size of the artery involved and the extent of collateral circulation. Commonly the arteries affected are those in the heart, abdomen and pelvis.

Narrowing of an artery

The tissues distal to the narrow point become ischaemic. The cells may receive enough blood to meet their minimum needs, but not enough to cope with an increase in metabolic rate, e.g. when muscle activity is increased. This causes acute cramp-like ischaemic pain. Cardiac muscle and skeletal muscles of the lower limb are most commonly affected. Ischaemic pain in the heart is called *angina pectoris* (p. 123), and in the lower limbs, *intermittent claudication*.

Occlusion of an artery

When an artery is completely blocked, the tissues it supplies rapidly undergo degeneration and die from *ischaemia*, which leads to infarction. If a major artery supplying a large amount of tissue is affected, the consequences are likely to be more severe than if the obstruction occurs in a minor vessel. If the tissue is well provided with a collateral circulation (such as the circulus arteriosus provides in the brain), tissue damage is less than if there are few collateral vessels (which may be the case in the heart).

When a coronary artery is occluded *myocardial infarction* (p. 124) occurs. Occlusion of arteries in the brain causes cerebral ischaemia and this leads to *cerebral infarction* (stroke).

Complications of atheroma

Thrombosis and infarction

If the fibrous cap overlying a plaque breaks down, platelets are activated by the damaged cells and a blood clot forms, blocking the artery and causing ischaemia and infarction. Emboli may break off, travel in the bloodstream and lodge in small arteries distal to the clot, causing small infarcts.

Haemorrhage

Plaques may become calcified, making the artery brittle, rigid and unresponsive to rises in blood pressure. They may rupture, causing haemorrhage.

Aneurysm

When the arterial wall is weakened by spread of the plaque between the layers of tissue, a local dilatation (aneurysm) may develop (see below). This may lead to thrombosis and embolism, or the aneurysm may rupture causing severe haemorrhage. The most common sites affected by atheroma are the aorta and the abdominal and pelvic arteries.

Arteriosclerosis

This is a progressive degeneration of arterial walls, associated with ageing and accompanied by hypertension.

In large and medium-sized arteries, the tunica media is infiltrated with fibrous tissue and calcium. This causes the vessels to become dilated, inelastic and tortuous (Fig. 5.58). Loss of elasticity increases systolic blood pressure, and the *pulse pressure* (the difference between systolic and diastolic pressure).

When small arteries (arterioles) are involved, their lumen is reduced because of a deposition of a substance called *hyaline material*, which also reduces the elasticity of the vessel wall. Because these arteries are the main determinants of peripheral resistance (p. 89), this narrowing increases peripheral resistance and blood pressure. Damage to small vessels has a disproportionate effect on blood flow, leading to ischaemia of tissues supplied by affected arteries. In the limbs, the resultant ischaemia predisposes to gangrene, which is particularly serious in people with diabetes mellitus.

117

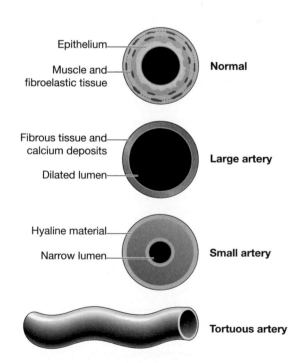

Figure 5.58 **Arteriosclerotic arteries.**

Senile arteriosclerosis. This is a condition affecting elderly people. Progressive loss of elasticity and reduced arterial lumen leads to cerebral ischaemia and loss of mental function. There may or may not be evidence of hypertension.

Aneurysms

Aneurysms are abnormal local dilatations of arteries, which vary considerably in size (Fig. 5.59). Predisposing factors include atheroma, hypertension and defective formation of collagen in the arterial wall.

Complications of aneurysm

If an aneurysm ruptures, haemorrhage follows, the consequences of which depend on the site and extent of the bleed. Rupture of the aorta is likely to be fatal, while bleeding into the subarachnoid space can also cause death, or permanent disability. Aneurysm damages the blood vessel endothelium, making it rougher than usual,

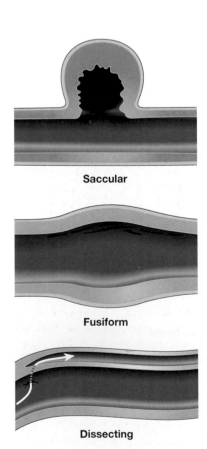

Saccular

Fusiform

Dissecting

Figure 5.59 Types of aneurysm.

which increases the risk of clot formation. Clots may block circulation locally, or elsewhere if they travel in the bloodstream as emboli. In addition, the swelling associated with the distended artery can cause pressure on local structures such as other blood vessels, nerves or organs.

Types of aneurysm

Fusiform or spindle-shaped distensions occur mainly in the abdominal aorta and less commonly in the iliac arteries. They are usually associated with atheromatous changes.

Saccular aneurysms bulge out on one side of the artery. When they occur in the relatively thin-walled arteries of the circulus arteriosus (circle of Willis) in the brain they are sometimes called 'berry' aneurysms. They may be congenital, or be associated with defective collagen production or with atheromatous changes.

Dissecting aneurysms occur mainly in the arch of the aorta, caused by infiltration of blood between the endothelium and tunica media, beginning at a site of endothelial damage.

Microaneurysms are fusiform or saccular aneurysms, occurring in small arteries and arterioles in the brain. They are associated with hypertension. Recurring small strokes (transient ischaemic attacks) are commonly due to thrombosis in the aneurysm or to haemorrhage when an aneurysm ruptures.

Venous thrombosis

The risk factors predisposing to a clot developing within a vein are discussed on page 115.

Venous thrombosis may be *superficial thrombophlebitis* or *deep vein thrombosis*.

Superficial thrombophlebitis

In this acute inflammatory condition a thrombus forms in a superficial vein and the tissue around the affected vein becomes red and painful. The most common causes are:

- intravenous infusion
- varicosities in the saphenous vein.

Deep vein thrombosis (DVT)

A thrombus forms in a deep vein commonly in the lower limb, pelvic or iliac veins, but occasionally in an upper limb. The thrombus may affect a long section of the vein and, after some days, fibrinolysis (p. 67) may enable recanalisation through the blockage. Deep vein thrombosis may be accompanied by pain and swelling, but is often asymptomatic.

The commonest complication of DVT is pulmonary embolism (p. 115)

Varicose veins

A varicosed vein is one that is so dilated that the valves do not close to prevent backward flow of blood. Such veins lose their elasticity, become elongated and tortuous, and fibrous tissue replaces the tunica media.

Predisposing factors

- Heredity – there appears to be a familial tendency.
- Gender – females are affected more than males.
- Pregnancy.
- Age – the progressive loss of elasticity in vein walls that accompanies increasing age leads to less efficient elastic recoil.
- Reduced efficiency of the skeletal muscle pump (p. 88), as in prolonged standing/sitting, or obesity, where excess adipose tissue around veins does not give adequate support.
- Pressure – because of their thin walls, veins are easily compressed by surrounding structures, leading to increased venous pressure distal to the site of compression.

Sites and effects of varicose veins

Varicose veins of the legs

When valves in anastomosing veins between deep and superficial leg veins become incompetent, the venous pressure in the superficial veins rises. In the long term they stretch and become chronically dilated because the superficial veins are less well supported by surrounding tissues than deeper ones. Such areas show through the skin as *varicose veins* (Fig. 5.60). The great and small saphenous veins and the anterior tibial veins are most commonly affected, causing aching and fatigue of the legs, especially during long periods of standing. These dilated, inelastic veins rupture easily if injured, and haemorrhage occurs.

The skin over a varicose vein may become poorly nourished due to stasis of blood, leading to the formation of *varicose ulcers,* usually on the medial aspects of the leg just above the ankle.

Haemorrhoids

Sustained pressure on the veins at the junction of the rectum and anus leads to increased venous pressure, valvular incompetence and the development of haemor-

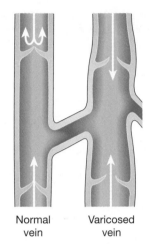
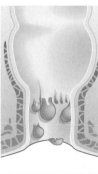
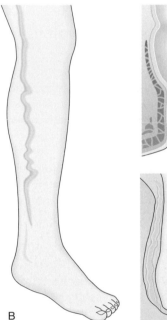
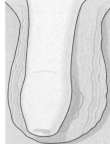

A Normal vein Varicosed vein

B

Figure 5.60 **A.** Normal and varicosed veins. **B.** Common sites for varicosities – the leg, scrotum (varicocele) and anus (haemorrhoids).

119

rhoids (piles, Fig. 5.60). The most common causes are chronic constipation, and the increased pressure in the pelvis towards the end of pregnancy. Slight bleeding may occur each time stools are passed and, in time, may cause anaemia. Severe haemorrhage is rare.

Scrotal varicocele

Each spermatic cord is surrounded by a plexus of veins that may become varicosed (Fig. 5.60), especially in men whose work involves standing for long periods. If the varicocele is bilateral, the increased temperature due to venous congestion may depress spermatogenesis and cause infertility.

Oesophageal varices

The veins involved are at the lower end of the oesophagus. When the venous pressure in the liver rises, there is a rise in pressure in the anastomosing veins between the left gastric vein and the azygos vein. Sustained pressure causes varicosities to develop in the oesophagus (see Fig. 12.47, p. 318). The commonest causes of increased portal vein pressure are cirrhosis of the liver and right-sided cardiac failure. If the pressure continues to rise, inelastic varicosed veins may rupture causing severe or possibly fatal haemorrhage.

Tumours of blood and lymph vessels

Angiomas

Angiomas are benign tumours of either blood vessels (haemangiomas) or lymph vessels (lymphangiomas). The latter rarely occur, so angioma is usually taken to mean haemangioma.

Haemangiomas. These are not true tumours, but are sufficiently similar to be classified as such. They consist of an excessive growth of blood vessels arranged in an uncharacteristic manner and interspersed with collagen fibres.

Capillary haemangiomas. Excess capillary growth interspersed with collagen in a localised area makes a dense, plexus-like network of tissue. Each haemangioma is supplied by only one blood vessel and if it thromboses, the haemangioma atrophies and disappears.

Capillary haemangiomas are usually present at birth and are seen as a purple or red mole or birthmark. They may be quite small at birth but grow at an alarming rate in the first few months, keeping pace with the growth of the child. After 1 to 3 years, atrophy may begin, and by the end of 5 years about 80% of tumours have disappeared.

Cavernous haemangiomas. Blood vessels larger than capillaries grow in excess of normal needs in a localised area and are interspersed with collagen fibres. They are dark red in colour and may be present in the skin, though more commonly in the liver. They grow slowly, do not regress and may become large and unsightly.

Oedema

Learning outcomes

After studying this section, you should be able to:

- define the term oedema
- describe the main causes of oedema
- relate the causes of oedema to relevant clinical problems
- explain the causes and consequences of excess fluid collecting in body cavities.

In oedema, excess tissue fluid accumulates, causing swelling. It may occur either in superficial tissues or deeper organs.

Sites of oedema

When oedema is present in the superficial tissues, *pitting* of the surface may be observed, i.e. an indentation in the skin remains after firm finger pressure has been applied. The sites at which superficial oedema is observed are influenced by gravity and the position of the individual. When the individual is in the standing or sitting position the oedema is observed in the lower limbs, beginning in the feet and ankles. Patients on bedrest tend to develop oedema in the sacral area. This may be described as *dependent oedema*.

In *pulmonary oedema*, venous congestion in the lungs, or increased pulmonary vessel permeability results in accumulation of fluid in the tissue spaces and in the alveoli. This reduces the area available for gaseous exchange and results in *dyspnoea* (breathlessness), cyanosis and expectoration of frothy sputum. The most common causes of pulmonary oedema are cardiac failure, inflammation or irritation of the lungs and excessive infusion of intravenous fluids.

Causes of oedema

Excess fluid accumulates in the tissues when some aspect of normal capillary fluid dynamics (p. 79) is deranged.

Increased venous hydrostatic (blood) pressure

Congestion of the venous circulation increases venous hydrostatic pressure, reducing the effect of osmotic pressure that draws fluid back into the capillary at the venous end. Excess fluid then remains in the tissues. This may be caused by heart failure, kidney disease or compression of a limb due to prolonged sitting or tight clothes.

Decreased plasma osmotic pressure

When there is depletion of plasma proteins, less fluid returns to the circulation at the venous end of the capillary (Fig. 5.61B). Causes include excessive protein loss in kidney disease (p. 349), and reduced plasma protein levels caused by e.g. liver failure or a protein-deficient diet.

Impaired lymphatic drainage

Some fluid returns to the circulation via the lymphatic system and when flow is impaired, oedema develops (Fig. 5.61C). Causes include malignancy that blocks lymph drainage, surgical removal of lymph nodes or the destruction of lymph nodes by chronic inflammation.

Increased small-vessel permeability

In inflammation (p. 371), chemical mediators increase small vessel permeability in the affected area. Plasma proteins then leave the circulation (Fig. 5.61D) and the increased tissue osmotic pressure draws fluid into the area causing swelling of the affected tissue. This type of oedema also occurs in allergic reactions (p. 380), e.g. anaphylaxis, asthma or hay fever.

Ascites and effusions

Ascites. This is the accumulation of excess fluid in the peritoneal cavity. The most common causes include liver failure (when plasma protein synthesis is reduced), obstruction of abdominal lymph nodes draining the peritoneal cavity, or inflammatory conditions. This includes malignant disease, because many tumours release pro-inflammatory mediators.

Pleural effusion. This is excess serous fluid in the pleural cavity. This is usually due to infection or inflammation of the pleura (p. 266), or to left ventricular failure, which increases pressure in the pulmonary circulation because the left ventricle is not able to pump out all the blood returning to it from the lungs.

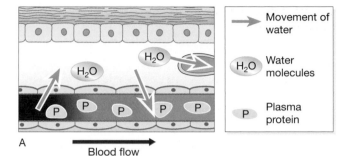

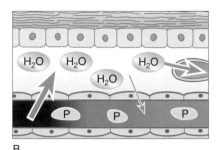

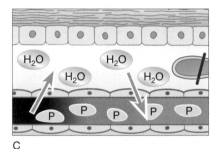

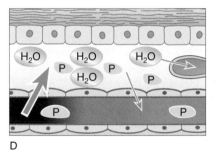

Figure 5.61 Capillary fluid dynamics. A. Normal. **B.** Effect of reduced plasma proteins. **C.** Effect of impaired lymphatic drainage. **D.** Effect of increased capillary permeability. Arrows indicate direction of movement of water.

121

Diseases of the heart

Learning outcomes

After studying this section, you should be able to:

- describe the consequences of failure of either or both sides of the heart

- explain the compensatory mechanisms that occur in heart failure

- explain the causes and consequences of faulty heart valve function

- define the term ischaemic heart disease

- discuss the main conditions associated with ischaemic heart disease

- describe rheumatic heart disease and its effects on cardiac function

- explain the underlying pathophysiology of pericarditis

- describe, with reference to standard ECG trace, the main cardiac arrhythmias

- describe the principal congenital cardiac abnormalities.

Cardiac failure

The heart is described as failing when the cardiac output is unable to maintain the circulation of sufficient blood to meet the needs of the body. In mild cases, cardiac output is adequate at rest and becomes inadequate only when increased cardiac output is required, e.g. in exercise. Heart failure may affect either side of the heart, but since both sides of the heart are part of one circuit, when one half of the pump begins to fail it frequently leads to increased strain on, and eventual failure of, the other side. The main clinical manifestations depend on which side of the heart is most affected. Left ventricular failure is more common than right, because of the greater workload of the left ventricle.

Compensatory mechanisms in heart failure

When heart failure happens acutely, the body has little time to make compensatory changes, but if the heart fails over a period of time the following changes are likely to occur in an attempt to maintain cardiac output and tissue perfusion, especially of vital organs.

- the cardiac muscle fibres enlarge and increase in number, which makes the walls of the chambers thicker

- the heart chambers enlarge

- decreased renal blood flow activates the renin–angiotensin–aldosterone system (p. 221), which leads to salt and water retention. This increases blood volume and cardiac workload. The direct vasoconstrictor action of angiotensin II increases peripheral resistance and puts further strain on the failing heart.

Acute cardiac failure

A sudden decrease in output of blood from both ventricles causes acute reduction in the oxygen supply to all the tissues. Recovery from the acute phase may be followed by chronic failure, or death may occur due to anoxia of vital centres in the brain. The commonest causes are:

- sudden interruption of the blood supply to the myocardium, which may cause ischaemia or tissue death

- pulmonary embolism, blocking blood flow through the pulmonary circulation – the heart fails because it has to pump against this obstruction

- severe cardiac arrhythmia, when the pumping action of the heart is badly impaired or effectively stopped

- rupture of a heart chamber or valve cusp; both greatly increase the cardiac effort required to maintain adequate output

- severe malignant hypertension, which greatly increases resistance to blood flow.

Chronic cardiac failure

This develops gradually and in the early stages there may be no symptoms because compensatory changes occur as described above. When further compensation is not possible there is a gradual decline in myocardial efficiency. Underlying causes include degenerative heart changes with advancing age, and many chronic conditions, e.g. anaemia, lung disease, hypertension or cardiac disease.

Right-sided (congestive) cardiac failure

The right ventricle fails when the pressure developed within it by the contracting myocardium is less than the force needed to push blood through the lungs.

When compensation has reached its limit, and the ventricle is not emptying completely, the right atrium and venae cavae become congested with blood and this is followed by congestion throughout the venous system. The organs affected first are the liver, spleen and kidneys. *Oedema* (p. 120) of the limbs and *ascites* (excess fluid in the peritoneal cavity) usually follow.

This problem may be caused by increased vascular resistance in the lungs, weakness of the myocardium and/or stenosis and incompetence of valves in the heart or great vessels.

Resistance to blood flow through the lungs

When this is increased the right ventricle has more work to do. It may be caused by:

- the formation of fibrous tissue following inflammation or chronic disease of the lungs
- back pressure of blood through the pulmonary circulation from the left side of the heart, e.g. in left ventricular failure, when the mitral valve is stenosed and/or incompetent.

Weakness of the myocardium

This may be caused by ischaemia following numerous small myocardial infarcts.

Left-sided (left ventricular) failure

This occurs when the pressure developed in the left ventricle by the contracting myocardium is less than the pressure in the aorta and the ventricle cannot then pump out all the blood it receives. Causes include ischaemic heart disease, which reduces the efficiency of the myocardium, and hypertension, when the heart's workload is increased because of raised systemic resistance. Disease of the mitral and/or aortic valves may prevent efficient emptying of the heart chambers, so that myocardial workload is increased.

Failure of the left ventricle leads to dilatation of the atrium and an increase in pulmonary blood pressure. This is followed by a rise in the blood pressure in the right side of the heart and eventually systemic venous congestion.

Congestion in the lungs leads to pulmonary oedema and dyspnoea, often most severe at night. This *paroxysmal nocturnal dyspnoea* may be due to raised blood volume as fluid from peripheral oedema is reabsorbed when the patient slips down in bed during sleep.

Disorders of heart valves

The heart valves prevent backflow of blood in the heart during the cardiac cycle. The left atrioventricular and aortic valves are subject to greater pressures than those on the right side and are therefore more susceptible to damage.

Distinctive heart sounds arise when the valves close during the cardiac cycle (p. 86). Damaged valves generate abnormal heart sounds called *murmurs*. A severe valve disorder causes heart failure. The most common causes of valve defects are rheumatic fever, fibrosis following inflammation and congenital abnormalities.

Stenosis

This is the narrowing of a valve opening, impeding blood flow through the valve. It occurs when inflammation and encrustations roughen the edges of the cusps so that they stick together, narrowing the valve opening. When healing occurs, fibrous tissue is formed which shrinks as it ages, increasing the stenosis and leading to incompetence.

Incompetence

Sometimes called *regurgitation*, this is a functional defect caused by failure of a valve to close completely, allowing blood to flow back into the ventricle when it relaxes.

Ischaemic heart disease

Ischaemia is due to the effects of atheroma, causing narrowing or occlusion of one or more branches of the coronary arteries. Atheromatous plaques (p. 116) cause narrowing. Occlusion may be by plaques alone, or plaques complicated by thrombosis. The overall effect depends on the size of the coronary artery involved and whether it is only narrowed or completely blocked. Narrowing of an artery leads to *angina pectoris*, and occlusion to myocardial infarction.

When atheroma develops slowly, a *collateral arterial blood supply* may have time to develop and effectively supplement or replace the original. This consists of the dilatation of normally occurring anastomotic arteries joining adjacent arteries. When sudden severe narrowing or occlusion of an artery occurs, the anastomotic arteries dilate but may not be able to supply enough blood to meet myocardial needs.

Angina pectoris

This is sometimes called *angina of effort* because the increased cardiac output required during extra physical effort causes severe chest pain, which may also radiate to the arms, neck and jaw. Other factors that may precipitate angina include cold weather and emotional states.

A narrowed coronary artery may supply sufficient blood to the myocardium to meet its needs during rest or moderate exercise but not when greatly increased cardiac output is needed, e.g. walking may be tolerated but not running. The thick, inflexible atheromatous artery wall is unable to dilate to allow for the increased blood flow needed by the more active myocardium, which then becomes ischaemic. In the early stages of angina, the chest pain stops when the cardiac output returns to its resting level soon after the extra effort stops.

Myocardial infarction

The myocardium may infarct (p. 115) when a branch of a coronary artery is occluded. The commonest cause is an atheromatous plaque complicated by thrombosis. The extent of myocardial damage depends on the size of the blood vessel and site of the infarct. The damage is permanent because cardiac muscle cannot regenerate, and the dead muscle is replaced with non-functional fibrous tissue. Speedy restoration of blood flow through the blocked artery using clot-dissolving (thrombolytic) drugs can greatly reduce the extent of the permanent damage and improve prognosis, but treatment must be started within a few hours of the infarction occurring. The effects and complications are greatest when the left ventricle is involved.

Myocardial infarction is usually accompanied by very severe crushing chest pain behind the sternum which, unlike angina pectoris, continues even when the individual is at rest.

Complications

These may be fatal and include:

- severe arrhythmias, especially *ventricular fibrillation* (p. 125), due to disruption of the cardiac conducting system
- cardiac failure, caused by impaired contraction of the damaged myocardium and, in severe cases, cardiogenic shock
- rupture of a ventricle wall, usually within 2 weeks of the original episode
- pulmonary or cerebral embolism originating from a mural clot within a ventricle, i.e. a clot that forms inside the heart over the infarct
- pericarditis
- angina pectoris
- recurrence.

Rheumatic heart disease

Rheumatic fever is an inflammatory illness that sometimes follows streptococcal throat infections, most commonly in children and young adults. It is an autoimmune disorder; the antibodies produced to combat the original infection damage connective tissues, including the heart, joints (p. 427) and skin.

Death rarely occurs in the acute phase, but after recovery there may be permanent damage to the heart valves, eventually leading to disability and possibly cardiac failure.

Effects on the endocardium

The endocardium becomes inflamed and oedematous and tiny pale areas called *Aschoff's bodies* appear which, when they heal, leave thick fibrous tissue. Thrombotic fibrous nodules consisting of platelets and fibrin form on the free borders of the cusps of the heart valves. When healing occurs, the fibrous tissue formed shrinks as it ages, distorting the shape of the cusps and causing stenosis and incompetence of the valve. The left atrioventricular (mitral) and aortic valves are commonly affected, the right atrioventricular (tricuspid) valve sometimes and the pulmonary valve rarely.

Effects on the myocardium

Aschoff's bodies form on the connective tissue between the cardiac muscle fibres. As in the endocardium, healing is accompanied by fibrosis that may interfere with myocardial contraction.

Effects on the pericardium

Inflammation leads to the accumulation of exudate in the pericardial cavity. Healing is accompanied by fibrous thickening of the pericardium and adhesions form between the two layers. In severe cases the layers may fuse, obliterating the cavity. Within this inelastic pericardium the heart may not be able to expand fully during diastole, leading to reduced cardiac output, generalised venous congestion and oedema.

Subclinical rheumatic heart disease

Valvular incompetence developing in older people who have a history of rheumatic fever many years previously is believed to be due to repeated subclinical attacks. These attacks are not associated with repeated episodes of sore throat, so it is assumed that the original disease has remained active in a subclinical form. In some cases there is no history of rheumatic fever.

Infective endocarditis

Pathogenic organisms (usually bacteria or fungi) in the blood may colonise any part of the endocardium, but the most common sites are on or near the heart valves and round the margins of congenital heart defects. These areas are susceptible to infection because they are exposed to fast-flowing blood that may cause mild trauma. This is a serious illness and often fatal unless adequately treated.

The main predisposing factors are bacteraemia, depressed immune response and heart abnormalities.

Bacteraemia

Microbes in the bloodstream, if not destroyed by phagocytes or antibodies, tend to adhere to platelets and form tiny infected emboli. Inside the heart, the emboli are most likely to settle on already damaged endocardium. Vegetations consisting of platelets and fibrin surround the microbes and seem to protect them from normal body defences and antibiotics. Because of this, infection may be caused by a wide range of microbes, including some that do not normally cause clinical infection. They normally originate from the skin or the mouth.

Depressed immune response

This enables low-virulence bacteria, viruses, yeasts and fungi to become established and cause infection. These are organisms always present in the body and the environment. Depression of the immune systems may be caused by HIV infection, malignant disease, cytotoxic drugs, radiotherapy or steroid therapy.

Heart abnormalities

The sites most commonly infected are already abnormal in some way. Pathogenic organisms present in the bloodstream cannot adhere to healthy endothelium, but if the endothelial lining of the cardiovascular system is damaged, infection is more likely. Often, the cardiac valves are involved, especially if damaged by rheumatic disease or congenital malformation. Other likely sites of infection include regions of cardiac abnormality, such as ventricular septal defect and patent ductus arteriosus. Prosthetic valves can also be a focus for infective growths.

Acute infective endocarditis

This is a severe febrile illness usually caused by high-virulence microbes, commonly *Staphylococcus aureus*. Vegetations grow rapidly and pieces may break off, becoming infected emboli. These settle in other organs where the microbes grow, destroying tissue and forming pus. The effects depend on the organ involved, e.g. brain or kidney infection may cause death in a few days. The causative microbes rapidly destroy heart valves, impairing their function and resulting in acute heart failure.

Subacute infective endocarditis

This endocarditis is usually caused by low-virulence microbes, e.g. non-haemolytic streptococci or some staphylococci. Infected emboli may settle in any organ but do not cause suppuration and rarely cause death. Microbes in the vegetations seem to be protected by surrounding platelets and fibrin from normal body defences and antibiotics. Healing by fibrosis further distorts the shape of the valve cusps, increasing the original stenosis and incompetence. Heart failure may develop later.

Cardiac arrhythmias

The heart rate is normally determined by intrinsic impulses generated in the SA node. The rhythm is determined by the route of impulse transmission through the conducting system. The heart rate is usually measured as the pulse, but to determine the rhythm, an electrocardiogram (ECG) is required (Fig. 5.62A). A *cardiac arrhythmia* is any disorder of heart rate or rhythm, and is the result of abnormal generation or conduction of impulses. The normal cardiac cycle (p. 86) gives rise to *normal sinus rhythm*, which has a rate between 60 and 100 beats per minute.

Sinus bradycardia. This is normal sinus rhythm below 60 beats per minute. This may occur during sleep and is common in athletes. It is an abnormality when it follows myocardial infarction or accompanies raised intracranial pressure (p. 177).

Sinus tachycardia. This is normal sinus rhythm above 100 beats per minute when the individual is at rest. This accompanies exercise and anxiety, but is an indicator of some disorders, e.g. fever, hyperthyroidism, some cardiac conditions.

Asystole

This occurs when there is no electrical activity in the ventricles and therefore no cardiac output. The ECG shows a flat line (Fig. 5.62B). Ventricular fibrillation and asystole cause sudden and complete loss of cardiac output, i.e. *cardiac arrest* and death.

Fibrillation

This is the contraction of the cardiac muscle fibres in a disorderly sequence. The chambers do not contract as a coordinated unit and the pumping action is disrupted.

In *atrial fibrillation*, contraction of the atria is uncoordinated and rapid, pumping is ineffective and stimulation of the AV node is disorderly. Ventricular contraction becomes rapid and rhythm and force irregular; although an adequate cardiac output and blood pressure may be maintained, the pulse is irregular. The causes of increased excitability and disorganised activity are not always clear but predisposing conditions include:

- ischaemic heart disease
- degenerative changes in the heart due to old age
- thyrotoxicosis
- rheumatic heart disease.

Ventricular fibrillation is a medical emergency that will swiftly lead to death if untreated, because the chaotic electrical activity within the ventricular walls cannot coordinate effective pumping action.

125

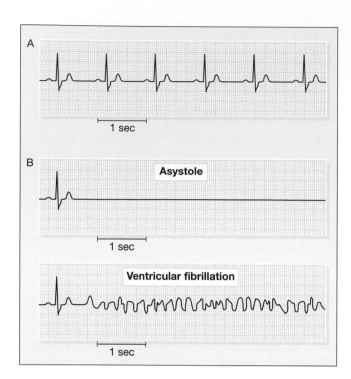

Figure 5.62 ECG traces: A. Normal sinus rhythm. **B.** Life-threatening arrhythmias.

Blood is not pumped from the heart into either the pulmonary or the systemic circulation. No pulses can be felt, consciousness is lost and breathing stops. The ECG shows an irregular chaotic trace with no recognisable wave pattern (Fig. 5.62B).

Heart block

Heart block occurs when normal impulse transmission is blocked or impaired. A common form involves obstruction of impulse transmission through the AV node, but (less commonly) conducting tissue in the atria or ventricles can also be affected. When the AV node is involved, the delay between atrial and ventricular contraction is increased. The severity depends on the extent of loss of stimulation of the AV node.

In *complete heart block*, ventricular contraction is entirely independent of impulses initiated by the SA node. Freed from the normal pacing action of the SA node, the ventricles are driven by impulses generated by the pacemaker activity of the AV node, resulting in slow, regular ventricular contractions and a heart rate of about 30 to 40 beats per minute. In this state the heart is unable to respond quickly to a sudden increase in demand by, e.g., muscular exercise. The most common causes are:

- acute ischaemic heart disease
- myocardial fibrosis following repeated infarctions or myocarditis

- drugs used to treat heart disease, e.g. digitalis, propranolol.

When heart block develops gradually there is some degree of adjustment in the body to reduced cardiac output but, if progressive, it eventually leads to death from cardiac failure and cerebral anoxia.

Congenital abnormalities

Abnormalities in the heart and great vessels at birth may be due to intrauterine developmental errors or to the failure of the heart and blood vessels to adapt to extrauterine life. Sometimes, there are no symptoms in early life and the abnormality is recognised only when complications appear.

Patent ductus arteriosus

Before birth the ductus arteriosus, joining the arch of the aorta and the pulmonary artery, allows blood to pass from the pulmonary artery to the aorta (Fig. 5.63). It carries blood pumped into the pulmonary trunk by the right ventricle into the aorta, bypassing the pulmonary circulation, which in the unborn child is not functional because the fetus derives his oxygen supply through the placenta. At birth, when the pulmonary circulation is established, the ductus arteriosus should close completely. If it remains patent, blood regurgitates from the aorta to the pulmonary artery where the pressure is lower, reducing the volume entering the systemic circula-

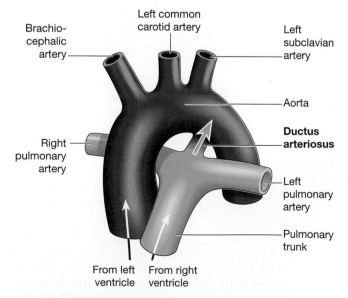

Figure 5.63 The ductus arteriosus in the fetus. The arrow indicates the direction of flow of blood from the pulmonary circulation into the aorta.

tion and increasing the volume of blood in the pulmonary circulation. This leads to pulmonary congestion and eventually cardiac failure.

Atrial septal defect

This is commonly known as 'hole in the heart'. Before birth, most oxygenated blood from the placenta enters the left atrium from the right atrium through the *foramen ovale* in the septum. There is a valve-like structure across the opening, consisting of two partly overlapping membranes. The 'valve' is open when the pressure in the right atrium is higher than in the left. This diverts blood flow from the right to the left side of the heart, bypassing the pulmonary circulation, which in the unborn child is not functional because the fetus derives his oxygen supply through the placenta. After birth, when the pulmonary circulation is established and the pressure in the left atrium is the higher, the two membranes come in contact, closing the 'valve'. Later the closure becomes permanent due to fibrosis (Fig. 5.64).

When the membranes do not overlap, an opening between the atria remains patent after birth. In many cases it is too small to cause symptoms in early life but they may appear later. In severe cases blood flows back to the right atrium from the left. This increases the right ventricular and pulmonary pressure, causing hypertrophy of the myocardium and eventually cardiac failure. As

pressure in the right atrium rises, blood flow through the defect may be reversed, but this is not an improvement because deoxygenated blood gains access to the general circulation.

Coarctation of the aorta

The most common site of coarctation (narrowing) of the aorta is between the left subclavian artery and ductus arteriosus. This leads to hypertension in the upper body (which is supplied by arteries arising from the aorta proximal to the narrowing) because increased force of contraction of the heart is needed to push the blood through the coarctation. There may be systemic hypotension.

Fallot's tetralogy

This is a characteristic combination of four congenital cardiac abnormalities, which causes cyanosis, growth retardation and exercise intolerance in babies and young children. The four abnormalities are:

- stenosis of the pulmonary artery at its point of origin, which increases right ventricular workload
- ventricular septal defect, i.e. an abnormal communicating hole between the two ventricles, just below the atrioventricular valves
- aortic misplacement, i.e. the origin of the aorta is displaced to the right so that it is immediately above the septal defect
- right ventricular hypertrophy to counteract the pulmonary stenosis.

Cardiac function is inadequate to meet the needs of the growing child; surgical correction carries a good prognosis.

127

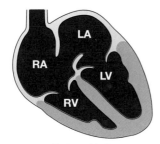

Before birth

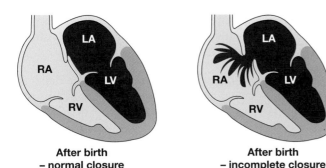

**After birth
– normal closure**

**After birth
– incomplete closure**

Figure 5.64 Atrioseptal valve: normal and defective closure after birth.

Disorders of blood pressure

Learning outcomes

After studying this section, you should be able to:

- explain the term hypertension
- define essential and secondary hypertension and list the main causes of the latter
- discuss the effects of prolonged hypertension on the body, including elevated blood pressure in the lungs
- describe the term hypotension.

Hypertension

The term hypertension is used to describe a level of blood pressure that, taking all other cardiovascular risk factors into account, would benefit the patient if reduced. It is therefore not possible to have a definitive blood pressure value that is classified as 'hypertension', but measurements above 140/90 mmHg are considered higher than 'normal'. Blood pressure tends to rise naturally with age. Arteriosclerosis (p. 117) may contribute to this, but is not the only factor.

Hypertension is described as *essential* (primary, idiopathic) or *secondary* to other diseases. Irrespective of the cause, hypertension commonly affects the kidneys (p. 349).

Essential hypertension

This means hypertension of unknown cause. It accounts for 95% of all cases and is subdivided according to the rate at which the disease progresses.

Benign (chronic) hypertension
The rise in blood pressure is usually slight to moderate and continues to rise slowly over many years. Sometimes complications, such as heart failure, cerebrovascular accident or myocardial infarction are the first indication of hypertension, but often the condition is symptomless and is only discovered during a routine examination.

Risk factors for hypertension include obesity, diabetes mellitus, family history, cigarette smoking, a sedentary lifestyle and high intakes of salt or alcohol. Stress may increase blood pressure, and there is a well-documented link between low birth weight and incidence of hypertension in later life.

Malignant (accelerated) hypertension
This is a rapid and aggressive acceleration of hypertensive disease. Diastolic pressure in excess of 120 mmHg is common. The effects are serious and quickly become apparent, e.g. haemorrhages into the retina, papillo-edema (oedema around the optic disc), encephalopathy (cerebral oedema) and progressive renal disease, leading to cardiac failure.

Secondary hypertension

Hypertension resulting from other diseases accounts for 5% of all cases.

Kidney disease
Raised blood pressure is a complication of many kidney diseases. In kidney disease, there is salt and water retention, sometimes with excessive renin activity.

Endocrine disorders
Adrenal cortex. Secretion of excess aldosterone and cortisol stimulates the retention of excess sodium and water by the kidneys, raising the blood volume and pressure. Oversecretion of aldosterone (Conn's syndrome) is due to a hormone-secreting tumour. Oversecretion of cortisol may be due to overstimulation of the gland by adrenocorticotrophic hormone secreted by the pituitary gland, or to a hormone-secreting tumour.

Adrenal medulla. Secretion of excess adrenaline (epinephrine) and noradrenaline (norepinephrine) raises blood pressure, e.g. phaeochromocytoma (p. 231).

Stricture of the aorta
Hypertension develops in branching arteries proximal to the site of a stricture, e.g *congenital coarctation* (p. 127).

Drug treatment
Hypertension may be a side-effect of some drugs, e.g. corticosteroids and oral contraceptives.

Effects and complications of hypertension

The effects of long-standing and progressively rising blood pressure are serious. Hypertension predisposes to atherosclerosis and has specific effects on particular organs (target organs).

Heart. The rate and force of cardiac contraction are increased to maintain the cardiac output against a sustained rise in arterial pressure. The left ventricle hypertrophies and begins to fail when compensation has reached its limit. This is followed by back pressure and accumulation of blood in the lungs (pulmonary congestion), hypertrophy of the right ventricle and eventually to right ventricular failure. Hypertension also predisposes to ischaemic heart disease (p. 123) and aneurysm formation (p. 118).

Brain. Stroke, caused by cerebral haemorrhage, is common, the effects depending on the position and size of the ruptured vessel. When a series of small blood vessels rupture, e.g. microaneurysms, at different times, there is progressive disability. Rupture of a large vessel causes extensive loss of function or death.

Kidneys. Essential hypertension causes kidney damage. If sustained for only a short time recovery may be complete. Otherwise the kidney damage causes further hypertension owing to activation of the renin–angiotensin–aldosterone system (p. 221), progressive loss of kidney function and kidney failure.

Blood vessels. High blood pressure damages blood vessels. The walls of small arteries become hardened, and in larger arteries, atheroma is accelerated. If other risk factors for vascular disease are present, such as diabetes or smoking, damage is more extensive. The vessel wall may become so badly weakened by these changes that an aneurysm develops, and as the blood vessels become progressively damaged and less compliant, hypertension worsens.

The capillaries of the retina and the kidneys are particularly susceptible to the effects of chronic hypertension, leading to retinal bleeding and reduced renal function.

Pulmonary hypertension

Normally, the pulmonary circulation is a low-pressure system, to prevent fluid being forced out of the pulmonary capillaries into the alveoli. When blood pressure rises, alveoli begin to fill with fluid, which blocks gas exchange. Rising pulmonary blood pressure may result from left-sided heart failure (p. 123), or other problems with left ventricular function, when blood accumulates in the pulmonary circulation because the left ventricle is not pumping efficiently. Lung disease can also increase in pulmonary blood pressure because of destruction of lung capillaries, e.g. in emphysema. Primary pulmonary hypertension, where there is no identifiable cause, is rare.

Hypotension

This usually occurs as a complication of other conditions, such as shock (p. 113) or Addison's disease (p. 113). Low blood pressure leads to inadequate blood supply to the brain. Depending on the cause, unconsciousness may be brief (fainting) or more prolonged, possibly causing death.

Postural hypotension syncope (fainting) is due to sudden reduction in blood pressure on standing up quickly from a sitting or lying position. It occurs most commonly in the elderly. It may be caused by delay in response of the baroreceptors in the carotid sinuses to the gravitational effects of standing up. It may also occur when patients are being treated with antihypertensive drugs, especially while the most appropriate dose is being established.

The lymphatic system

6

All body tissues are bathed in tissue fluid, consisting of the diffusible constituents of blood and waste materials from cells. Some tissue fluid returns to the capillaries at their venous end and the remainder diffuses through the more permeable walls of the lymph capillaries, forming *lymph*.

Lymph passes through vessels of increasing size and a varying number of *lymph nodes* before returning to the blood. The lymphatic system (Fig. 6.1) consists of:

- lymph
- lymph vessels

- lymph nodes
- lymph organs, e.g. spleen and thymus
- diffuse lymphoid tissue, e.g. tonsils
- bone marrow.

Functions of the lymphatic system include the following.

Tissue drainage. Every day, around 21 litres of fluid from plasma, carrying dissolved substances and some plasma protein, escape from the arterial end of the capillaries and into the tissues. Most of this fluid is returned directly to

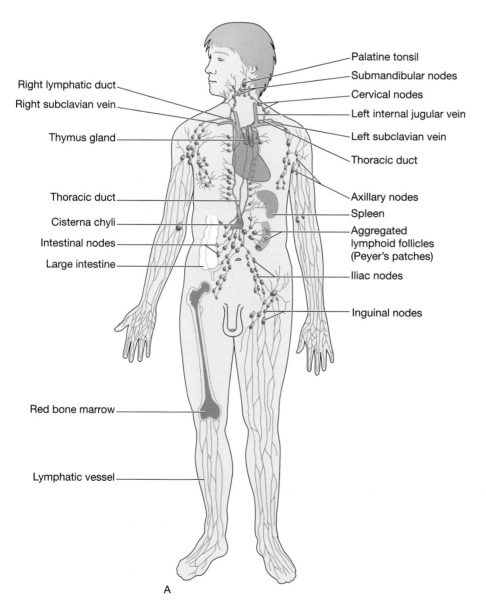

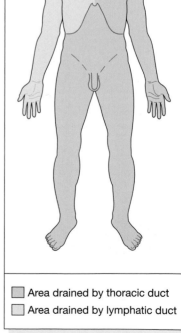

Area drained by thoracic duct
Area drained by lymphatic duct

A   B

Figure 6.1 A. Major parts of the lymphatic system. B. Regional drainage of lymph.

the bloodstream via the capillary at its venous end, but 3–4 litres of fluid are drained away by the lymphatic vessels. Without this, the tissues would rapidly become waterlogged, and the cardiovascular system would begin to fail as the blood volume falls.

Absorption in the small intestine. Fat and fat-soluble materials, e.g. the fat-soluble vitamins, are absorbed into the central lacteals (lymphatic vessels) of the villi.

Immunity. The lymphatic organs are concerned with the production and maturation of lymphocytes, the white blood cells responsible for immunity. Bone marrow is therefore considered to be lymphatic tissue, since lymphocytes are produced there.

Lymph

Learning outcome

After studying this section, you should be able to:

■ describe the composition and the main functions of lymph.

Lymph is a clear watery fluid, similar in composition to plasma, with the important exception of plasma proteins, and identical in composition to interstitial fluid. Lymph transports the plasma proteins that seep out of the capillary beds back to the bloodstream. It also carries away larger particles, e.g. bacteria and cell debris from damaged tissues, which can then be filtered out and destroyed by the lymph nodes. Lymph contains lymphocytes, which circulate in the lymphatic system allowing them to patrol the different regions of the body. In the lacteals of the small intestine, fats absorbed into the lymphatics give the lymph (now called *chyle*), a milky appearance.

Lymph vessels

Learning outcome

After studying this section, you should be able to:

■ identify the locations and functions of the main lymphatic vessels of the body.

Lymph capillaries

These originate as blind-end tubes in the interstitial spaces (Fig. 6.2). They have the same structure as blood capillaries, i.e. a single layer of endothelial cells, but their walls are more permeable to all interstitial fluid constituents, including proteins and cell debris. The tiny capillaries join up to form larger lymph vessels.

Nearly all tissues have a network of lymphatic vessels, the exceptions being the central nervous system, the bones and the most superficial layers of the skin.

Larger lymph vessels

The walls of lymph vessels are about the same thickness as those of small veins and have the same layers of tissue, i.e. a fibrous covering, a middle layer of smooth muscle and elastic tissue and an inner lining of endothelium. Lymph vessels have numerous cup-shaped valves to ensure that lymph flows in one way only, i.e. towards the thorax (Fig. 6.3). There is no 'pump', like the heart, involved in the onward movement of lymph but the muscle layer in the walls of the large lymph vessels has an intrinsic ability to contract rhythmically (the lymphatic pump).

In addition, any structure that periodically compresses the lymphatic vessels can assist in the movement of lymph along the vessels, commonly including the contraction of adjacent muscles and the pulsation of large arteries.

Lymph vessels become larger as they join together, eventually forming two large ducts, the *thoracic duct* and *right lymphatic duct*, which empty lymph into the subclavian veins.

133

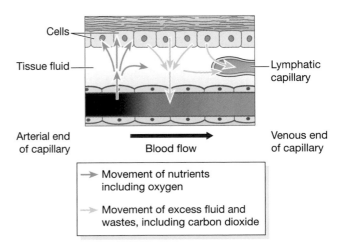

Figure 6.2 **The origin of a lymph capillary.**

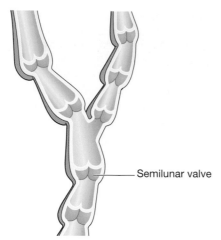

Figure 6.3 A lymph vessel cut open to show valves.

Thoracic duct

This duct begins at the *cisterna chyli*, which is a dilated lymph channel situated in front of the bodies of the first two lumbar vertebrae. The duct is about 40 cm long and opens into the left subclavian vein in the root of the neck. It drains lymph from both legs, the pelvic and abdominal cavities, the left half of the thorax, head and neck and the left arm (Fig. 6.1A and B).

Right lymphatic duct

This is a dilated lymph vessel about 1 cm long. It lies in the root of the neck and opens into the right subclavian vein. It drains lymph from the right half of the thorax, head and neck and the right arm (Fig. 6.1A and B).

Lymphatic organs and tissues

Learning outcomes

After studying this section, you should be able to:

■ compare and contrast the structure and functions of a typical lymph node with that of the spleen

■ describe the location, structure and function of the thymus gland

■ describe the location, structure and function of mucosa-associated lymphatic tissue (MALT).

Lymph nodes

Lymph nodes are oval or bean-shaped organs that lie, often in groups, along the length of lymph vessels. The lymph drains through a number of nodes, usually 8 to 10, before returning to the venous circulation. These nodes vary considerably in size: some are as small as a pin head and the largest are about the size of an almond.

Structure of lymph nodes

Lymph nodes (Fig. 6.4) have an outer capsule of fibrous tissue that dips down into the node substance forming partitions, or *trabeculae*. The main substance of the node consists of reticular and lymphatic tissue containing many lymphocytes and macrophages.

As many as four or five *afferent* lymph vessels may enter a lymph node while only one *efferent* vessel carries lymph away from the node. Each node has a concave surface called the *hilum* where an artery enters and a vein and the efferent lymph vessel leave.

The large numbers of lymph nodes situated in strategic positions throughout the body are arranged in deep and superficial groups.

Lymph from the head and neck passes through deep and superficial *cervical nodes* (Fig. 6.5).

Lymph from the upper limbs passes through nodes situated in the elbow region, then through the deep and superficial *axillary nodes*.

Lymph from organs and tissues in the thoracic cavity drains through groups of nodes situated close to the

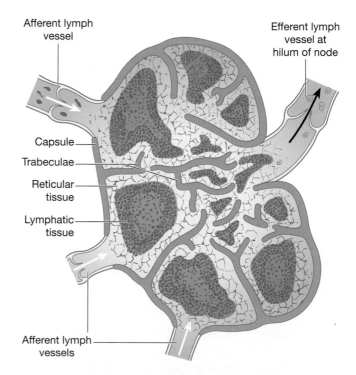

Figure 6.4 Section through a lymph node. Arrows indicate the direction of lymph flow.

been cleared of foreign matter and cell debris. In some cases where phagocytosis of microbes is incomplete they may stimulate inflammation and enlargement of the node (*lymphadenopathy*).

Proliferation of lymphocytes

Activated T- and B-lymphocytes multiply in lymph nodes. Antibodies produced by sensitised B-lymphocytes enter lymph and blood draining the node.

Spleen

The spleen (Fig. 6.6) contains reticular and lymphatic tissue and is the largest lymph organ.

The spleen lies in the left hypochondriac region of the abdominal cavity between the fundus of the stomach and the diaphragm. It is purplish in colour and varies in size in different individuals, but is usually about 12 cm long, 7 cm wide and 2.5 cm thick. It weighs about 200 g.

Organs associated with the spleen

Superiorly and posteriorly	– diaphragm
Inferiorly	– left colic flexure of the large intestine
Anteriorly	– fundus of the stomach
Medially	– pancreas and the left kidney
Laterally	– separated from the 9th, 10th and 11th ribs and the intercostal muscles by the diaphragm

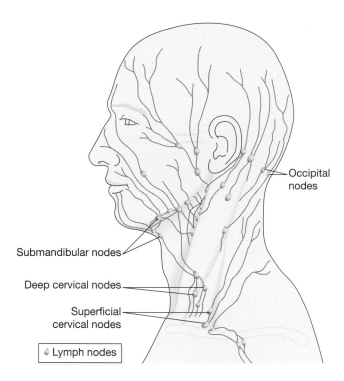

Figure 6.5 Some lymph nodes of the face and neck.

mediastinum, large airways, oesophagus and chest wall. Most of the lymph from the breast passes through the axillary nodes.

Lymph from the pelvic and abdominal cavities passes through many lymph nodes before entering the cisterna chyli. The abdominal and pelvic nodes are situated mainly in association with the blood vessels supplying the organs and close to the main arteries, i.e. the aorta and the external and internal iliac arteries.

The lymph from the lower limbs drains through deep and superficial nodes including groups of nodes behind the knee and in the groin (inguinal nodes).

Functions of lymph nodes

Filtering and phagocytosis

Lymph is filtered by the reticular and lymphoid tissue as it passes through lymph nodes. Particulate matter may include microbes, dead and live phagocytes containing ingested microbes, cells from malignant tumours, worn-out and damaged tissue cells and inhaled particles. Organic material is destroyed in lymph nodes by macrophages and antibodies. Some inorganic inhaled particles cannot be destroyed by phagocytosis. These remain inside the macrophages, either causing no damage or killing the cell. Material not filtered out and dealt with in one lymph node passes on to successive nodes and by the time lymph enters the blood it has usually

135

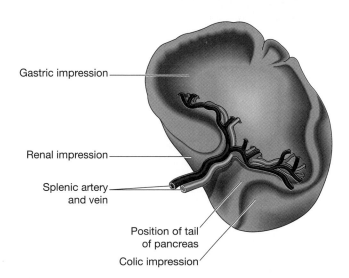

Figure 6.6 The spleen.

Structure (Fig. 6.7)

The spleen is slightly oval in shape with the hilum on the lower medial border. The anterior surface is covered with peritoneum. It is enclosed in a fibroelastic capsule that dips into the organ, forming trabeculae. The cellular material, consisting of lymphocytes and macrophages, is called *splenic pulp*, and lies between the trabeculae. *Red pulp* is the part suffused with blood and *white pulp* consists of areas of lymphatic tissue where there are sleeves of lymphocytes and macrophages around blood vessels.

The structures entering and leaving the spleen at the hilum are:

- splenic artery, a branch of the coeliac artery
- splenic vein, a branch of the portal vein
- lymph vessels (efferent only)
- nerves.

Blood passing through the spleen flows in sinuses, which have distinct pores between the endothelial cells, allowing it to come into close association with splenic pulp.

Functions

Phagocytosis

As described previously (p. 62), old and abnormal erythrocytes are destroyed in the spleen, and the breakdown products, bilirubin and iron, are transported to the liver via the splenic and portal veins. Other cellular material, e.g. leukocytes, platelets and microbes, is phagocytosed in the spleen. Unlike lymph nodes, the spleen has no afferent lymphatics entering it, so it is not exposed to diseases spread by lymph.

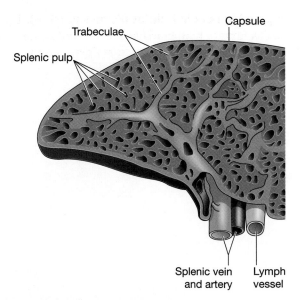

Figure 6.7 A section through the spleen.

Storage of blood

The spleen contains up to 350 ml of blood, and in response to sympathetic stimulation can rapidly return most of this volume to the circulation, e.g. in haemorrhage.

Immune response

The spleen contains T- and B-lymphocytes, which are activated by the presence of antigens, e.g. in infection. Lymphocyte proliferation during serious infection can cause enlargement of the spleen (*splenomegaly*).

Erythropoiesis

The spleen and liver are important sites of fetal blood cell production, and the spleen can also fulfil this function in adults in times of great need.

Thymus gland

The thymus gland lies in the upper part of the mediastinum behind the sternum and extends upwards into the root of the neck (Fig. 6.8). It weighs about 10 to 15 g at birth and grows until puberty, when it begins to atrophy. Its maximum weight, at puberty, is between 30 and 40 g and by middle age it has returned to approximately its weight at birth.

Organs associated with the thymus

Anteriorly – sternum and upper four costal cartilages
Posteriorly – aortic arch and its branches, brachiocephalic veins, trachea
Laterally – lungs
Superiorly – structures in the root of the neck
Inferiorly – heart

Structure

The thymus consists of two lobes joined by areolar tissue. The lobes are enclosed by a fibrous capsule which dips into their substance, dividing them into lobules that consist of an irregular branching framework of epithelial cells and lymphocytes.

Function

Lymphocytes originate from pluripotent stem cells in red bone marrow. Those that enter the thymus develop into activated T-lymphocytes (p. 375).

Thymic processing produces mature T-lymphocytes that can distinguish 'self' tissue from foreign tissue, and also provides each T-lymphocyte with the ability to react to only one specific antigen from the millions it will encounter (p. 375). T-lymphocytes then leave the thymus and enter the blood. Some enter lymphoid tissues and

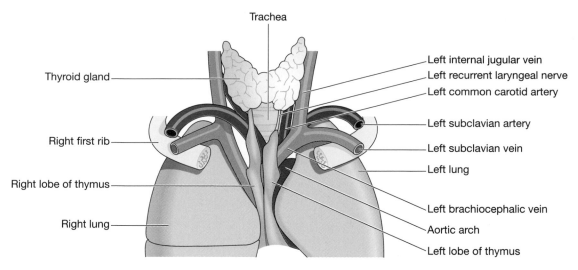

Trachea

Thyroid gland

Right first rib

Right lobe of thymus

Right lung

Left internal jugular vein
Left recurrent laryngeal nerve
Left common carotid artery

Left subclavian artery

Left subclavian vein

Left lung

Left brachiocephalic vein

Aortic arch

Left lobe of thymus

Figure 6.8 The thymus gland in the adult, and related structures.

others circulate in the bloodstream. T-lymphocyte production, although most prolific in youth, probably continues throughout life from a resident population of thymic stem cells.

The maturation of the thymus and other lymphoid tissue is stimulated by *thymosin*, a hormone secreted by the epithelial cells that form the framework of the thymus gland. Involution of the gland begins in adolescence and, with increasing age, the effectiveness of the T-lymphocyte response to antigens declines.

Mucosa-associated lymphoid tissue (MALT)

Throughout the body, at strategically placed locations, are collections of lymphoid tissue which, unlike the spleen and thymus, are not enclosed within a capsule. They contain B- and T-lymphocytes, which have migrated from bone marrow and the thymus, and are important in the early detection of invaders. However, as they have no afferent lymphatic vessels, they do not filter lymph, and are therefore not exposed to diseases spread by lymph. MALT is found throughout the gastrointestinal tract, in the respiratory tract and in the genitourinary tract, all systems of the body exposed to the external environment.

The main groups of MALT are the tonsils and Peyer's patches.

Tonsils. These are located in the mouth and throat, and will therefore destroy swallowed and inhaled antigens (see also p. 241).

Aggregated lymphoid follicles (Peyer's patches). These large collections of lymphoid tissue are found in the small intestine, and intercept swallowed antigens (p. 302).

137

Lymph vessel pathology

Learning outcomes

After studying this section, you should be able to:

■ explain the role of lymphatic vessels in the spread of infectious and malignant disease

■ discuss the main causes and consequences of lymphatic obstruction.

The main involvements of lymph vessels are in relation to the spread of disease in the body, and the effects of lymphatic obstruction.

Spread of disease

The materials most commonly spread via the lymph vessels from their original site to the circulating blood are fragments of tumours and infected material.

Tumour fragments

Tumour cells may enter a lymph capillary draining a tumour, or a larger vessel if a tumour has eroded its wall. Cells from a malignant tumour, if not phagocytosed, settle and multiply in the first lymph node they encounter. Later, there may be further spread to other lymph nodes, to the bloodstream and to other parts of the body via the blood. In this sequence of events, each new metastatic tumour becomes a source of malignant cells that may spread by the same routes.

Infection

Infected material may enter lymph vessels either at their origin in the interstitial spaces, or through the walls of larger vessels invaded by microbes when infection spreads locally. If phagocytosis is not effective the infection may spread from node to node, and eventually reach the bloodstream.

Lymphangitis (infection of lymph vessel walls). This occurs in some acute bacterial infections in which the microbes in the lymph draining from the area infect and spread along the walls of lymph vessels, e.g. in acute *Streptococcus pyogenes* infection of the hand, a red line may be seen extending from the hand to the axilla. This is caused by an inflamed superficial lymph vessel and adjacent tissues. The infection may be stopped at the first lymph node or spread through the lymph drainage network to the blood.

Lymphatic obstruction

When a lymph vessel is obstructed, lymph accumulates distal to the obstruction (*lymphoedema*). The amount of resultant swelling and the size of the area affected depend on the size of the vessel involved. Lymphoedema usually leads to low-grade inflammation and fibrosis of the lymph vessel and further lymphoedema. The most common causes are tumours and following surgical removal of lymph nodes.

Tumours

A tumour may grow into, and block, a lymph vessel or node, obstructing the flow of lymph. A large tumour outside the lymphatic system may cause sufficient pressure to stop the flow of lymph.

Surgery

In some surgical procedures lymph nodes are removed because cancer cells may have already spread to them. This aims to prevent growth of secondary tumours in local lymph nodes and further spread of the disease via the lymphatic system, e.g. axillary nodes may be removed during mastectomy.

Diseases of lymph nodes

Learning outcomes

After studying this section, you should be able to:

■ describe the term lymphadenitis, listing its primary causes

■ describe the effects of the two main forms of lymphoma

■ explain why secondary disease of the lymph nodes in commonly found in individuals with cancer.

Lymphadenitis

Acute lymphadenitis (acute infection of lymph nodes) is usually caused by microbes transported in lymph from other areas of infection. The nodes become inflamed, enlarged and congested with blood, and chemotaxis attracts large numbers of phagocytes. If lymph node defences (phagocytes and antibody production) are overwhelmed, the infection can cause abscess formation within the node. Adjacent tissues may become involved, and infected materials transported through other nodes and into the blood.

Acute lymphadenitis is secondary to a number of conditions.

Infectious mononucleosis (glandular fever)

This is a highly contagious viral infection, usually of young adults, spread by direct contact. During the incubation period of 7 to 10 days, viruses multiply in the epithelial cells of the pharynx. They subsequently spread to cervical lymph nodes, then to lymphoid tissue throughout the body.

Clinical features include tonsillitis, lymphadenopathy and splenomegaly. A common complication is myalgic encephalitis (chronic fatigue syndrome, p. 184). Clinical or subclinical infection confers life-long immunity.

Other diseases

Minor lymphadenitis accompanies many infections and indicates the mobilisation of normal protective mechanisms. More serious infection occurs in, e.g. measles, typhoid and cat-scratch fever, and wound or skin infections. Chronic lymphadenitis occurs following unresolved acute infections, in tuberculosis, syphilis and some low-grade infections.

Lymphomas

These are malignant tumours of lymphoid tissue and are classified as either Hodgkin's or non-Hodgkin lymphomas.

Hodgkin's disease

In this disease there is progressive, painless enlargement of lymph nodes throughout the body, as lymphoid tissue within them proliferates. The superficial lymph nodes in the neck are often the first to be noticed. The disease is malignant and the cause is unknown. The prognosis varies considerably but the pattern of spread is predictable because the disease spreads to adjacent nodes and to other tissues in a consistent way. The effectiveness of treatment depends largely on the stage of the disease at which it begins. The disease leads to reduced immunity, because lymphocyte function is depressed, and recurrent infection is therefore common. As lymph nodes enlarge, they may compress adjacent tissues and organs. Anaemia and changes in leukocyte numbers occur if the bone marrow is involved.

Non-Hodgkin lymphomas

These tumours, e.g. *multiple myeloma* and *Burkitt's lymphoma*, may occur in any lymphoid tissue and in bone marrow. They are classified according to the type of cell involved and the degree of malignancy, i.e. low, intermediate or high grade. Low-grade tumours consist of well-differentiated cells and slow progress of the disease, death occurring after a period of years. High-grade lymphomas consist of poorly differentiated cells and rapid progress of the disease, death occurring in weeks or months. Some low- or intermediate-grade tumours change their status to high grade with increased rate of progress.

The expanding lymph nodes may compress adjacent tissues and organs. Immunological deficiency leads to increased incidence of infections, and if the bone marrow or spleen (or both) is involved there may be varying degrees of anaemia and leukopenia.

Malignant neoplastic metastases

Metastatic tumours develop in lymph nodes in any part of the body. Lymph from a tumour may contain cancer cells that are filtered out by the lymph nodes. If not phagocytosed, they multiply, forming metastatic tumours. Nodes nearest the primary tumour are affected first but there may be further spread through the sequence of nodes, eventually reaching the bloodstream.

Disorders of the spleen

139

Learning outcome

After studying this section, you should be able to:

■ identify the main causes of splenomegaly.

Splenomegaly

This is enlargement of the spleen, and is usually secondary to other conditions, e.g. infections, circulatory disorders, blood diseases, malignant neoplasms.

Infections

The spleen may be infected by blood-borne microbes or by local spread of infection. The red pulp becomes congested with blood and there is an accumulation of phagocytes and plasma cells. Acute infections are rare.

Chronic infections. Some chronic non-pyogenic infections cause splenomegaly, but this is usually less severe than in the case of acute infections. The most commonly occurring primary infections include:

• tuberculosis
• typhoid fever

- malaria
- brucellosis (undulant fever)
- infectious mononucleosis.

Circulatory disorders

Splenomegaly due to congestion of blood occurs when the flow of blood through the liver is impeded by, e.g., fibrosis in cirrhosis of liver, or portal venous congestion in right-sided heart failure.

Blood diseases

Splenomegaly may be caused by blood disorders. The spleen enlarges to deal with the extra workload associated with removing damaged, worn out and abnormal blood cells in, e.g., haemolytic and macrocytic anaemia, polycythaemia and chronic myeloid leukaemia.

Splenomegaly may itself cause blood disorders. When the spleen is enlarged for any reason, especially in portal hypertension, excessive and premature haemolysis of red cells or phagocytosis of normal white cells and platelets leads to marked anaemia, leukopenia and thrombocytopenia.

Tumours

Benign and primary malignant tumours of the spleen are rare but blood-spread tumour fragments from elsewhere in the body may cause metastatic tumours. Splenomegaly caused by infiltration of malignant cells is characteristic of some conditions, especially chronic leukaemia, Hodgkin's disease and non-Hodgkin lymphoma.

Diseases of the thymus gland

Learning outcome

After studying this section, you should be able to:

- describe the principal disorders of the thymus gland.

Enlargement of the gland is associated with some autoimmune diseases, such as thyrotoxicosis and Addison's disease.

Tumours are rare, although pressure caused by enlargement of the gland may damage or interfere with the functions of adjacent structures, e.g. the trachea, oesophagus or veins in the neck.

In myasthenia gravis (p. 381), most patients have either thymic hyperplasia (the majority) or thymoma (a minority).

The nervous system

7

The nervous system detects and responds to changes inside and outside the body. Together with the endocrine system, it controls important aspects of body function and maintains homeostasis. Nervous system stimulation provides an immediate response while endocrine activity is, in the main, slower and more prolonged (Ch. 9).

The nervous system consists of the brain, the spinal cord and peripheral nerves. The structure and organisation of the tissues that form these components enables rapid communication between different parts of the body.

Response to changes in the internal environment regulates involuntary functions, such as blood pressure and digestive activity. Response to changes in the external environment maintains posture and other voluntary activities.

For descriptive purposes the parts of the nervous system are grouped as follows:

- the *central nervous system* (CNS), consisting of the brain and the spinal cord

- the *peripheral nervous system* (PNS) consisting of all the nerves outside the brain and spinal cord.

The PNS comprises paired cranial and sacral nerves – some of these are sensory (afferent), some are motor (efferent) and some mixed. It is useful to consider two functional parts within the PNS:

- the sensory division
- the motor division (Fig. 7.1).

In turn the motor division is involved in activities that are:

- *voluntary* – the somatic nervous system (movement of voluntary muscles)
- *involuntary* – the autonomic nervous system (functioning of smooth and cardiac muscle and glands). The autonomic nervous system has two parts: *sympathetic* and *parasympathetic*.

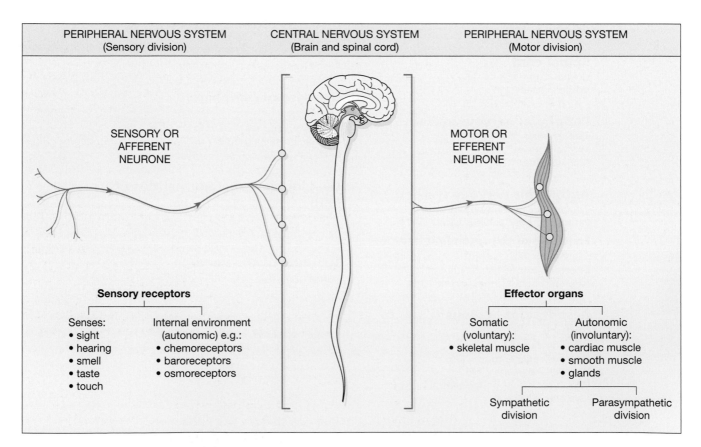

Figure 7.1 Functional components of the nervous system.

Neurones

Learning outcomes

After studying this section you should be able to:

- describe the structure of a myelinated neurone

- compare and contrast the transmission of impulses in myelinated and unmyelinated neurones

- state the functions of sensory and motor nerves

- explain the events that occur following release of a neurotransmitter at a synapse

- name common neurotransmitters.

The nervous system consists of a vast number of cells called *neurones* (Fig. 7.2), supported by a special type of connective tissue, *neuroglia*. Each neurone consists of a *cell body* and its processes, one *axon* and many *dendrites*. Neurones are commonly referred to as nerve cells. Bundles of axons bound together are called *nerves*.

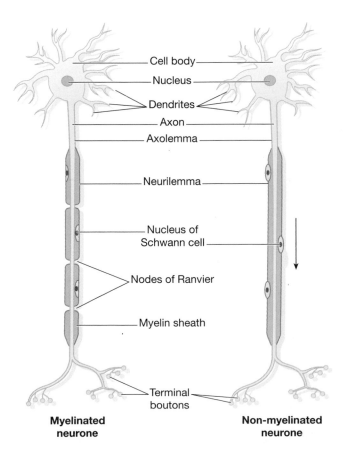

Myelinated neurone **Non-myelinated neurone**

Figure 7.2 The structure of neurones. Arrow indicates direction of impulse conduction.

Neurones cannot divide, and for survival they need a continuous supply of oxygen and glucose. Unlike many other cells, neurones can synthesise chemical energy (ATP) only from glucose. The effects of damage to neurones are described on page 175.

The physiological 'units' of the nervous system are *nerve impulses*, or *action potentials*, which are akin to tiny electrical charges. However, unlike ordinary electrical wires, the neurones are actively involved in conducting nerve impulses. In effect the initial strength of the impulse is maintained throughout the length of the neurone.

Some neurones initiate nerve impulses while others act as 'relay stations' where impulses are passed on and sometimes redirected.

Properties of neurones

Neurones have the characteristics of *irritability* and *conductivity*.

Irritability is the ability to initiate nerve impulses in response to stimuli from:

- outside the body, e.g. touch, light waves
- inside the body, e.g. a change in the concentration of carbon dioxide in the blood alters respiration; a thought may result in voluntary movement.

In the body this stimulation may be described as partly electrical and partly chemical–electrical in that motor neurones and sensory nerve endings initiate nerve impulses, and chemical in the transmission of impulses between one neurone and the next or between a neurone and an effector organ.

Conductivity means the ability to transmit an impulse.

Cell bodies

Nerve cells vary considerably in size and shape but they are all too small to be seen by the naked eye. Cell bodies form the *grey matter* of the nervous system and are found at the periphery of the brain and in the centre of the spinal cord. Groups of cell bodies are called *nuclei* in the central nervous system and *ganglia* in the peripheral nervous system. An important exception is the basal ganglia (nuclei) situated within the cerebrum (p. 154).

Axons and dendrites

Axons and dendrites are extensions of cell bodies and form the *white matter* of the nervous system. Axons are found deep in the brain and in groups, called *tracts*, at the periphery of the spinal cord. They are referred to as *nerves* or *nerve fibres* outside the brain and spinal cord.

Axons

Each nerve cell has only one axon, carrying nerve impulses away from the cell body. They are usually longer than the dendrites, sometimes as long as 100 cm.

Structure of an axon

The membrane of the axon is called the *axolemma* and it encloses the cytoplasmic extension of the cell body.

Large axons and those of peripheral nerves are surrounded by a *myelin sheath* (Fig. 7.3A). This consists of a series of *Schwann cells* arranged along the length of the axon. Each one is wrapped around the axon so that it is covered by a number of concentric layers of Schwann cell plasma membrane. Between the layers of plasma membrane there is a small amount of fatty substance called *myelin*. The outermost layer of Schwann cell plasma membrane is sometimes called the *neurilemma*. There are tiny areas of exposed axolemma between adjacent Schwann cells, called *nodes of Ranvier,* which assist the rapid transmission of nerve impulses in myelinated neurones.

Postganglionic fibres and some small fibres in the central nervous system are *non-myelinated*. In this type a number of axons are embedded in Schwann cell plasma membranes (Fig. 7.3B). The adjacent Schwann cells are in close association and there is no exposed axolemma. The speed of transmission of nerve impulses is significantly slower in non-myelinated fibres.

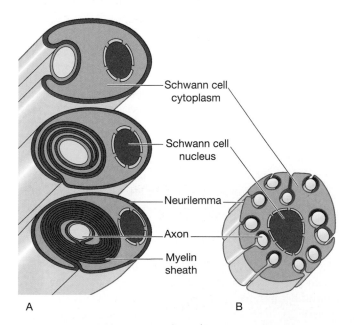

Figure 7.3 Nerve fibres. A. Myelinated. B. Non-myelinated.

Schwann cell cytoplasm

Schwann cell nucleus

Neurilemma

Axon

Myelin sheath

A
B

Dendrites

The dendrites are the many short processes that receive and carry incoming impulses towards cell bodies. They have the same structure as axons but are usually shorter and branching. In motor neurones they form part of synapses (see Fig. 7.7A) and in sensory neurones they form the sensory receptors that respond to specific stimuli.

The nerve impulse (action potential)

An impulse is initiated by stimulation of sensory nerve endings or by the passage of an impulse from another nerve. Transmission of the impulse, or action potential, is due to movement of ions across the nerve cell membrane. In the resting state the nerve cell membrane is *polarised* due to differences in the concentrations of ions across the plasma membrane. This means that there is a different electrical charge on each side of the membrane, which is called the *resting membrane potential*. At rest the charge on the outside is positive and inside it is negative. The principal ions involved are:

- sodium (Na^+), the main extracellular cation
- potassium (K^+), the main intracellular cation.

In the resting state there is a continual tendency for these ions to diffuse along their concentration gradients, i.e. K^+ outwards and Na^+ into cells. When stimulated, the permeability of the nerve cell membrane to these ions changes. Initially Na^+ floods into the neurone from the ECF causing *depolarisation*, creating a *nerve impulse* or *action potential*. Depolarisation is very rapid, enabling the conduction of a nerve impulse along the entire length of a neurone in a few milliseconds (ms). It passes from the point of stimulation in one direction only, i.e. away from the point of stimulation towards the area of resting potential. The one-way direction of transmission is ensured because following depolarisation it takes time for *repolarisation* to occur.

During this process K^+ floods out of the neurone and the movement of these ions returns the membrane potential to its resting state. This is called the *refractory period* during which restimulation is not possible. As the neurone returns to its original resting state, the action of the *sodium–potassium pump* expels Na^+ from the cell in exchange for K^+ (see p. 33).

In myelinated neurones, the insulating properties of the myelin sheath prevent the movement of ions. Therefore electrical changes across the membrane can only occur at the gaps in the myelin sheath, i.e. at the nodes of Ranvier. When an impulse occurs at one node, depolarisation passes along the myelin sheath to the next node so that the flow of current appears to 'leap' from one node to the next. This is called *saltatory conduction* (Fig. 7.4).

The speed of conduction depends on the diameter of the neurone: the larger the diameter, the faster the conduction. Myelinated fibres conduct impulses faster than unmyelinated fibres because saltatory conduction is faster than complete conduction, or *simple propagation* (Fig. 7.5). The fastest fibres can conduct impulses to, e.g., skeletal muscles at a rate of 130 metres per second while the slowest impulses travel at 0.5 metres per second.

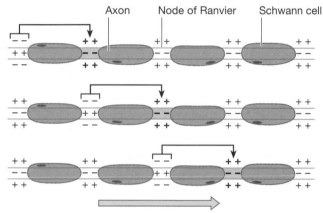

Direction of transmission of nerve impulse

Figure 7.4 Saltatory conduction of an impulse in a myelinated nerve fibre.

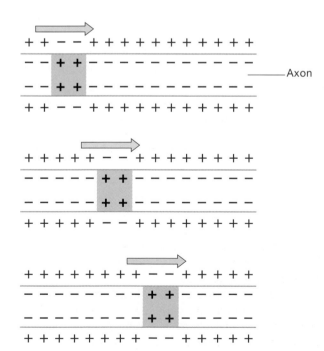

Figure 7.5 Simple propagation of an impulse in a non-myelinated nerve fibre. Arrows indicate the direction of impulse transmission.

Types of nerves (see Fig. 7.1)

Sensory or afferent nerves

When action potentials are generated by sensory receptors on the dendrites of these neurones, they are transmitted to the spinal cord by the sensory nerve fibres. The impulses may then pass to the brain or to connector neurones of reflex arcs in the spinal cord (see p. 160).

Sensory receptors

Specialised endings of sensory neurones respond to different stimuli (changes) inside and outside the body.

Somatic, cutaneous or *common senses.* These originate in the skin. They are: pain, touch, heat and cold. Sensory nerve endings in the skin are fine branching filaments without myelin sheaths (Fig. 7.6). When stimulated, an impulse is generated and transmitted by the sensory nerves to the brain where the sensation is perceived.

Proprioceptor senses. These originate in muscles and joints and contribute to the maintenance of balance and posture.

Special senses. These are sight, hearing, balance, smell and taste (see Ch. 8).

Autonomic afferent nerves. These originate in internal organs, glands and tissues, e.g. baroreceptors, chemoreceptors, and are associated with reflex regulation of involuntary activity and visceral pain.

Motor or efferent nerves

Motor nerves originate in the brain, spinal cord and autonomic ganglia. They transmit impulses to the effector organs: muscles and glands. There are two types:

- *somatic nerves* – involved in voluntary and reflex skeletal muscle contraction

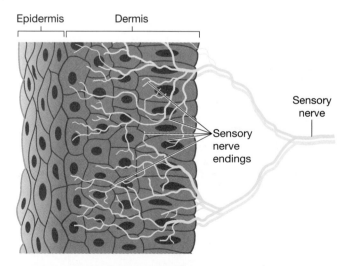

Figure 7.6 Sensory nerve endings in the skin.

145

- *autonomic nerves* (sympathetic and parasympathetic) – involved in cardiac and smooth muscle contraction and glandular secretion.

Mixed nerves

In the spinal cord, sensory and motor nerves are arranged in separate groups, or *tracts*. Outside the spinal cord, when sensory and motor nerves are enclosed within the same sheath of connective tissue they are called *mixed nerves*.

The synapse and neurotransmitters

There is always more than one neurone involved in the transmission of a nerve impulse from its origin to its destination, whether it is sensory or motor. There is no physical contact between these neurones. The point at which the nerve impulse passes from one to another is the *synapse* (Fig. 7.7). At its free end, the axon of the *presynaptic neurone* breaks up into minute branches that

terminate in small swellings called *synaptic knobs*, or terminal boutons. These are in close proximity to the dendrites and the cell body of the *postsynaptic neurone*. The space between them is the *synaptic cleft*. In the ends of synaptic knobs are spherical *synaptic vesicles*, containing a chemical, the *neurotransmitter*, which is released into synaptic clefts. Neurotransmitters are synthesised by nerve cells, actively transported along the axons and stored in the synaptic vesicles. They are released by exocytosis in response to the action potential and diffuse across the synaptic cleft. They act on specific receptor sites on the postsynaptic membranes. Their action is short lived, because immediately they have stimulated the postsynaptic neurone or effector organ, such as a muscle fibre, they are either inactivated by enzymes or taken back into the synaptic knob. Knowledge of the action of the common neurotransmitters is important because some drugs mimic, neutralise or prolong their effect. Usually neurotransmitters have an excitatory effect at the synapse but they are sometimes inhibitory.

The neurotransmitters in the brain and spinal cord include *noradrenaline (norepinephrine), adrenaline (epinephrine), dopamine, histamine, serotonin, gamma aminobutyric acid (GABA)* and *acetylcholine*. Other substances, such as enkephalins, endorphins and substance P, have specialised roles in, for example, transmission of pain signals. Figure 7.8 summarises the neurotransmitters of the peripheral nervous system.

Somatic nerves carry impulses directly to the synapses at skeletal muscles: the neuromuscular junctions (p. 416). In the autonomic nervous system, efferent impulses travel along two nerves (preganglionic and postganglionic) and across two synapses to the effector organs, e.g. smooth muscle and glands, in both the sympathetic and the parasympathetic divisions.

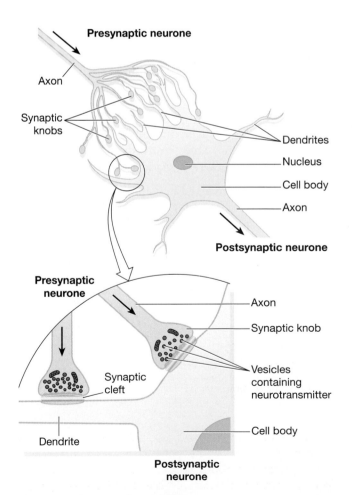

Figure 7.7 Diagram of a synapse.

Central nervous system

Learning outcomes

After studying this section you should be able to:

- outline the functions of 4 types of neuroglial cells
- describe the structure of the meninges
- describe the flow of cerebrospinal fluid in the brain
- list the functions of cerebrospinal fluid.

The central nervous system consists of the brain and the spinal cord.

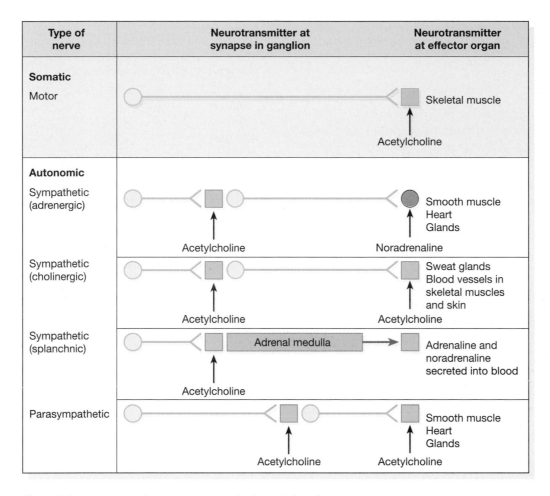

Figure 7.8 **Neurotransmitters at synapses in the peripheral nervous system.**

Neuroglia

The neurones of the central nervous system are supported by four types of non-excitable *glial cells* that make up a quarter to a half of the volume of brain tissue. Unlike nerve cells, these continue to replicate throughout life. They are *astrocytes, oligodendrocytes, microglia* and *ependymal cells*.

Astrocytes

These cells form the main supporting tissue of the central nervous system. They are star shaped with fine branching processes and they lie in a mucopolysaccharide ground substance. At the free ends of some of the processes there are small swellings called *foot processes*. Astrocytes are found in large numbers adjacent to blood vessels with their foot processes forming a sleeve round them. This means that the blood is separated from the neurones by the capillary wall and a layer of astrocyte foot processes which together constitute the *blood–brain barrier* (Fig. 7.9). Their functions are analogous to those of fibroblasts elsewhere in the body.

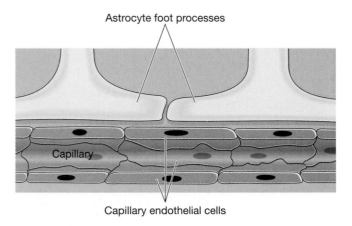

Figure 7.9 **Blood–brain barrier.**

The blood–brain barrier is a selective barrier that protects the brain from potentially toxic substances and chemical variations in the blood, e.g. after a meal. Oxygen, carbon dioxide, alcohol, barbiturates, glucose and lipophilic substances quickly cross the barrier into the brain. Some large molecules, drugs, inorganic ions and amino acids pass slowly from the blood to the brain.

Oligodendrocytes

These cells are smaller than astrocytes and are found:

- in clusters round nerve cell bodies in grey matter where they are thought to have a supportive function
- adjacent to, and along the length of, myelinated nerve fibres.

The oligodendrocytes form and maintain myelin, having the same functions as Schwann cells in peripheral nerves.

Microglia

These cells are derived from monocytes that migrate from the blood into the nervous system before birth. They are found mainly in the area of blood vessels. They enlarge and become phagocytic, removing microbes and damaged tissue, in areas of inflammation and cell destruction.

Ependymal cells

These cells form the epithelial lining of the ventricles of the brain and the central canal of the spinal cord. Those cells that form the choroid plexuses of the ventricles secrete cerebrospinal fluid.

The meninges

The brain and spinal cord are completely surrounded by three layers of tissue, the *meninges*, lying between the skull and the brain, and between the vertebral foramina and the spinal cord. Named from outside inwards they are the:

- dura mater
- arachnoid mater
- pia mater (Fig. 7.10).

The dura and arachnoid maters are separated by a potential space, the *subdural space*. The arachnoid and pia maters are separated by the *subarachnoid space*, containing *cerebrospinal fluid*.

Dura mater

The cerebral dura mater consists of two layers of dense fibrous tissue. The outer layer takes the place of the periosteum on the inner surface of the skull bones and the inner layer provides a protective covering for the brain. There is only a potential space between the two layers except where the inner layer sweeps inwards between the cerebral hemispheres to form the *falx cerebri*; between the cerebellar hemispheres to form the *falx cerebelli*; and between the cerebrum and cerebellum to form the *tentorium cerebelli*.

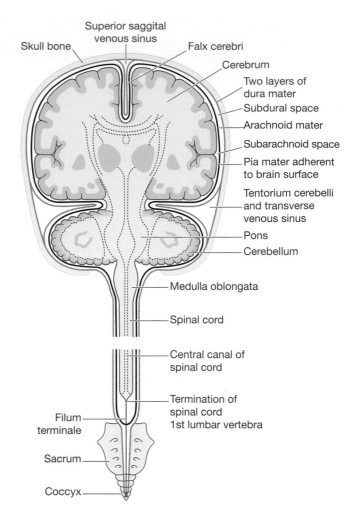

Figure 7.10 The meninges covering the brain and spinal cord.

Venous blood from the brain drains into venous sinuses between the layers of dura mater. The *superior sagittal sinus* is formed by the falx cerebri, and the tentorium cerebelli forms the *straight* and *transverse sinuses* (see Figs 5.36 and 5.37, pp. 99 and 100).

Spinal dura mater forms a loose sheath round the spinal cord, extending from the foramen magnum to the second sacral vertebra. Thereafter it encloses the *filum terminale* and fuses with the periosteum of the coccyx. It is an extension of the inner layer of cerebral dura mater and is separated from the periosteum of the vertebrae and ligaments within the neural canal by the *epidural* or *extradural* space, containing blood vessels and areolar tissue. It is attached to the foramen magnum and, by a number of fibrous slips, to the posterior longitudinal ligament at intervals along its length. Nerves entering and leaving the spinal cord pass through the epidural space. These attachments stabilise the spinal cord in the neural canal. Dyes, used for diagnostic purposes, and local anaesthetics or analgesics to relieve pain, may be injected into the epidural space.

Arachnoid mater

This is a layer of fibrous tissue that lies between the dura and pia maters. It is separated from the dura mater by the *subdural space*, and from the pia mater by the *subarachnoid space*, containing *cerebrospinal fluid*. The arachnoid mater passes over the convolutions of the brain and accompanies the inner layer of dura mater in the formation of the falx cerebri, tentorium cerebelli and falx cerebelli. It continues downwards to envelop the spinal cord and ends by merging with the dura mater at the level of the 2nd sacral vertebra.

Pia mater

This is a delicate layer of connective tissue containing many minute blood vessels. It adheres to the brain, completely covering the convolutions and dipping into each fissure. It continues downwards surrounding the spinal cord. Beyond the end of the cord it continues as the *filum terminale*, pierces the arachnoid tube and goes on, with the dura mater, to fuse with the periosteum of the coccyx.

Ventricles of the brain and the cerebrospinal fluid

Within the brain there are four irregular-shaped cavities, or *ventricles*, containing *cerebrospinal fluid* (CSF) (Fig. 7.11). They are:

- right and left lateral ventricles
- third ventricle
- fourth ventricle.

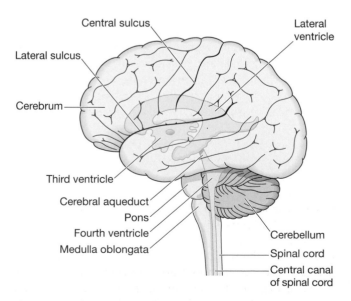

Figure 7.11 The positions of the ventricles of the brain (in yellow) superimposed on its surface. Viewed from the left side.

Labels: Central sulcus, Lateral sulcus, Cerebrum, Third ventricle, Cerebral aqueduct, Pons, Fourth ventricle, Medulla oblongata, Lateral ventricle, Cerebellum, Spinal cord, Central canal of spinal cord

The lateral ventricles

These cavities lie within the cerebral hemispheres, one on each side of the median plane just below the corpus callosum. They are separated from each other by a thin membrane, the septum lucidum, and are lined with ciliated epithelium. They communicate with the third ventricle by *interventricular foramina*.

The third ventricle

The third ventricle is a cavity situated below the lateral ventricles between the two parts of the thalamus. It communicates with the fourth ventricle by a canal, the *cerebral aqueduct*.

The fourth ventricle

The fourth ventricle is a diamond-shaped cavity situated below and behind the third ventricle, between the *cerebellum* and *pons*. It is continuous below with the *central canal* of the spinal cord and communicates with the subarachnoid space by foramina in its roof. Cerebrospinal fluid enters the subarachnoid space through these openings and through the open distal end of the central canal of the spinal cord.

Cerebrospinal fluid (CSF)

Cerebrospinal fluid is secreted into each ventricle of the brain by *choroid plexuses*. These are vascular areas where there is a proliferation of blood vessels surrounded by ependymal cells in the lining of ventricle walls. CSF passes back into the blood through tiny diverticula of arachnoid mater, called *arachnoid villi* (arachnoid granulations), which project into the venous sinuses. The movement of CSF from the subarachnoid space to venous sinuses depends upon the difference in pressure on each side of the walls of the arachnoid villi, which act as one-way valves. When CSF pressure is higher than venous pressure CSF passes into the blood and when the venous pressure is higher the arachnoid villi collapse, preventing the passage of blood constituents into the CSF. There may also be some reabsorption of CSF by cells in the walls of the ventricles.

From the roof of the fourth ventricle CSF flows through foramina into the subarachnoid space and completely surrounds the brain and spinal cord (Fig. 7.12). There is no intrinsic system of CSF circulation but its movement is aided by pulsating blood vessels, respiration and changes of posture.

CSF is secreted continuously at a rate of about 0.5 ml per minute, i.e. 720 ml per day. The volume remains fairly constant at about 120 ml, which means that absorption keeps pace with secretion. CSF pressure may be measured using a vertical tube attached to a lumbar puncture needle. It remains fairly constant at about 10 cm H_2O

149

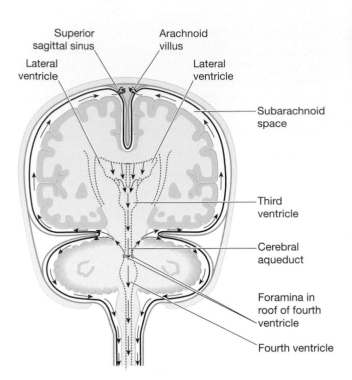

Superior sagittal sinus — Arachnoid villus

Lateral ventricle — Lateral ventricle

Subarachnoid space

Third ventricle

Cerebral aqueduct

Foramina in roof of fourth ventricle

Fourth ventricle

Figure 7.12 Arrows showing the flow of cerebrospinal fluid.

when the individual is lying on his side and about 30 cm H_2O when sitting up. If the brain is enlarged by, e.g. haemorrhage or tumour, some compensation is made by a reduction in the amount of CSF. When the volume of brain tissue is reduced, such as in degeneration or atrophy, the volume of CSF is increased. CSF is a clear, slightly alkaline fluid with a specific gravity of 1.005, consisting of:

- water
- mineral salts
- glucose
- plasma proteins: small amounts of albumin and globulin
- creatinine ⎫
- urea ⎭ small amounts
- a few leukocytes.

Functions of cerebrospinal fluid

- It supports and protects the brain and spinal cord.
- It maintains a uniform pressure around these delicate structures.
- It acts as a cushion and shock absorber between the brain and the cranial bones.
- It keeps the brain and spinal cord moist and there may be interchange of substances between CSF and nerve cells, such as nutrients and waste products.

Brain

The brain constitutes about one-fiftieth of the body weight and lies within the cranial cavity. The parts are (Fig. 7.13):

- cerebrum
- midbrain
- pons ⎫
- medulla oblongata ⎭ the brain stem
- cerebellum.

Blood supply to the brain

The circulus arteriosus and its contributing arteries (see Fig. 5.33, p. 99) play a vital role in maintaining a constant supply of oxygen and glucose to the brain even when a contributing artery is narrowed or the head is moved. The brain receives about 15% of the cardiac output, approximately 750 ml of blood per minute. Autoregulation keeps blood flow to the brain constant by adjusting the diameter of the arterioles across a wide range of arterial blood pressure (about 65–140 mmHg) with changes occurring only outside these limits.

Cerebrum

This is the largest part of the brain and it occupies the anterior and middle cranial fossae (see Fig. 16.9, p. 391). It is divided by a deep cleft, the *longitudinal cerebral fissure*, into *right* and *left cerebral hemispheres*, each containing one of the lateral ventricles. Deep within the brain

For descriptive purposes each hemisphere of the cerebrum is divided into *lobes* which take the names of the bones of the cranium under which they lie:

- frontal
- parietal
- temporal
- occipital.

The boundaries of the lobes are marked by deep sulci. These are the *central, lateral* and *parieto-occipital sulci* (Fig. 7.14).

Interior of the cerebrum (Fig. 7.15)

The surface of the cerebral cortex is composed of grey matter (nerve cell bodies). Within the cerebrum the lobes are connected by masses of nerve fibres, or *tracts*, which

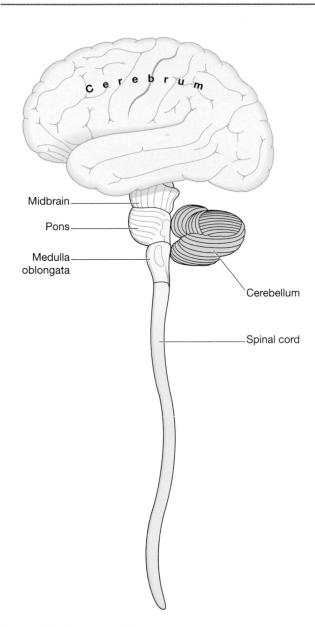

Figure 7.13 The parts of the central nervous system.

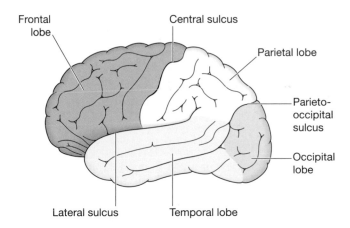

Figure 7.14 The lobes and principal sulci of the cerebrum. Viewed from the left side.

151

the hemispheres are connected by a mass of white matter (nerve fibres) called the *corpus callosum*. The falx cerebri is formed by the dura mater (see Fig. 7.10). It separates the two hemispheres and penetrates to the depth of the corpus callosum. The superficial (peripheral) part of the cerebrum is composed of nerve cell bodies or grey matter, forming the *cerebral cortex*, and the deeper layers consist of nerve fibres or white matter.

The cerebral cortex shows many infoldings or furrows of varying depth. The exposed areas of the folds are the *gyri* or *convolutions* and these are separated by *sulci* (fissures). These convolutions greatly increase the surface area of the cerebrum.

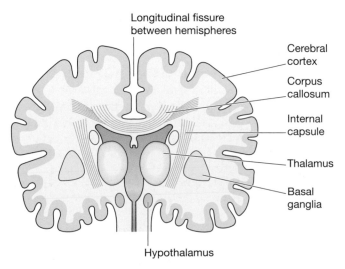

Figure 7.15 A section of the cerebrum showing some connecting nerve fibres.

make up the white matter of the brain. The afferent and efferent fibres linking the different parts of the brain and spinal cord are as follows.

- *Association (arcuate) tracts* connect different parts of a cerebral hemisphere by extending from one gyrus to another, some of which are adjacent and some distant.
- *Commissural tracts* connect corresponding areas of the two cerebral hemispheres; the largest and most important commissure is the *corpus callosum.*
- *Projection tracts* connect the cerebral cortex with grey matter of lower parts of the brain and with the spinal cord, e.g. the internal capsule.

The *internal capsule* is an important projection tract that lies deep within the brain between the basal ganglia (nuclei) and the thalamus. Many nerve impulses passing to and from the cerebral cortex are carried by fibres that form the internal capsule. Motor fibres within the internal capsule form the *pyramidal tracts* (corticospinal tracts) that cross over (decussate) at the medulla oblongata.

Functions of the cerebral cortex

There are three main varieties of activity associated with the cerebral cortex:

- mental activities involved in memory, intelligence, sense of responsibility, thinking, reasoning, moral sense and learning are attributed to the *higher centres*
- sensory perception, including the perception of pain, temperature, touch, sight, hearing, taste and smell
- initiation and control of skeletal (voluntary) muscle contraction.

Functional areas of the cerebral cortex

(Fig. 7.16)

The main functional areas of the cerebral cortex have been identified but it is unlikely that any area is associated exclusively with only one function. Except where specially mentioned, the different areas are active in both hemispheres; however, there is some variation between individuals. There are different types of functional areas:

- motor, which direct skeletal (voluntary) muscle movements
- sensory, which receive and decode sensory impulses enabling sensory perception
- association, which are concerned with integration and processing of complex mental functions such as intelligence, memory, reasoning, judgement and emotions.

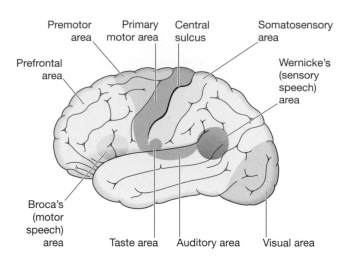

Figure 7.16 The cerebrum showing the main functional areas.

In general, motor impulses leave from the anterior part of each cerebral hemisphere while sensory impulses arrive at the posterior part, i.e. areas behind the central sulcus.

Motor areas of the cerebral cortex

The primary motor area. This lies in the frontal lobe immediately anterior to the central sulcus. The cell bodies are pyramid shaped (Betz's cells) and they initiate the contraction of skeletal muscles. A nerve fibre (the upper motor neurone) from a Betz's cell passes downwards through the internal capsule to the medulla oblongata where it crosses to the opposite side then descends in the spinal cord. At the appropriate level in the spinal cord the nerve impulse crosses a synapse to stimulate a second neurone (the lower motor neurone) that terminates at the motor end-plate of a muscle fibre (Fig. 7.17). This means that the motor area of the right hemisphere of the cerebrum controls voluntary muscle movement on the left side of the body and vice versa. Damage to either of these neurones may result in paralysis.

In the motor area of the cerebrum the body is represented upside down, i.e. the uppermost cells control the feet and those in the lowest part control the head, neck, face and fingers (Fig. 7.18A). The sizes of the areas of cortex representing different parts of the body are proportional to the complexity of movement of the body part, not to its size. Figure 7.18A shows that, in comparison with the trunk, the hand, foot, tongue and lips are represented by large cortical areas.

Broca's (motor speech) area. This is situated in the frontal lobe just above the lateral sulcus and controls muscle movements necessary for speech. It is dominant in the left hemisphere in right-handed people and vice versa.

152

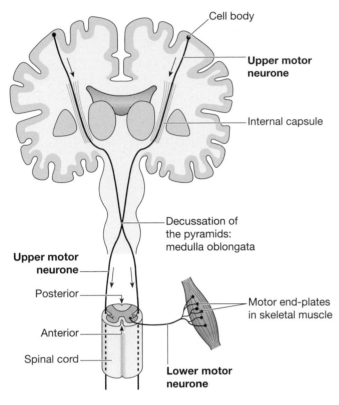

Figure 7.17 The motor nerve pathways: upper and lower motor neurones.

Sensory areas of the cerebral cortex

The somatosensory area. This is the area immediately behind the central sulcus. Here sensations of pain, temperature, pressure and touch, awareness of muscular movement and the position of joints are perceived. The somatosensory area of the right hemisphere receives impulses from the left side of the body and vice versa. The size of the cortical areas representing different parts of the body (Fig. 7.18B) is proportional to the extent of sensory innervation, e.g. the large area for the face is consistent with the extensive sensory nerve supply by the three branches of the trigeminal nerves (5th cranial nerves).

The auditory (hearing) area. This lies immediately below the lateral sulcus within the temporal lobe. The nerve cells receive and interpret impulses transmitted from the inner ear by the cochlear (auditory) part of the vestibulocochlear nerves (8th cranial nerves).

The olfactory (smell) area. This lies deep within the temporal lobe where impulses from the nose, transmitted via the olfactory nerves (1st cranial nerves), are received and interpreted.

The taste area. This lies just above the lateral sulcus in the deep layers of the somatosensory area. Here, impulses from sensory receptors in taste buds are received and perceived as taste.

153

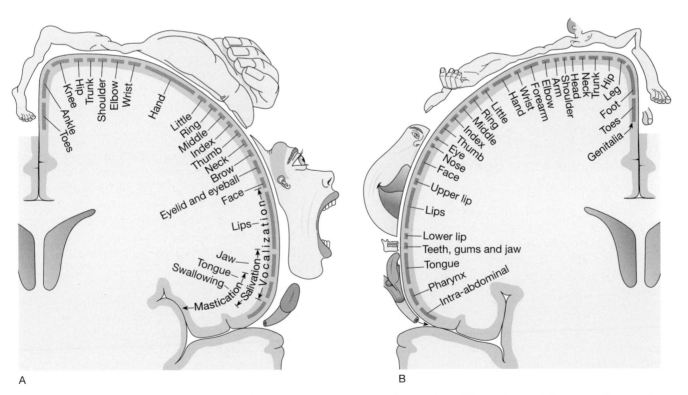

A

B

Figure 7.18 A. The *motor homunculus* showing how the body is represented in the motor area of the cerebrum. **B.** The *sensory homunculus* showing how the body is represented in the sensory area of the cerebrum. (Both **A** and **B** are from Penfield W, Rasmussen T 1950 The cerebral cortex of man. Macmillan, New York. © 1950 Macmillan Publishing Co., renewed 1978 Theodore Rasmussen.)

The visual area. This lies behind the parieto-occipital sulcus and includes the greater part of the occipital lobe. The optic nerves (2nd cranial nerves) pass from the eye to this area, which receives and interprets the impulses as visual impressions.

Association areas

These are connected to each other and other areas of the cerebral cortex by association tracts and some are outlined below. They receive, coordinate and interpret impulses from the sensory and motor cortices permitting higher cognitive abilities and, although Figure 7.19 depicts some of the areas involved, their functions are much more complex.

The premotor area. This lies in the frontal lobe immediately anterior to the motor area. The neurones here coordinate movement initiated by the primary motor cortex, ensuring that learned patterns of movement can be repeated. For example, in tying a shoelace or writing, many muscles contract but the movements must be coordinated and carried out in a particular sequence. Such a pattern of movement, when established, is described as *manual dexterity.*

The prefrontal area. This extends anteriorly from the premotor area to include the remainder of the frontal lobe. It is a large area and is more highly developed in humans than in other animals. Intellectual functions controlled here include perception and comprehension of the passage of time, the ability to anticipate consequences of events and the normal management of emotions.

Wernicke's (sensory speech) area. This is situated in the temporal lobe adjacent to the parieto-occipitotemporal area. It is here that the spoken word is perceived, and comprehension and intelligence are based. Understanding language is central to higher mental functions as they are language based. This area is dominant in the left hemisphere in right-handed people and vice versa.

The parieto-occipitotemporal area. This lies behind the somatosensory area and includes most of the parietal lobe. Its functions are thought to include spatial awareness, interpreting written language and the ability to name objects (Fig. 7.19). It has been suggested that objects can be recognised by touch alone because of the knowledge from past experience (memory) retained in this area.

Other areas of the cerebrum

Deep within the cerebral hemispheres there are groups of cell bodies called *nuclei*, the exception being those that form the basal ganglia, which act as relay stations where impulses are passed from one neurone to the next in a chain. Important masses of grey matter include the:

- basal ganglia
- thalamus
- hypothalamus.

Basal ganglia. These are areas of grey matter, lying deep within the cerebral hemispheres, with connections to the cerebral cortex and thalamus. The basal ganglia form part of the extrapyramidal tracts and are involved in initiation and fine control of complex movement, and learned coordinated activities. If control is inadequate or absent, movements are jerky, clumsy and uncoordinated.

Thalamus. The thalamus consists of two masses of nerve cells and fibres situated within the cerebral hemispheres just below the corpus callosum, one on each side of the third ventricle. Sensory input from the skin, viscera and special sense organs is relayed to the thalamus before redistribution to the cerebrum.

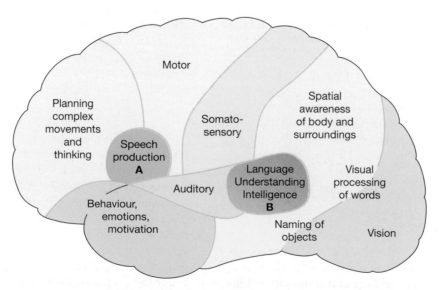

Figure 7.19 Areas of the cerebral cortex involved in higher mental functions. A. Broca's area. B. Wernicke's area.

Hypothalamus. The hypothalamus is composed of a number of groups of nerve cells. It is situated below and in front of the thalamus, immediately above the *pituitary gland*. The hypothalamus is linked to the posterior lobe of the pituitary gland by nerve fibres and to the anterior lobe by a complex system of blood vessels. Through these connections, the hypothalamus controls the output of hormones from both lobes of the gland (see p. 213).

Other functions of the hypothalamus include control of:

- the autonomic nervous system (p. 170)
- appetite and satiety
- thirst and water balance
- body temperature (p. 361)
- emotional reactions, e.g. pleasure, fear, rage
- sexual behaviour including mating and child rearing
- biological clocks or circadian rhythms, e.g. sleeping and waking cycles, body temperature and secretion of some hormones.

Brain stem

Midbrain

The midbrain is the area of the brain situated around the cerebral aqueduct between the cerebrum above and the *pons* below. It consists of nuclei and nerve fibres (tracts), which connect the cerebrum with lower parts of the brain and with the spinal cord. The nuclei act as relay stations for the ascending and descending nerve fibres.

Pons

The pons is situated in front of the cerebellum, below the midbrain and above the medulla oblongata. It consists mainly of nerve fibres (white matter) that form a bridge between the two hemispheres of the cerebellum, and of fibres passing between the higher levels of the brain and the spinal cord. There are nuclei within the pons that act as relay stations and some of these are associated with the cranial nerves. Others form the *pneumotaxic* and *apnoustic centres* that operate in conjunction with the respiratory centre in the medulla oblongata.

The anatomical structure of the pons differs from that of the cerebrum in that the cell bodies (grey matter) lie deeply and the nerve fibres are on the surface.

Medulla oblongata

The medulla oblongata, or simply the medulla, extends from the pons above and is continuous with the spinal cord below. It is about 2.5 cm long and it lies just within the cranium above the foramen magnum. Its anterior and posterior surfaces are marked by central fissures. The outer aspect is composed of white matter, which passes between the brain and the spinal cord, and grey matter, which lies centrally. Some cells constitute relay stations for sensory nerves passing from the spinal cord to the cerebrum.

The vital centres, consisting of groups of cells (nuclei) associated with autonomic reflex activity, lie in its deeper structure. These are the:

- cardiovascular centre
- respiratory centre
- reflex centres of vomiting, coughing, sneezing and swallowing.

The medulla oblongata has several special features:

- *Decussation (crossing) of the pyramids.* In the medulla, motor nerves descending from the motor area in the cerebrum to the spinal cord in the pyramidal (corticospinal) tracts cross from one side to the other. This means that the left hemisphere of the cerebrum controls the right half of the body, and vice versa. These tracts are the main pathway for impulses to skeletal (voluntary) muscles.
- *Sensory decussation.* Some of the sensory nerves ascending to the cerebrum from the spinal cord cross from one side to the other in the medulla. Others decussate at lower levels, i.e. in the spinal cord.
- *The cardiovascular centre* (CVC) controls the rate and force of cardiac contraction (p. 91). It also controls blood pressure (p. 90). Within the CVC, other groups of nerve cells forming the *vasomotor centre* (p. 91) control the diameter of the blood vessels, especially the small arteries and arterioles, which have a large proportion of smooth muscle fibres in their walls. The vasomotor centre is stimulated by the arterial baroreceptors, body temperature and emotions such as sexual excitement and anger. Pain usually causes vasoconstriction although severe pain may cause vasodilatation, a fall in blood pressure and fainting.
- *The respiratory centre* controls the rate and depth of respiration. From here, nerve impulses pass to the phrenic and intercostal nerves which stimulate contraction of the diaphragm and intercostal muscles, thus initiating inspiration. It functions in close association with the pnuemotaxic and apneustic centres in the pons (see p. 255).
- *Reflex centres.* Irritants present in the stomach or respiratory tract stimulate the medulla oblongata, activating the reflex centres. The vomiting, coughing or sneezing reflexes then attempt to expel the irritant.

155

Reticular formation

The reticular formation is a collection of neurones in the core of the brain stem, surrounded by neural pathways that conduct ascending and descending nerve impulses between the brain and the spinal cord. It has a vast number of synaptic links with other parts of the brain and is therefore constantly receiving 'information' being transmitted in ascending and descending tracts.

Functions

The reticular formation is involved in:

- coordination of skeletal muscle activity associated with voluntary motor movement and the maintenance of balance
- coordination of activity controlled by the autonomic nervous system, e.g. cardiovascular, respiratory and gastrointestinal activity
- selective awareness that functions through the *reticular activating system* (RAS), which selectively blocks or passes sensory information to the cerebral cortex, e.g. the slight sound made by a sick child moving in bed may arouse his mother but the noise of regularly passing trains may be suppressed.

Cerebellum

The cerebellum (Fig. 7.20) is situated behind the pons and immediately below the posterior portion of the cerebrum occupying the posterior cranial fossa. It is ovoid in shape and has two hemispheres, separated by a narrow median strip called the *vermis*. Grey matter forms the surface of the cerebellum, and the white matter lies deeply.

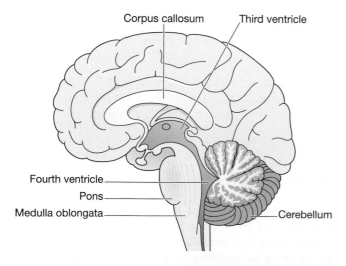

Figure 7.20 The cerebellum and associated structures.

Corpus callosum — Third ventricle
Fourth ventricle
Pons
Medulla oblongata
Cerebellum

Functions

The cerebellum is concerned with the coordination of voluntary muscular movement, posture and balance. Cerebellar activity is not under voluntary control. The cerebellum controls and coordinates the movements of various groups of muscles ensuring smooth, even, precise actions. It coordinates activities associated with the *maintenance of posture, balance* and *equilibrium*. The sensory input for these functions is derived from the muscles and joints, the eyes and the ears. *Proprioceptor impulses* from the muscles and joints indicate their position in relation to the body as a whole, and those impulses from the eyes and the semicircular canals in the ears provide information about the position of the head in space. Impulses from the cerebellum influence the contraction of skeletal muscle so that balance and posture are maintained.

The cerebellum may also have a role in learning and language processing.

Damage to the cerebellum results in clumsy uncoordinated muscular movement, staggering gait and inability to carry out smooth, steady, precise movements.

Spinal cord

Learning outcomes

After studying this section you should be able to:

- describe the gross structure of the spinal cord
- state the functions of the sensory (afferent) nerve tracts in the spinal cord
- state the functions of the motor (efferent) nerve tracts in the spinal cord
- explain the events of a simple reflex arc.

The spinal cord is the elongated, almost cylindrical part of the central nervous system, which is suspended in the vertebral canal surrounded by the meninges and cerebrospinal fluid (Fig. 7.21). It is continuous above with the medulla oblongata and extends from the upper border of the atlas to the lower border of the 1st lumbar vertebra (Fig. 7.22). It is approximately 45 cm long in adult males, and is about the thickness of the little finger. When a specimen of cerebrospinal fluid is required it is taken from the subarachnoid space at a point below the end of the cord, i.e. below the level of the 2nd lumbar vertebra. This procedure is called *lumbar puncture*.

Except for the cranial nerves, the spinal cord is the nervous tissue link between the brain and the rest of

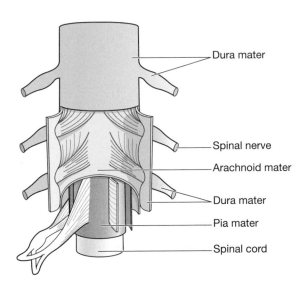

Figure 7.21 The meninges covering the spinal cord. Each cut away to show the underlying layers.

the body (Fig. 7.23). Nerves conveying impulses from the brain to the various organs and tissues descend through the spinal cord. At the appropriate level they leave the cord and pass to the structure they supply. Similarly, sensory nerves from organs and tissues enter and pass upwards in the spinal cord to the brain.

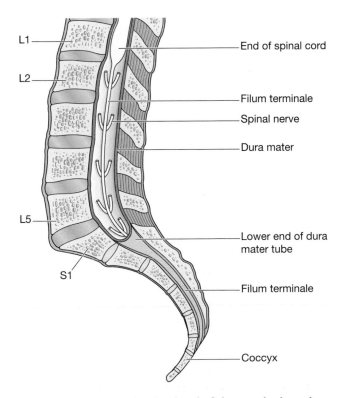

Figure 7.22 Section of the distal end of the vertebral canal.

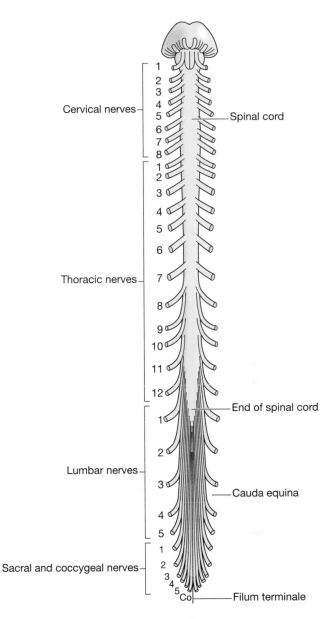

Figure 7.23 The spinal cord and spinal nerves.

157

Some activities of the spinal cord are independent of the brain, i.e. *spinal reflexes*. To facilitate these, there are extensive neurone connections between sensory and motor neurones at the same or different levels in the cord.

The spinal cord is incompletely divided into two equal parts, anteriorly by a short, shallow *median fissure* and posteriorly by a deep narrow septum, the *posterior median septum*.

A cross-section of the spinal cord shows that it is composed of grey matter in the centre surrounded by white matter supported by neuroglia. Figure 7.24 shows the parts of the spinal cord and the nerve roots on one side. The other side is the same.

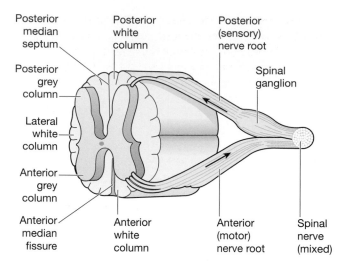

Figure 7.24 A section of the spinal cord showing nerve roots on one side.

Grey matter

The arrangement of grey matter in the spinal cord resembles the shape of the letter H, having *two posterior, two anterior* and *two lateral columns*. The area of grey matter lying transversely is the *transverse commissure* and it is pierced by the central canal, an extension from the fourth ventricle, containing cerebrospinal fluid. The nerve cell bodies may be:

- *sensory neurones*, which receive impulses from the periphery of the body
- *lower motor neurones*, which transmit impulses to the skeletal muscles
- *connector neurones*, linking sensory and motor neurones, at the same or different levels, which form spinal reflex arcs.

At each point where nerve impulses are passed from one neurone to another, there is a synaptic cleft and a neurotransmitter.

Posterior columns of grey matter

These are composed of cell bodies that are stimulated by sensory impulses from the periphery of the body. The nerve fibres of these cells contribute to the formation of the white matter of the cord and transmit the sensory impulses upwards to the brain.

Anterior columns of grey matter

These are composed of the cell bodies of the lower motor neurones that are stimulated by the upper motor neurones or the connector neurones linking the anterior and posterior columns to form reflex arcs.

The posterior root (spinal) ganglia are formed by the cell bodies of the sensory nerves.

White matter

The white matter of the spinal cord is arranged in three *columns* or *tracts*; anterior, posterior and lateral. These tracts are formed by sensory nerve fibres ascending to the brain, motor nerve fibres descending from the brain and fibres of connector neurones.

Tracts are often named according to their points of origin and destination, e.g. spinothalamic, corticospinal.

Sensory nerve tracts in the spinal cord

Neurones that transmit impulses towards the brain are sensory, and also known as afferent or ascending neurones. There are two main sources of sensation transmitted to the brain via the spinal cord.

1. *The skin.* Sensory receptors (nerve endings) in the skin, called *cutaneous receptors*, are stimulated by pain, heat, cold and touch, including pressure. Nerve impulses generated are conducted by three neurones to the sensory area in the *opposite hemisphere of the cerebrum* where the sensation and its location are perceived (Fig. 7.25). Crossing to the other side, or decussation, occurs either at the level of entry into the cord or in the medulla.
2. *The tendons, muscles and joints.* Sensory receptors are specialised nerve endings in these structures, called *proprioceptors*, and they are stimulated by stretch. Together with impulses from the eyes and the ears they are associated with the maintenance of balance and posture and with perception of the position of the body in space. These nerve impulses have two destinations:
   - by a three-neurone system, the impulses reach the sensory area of the opposite hemisphere of the cerebrum
   - by a two-neurone system, the nerve impulses reach the cerebellar hemisphere on the same side.

Table 7.1 provides further information about the origins, routes of transmission and the destinations of sensory nerve impulses.

Motor nerve tracts in the spinal cord

Neurones that transmit nerve impulses away from the brain are motor (efferent or descending) neurones. Motor neurone stimulation results in:

- contraction of skeletal (voluntary) muscle
- contraction of smooth (involuntary) muscle, cardiac

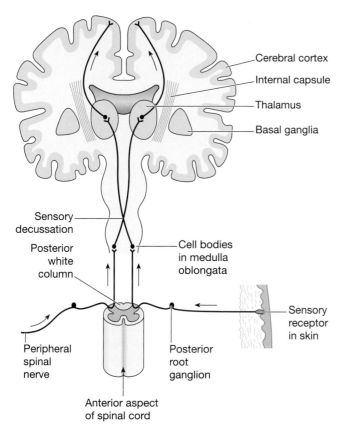

Figure 7.25 A sensory nerve pathway from the skin to the cerebrum.

muscle and the secretion by glands controlled by nerves of the autonomic nervous system (p. 170).

Voluntary muscle movement

The contraction of the muscles that move the joints is, in the main, under conscious (voluntary) control, which means that the stimulus to contract originates at the level

of consciousness in the cerebrum. However, some nerve impulses that affect skeletal muscle contraction are initiated in the midbrain, brain stem and cerebellum. This involuntary activity is associated with coordination of muscle activity, e.g. when very fine movement is required and in the maintenance of posture and balance.

Efferent nerve impulses are transmitted from the brain to other parts of the body via bundles of nerve fibres (tracts) in the spinal cord. The *motor pathways* from the brain to the muscles are made up of two neurones (see Fig. 7.17). These pathways, or tracts, are either:

- pyramidal (corticospinal)
- extrapyramidal.

The motor fibres that form the pyramidal tracts travel through the internal capsule and are the main pathway for impulses to skeletal muscles. Those motor fibres that do not pass through the internal capsule form the extrapyramidal tracts and have connections with many parts of the brain including the basal ganglia and the thalamus.

The upper motor neurone. This has its cell body (Betz's cell) in the primary motor area of the cerebrum. The axons pass through the internal capsule, pons and medulla. In the spinal cord they form the lateral corticospinal tracts of white matter and the fibres synapse with the cell bodies of the lower motor neurones in the anterior columns of grey matter. The axons of the upper motor neurones make up the pyramidal tracts and decussate in the medulla oblongata, forming the pyramids.

The lower motor neurone. This has its cell body in the anterior horn of grey matter in the spinal cord. Its axon emerges from the spinal cord by the anterior root, joins with the incoming sensory fibres and forms the mixed

159

Receptor	Route		Destination
Table 7.1 Sensory nerve impulses: origins, routes, destinations			
Pain, touch, temperature	Neurone 1 – to spinal cord by posterior root		
	Neurone 2 – decussation on entering spinal cord then in anterolateral spinothalamic tract to thalamus		
	Neurone 3 –		to parietal lobe of cerebrum
Touch, proprioceptors	Neurone 1 – to medulla in posterior spinothalamic tract		
	Neurone 2 – decussation in medulla, transmission to thalamus		
	Neurone 3 –		to parietal lobe of cerebrum
Proprioceptors	Neurone 1 – to spinal cord		
	Neurone 2 –		no decussation, to cerebellum in posterior spinocerebellar tract

Table 7.2 Extrapyramidal upper motor neurones: origins and tracts

Origin	Name of tract	Site in spinal cord	Functions
Midbrain and pons	Rubrospinal tract decussates in brain stem	Lateral column	Control of skilled muscle movement
Reticular formation	Reticulospinal tract does not decussate	Lateral column	Coordination of muscle movement
Midbrain and pons	Tectospinal tract decussates in midbrain	Anterior column	Maintenance of posture and balance
Midbrain and pons	Vestibulospinal tract, some fibres decussate in the cord	Anterior column	

spinal nerve that passes through the intervertebral foramen. Near its termination in muscle the axon branches into a variable number of tiny fibres that form motor end-plates, each of which is in close association with a sensitive area on the wall of a muscle fibre. The motor end-plates of each nerve and the muscle fibres they supply form a *motor unit* (see Fig. 16.53, p. 416). The neurotransmitter that conveys the nerve impulse across the neuromuscular junction (synapse) to stimulate the muscle fibre is *acetylcholine*. Motor units contract as a whole and the strength of contraction of a muscle depends on the number of motor units in action at any time.

The lower motor neurone is the *final common pathway* for the transmission of nerve impulses to skeletal muscles. The cell body of this neurone is influenced by a number of upper motor neurones originating from various sites in the brain and by some neurones which begin and end in the spinal cord. Some of these neurones stimulate the cell bodies of the lower motor neurone while others have an inhibiting effect. The outcome of these influences is smooth, coordinated muscle movement, some of which is voluntary and some involuntary.

Involuntary muscle movement
Upper motor neurones. These have their cell bodies in the brain at a level *below* the cerebrum, i.e. in the midbrain, brain stem, cerebellum or spinal cord. They influence muscle activity that maintains posture and balance, coordinates skeletal muscle movement and controls muscle tone.

Table 7.2 shows details of the area of origin of these neurones and the tracts which their axons form before reaching the cell body of the lower motor neurone in the spinal cord.

Spinal reflexes. These consist of three elements:

- sensory neurones
- connector neurones in the spinal cord
- lower motor neurones.

In the simplest *reflex arc* there is only one of each (Fig. 7.26). A *reflex action* is an involuntary and immediate motor response to a sensory stimulus. Many connector and motor neurones may be stimulated by afferent impulses from a small area of skin, e.g. the pain impulses

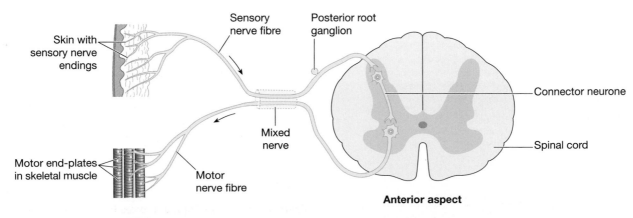

Figure 7.26 A simple reflex arc involving one side only.

initiated by touching a very hot surface with the finger are transmitted to the spinal cord by sensory fibres in mixed nerves. These stimulate many connector and lower motor neurones in the spinal cord, which results in the contraction of many skeletal muscles of the hand, arm and shoulder, and the removal of the finger. Reflex action takes place very quickly, in fact, the motor response may have occurred simultaneously with the perception of the pain in the cerebrum. Reflexes of this type are invariably protective but they can on occasion be inhibited. For example, if it is a precious plate that is very hot when lifted every effort will be made to overcome the pain to prevent dropping it!

Stretch reflexes. Only two neurones are involved. The cell body of the lower motor neurone is stimulated directly by the sensory neurone, with no connector neurone in between. The *knee jerk* is one example, but this type of reflex can be demonstrated at any point where a stretched tendon crosses a joint. By tapping the tendon just below the knee when it is bent, the sensory nerve endings in the tendon and in the thigh muscles are stretched. This initiates a nerve impulse that passes into the spinal cord to the cell body of the lower motor neurone in the anterior column of grey matter on the same side. As a result the thigh muscles suddenly contract and the foot kicks forward. This is used as a test of the integrity of the reflex arc. This type of reflex has a protective function – it prevents excessive joint movement that may damage tendons, ligaments and muscles.

Autonomic reflexes. These include e.g. the pupillary light reflex when the pupil immediately constricts, in response to bright light, preventing retinal damage.

Peripheral nervous system

Learning outcomes

After studying this section you should be able to:

- state the origins of the paired spinal nerves
- outline the function of a nerve plexus
- list the spinal nerves entering each plexus and the main nerves emerging from it
- describe the areas innervated by the thoracic nerves
- outline the functions of the 12 cranial nerves.

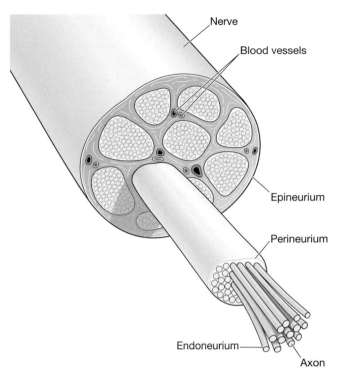

Figure 7.27 Transverse section of a peripheral nerve showing the protective coverings.

This part of the nervous system consists of:

- 31 pairs of spinal nerves
- 12 pairs of cranial nerves
- the autonomic nervous system.

Most of the nerves of the peripheral nervous system are composed of sensory nerve fibres conveying afferent impulses from sensory organs to the brain, and motor nerve fibres conveying efferent impulses from the brain to the effector organs, e.g. skeletal muscles, smooth muscle and glands.

Each nerve consists of numerous nerve fibres collected into bundles. Each bundle has several coverings of protective connective tissue (Fig. 7.27).

- *Endoneurium* is a delicate tissue, surrounding each individual fibre, which is continuous with the septa that pass inwards from the perineurium.
- *Perineurium* is a smooth connective tissue, surrounding each *bundle* of fibres.
- *Epineurium* is the fibrous tissue which surrounds and encloses a number of bundles of nerve fibres. Most large nerves are covered by epineurium.

Spinal nerves

There are 31 pairs of spinal nerves that leave the vertebral canal by passing through the intervertebral foramina

161

formed by adjacent vertebrae. They are named and grouped according to the vertebrae with which they are associated (see Fig. 7.23):

- 8 cervical
- 12 thoracic
- 5 lumbar
- 5 sacral
- 1 coccygeal.

Although there are only seven cervical vertebrae, there are eight nerves because the first pair leaves the vertebral canal between the occipital bone and the atlas and the eighth pair leave below the last cervical vertebra. Thereafter the nerves are given the name and number of the vertebra immediately *above*.

The lumbar, sacral and coccygeal nerves leave the spinal cord near its termination at the level of the first lumbar vertebra, and extend downwards inside the vertebral canal in the subarachnoid space, forming a sheaf of nerves which resembles a horse's tail, the *cauda equina* (see Fig. 7.23). These nerves leave the vertebral canal at the appropriate lumbar, sacral or coccygeal level, depending on their destination.

Nerve roots (Fig. 7.28)

The spinal nerves arise from both sides of the spinal cord and emerge through the intervertebral foramina (see Fig 16.24, p, 398). Each nerve is formed by the union of a *motor* (anterior) and a *sensory* (posterior) *nerve root* and is, therefore, a *mixed nerve*. Thoracic and upper lumbar (L1 and L2) spinal nerves have a contribution from the sympathetic part of the autonomic nervous system in the form of a *preganglionic fibre*.

Chapter 16 describes the bones and muscles mentioned in the following section. Bones and joints are supplied by adjacent nerves.

The *anterior nerve root* consists of motor nerve fibres, which are the axons of the lower motor neurones from the anterior column of grey matter in the spinal cord and, in the thoracic and lumbar regions, *sympathetic nerve fibres*, which are the axons of cells in the lateral columns of grey matter.

The *posterior nerve root* consists of sensory nerve fibres. Just outside the spinal cord there is a *spinal ganglion* (posterior root ganglion), consisting of a little cluster of cell bodies. Sensory nerve fibres pass through these ganglia before entering the spinal cord. The area of skin whose sensory receptors contribute to each nerve is called a *dermatome* (see Figs 7.33 and 7.37).

For a very short distance after leaving the spinal cord the nerve roots have a covering of *dura* and *arachnoid maters*. These terminate before the two roots join to form the mixed spinal nerve. The nerve roots have no covering of pia mater.

Branches

Immediately after emerging from the intervertebral foramen, spinal nerves divide into branches, or *rami*: a ramus communicans, a posterior ramus and an anterior ramus.

The *rami communicante* are part of preganglionic sympathetic neurones of the autonomic nervous system.

The *posterior rami* pass backwards and divide into medial and lateral branches to supply skin and muscles of relatively small areas of the posterior aspect of the head, neck and trunk.

The *anterior rami* supply the anterior and lateral aspects of the neck, trunk and the upper and lower limbs.

Plexuses

In the cervical, lumbar and sacral regions the anterior rami unite near their origins to form large masses of nerves, or *plexuses*, where nerve fibres are regrouped and rearranged before proceeding to supply skin, bones, muscles and joints of a particular area (Fig. 7.29). This means that these structures have a nerve supply from more than one spinal nerve and therefore damage to one spinal nerve does not cause loss of function of a region.

In the thoracic region the anterior rami do not form plexuses.

There are five large plexuses of mixed nerves formed on each side of the vertebral column. They are the:

- cervical plexuses
- brachial plexuses
- lumbar plexuses
- sacral plexuses
- coccygeal plexuses.

Cervical plexus (Fig. 7.30)

This is formed by the anterior rami of the first four cervical nerves. It lies opposite the 1st, 2nd, 3rd and 4th

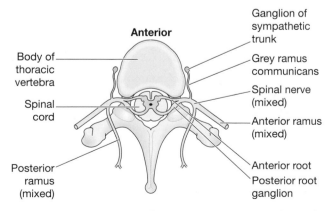

Figure 7.28 The relationship between sympathetic and mixed spinal nerves. Sympathetic nerves in green.

Anterior

Ganglion of sympathetic trunk

Grey ramus communicans

Spinal nerve (mixed)

Anterior ramus (mixed)

Anterior root

Posterior root ganglion

Body of thoracic vertebra

Spinal cord

Posterior ramus (mixed)

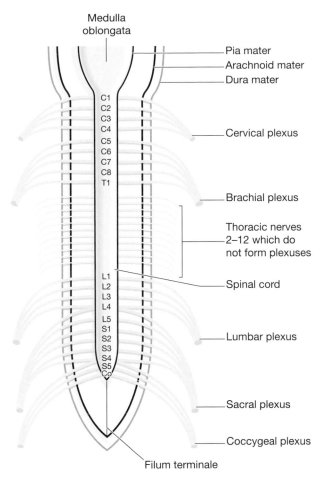

Figure 7.29 The meninges covering the spinal cord, spinal nerves and the plexuses they form.

cervical vertebrae under the protection of the sterno-cleidomastoid muscle.

The superficial branches supply the structures at the back and side of the head and the skin of the front of the neck to the level of the sternum.

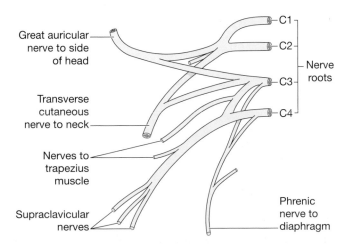

Figure 7.30 The cervical plexus. Anterior view.

The deep branches supply muscles of the neck, e.g. the sternocleidomastoid and the trapezius.

The phrenic nerve originates from cervical roots 3, 4 and 5 and passes downwards through the thoracic cavity in front of the root of the lung to supply the diaphragm with impulses that stimulate contraction, initiating inspiration.

Brachial plexus

The anterior rami of the lower four cervical nerves and a large part of the first thoracic nerve form the brachial plexus. Figure 7.31 shows its formation and the nerves that emerge from it. The plexus is situated in the neck and shoulder above and behind the subclavian vessels and in the axilla.

The branches of the brachial plexus supply the skin and muscles of the upper limbs and some of the chest muscles. Five large nerves and a number of smaller ones emerge from this plexus, each with a contribution from more than one nerve root, containing sensory, motor and autonomic fibres:

- axillary (circumflex) nerve: C5, 6
- radial nerve: C5, 6, 7, 8, T1
- musculocutaneous nerve: C5, 6, 7
- median nerve: C5, 6, 7, 8, T1
- ulnar nerve: C7, 8, T1
- medial cutaneous nerve: C8, T1.

The axillary (circumflex) nerve winds round the humerus at the level of the surgical neck. It then breaks up into

163

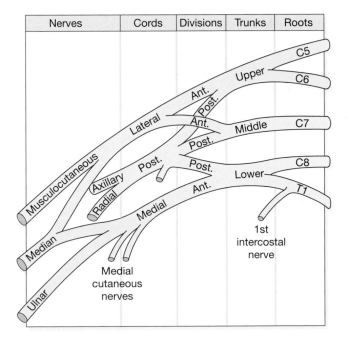

Figure 7.31 The brachial plexus. Anterior view. Ant = anterior, Post = posterior.

minute branches to supply the deltoid muscle, shoulder joint and overlying skin.

The radial nerve is the largest branch of the brachial plexus. It supplies the triceps muscle behind the humerus, crosses in front of the elbow joint then winds round to the back of the forearm to supply extensors of the wrist and finger joints. It continues into the back of the hand to supply the skin of the thumb, the first two fingers and the lateral half of the third finger.

The musculocutaneous nerve passes downwards to the lateral aspect of the forearm. It supplies the muscles of the upper arm and the skin of the forearm.

The median nerve passes down the midline of the arm in close association with the brachial artery. It passes in front of the elbow joint then down to supply the muscles of the front of the forearm. It continues into the hand where it supplies small muscles and the skin of the front of the thumb, the first two fingers and the lateral half of the third finger. It gives off no branches above the elbow.

The ulnar nerve descends through the upper arm lying medial to the brachial artery. It passes behind the medial epicondyle of the humerus to supply the muscles on the ulnar aspect of the forearm. It continues downwards to supply the muscles in the palm of the hand and the skin of the whole of the little finger and the medial half of the third finger. It gives off no branches above the elbow.

The main nerves of the arm are presented in Figure 7.32. The distribution and origins of the cutaneous sensory nerves of the arm, i.e. the dermatomes, are shown in Figure 7.33.

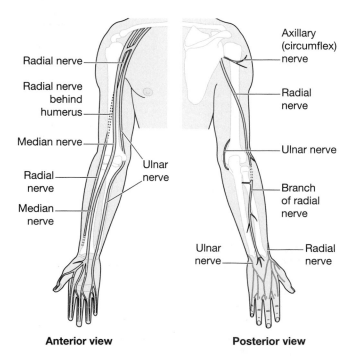

Figure 7.32 The main nerves of the arm.

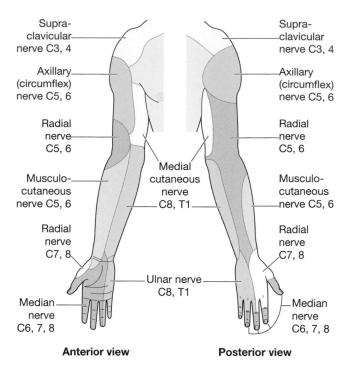

Figure 7.33 The distribution and origins of the cutaneous nerves of the arm.

Lumbar plexus (Figs 7.34, 7.36 and 7.37)

The lumbar plexus is formed by the anterior rami of the first three and part of the fourth lumbar nerves. The plexus is situated in front of the transverse processes of the lumbar vertebrae and behind the psoas muscle. The main branches, and their nerve roots are:

- iliohypogastric nerve: L1
- ilioinguinal nerve: L1
- genitofemoral: L1, 2
- lateral cutaneous nerve of thigh: L2, 3
- femoral nerve: L2, 3, 4
- obturator nerve: L2, 3, 4
- lumbosacral trunk: L4, (5).

The iliohypogastric, ilioinguinal and *genitofemoral nerves* supply muscles and the skin in the area of the lower abdomen, upper and medial aspects of the thigh and the inguinal region.

The lateral cutaneous nerve of the thigh supplies the skin of the lateral aspect of the thigh including part of the anterior and posterior surfaces.

The femoral nerve is one of the larger branches. It passes behind the inguinal ligament to enter the thigh in close association with the femoral artery. It divides into cutaneous and muscular branches to supply the skin and the muscles of the front of the thigh. One branch, the *saphenous nerve*, supplies the medial aspect of the leg, ankle and foot.

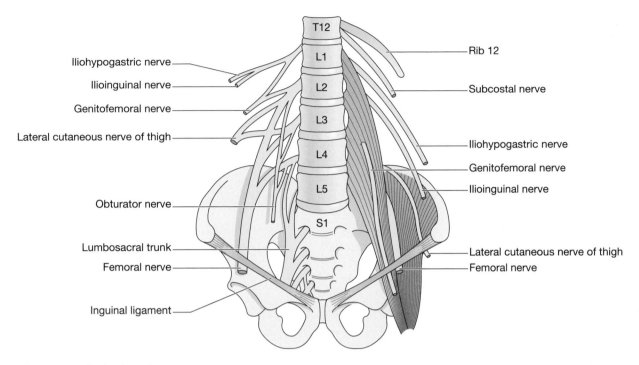

Iliohypogastric nerve
Ilioinguinal nerve
Genitofemoral nerve
Lateral cutaneous nerve of thigh
Obturator nerve
Lumbosacral trunk
Femoral nerve
Inguinal ligament

T12
L1
L2
L3
L4
L5
S1

Rib 12
Subcostal nerve
Iliohypogastric nerve
Genitofemoral nerve
Ilioinguinal nerve
Lateral cutaneous nerve of thigh
Femoral nerve

Figure 7.34 **The lumbar plexus.**

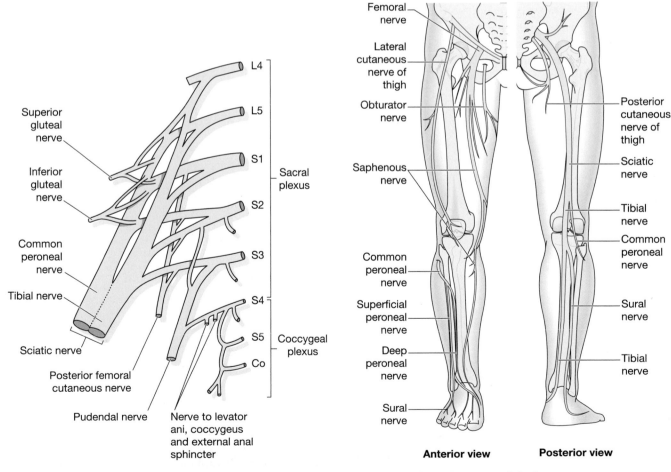

Superior gluteal nerve
Inferior gluteal nerve
Common peroneal nerve
Tibial nerve
Sciatic nerve
Posterior femoral cutaneous nerve
Pudendal nerve
Nerve to levator ani, coccygeus and external anal sphincter

L4
L5
S1
S2
S3
S4
S5
Co

Sacral plexus

Coccygeal plexus

Figure 7.35 **Sacral and coccygeal plexuses.**

Femoral nerve
Lateral cutaneous nerve of thigh
Obturator nerve
Saphenous nerve
Common peroneal nerve
Superficial peroneal nerve
Deep peroneal nerve
Sural nerve

Posterior cutaneous nerve of thigh
Sciatic nerve
Tibial nerve
Common peroneal nerve
Sural nerve
Tibial nerve

Anterior view   **Posterior view**

Figure 7.36 **The main nerves of the leg.**

165

The obturator nerve supplies the adductor muscles of the thigh and skin of the medial aspect of the thigh. It ends just above the level of the knee joint.

The lumbosacral trunk descends into the pelvis and makes a contribution to the sacral plexus.

Sacral plexus (Figs 7.35, 7.36 and 7.37)

The sacral plexus is formed by the anterior rami of the lumbosacral trunk and the first, second and third sacral nerves. The lumbosacral trunk is formed by the fifth and part of the fourth lumbar nerves. It lies in the posterior wall of the pelvic cavity.

The sacral plexus divides into a number of branches, supplying the muscles and skin of the pelvic floor, muscles around the hip joint and the pelvic organs. In addition to these it provides the *sciatic nerve*, which contains fibres from L4 and 5 and S1–3.

The sciatic nerve is the largest nerve in the body. It is about 2 cm wide at its origin. It passes through the greater sciatic foramen into the buttock then descends through the posterior aspect of the thigh supplying the hamstring muscles. At the level of the middle of the femur it divides to form the *tibial* and the *common peroneal nerves*.

The tibial nerve descends through the popliteal fossa to the posterior aspect of the leg where it supplies muscles and skin. It passes under the medial malleolus to supply muscles and skin of the sole of the foot and toes. One of the main branches is the *sural nerve*, which supplies the tissues in the area of the heel, the lateral aspect of the ankle and a part of the dorsum of the foot.

The common peroneal nerve descends obliquely along the lateral aspect of the popliteal fossa, winds round the neck of the fibula into the front of the leg where it divides into the *deep peroneal* (anterior tibial) and the *superficial peroneal* (musculocutaneous) nerves. These nerves supply the skin and muscles of the anterior aspect of the leg and the dorsum of the foot and toes.

The pudendal nerve (S2, 3, 4) – the perineal branch supplies the external anal sphincter, the external urethral sphincter and adjacent skin. Figures 7.36 and 7.37 show

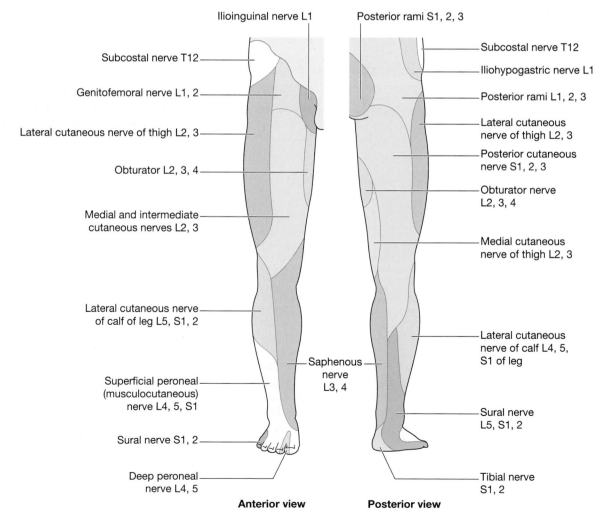

Figure 7.37 Distribution and origins of the cutaneous nerves of the leg.

the main nerves of the leg, the dermatomes and the origins of the main nerves.

Coccygeal plexus (Fig. 7.35)

The coccygeal plexus is a very small plexus formed by part of the fourth and fifth sacral and the coccygeal nerves. The nerves from this plexus supply the skin around the coccyx and anal area.

Thoracic nerves

The thoracic nerves *do not* intermingle to form plexuses. There are 12 pairs and the first 11 are the *intercostal nerves*. They pass between the ribs supplying them, the intercostal muscles and overlying skin. The 12th pair comprise the *subcostal nerves*. The 7th to the 12th thoracic nerves also supply the muscles and the skin of the posterior and anterior abdominal walls (Fig. 7.38).

Cranial nerves (Fig. 7.39)

There are 12 pairs of cranial nerves originating from nuclei in the inferior surface of the brain, some sensory, some motor and some mixed. Their names and numbers are:

I.	Olfactory:	sensory
II.	Optic:	sensory
III.	Oculomotor:	motor
IV.	Trochlear:	motor
V.	Trigeminal:	mixed
VI.	Abducent:	motor
VII.	Facial:	mixed
VIII.	Vestibulocochlear (auditory):	sensory
IX.	Glossopharyngeal:	mixed
X.	Vagus:	mixed
XI.	Accessory:	motor
XII.	Hypoglossal:	motor.

I. Olfactory nerves (sensory)

These are the nerves of the *sense of smell*. Their sensory receptors and fibres originate in the upper part of the mucous membrane of the nasal cavity, pass upwards through the cribriform plate of the ethmoid bone and then go to the *olfactory bulb* (see Fig. 8.23, p. 204). The nerves then proceed backwards as the olfactory tract, to the area for the perception of smell in the temporal lobe of the cerebrum.

II. Optic nerves (sensory)

These are the nerves of the *sense of sight*. The fibres originate in the retinae of the eyes and they combine to form the optic nerves (see Fig. 8.13, p. 198). They are directed backwards and medially through the posterior part of the orbital cavity. They then pass through the *optic foramina* of the sphenoid bone into the cranial cavity and join at the *optic chiasma*. The nerves proceed backwards as the *optic tracts* to the *lateral geniculate bodies* of the

167

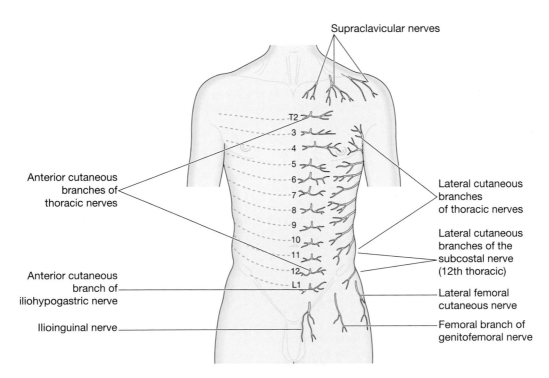

Figure 7.38 Segmental distribution of the thoracic cutaneous nerves.

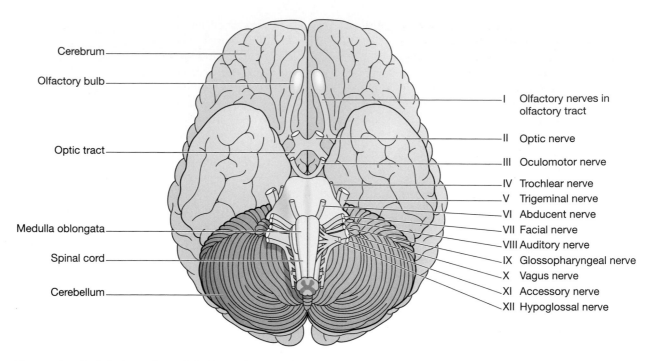

Figure 7.39 The inferior surface of the brain showing the cranial nerves.

thalamus. Impulses pass from these to the centre for sight in the occipital lobes of the cerebrum and to the cerebellum. In the occipital lobe sight is perceived, and in the cerebellum the impulses from the eyes contribute to the maintenance of balance, posture and orientation of the head in space.

III. Oculomotor nerves (motor)

These nerves arise from nuclei near the cerebral aqueduct. They supply:

- four of the six extrinsic muscles, which move the eyeball, i.e. the *superior, medial* and *inferior recti* and the *inferior oblique muscle* (see Table 8.1, p. 202)
- the intrinsic (intraocular) muscles:
  - *ciliary muscles*, which alter the shape of the lens, changing its refractive power
  - *circular muscles* of the iris, which constrict the pupil
- the *levator palpebrae muscles*, which raise the upper eyelids.

IV. Trochlear nerves (motor)

These nerves arise from nuclei near the cerebral aqueduct. They supply the *superior oblique muscles* of the eyes.

V. Trigeminal nerves (mixed)

These nerves contain motor and sensory fibres and are among the largest of the cranial nerves. They are the chief sensory nerves for the face and head (including the oral and nasal cavities and teeth), receiving impulses of pain,

temperature and touch. The motor fibres stimulate the muscles of mastication.

As the name suggests, there are three main branches of the trigeminal nerves. The dermatomes innervated by the sensory fibres on the right side are shown in Figure 7.40.

The ophthalmic nerves are sensory only and supply the lacrimal glands, conjunctiva of the eyes, forehead, eyelids, anterior aspect of the scalp and mucous membrane of the nose.

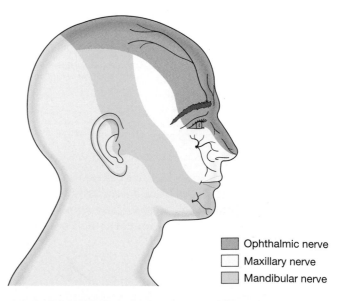

Ophthalmic nerve
Maxillary nerve
Mandibular nerve

Figure 7.40 The cutaneous distribution of the main branches of the right trigeminal nerve.

The maxillary nerves are sensory only and supply the cheeks, upper gums, upper teeth and lower eyelids.

The mandibular nerves contain both sensory and motor fibres. These are the largest of the three divisions and they supply the teeth and gums of the lower jaw, pinnae of the ears, lower lip and tongue. The motor fibres supply the muscles of mastication.

VI. Abducent nerves (motor)

These nerves arise from nuclei lying under the floor of the fourth ventricle. They supply the *lateral rectus muscles* of the eyeballs.

VII. Facial nerves (mixed)

These nerves are composed of both motor and sensory nerve fibres, arising from nuclei in the lower part of the pons. The motor fibres supply the muscles of facial expression. The sensory fibres convey impulses from the taste buds in the anterior two-thirds of the tongue to the taste perception area in the cerebral cortex (see Fig. 7.16).

VIII. Vestibulocochlear (auditory) nerves (sensory)

These nerves are composed of two distinct sets of fibres, vestibular nerves and cochlear nerves.

The vestibular nerves arise from the semicircular canals of the inner ear and convey impulses to the cerebellum. They are associated with the maintenance of posture and balance.

The cochlear nerves originate in the spiral organ (of Corti) in the inner ear and convey impulses to the hearing areas in the cerebral cortex where sound is perceived.

IX. Glossopharyngeal nerves (mixed)

The motor fibres arise from nuclei in the medulla oblongata and stimulate the muscles of the tongue and pharynx and the secretory cells of the parotid (salivary) glands.

The sensory fibres convey impulses to the cerebral cortex from the posterior third of the tongue, the tonsils and pharynx and from taste buds in the tongue and pharynx. These nerves are essential for the swallowing and gag reflexes.

X. Vagus nerves (mixed) (Fig. 7.41)

These nerves have a more extensive distribution than any other cranial nerves. They pass down through the neck into the thorax and the abdomen. These nerves form an important part of the parasympathetic nervous system (see Fig. 7.43).

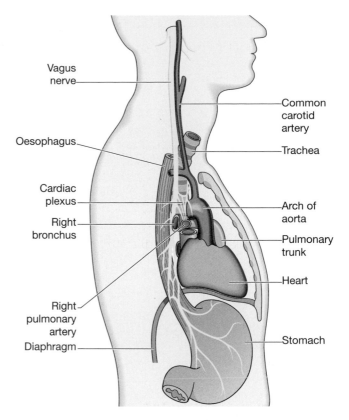

Figure 7.41 The position of the vagus nerve in the thorax viewed from the right side.

The motor fibres arise from nuclei in the medulla and supply the smooth muscle and secretory glands of the pharynx, larynx, trachea, heart, oesophagus, stomach, intestines, exocrine pancreas, gall bladder, bile ducts, spleen, kidneys, ureter and blood vessels in the thoracic and abdominal cavities.

The sensory fibres convey impulses from the membranes lining the same structures to the brain.

XI. Accessory nerves (motor)

These nerves arise from nuclei in the medulla oblongata and in the spinal cord. The fibres supply the *sternocleidomastoid* and *trapezius muscles*. Branches join the vagus nerves and supply the *pharyngeal* and *laryngeal muscles*.

XII. Hypoglossal nerves (motor)

These nerves arise from nuclei in the medulla oblongata. They supply the muscles of the tongue and muscles surrounding the hyoid bone and contribute to swallowing and speech.

169

Autonomic nervous system

After studying this section you should be able to:

- identify the two divisions of the autonomic nervous system

- compare and contrast the structures and neurotransmitters of the two divisions

- compare and contrast the effects of stimulation of the two divisions on body systems

- explain how referred pain occurs.

The autonomic or involuntary part of the nervous system (Fig. 7.1) controls the 'automatic' functions of the body, i.e. initiated in the brain below the level of the cerebrum. Although stimulation does not occur voluntarily, the individual may be conscious of its effects, e.g. an increase in their heart rate.

The effects of autonomic activity are rapid and the effector organs are:

- smooth muscle, e.g. changes in airway or blood vessel diameter
- cardiac muscle, e.g. changes in rate and force of the heartbeat
- glands, e.g. increasing or decreasing gastrointestinal secretions.

The *efferent (motor) nerves* of the autonomic nervous system arise from nerve cells in the brain and emerge at various levels between the midbrain and the sacral region of the spinal cord. Many of them travel within the same nerve sheath as the peripheral nerves of the central nervous system to reach the organs that they innervate.

The autonomic nervous system is separated into two divisions:

- *sympathetic* (thoracolumbar outflow)
- *parasympathetic* (craniosacral outflow).

The two divisions have both structural and functional differences. They normally work in an opposing manner, enabling or restoring balance of involuntary functions. Sympathetic activity tends to predominate in stressful situations and parasympathetic activity during rest.

Each division has two efferent neurones in its peripheral pathways between the central nervous system and effector organs. These are:

- the preganglionic neurone
- the postganglionic neurone.

The cell body of the preganglionic neurone is in the brain or spinal cord. Its axon terminals synapse with the cell body of the postganglionic neurone in an *autonomic ganglion* outside the central nervous system. The postganglionic neurone conducts impulses to the effector organ (see Fig. 7.8).

Sympathetic nervous system

Neurones convey impulses from their origin in the hypothalamus, reticular formation and medulla oblongata to effector organs and tissues (Fig. 7.42). The first neurone has its cell body in the brain and its fibre extends into the spinal cord. The preganglionic and postganglionic neurones then conduct sympathetic impulses to effector organs.

The preganglionic neurone. This has its cell body in the *lateral column of grey matter* in the spinal cord between the levels of the 1st thoracic and 2nd or 3rd lumbar vertebrae. The nerve fibre of this cell leaves the cord by the anterior root and terminates at a synapse in one of the ganglia either in the *lateral chain of sympathetic ganglia* or passes through it to one of the *prevertebral ganglia* (see below). Acetylcholine is the neurotransmitter at sympathetic ganglia.

The postganglionic neurone. This has its cell body in a ganglion and terminates in the organ or tissue supplied. Noradrenaline (norepinephrine) is usually the neurotransmitter at sympathetic effector organs. The major exception is that there is no parasympathetic supply to the sweat glands, the skin and blood vessels of skeletal muscles. These structures are supplied by only sympathetic postganglionic neurones, which usually have acetylcholine as their neurotransmitter (see Fig. 7.8). They have, therefore, the effects of both sympathetic and parasympathetic nerve supply (Fig. 7.42).

Sympathetic ganglia
The lateral chains of sympathetic ganglia. These are chains of ganglia that extend from the upper cervical level to the sacrum, one chain lying on each side of the bodies of the vertebrae. The ganglia are attached to each other by nerve fibres. Preganglionic neurones that emerge from the cord may synapse with the cell body of the postganglionic neurone at the same level or they may pass up or down the chain through one or more ganglia before synapsing. For example, the nerve that dilates the pupil of the eye leaves the cord at the level of the 1st thoracic vertebra and passes up the chain to the superior cervical ganglion before it synapses with the cell body of

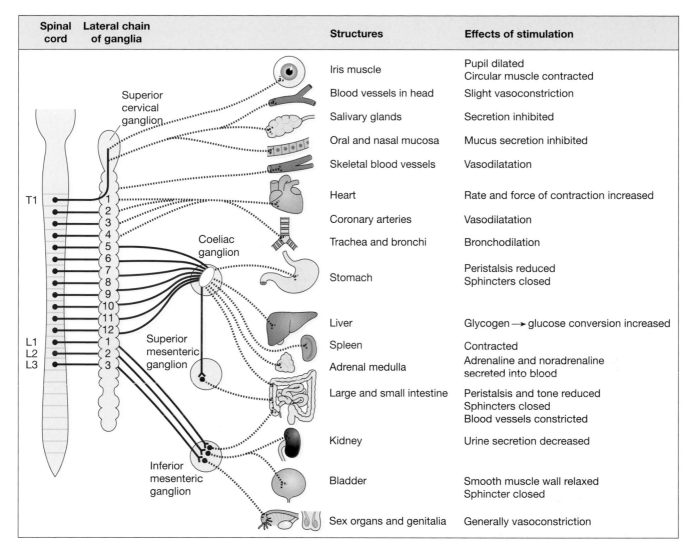

Spinal cord	Lateral chain of ganglia		Structures	Effects of stimulation
			Iris muscle	Pupil dilated Circular muscle contracted
			Blood vessels in head	Slight vasoconstriction
			Salivary glands	Secretion inhibited
			Oral and nasal mucosa	Mucus secretion inhibited
			Skeletal blood vessels	Vasodilatation
			Heart	Rate and force of contraction increased
			Coronary arteries	Vasodilatation
			Trachea and bronchi	Bronchodilation
			Stomach	Peristalsis reduced Sphincters closed
			Liver	Glycogen → glucose conversion increased
			Spleen	Contracted
			Adrenal medulla	Adrenaline and noradrenaline secreted into blood
			Large and small intestine	Peristalsis and tone reduced Sphincters closed Blood vessels constricted
			Kidney	Urine secretion decreased
			Bladder	Smooth muscle wall relaxed Sphincter closed
			Sex organs and genitalia	Generally vasoconstriction

Figure 7.42 The sympathetic outflow, the main structures supplied and the effects of stimulation. Solid red lines – preganglionic fibres; broken lines – postganglionic fibres. There is a right and left lateral chain of ganglia.

the postsynaptic neurone. The postganglionic neurones then pass to the eyes.

The arrangement of the ganglia allows excitation of nerves at multiple levels very quickly, providing a rapid and widespread sympathetic response.

Prevertebral ganglia. There are three prevertebral ganglia situated in the abdominal cavity close to the origins of arteries of the same names:

- coeliac ganglion
- superior mesenteric ganglion
- inferior mesenteric ganglion.

The ganglia consist of nerve cell bodies rather diffusely distributed among a network of nerve fibres that form plexuses. Preganglionic sympathetic fibres pass through the lateral chain to reach these ganglia.

Parasympathetic nervous system

Two neurones (preganglionic and postganglionic) are involved in the transmission of impulses from their source to the effector organ (Fig. 7.43). The neurotransmitter at both synapses is acetylcholine.

The preganglionic neurone. This is usually long in comparison to its counterpart in the sympathetic nervous system and has its cell body either in the brain or in the spinal cord. Those originating in the brain are the cranial

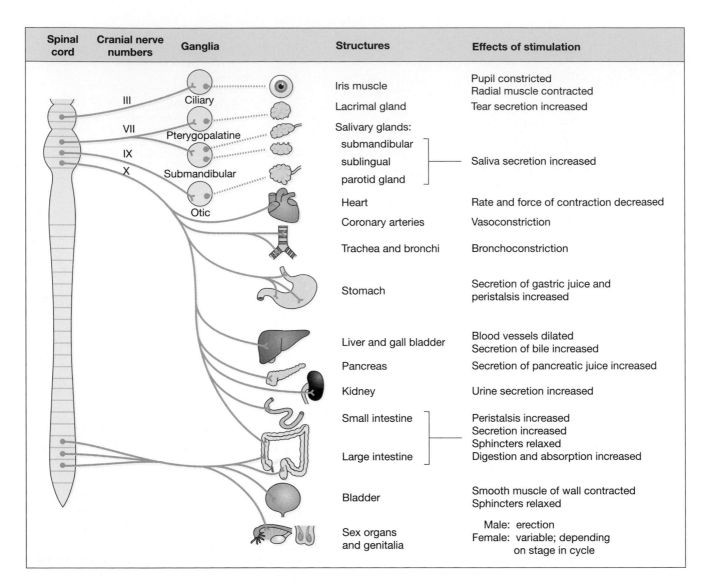

Spinal cord	Cranial nerve numbers	Ganglia	Structures	Effects of stimulation
	III	Ciliary	Iris muscle	Pupil constricted Radial muscle contracted
	VII	Pterygopalatine	Lacrimal gland	Tear secretion increased
	IX	Submandibular	Salivary glands: submandibular sublingual parotid gland	Saliva secretion increased
	X	Otic	Heart	Rate and force of contraction decreased
			Coronary arteries	Vasoconstriction
			Trachea and bronchi	Bronchoconstriction
			Stomach	Secretion of gastric juice and peristalsis increased
			Liver and gall bladder	Blood vessels dilated Secretion of bile increased
			Pancreas	Secretion of pancreatic juice increased
			Kidney	Urine secretion increased
			Small intestine	Peristalsis increased Secretion increased Sphincters relaxed
			Large intestine	Digestion and absorption increased
			Bladder	Smooth muscle of wall contracted Sphincters relaxed
			Sex organs and genitalia	Male: erection Female: variable; depending on stage in cycle

Figure 7.43 The parasympathetic outflow, the main structures supplied and the effects of stimulation. Solid blue lines – preganglionic fibres; broken lines – postganglionic fibres. Where there are no broken lines, the postganglionic neurone is in the wall of the structure.

nerves III, VII, IX and X, arising from nuclei in the midbrain and brain stem, and their nerve fibres terminate outside the brain. The cell bodies of the *sacral outflow* are in the lateral columns of grey matter at the distal end of the spinal cord. Their fibres leave the cord in sacral segments 2, 3 and 4 and synapse with postganglionic neurones in the walls of pelvic organs.

The postganglionic neurone. This is usually very short and has its cell body either in a ganglion or, more often, in the wall of the organ supplied.

Functions of the autonomic nervous system

The autonomic nervous system is involved in many complex reflex activities which, like the reflexes described previously, depend on sensory input to the brain or spinal cord, and on motor output. In this case the reflex action is rapid contraction, or inhibition of contraction, of involuntary (smooth and cardiac) muscle or glandular secretion. These reflexes are coordinated subconsciously in the brain, i.e. below the level of the cerebrum. Some sensory input does reach consciousness and may result in temporary inhibition of the reflex action, e.g. reflex micturition can be inhibited temporarily.

The majority of the organs of the body are supplied by both sympathetic and parasympathetic nerves, which have opposite effects that are finely balanced to ensure their optimum functioning.

Sympathetic stimulation prepares the body to deal with exciting and stressful situations, e.g. strengthening its defences in times of danger and in extremes of environmental temperature. A range of emotional states, e.g. fear, embarrassment and anger, also cause sympathetic stimulation. The adrenal glands are stimulated to secrete the hormones adrenaline (epinephrine) and noradrenaline (norepinephrine) into the bloodstream. These hormones potentiate and sustain the effects of sympathetic stimulation. It is sometimes said that sympathetic stimulation mobilises the body for 'fight or flight'.

Parasympathetic stimulation has a tendency to slow down body processes except digestion and absorption of food and the functions of the genitourinary systems. Its general effect is that of a 'peace maker' allowing restoration processes to occur quietly and peacefully.

Normally the two systems function together maintaining a regular heartbeat, normal temperature and an internal environment compatible with the immediate external surroundings.

Effects of autonomic stimulation

Cardiovascular system

Sympathetic stimulation

- Accelerates firing of the sinoatrial node in the heart, increasing the rate and force of the heartbeat.
- Dilates the coronary arteries, increasing the blood supply to cardiac muscle.
- Dilates the blood vessels supplying skeletal muscle, increasing the supply of oxygen and nutritional materials and the removal of metabolic waste products, thus increasing the capacity of the muscle to work.
- Raises peripheral resistance and blood pressure by constricting the small arteries and arterioles in the skin. In this way an increased blood supply is available for highly active tissue, such as skeletal muscle, heart, and brain.
- Constricts the blood vessels in the secretory glands of the digestive system. This raises the volume of blood available for circulation in dilated blood vessels.
- Accelerates blood coagulation because of vasoconstriction.

Parasympathetic stimulation

- Decreases the rate and force of the heartbeat.
- Constricts the coronary arteries reducing the blood supply to cardiac muscle.

The parasympathetic nervous system exerts little or no effect on blood vessels except the coronary arteries.

Respiratory system

Sympathetic stimulation

This causes smooth muscle relaxation and therefore dilatation of the airways, especially the bronchioles, allowing a greater amount of air to enter the lungs at each inspiration, and increases the respiratory rate. In conjunction with the increased heart rate, the oxygen intake and carbon dioxide output of the body are increased to deal with 'fight or flight' situations.

Parasympathetic stimulation

Produces contraction of smooth muscle in airway walls causing their constriction, e.g. bronchioles and bronchi.

Digestive and urinary systems

Sympathetic stimulation

- *The liver* increases conversion of glycogen to glucose, making more carbohydrate immediately available to provide energy.
- *The stomach* and *small intestine*. Smooth muscle contraction (peristalsis) and secretion of digestive juices are inhibited, delaying digestion, onward movement and absorption of food, and the tone of sphincter muscles is increased.
- *The adrenal (suprarenal) glands* are stimulated to secrete adrenaline (epinephrine) and noradrenaline (norepinephrine) which potentiate and sustain the effects of sympathetic stimulation.
- *Urethral* and *anal sphincters*. The muscle tone of the sphincters is increased, inhibiting micturition and defecation.
- *The bladder wall* relaxes.
- *The metabolic rate* is greatly increased.

Parasympathetic stimulation

- *The liver*. Conversion of glucose to glycogen and secretion of bile are increased.
- *The stomach* and *small intestine*. Motility and secretion are increased together with the rate of digestion and absorption of food.
- *The pancreas*. The secretion of pancreatic juice and the hormone insulin are increased.
- *Urethral* and *anal sphincters*. Relaxation of the internal urethral sphincter is accompanied by contraction of

173

the muscle of the bladder wall, and micturition occurs. Similar relaxation of the internal anal sphincter is accompanied by contraction of the muscle of the rectum, and defecation occurs. In both cases there is voluntary relaxation of the external sphincters.

- *The adrenal glands.* No effect known.

Eye

Sympathetic stimulation

This causes contraction of the radiating muscle fibres of the iris, dilating the pupil. Retraction of the levator palpebrae muscles occurs, opening the eyes wide and giving the appearance of alertness and excitement. The ciliary muscle that adjusts the thickness of the lens is slightly relaxed facilitating distant vision.

Parasympathetic stimulation

This contracts the circular muscle fibres of the iris, constricting the pupil. The eyelids tend to close, giving the appearance of sleepiness.

Skin

Sympathetic stimulation

- Increases sweat secretion, leading to increased heat loss from the body.
- Contracts the arrector pili (the muscles in the hair follicles of the skin), giving the appearance of 'goose flesh'.
- Constricts the peripheral blood vessels increasing blood supply available to active organs, e.g. the heart and skeletal muscle.

There is no parasympathetic nerve supply to the skin. Some sympathetic fibres are adrenergic, causing vasoconstriction, and some are cholinergic, causing vasodilatation (see Fig. 7.8, p. 147).

Afferent impulses from viscera

Sensory fibres from the viscera travel with autonomic fibres and are sometimes called *autonomic afferents*. The impulses they transmit are associated with:

- visceral reflexes, usually at an unconscious level, e.g. cough, blood pressure (baroreceptors)
- sensation of, e.g., hunger, thirst, nausea, sexual sensation, rectal and bladder distension
- visceral pain.

Visceral pain

Normally the viscera are insensitive to cutting, burning and crushing. However, a sensation of dull, poorly located pain is experienced when:

- visceral nerves are stretched
- a large number of fibres are stimulated
- there is ischaemia and local accumulation of metabolites
- the sensitivity of nerve endings to painful stimuli is increased, e.g. during inflammation.

If the cause of the pain, e.g. inflammation, affects the parietal layer of a serous membrane (pleura, peritoneum) the pain is acute and easily located over the site of inflammation. This is because the peripheral spinal (somatic) nerves that innervate the superficial tissues also innervate the parietal layer of serous membrane. They transmit the impulses to the cerebral cortex where *somatic pain* is perceived and accurately located. Appendicitis is an example of this type of pain. Initially it is dull and vaguely located around the midline of the abdomen. As the condition progresses the parietal peritoneum becomes involved and acute pain is clearly located in the right iliac fossa, i.e. over the appendix.

Referred pain (Fig. 7.44)

In some cases of visceral disease, pain may be perceived to occur in superficial tissues remote from its site of origin, i.e. referred pain. This occurs when sensory fibres

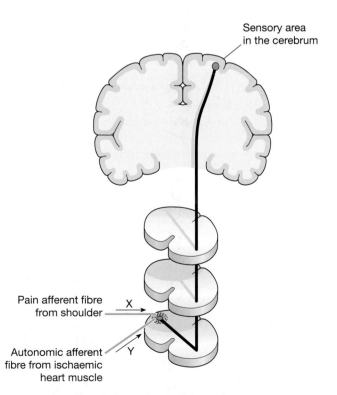

Figure 7.44 Referred pain. Ischaemic heart tissue generates impulses in nerve Y that then stimulate nerve X and pain is perceived in the shoulder.

Table 7.3 Referred pain	
Tissue of origin of pain	**Site of referred pain**
Heart	Left shoulder
Liver Biliary tract }	Right shoulder
Kidney Ureter }	Loin and groin
Uterus	Low back
Male genitalia	Low abdomen
Prolapsed intervertebral disc	Leg

from the affected organ enter the same segment of the spinal cord as somatic nerves, i.e. those from the superficial tissues. It is believed that the sensory nerve from the damaged organ stimulates the closely associated nerve in the spinal cord and it transmits the impulses to the sensory area in the cerebral cortex where the pain is perceived as originating in the area supplied by the somatic nerve. Examples of referred pain are given in Table 7.3.

Response of nervous tissue to injury

Learning outcome

After studying this section you should be able to:

■ outline the response of nervous tissue to injury.

Neurone damage

Damage to nerve cell bodies or their processes can either lead to rapid necrosis with sudden acute functional failure, or to slow atrophy with gradually increasing dysfunction. These changes are associated with:

- hypoxia and anoxia
- nutritional deficiencies
- poisons, e.g. organic lead
- trauma

- infections
- ageing
- hypoglycaemia.

Neurone regeneration (Fig. 7.45)

Neurones of the brain, spinal cord and ganglia reach maturity a few weeks after birth and are not normally replaced when they are damaged or die.

The axons of *peripheral nerves* may regenerate if the cell body remains intact. Distal to the damage, the axon and myelin sheath disintegrate and are removed by macrophages, but the Schwann cells survive and proliferate within the neurilemma. The live proximal part of the axon grows along the original track (about 1.5 mm per day), provided the two parts of neurilemma are correctly positioned and in close apposition. Restoration of function depends on the re-establishment of satisfactory connections with the end organ. When the neurilemma is out of position or destroyed, the sprouting

175

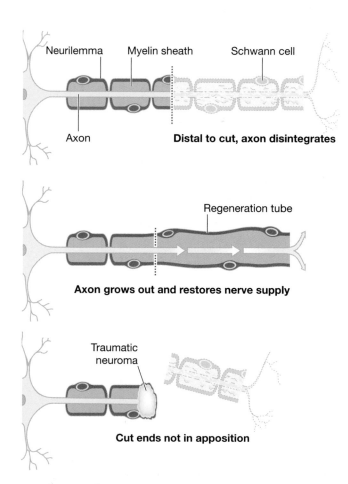

Figure 7.45 Regrowth of peripheral nerves following injury.

axons and Schwann cells form a tumour-like cluster (*traumatic neuroma*) producing severe pain, e.g. following some fractures and amputation of limbs.

Neuroglial damage

Astrocytes

When severely damaged, astrocytes undergo necrosis and disintegrate. In less severe and chronic conditions there is proliferation of astrocyte processes and later cell atrophy (*gliosis*). This process occurs in many diseases and is analogous to fibrosis in other tissues.

Oligodendrocytes

These cells form and maintain myelin, having the same functions as Schwann cells in peripheral nerves. They increase in number around degenerating neurones and are destroyed in demyelinating diseases such as *multiple sclerosis* (p. 184).

Microglia

Microglia are derived from monocytes that migrate from the blood into the nervous system before birth, and are found mainly around blood vessels. Where there is inflammation and cell destruction the microglia increase in size and become phagocytic.

Effects of poisons on the central nervous system

Many chemical substances encountered either as drugs or in the environment damage the nervous system. Neurone function may be disturbed either by damage to the neurone itself or be secondary to dysfunction of other organs, e.g. liver, kidneys. The outcome depends on the toxicity of the substance, the dose and the duration of exposure, ranging from minor short-term neurological disturbance to encephalopathy, which may cause coma and death.

Disorders of the brain

Learning outcomes

After studying this section you should be able to:

- list three causes of raised intracranial pressure (ICP)

- relate the effects of raised ICP to the functions of the brain and changes in vital signs

- outline how the brain is damaged during different types of head injury

- describe four complications of head injury

- explain the effects of cerebral hypoxia and stroke

- outline the causes and effects of dementia

- relate the pathology of Parkinson's disease to its effects on body function.

Increased intracranial pressure

This is a very serious complication of many conditions. The cranium forms a rigid cavity enclosing:

- the brain
- cerebral blood vessels and blood
- cerebrospinal fluid (CSF).

An increase in volume of any one of these will lead to raised intracranial pressure (ICP).

Sometimes its effects are more serious than the condition causing it, e.g. by disrupting the blood supply or distorting the shape of the brain especially if the ICP rises rapidly. A slow rise in ICP allows time for com-

pensatory adjustment to be made, i.e. a slight reduction in the volume of circulating blood and of CSF. The slower the rise in ICP, the more effective is the compensation.

Rising ICP is accompanied by bradycardia and hypertension. As it reaches its limit a further small increase in pressure is followed by a sudden and usually serious reduction in the cerebral blood flow. The result is hypoxia and a rise in carbon dioxide levels, causing arteriolar dilatation, which further increases ICP. This leads to progressive loss of functioning neurones, which exacerbates bradycardia and hypertension. Further cerebral hypoxia causes *vasomotor paralysis* and death.

The causes of increased ICP are described on the following pages and include:

- cerebral oedema
- hydrocephalus, the accumulation of excess CSF
- expanding lesions inside the skull, also known as space-occupying lesions
  - haemorrhage, haematoma (traumatic or spontaneous)
  - tumours (primary or secondary).

Expanding lesions may occur in the brain or in the meninges and they can damage the brain in various ways (Fig. 7.46).

Effects of increased ICP

Displacement of the brain

Lesions causing displacement are usually one sided but may affect both sides. Such lesions may cause:

- *herniation* (displacement of part of the brain from its usual compartment) of the cerebral hemisphere between the corpus callosum and the free border of the falx cerebri on the same side

177

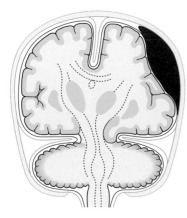

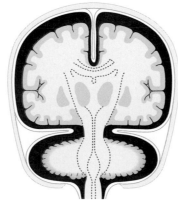

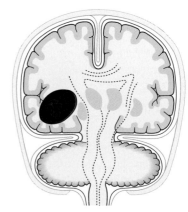

A Subdural haematoma   B Subarachnoid haemorrhage   C Tumour or intracerebral haemorrhage

Figure 7.46 Effects of different types of expanding lesions inside the skull: A. Subdural haematoma. B. Subarachnoid haemorrhage. C. Tumour or intracerebral haemorrhage.

- herniation of the midbrain between the pons and the free border of the tentorium cerebelli on the same side
- compression of the subarachnoid space and flattening of the cerebral convolutions
- distortion of the shape of the ventricles and their ducts
- herniation of the cerebellum through the foramen magnum
- protrusion of the medulla oblongata through the foramen magnum ('*coning*').

Obstruction of the flow of cerebrospinal fluid

The ventricles or their ducts may be pushed out of position or a duct obstructed. The effects depend on the position of the lesion, e.g. compression of the aqueduct of the midbrain causes dilatation of the lateral ventricles and the third ventricle, further increasing the ICP.

Vascular damage

There may be stretching or compression of blood vessels, causing:

- haemorrhage when stretched blood vessels rupture
- ischaemia and infarction due to compression of blood vessels
- papilloedema (oedema round the optic disc) due to compression of the retinal vein in the optic nerve sheath where it crosses the subarachnoid space.

Neural damage

The vital centres in the medulla oblongata may be damaged when the increased ICP causes 'coning'. Stretching may damage cranial nerves, especially the oculomotor (III) and the abducent (VI), causing disturbances of eye movement and accommodation.

Bone changes

Prolonged increase of ICP causes bony changes, e.g.:

- erosion, especially of the sphenoid
- stretching and thinning before ossification is complete.

Cerebral oedema

There is movement of fluid from its normal compartment when oedema develops (p. 120). Cerebral oedema occurs when there is excess fluid in brain cells and/or in the interstitial spaces, causing increased intracranial pressure. *Vasogenic oedema* occurs when there is excess fluid in the interstitial spaces due to increased capillary wall permeability. Oedema develops as plasma proteins pass from the capillaries into the interstitial spaces drawing water with them. *Cytotoxic oedema* occurs when neurones

and neuroglial cells contain excess water due to disruption of the sodium–potassium pump (p. 33) that maintains normal levels of these electrolytes on each side of the plasma membrane. There is accumulation of intracellular Na^+ followed by osmotic movement of water and swelling. The permeability of capillary walls is normal. Cerebral oedema is associated with:

- traumatic injury
- haemorrhage
- infections, abscesses
- hypoxia
- local ischaemia or infarcts
- tumours
- inflammation of the brain or meninges
- hypoglycaemia.

Hydrocephalus

In this condition the volume of CSF is abnormally high and is usually accompanied by increased ICP. An obstruction to CSF flow (see Fig. 7.12) is the most common cause. It is described as *communicating* when there is free flow of CSF from the ventricular system to the subarachnoid space and *non-communicating* when there is not, i.e. there is obstruction in the system of ventricles, foramina or ducts.

Enlargement of the head occurs in children when ossification of the cranial bones is incomplete but, in spite of this, the ventricles dilate and cause stretching and thinning of the brain. After ossification is complete, hydrocephalus leads to a marked increase in ICP and destruction of neural tissue.

Primary hydrocephalus

In this condition there is accumulation of CSF accompanied by dilatation of the ventricles. It is usually caused by obstruction to the flow of CSF but is occasionally due to malabsorption of CSF by the arachnoid villi. It may be communicating or non-communicating. Without treatment, permanent brain damage occurs.

Congenital primary hydrocephalus is due to malformation of the ventricles, foramina or ducts, usually at a narrow point.

Acquired primary hydrocephalus is caused by lesions that obstruct the circulation of the CSF, usually expanding lesions, e.g. tumours, haematomas or adhesions between arachnoid and pia maters, following meningitis.

Secondary hydrocephalus

Compensatory increases in the amount of CSF and ventricle capacity occur when there is atrophy of brain tissue, e.g. in dementia and following cerebral infarcts. There may not be a rise in ICP.

Head injuries

The brain may be injured by a blow to the head or movement of the brain during sudden acceleration or deceleration of the head. The damage to the brain may be serious even when there is no outward sign of injury.

Blow to the head

At the site of injury there may be:

- a scalp wound, with haemorrhage between scalp and skull bones
- damage to the underlying meninges and/or brain with local haemorrhage inside the skull
- depressed fracture of the skull, causing local damage to the underlying meninges and brain tissue
- temporal bone fracture, making an opening between the middle ear and the meninges
- fracture involving the air sinuses of the sphenoid, ethmoid or frontal bones, making an opening between the nose and the meninges.

Acceleration–deceleration injuries

Because the brain floats relatively freely in 'a cushion' of CSF, sudden acceleration or deceleration has an inertia effect, i.e. there is delay between the movement of the head and the corresponding movement of the brain. During this period the brain may be compressed and damaged at the site of impact. In 'contre coup' injuries, brain damage is more severe on the side opposite to the site of impact. Other injuries include:

- nerve cell damage, usually to the frontal and parietal lobes, due to movement of the brain over the rough surface of bones of the base of the skull
- nerve fibre damage due to stretching, especially following rotational movement
- haemorrhage due to rupture of blood vessels in the subarachnoid space on the side opposite the impact or more diffuse small haemorrhages, following rotational movement.

Complications of head injury

If the individual survives the immediate effects, complications may develop hours or days later. Sometimes they are the first indication of serious damage caused by a seemingly trivial injury. Their effects may be to increase ICP, damage brain tissue or provide a route of entry for microbes.

Traumatic intracranial haemorrhage

Haemorrhage may occur causing secondary brain damage at the site of injury, on the opposite side of the brain or diffusely throughout the brain. If bleeding continues, the expanding haematoma damages the brain and increases the ICP.

Extradural haemorrhage. This may follow a direct blow that may or may not cause a fracture. The individual may recover quickly and indications of increased ICP appear only several hours later as the haematoma grows and the outer layer of dura mater (periosteum) is stripped off the bone. The haematoma grows rapidly when arterial blood vessels are damaged. In children there is rarely a fracture because the skull bones are still soft and the joints have not fused. The haematoma usually remains localised.

Acute subdural haemorrhage. This is due to haemorrhage from small veins in the dura mater or from larger veins between the layers of dura mater before they enter the venous sinuses. The blood may spread in the subdural space over one or both hemispheres (Fig. 7.46B). There may be concurrent subarachnoid haemorrhage, especially when there are extensive brain contusions and lacerations.

Chronic subdural haemorrhage. This may occur weeks or months after minor injuries and sometimes there is no history of injury. It occurs most commonly in people in whom there is some cerebral atrophy, e.g. older people and in alcoholism. Evidence of increased ICP may be delayed when brain volume is reduced. The haematoma formed gradually increases in size owing to repeated small haemorrhages and causes mild chronic inflammation and accumulation of inflammatory exudate. In time it is isolated by a wall of fibrous tissue.

Intracerebral haemorrhage and cerebral oedema. These occur following contusions, lacerations and shearing injuries associated with acceleration and deceleration, especially rotational movements.

Cerebral oedema (p. 178) is a common complication of contusions of the brain, leading to increased ICP, hypoxia and further brain damage.

Meningitis

Inflammation of the meninges may occur following a compound fracture of the skull that is accompanied by leakage of CSF and blood from the site, providing a route of entry for microbes. The escape of CSF and blood may be through the:

- skin, in compound fractures of the skull
- middle ear, in fractures of the temporal bone (CSF otorrhoea)
- nose, in fractures of sphenoid, ethmoid or frontal bones when the air sinuses are involved (CSF rhinorrhoea).

Post-traumatic epilepsy

This is usually characterised by seizures (fits) and may develop in the first week or several months after injury. Early development is most common after severe injuries, although in children the injury itself may have appeared trivial. After depressed fractures or large haematomas epilepsy tends to develop later.

Persistent vegetative state

In this condition there is severe brain damage that results in unconsciousness but the vital centres that control homeostasis remain intact, e.g. breathing, blood pressure.

Cerebral hypoxia

Hypoxia may be due to:

- disturbances in the autoregulation of blood supply to the brain
- conditions affecting cerebral blood vessels.

When the mean blood pressure falls below about 60 mmHg, the autoregulating mechanisms that control the blood flow to the brain by adjusting the diameter of the arterioles fail. The consequent rapid decrease in the cerebral blood supply leads to hypoxia and lack of glucose. If severe hypoxia is sustained for more than a few minutes there is irreversible brain damage. The neurones are affected first, then the neuroglial cells and later the meninges and blood vessels. Conditions in which autoregulation breaks down include:

- cardiorespiratory arrest
- sudden severe hypotension
- carbon monoxide poisoning
- hypercapnia (excess blood carbon dioxide)
- drug overdosage with, e.g., opioid analgesics, hypnotics.

Conditions affecting cerebral blood vessels that may lead to hypoxia include:

- occlusion of a cerebral artery by, e.g. a rapidly expanding intracranial lesion, atheroma, thrombosis or embolism (Ch. 4)
- arterial stenosis that occurs in arteritis, e.g. polyarteritis nodosa, syphilis, diabetes, degenerative changes in older people.

If the individual survives the initial episode of ischaemia then infarction, necrosis and loss of function of the affected area of brain may occur.

Stroke (cerebrovascular disease)

This condition is a common cause of death and disability, especially in older people. Predisposing factors include:

- hypertension
- atheroma
- cigarette smoking
- diabetes mellitus.

It occurs when blood flow to the brain is suddenly interrupted, causing hypoxia. The effects include paralysis of a limb or one side of the body and disturbances of speech and vision. The nature and extent of damage depends on the size and location of the affected blood vessels. The main causes are cerebral infarction (approx 85%) and spontaneous intracranial haemorrhage (15%).

Cerebral infarction

This is caused by atheroma complicated by thrombosis (p. 117) or blockage of an artery by an embolus from, e.g., infective endocarditis. When complete recovery occurs within 24 hours, the event is called a *transient ischaemic attack* (TIA). Recurrence or *completed stroke* associated with permanent damage may follow.

Spontaneous intracranial haemorrhage

The haemorrhage may be into the subarachnoid space or intracerebral (Fig. 7.47). It is commonly associated with an aneurysm or hypertension. In each case the escaped blood may cause arterial spasm, leading to ischaemia, infarction, fibrosis (gliosis) and hypoxic brain

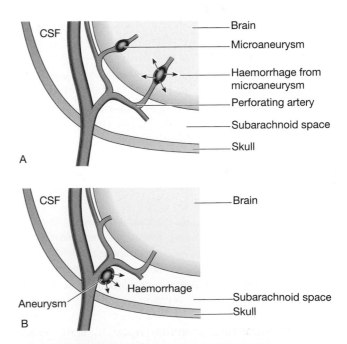

Figure 7.47 Types of haemorrhage causing stroke:
A. Intracerebral. B. Subarachnoid.

damage. A severe haemorrhage may be instantly fatal while repeated small haemorrhages have a cumulative effect in extending brain damage (*multi-infarct dementia*).

Intracerebral haemorrhage

Prolonged hypertension leads to the formation of multiple microaneurysms in the walls of very small arteries in the brain. Rupture of one or more of these, due to continuing rise in blood pressure, is usually the cause of intracerebral haemorrhage. The most common sites are branches of the middle cerebral artery in the region of the internal capsule and the basal ganglia.

Severe haemorrhage. This causes compression and destruction of tissue, a sudden increase in ICP and distortion and herniation of the brain. Death follows when the vital centres in the medulla oblongata are damaged by haemorrhage or if there is coning due to increased ICP.

Less severe haemorrhage. This causes paralysis and loss of sensation of varying severity, affecting the side of the body opposite the haemorrhage. If the bleeding stops and does not recur a fluid-filled cyst develops, i.e. the haematoma is walled off by gliosis, the blood clot is gradually absorbed and the cavity filled with tissue exudate. When the ICP returns to normal some function may be restored, e.g. speech and movement of limbs.

Subarachnoid haemorrhage

This is usually due to rupture of a berry aneurysm on one of the major cerebral arteries, or bleeding from a congenitally malformed blood vessel (Fig. 7.47B). The blood may remain localised but usually spreads in the subarachnoid space round the brain and spinal cord, causing a general increase in ICP without distortion of the brain (Fig. 7.46B). The irritant effect of the blood may cause arterial spasm, leading to ischaemia, infarction, gliosis and the effects of localised brain damage. It occurs most commonly in middle life, but occasionally in young people owing to rupture of a malformed blood vessel. This condition is often fatal or results in permanent disability.

Dementia

Dementia is caused by progressive, irreversible degeneration and atrophy of the cerebral cortex and results in mental deterioration, usually over several years. There is gradual impairment of memory (especially short term), intellect and reasoning. Emotional lability and personality change may also occur.

Alzheimer's disease

This condition is the commonest form of dementia; the aetiology is unknown although genetic factors may be involved. Females are affected twice as often as males and it usually affects those over 60 years, the incidence increasing with age. There is progressive atrophy of the cerebral cortex accompanied by deteriorating mental functioning. Death usually occurs between 2 and 8 years after onset.

Huntington's disease (chorea)

This usually manifests itself between the ages of 30 and 50 years. It is inherited as an autosomal dominant disorder (see p. 437) associated with deficient production of the neurotransmitter gamma aminobutyric acid (GABA). By the time of onset, the individual may have passed the genetic abnormality on to their children. Extrapyramidal changes cause *chorea*, rapid uncoordinated jerking movements of the limbs and involuntary twitching of the facial muscles. As the disease progresses, cortical atrophy causes personality changes and dementia.

Secondary dementias

Dementia may occur in association with other diseases:

- cerebrovascular disease – multi-infarct dementia
- infections, e.g. neurosyphilis, human immunodeficiency virus (HIV), Creutzfeldt–Jakob disease
- cerebral trauma
- chronic misuse of alcohol and some drugs
- vitamin B deficiencies
- effects of metabolic disorders, e.g. hypothyroidism, uraemia, liver failure.

Parkinson's disease

In this disease there is gradual degeneration of dopamine-releasing neurones in the extrapyramidal system. This leads to lack of control and coordination of muscle movement resulting in:

- fixed muscle tone causing expressionless facial features, rigidity of voluntary muscles causing the slow and characteristic stiff shuffling gait and stooping posture
- muscle tremor of extremities, e.g. 'pill rolling' movement of the fingers.

Onset is usually between 45 and 60 years. The cause is usually unknown but some cases are associated with repeated trauma as in, e.g., 'punch drunk' boxers; tumours

181

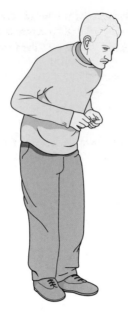

Figure 7.48 Typical posture of Parkinson's disease.

causing midbrain compression; drugs, e.g. pheno-thiazines; heavy metal poisoning. There is progressive physical disability but the intellect is not impaired (Fig. 7.48).

Infections of the central nervous system

Learning outcome

After studying this section you should be able to:

■ describe common infections of the nervous system and their effects on body function.

The brain and spinal cord are relatively well protected from microbial infection by the blood–brain barrier.

The microbes usually involved are bacteria and viruses, occasionally protozoa and fungi. The infection may originate in the meninges (*meningitis*) or in the brain (*encephalitis*), then spread from one site to the other.

Bacterial infections

Entry of bacteria into the CNS may be:

- direct – through a skull fracture or through the skull bones from e.g. middle ear infections, mastoiditis

- blood-borne – from infection elsewhere in the body e.g. septicaemia, bacterial endocarditis (p. 124)
- iatrogenic – introduced during an invasive procedure e.g. lumbar puncture.

Bacterial meningitis

The term 'meningitis' usually refers to inflammation of the subarachnoid space and is most commonly transmitted through contact with an infected individual. Bacterial meningitis is usually preceded by a mild upper respiratory tract infection during which a few bacteria enter the bloodstream and are carried to the meninges. Common microbes include:

- *Haemophilus influenzae* in children between the ages of 2 and 5 years
- *Neisseria meningitidis* in those between 5 and 30 years
- *Streptococcus pneumoniae* in people over 30 years.

Other pathogenic bacteria can also cause meningitis, e.g. those causing tuberculosis (p. 262) and syphilis.

Meningitis can also affect the dura mater especially when spread is direct through a skull fracture or from a local infection. In this type, an extradural or sub-dural abscess may form and cause further spread if it ruptures.

The onset is usually sudden with severe headache, neck stiffness, photophobia (intolerance of bright light) and fever. This is sometimes accompanied by a petechial rash. CSF appears cloudy owing to the presence of many bacteria and neutrophils. Mortality and morbidity rates are considerable.

Viral infections

Entry of viruses into the CNS is usually blood-borne from viral infection elsewhere in the body and, less commonly, through the nervous system. In the latter situation, *neurotropic viruses*, i.e. those with an affinity for the nervous system, travel along peripheral nerve from a site elsewhere, e.g. poliovirus. They enter the body via:

- the alimentary tract, e.g. poliomyelitis
- the respiratory tract, e.g. shingles
- skin abrasions, e.g. rabies.

The effects of viral infections vary according to the site and the amount of tissue destroyed. Viruses may damage neurones by:

- multiplying within them
- stimulating an immune reaction which may explain why signs of some infections do not appear until there is a high antibody titre, 1 to 2 weeks after infection.

Viral meningitis

This is the most common form of meningitis and is usually a relatively mild infection followed by complete recovery.

Viral encephalitis

Viral encephalitis is rare and not always associated with a recent viral infection. Most cases are mild and recovery is usually complete. It may affect a wide variety of sites and, as nerve cells are not replaced, loss of function reflects the extent of damage. In severe infection neurones and neuroglia may be affected, followed by necrosis and gliosis. Early senility may develop or, if vital centres in the medulla oblongata are involved, death may ensue.

Herpes simplex encephalitis. This is the most common type of encephalitis in the UK. It is an acute, often fatal, condition causing necrosis of areas of the cerebrum, usually the temporal lobes. If the patient survives the initial acute phase there may be residual dysfunction, e.g. behavioural disturbance and loss of memory.

Herpes zoster (shingles)

Herpes zoster viruses cause chickenpox (varicella) mainly in children and shingles (zoster) in adults. Susceptible children may contract chickenpox from a person with shingles but not the reverse. Adults infected with the viruses may show no immediate signs of disease. The viruses remain dormant in posterior root ganglia of the spinal nerves then become active years later, causing shingles. Reactivation may be either spontaneous or associated with the following factors:

- depression of the immune system, e.g. by drugs, old age, AIDS
- exposure of the dermatome to irradiation, e.g. sun, X-rays.

The posterior root ganglion becomes acutely inflamed. From there the viruses pass along the sensory nerve to the surface tissues supplied, e.g. skin, cornea. The infection is usually unilateral and the most common sites are:

- nerves supplying the trunk, sometimes two or three adjacent dermatomes (Fig. 7.38)
- the ophthalmic division of the trigeminal nerve (Fig. 7.40), causing *trigeminal neuralgia*, and, if vesicles form on the cornea, there may be ulceration, scarring and residual interference with vision.

Affected tissues become inflamed and vesicles, containing serous fluid and viruses, develop along the course of the nerve. This is accompanied by persistent pain and hypersensitivity to touch (*hyperaesthesia*). Recovery is usually slow and there may be some loss of sensation, depending on the severity of the disease.

Poliomyelitis

This disease is usually caused by *polioviruses* and, occasionally, by other *enteroviruses*. The infection is spread by food contaminated by infected faecal matter and initially, viral multiplication occurs in the alimentary tract. The viruses are then blood-borne to the nervous system and invade anterior horn cells in the spinal cord. Usually there is a mild febrile illness with no indication of nerve damage. In mild cases there is complete recovery but there is permanent disability in many others. Paralytic disease is believed to be precipitated by muscular exercise during the early febrile stage. Irreversible damage to lower motor neurones causes muscle paralysis which, in the limbs, may lead to deformity because of the unopposed tonal contraction of antagonistic muscles. Death may occur owing to respiratory paralysis. Vaccination programmes have now almost eradicated this disease in developed countries.

Rabies

All warm-blooded animals are susceptible to the rabies virus, which is endemic in many countries but not in the UK. The main reservoirs of virus are wild animals, some of which may be carriers. These may infect domestic pets which then become the main source of human infection. The viruses multiply in the salivary glands and are present in large numbers in saliva. They enter the body through skin abrasions and are believed to travel to the brain along peripheral nerves. The incubation period varies from about 2 weeks to several months, possibly reflecting the distance viruses travel between the site of entry and the brain. Extensive damage to the basal ganglia, midbrain, medulla oblongata and the posterior root ganglia of the peripheral nerves causes meningeal irritation, extreme hyperaesthesia, muscle spasm and convulsions. *Hydrophobia* (hatred of water) and overflow of saliva from the mouth are due to painful spasm of the throat muscles that inhibits swallowing. In the advanced stages muscle spasm may alternate with flaccid paralysis and death is usually due to respiratory muscle spasm or paralysis.

Not all people exposed to the virus contract rabies, but in those who do, the mortality rate is high.

Human immunodeficiency virus (HIV)

The brain is often affected in individuals with AIDS (p. 382) resulting in opportunistic infection and dementia.

Creutzfeldt–Jakob disease

This infective condition may be caused by a 'slow' virus, the nature and transmission of which is poorly understood. It is thought to be via a heat-resistant transmissible particle known as a *prion protein*. It is a rapidly progressive form of dementia for which there is no known treatment so the condition is always fatal.

Myalgic encephalitis (ME)

This condition is also known as post-viral syndrome or chronic fatigue syndrome. It affects mostly teenagers and young adults and the aetiology is unknown. Sometimes the condition follows a viral illness. The effects include malaise, severe fatigue, poor concentration and myalgia. Recovery is usually spontaneous but sometimes results in chronic disability.

Demyelinating diseases

Learning outcome

After studying this section you should be able to:

- explain how the signs and symptoms of demyelinating disease are related to pathological changes in the nervous system.

These diseases are caused either by injury to axons or by disorders of cells that secrete myelin, i.e. oligodendrocytes and Schwann cells.

Multiple sclerosis (MS)

In this disease there are areas of demyelinated white matter, called *plaques*, irregularly distributed throughout the brain and spinal cord. Grey matter in the brain and spinal cord may also be affected because of the arrangement of satellite oligodendrocytes round cell bodies. In the early stages there may be little damage to axons.

It usually develops between the ages of 20 and 40 years. The actual cause(s) of MS are not known but several factors seem to be involved.

Environment before adolescence is implicated because the disease is most prevalent in people who spend their preadolescent years in temperate climates, and those who move to other climates after that age retain their susceptibility to MS. People from equatorial areas moving into a temperate climate during adolescence or later life appear not to be susceptible.

Genetic factors are implicated too as there is an increased incidence of MS among siblings, especially identical twins, and parents of patients.

Immune factors are also thought to be involved.

Effects of multiple sclerosis

Neuronal damage leads to a variety of dysfunctions, depending on the sites and sizes of demyelinated plaques. Plaques damage white matter leading to upper motor neurone dysfunction causing:

- weakness of skeletal muscles and sometimes paralysis
- lack of coordination and movement
- disturbed sensation, e.g. burning or pins and needles
- incontinence of urine
- visual disturbances especially blurring and double vision. The optic nerves are commonly affected early in the disease.

The disease pattern is usually one of relapses and remissions of widely varying duration. Each relapse causes further loss of nervous tissue and progressive dysfunction. In some cases there may be chronic progression without remission, or acute disease rapidly leading to death.

Acute disseminated encephalomyelitis

This is a rare but serious condition that may occur:

- during or very soon after a viral infection, e.g. measles, chickenpox, mumps, respiratory tract infection
- following primary immunisation against viral diseases, mainly in older children and adults.

The cause of the acute diffuse demyelination is not known. It has been suggested that an autoimmune effect on myelin is triggered either by viruses during a viral infection such as measles, or by an immune response to vaccines. The effects vary considerably, according to the distribution and degree of demyelination and are similar to those of MS. The early febrile state may progress to paralysis and coma. Most patients survive the initial phase and recover with no residual dysfunction but some have severe neurological impairment.

Diseases of the spinal cord

Learning outcome

After studying this section you should be able to:

- explain how disorders of the spinal cord cause abnormal function.

Because space in the neural canal and intervertebral foramina is limited, any condition that distorts their shape or reduces the space may damage the spinal cord or peripheral nerve roots, or cause ischaemia by compressing blood vessels. Such conditions include:

- fracture and/or dislocation of vertebrae
- tumours of the meninges or vertebrae
- prolapsed intervertebral disc.

The effects of disease or injury depend on the severity of the damage, the type and position of the neurones involved, i.e. motor, sensory, proprioceptor, autonomic, connector neurones in reflex arcs in the spinal cord or in peripheral nerves.

Motor neurones

Upper motor neurone (UMN) lesions
Lesions of the UMNs above the level of the decussation of the pyramids affect the opposite side of the body, e.g. haemorrhage or infarction in the internal capsule of one hemisphere causes paralysis of the opposite side of the body. Lesions below the decussation level affect the same side of the body. The lower motor neurones are released from cortical control and muscle tone is increased (Table 7.4).

Lower motor neurone (LMN) lesions
The cell bodies of LMNs are in the spinal cord and the axons are part of peripheral nerves. Lesions of LMNs lead to weakness or paralysis of the effector muscles they supply.

Table 7.4 gives a summary of the effects of damage to the motor neurones. The parts of the body affected depend on which neurones have been damaged and their site in the brain, spinal cord or peripheral nerve.

Table 7.4 Summary of effects of damage to motor neurones

Upper motor neurone	Lower motor neurone
Muscle weakness and spastic paralysis	Muscle weakness and flaccid paralysis
Exaggerated tendon reflexes	Absence of tendon reflexes
Muscle twitching	Muscle wasting Contracture of muscles Impaired circulation

Motor neurone disease

This is a chronic progressive degeneration of motor neurones, occurring more commonly in men over 50 years of age. The cause is not known. Motor neurones in the cerebral cortex, brain stem and anterior horns of the spinal cord are destroyed and replaced by gliosis. Early effects are usually weakness and twitching of the small muscles of the hand, and muscles of the arm and shoulder girdle. The legs are affected later. Death occurs within 3–5 years and is usually due to respiratory difficulties or complications of immobility.

Sensory neurones

The sensory functions lost as a result of disease or injury depend on which neurones have been damaged. Spinal cord damage leads to loss of sensation and cerebellar function. Peripheral nerve damage leads to loss of reflex activity, loss of sensation and of cerebellar function.

Mixed motor and sensory conditions

Subacute combined degeneration of the spinal cord

This condition most commonly occurs as a complication of pernicious anaemia (p. 69). Vitamin B_{12} is associated with the formation and maintenance of myelin by Schwann cells and oligodendrocytes. Although degeneration of the spinal cord may be apparent before the anaemia, it is arrested by treatment with vitamin B_{12}.

The degeneration of nerve fibre myelin occurs in the posterior and lateral columns of white matter in the spinal cord, especially in the upper thoracic and lower cervical regions. Less frequently the changes occur in the posterior root ganglia and peripheral nerves. Demyelination of proprioceptor fibres (sensory) leads to ataxia and involvement of upper motor neurones leads to increased muscle tone and spastic paralysis. Without treatment, the outcome is death within 5 years.

Compression of the spinal cord and nerve roots

The causes include:

- prolapsed intervertebral disc
- syringomyelia
- tumours: metastatic, meningeal or nerve sheath
- fractures with displacement of bone fragments.

Prolapsed intervertebral disc (Fig. 7.49)
This is the most common cause of compression of the spinal cord and/or nerve roots. The vertebral bodies

185

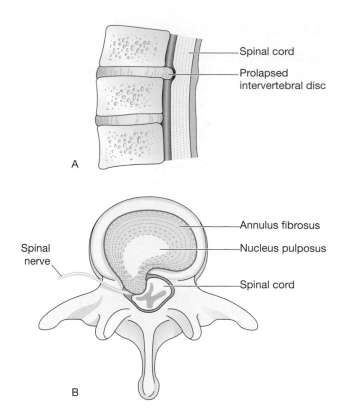

A

B

Figure 7.49 Prolapsed intervertebral disc. A. Viewed from the side. **B.** Viewed from above.

Labels in figure:
- Spinal cord
- Prolapsed intervertebral disc
- Annulus fibrosus
- Nucleus pulposus
- Spinal cord
- Spinal nerve

186

are separated by the intervertebral discs, each consisting of an outer rim of cartilage, the *annulus fibrosus*, and a central core of soft gelatinous material, the *nucleus pulposus*.

Prolapse of a disc is herniation of the nucleus pulposus, causing the annulus fibrosus and the posterior longitudinal ligament to protrude into the neural canal. It is most common in the lumbar region usually below the level of the spinal cord, i.e. below L2, and therefore affects nerve roots only. If it occurs in the cervical region, the cord may also be compressed. Herniation may occur suddenly, typically in young adults during strenuous exercise or exertion, or progressively in older people when bone disease or degeneration of the disc leads to rupture during minimal exercise. The hernia may be:

- one sided, causing pressure damage to a nerve root
- midline, compressing the spinal cord, the anterior spinal artery and possibly bilateral nerve roots.

The outcome depends upon the size of the hernia and the length of time the pressure is applied. Small herniations cause local pain due to pressure on the nerve endings in the posterior longitudinal ligament.

Large herniations may cause:

- unilateral or bilateral paralysis
- acute or chronic pain perceived to originate from the area supplied by the compressed sensory nerve, e.g. in the leg or foot
- compression of the anterior spinal artery, causing ischaemia and possibly necrosis of the spinal cord
- local muscle spasm due to pressure on motor nerves.

Syringomyelia

This dilatation (syrinx) of the central canal of the spinal cord occurs most commonly in the cervical region and is associated with congenital abnormality of the distal end of the fourth ventricle. As the central canal dilates, pressure causes progressive damage to sensory and motor neurones.

Early effects include *dissociated anaesthesia*, i.e. insensibility to heat and pain, due to compression of the sensory fibres that cross the cord immediately they enter. In the long term there is destruction of motor and sensory tracts, leading to spastic paralysis and loss of sensation and reflexes.

Tumours and displaced fragments of fractured vertebrae

These may affect the spinal cord and nerve roots at any level. The pressure damage initially causes pain and later, if the pressure is not relieved, there may be loss of sensation and paralysis. The areas affected depend on the site of pressure.

Diseases of peripheral nerves

Learning outcomes

After studying this section you should be able to:

- compare and contrast the causes and effects of polyneuropathies and mononeuropathies

- describe the effects of Guillain–Barré syndrome and Bell's palsy.

Peripheral neuropathy

This is a group of diseases of peripheral nerves not associated with inflammation. They are classified as:

- polyneuropathy: several nerves are affected
- mononeuropathy: a single nerve is usually affected.

Polyneuropathy

Damage to a number of nerves and their myelin sheaths occurs in association with other disorders, e.g.:

- nutritional deficiencies, e.g. vitamins B_1, B_6, B_{12}
- metabolic disorders, e.g. diabetes mellitus, renal failure, hepatic failure, carcinoma
- toxic reactions to, e.g., alcohol, lead, arsenic, mercury, carbon tetrachloride, aniline dyes and some drugs, such as phenytoin, isoniazid
- infections, e.g. influenza, measles, typhoid fever, diphtheria, leprosy.

The long nerves are usually affected first, e.g. those supplying the feet and legs. The outcome depends upon the cause of the neuropathy and the extent of the damage.

Mononeuropathy

Usually only one nerve is damaged and the most common cause is ischaemia due to pressure. Examples include:

- pressure applied to cranial nerves in cranial bone foramina due to distortion of the brain by increased ICP
- compression of a nerve in a confined space caused by surrounding inflammation and oedema, e.g. the median nerve in carpal tunnel syndrome (see p. 430)
- external pressure on a nerve, e.g. an unconscious person lying with an arm hanging over the side of a bed or trolley
- compression of the axillary (circumflex) nerve by ill-fitting crutches
- trapping of a nerve between the broken ends of a bone
- ischaemia due to thrombosis of blood vessels supplying a nerve.

The resultant dysfunction depends on the site and extent of the injury.

Guillain–Barré syndrome

Also known as acute inflammatory polyneuropathy, this is sudden, acute, progressive, bilateral ascending muscular weakness or paralysis. It begins in the lower limbs and spreads to the arms, trunk and cranial nerves. It usually occurs 1 to 3 weeks after an upper respiratory tract infection. There is widespread inflammation accompanied by some demyelination of spinal, peripheral and cranial nerves and the spinal ganglia. Paralysis may affect all the limbs and the respiratory muscles. Patients who survive the acute phase usually recover completely in weeks or months.

Bell's palsy

Compression of a facial nerve in the temporal bone foramen causes paralysis of facial muscles with drooping and loss of facial expression on the affected side. The immediate cause is inflammation and oedema of the nerve. The underlying cause is unknown although viruses may be involved. The onset may be sudden or develop over several hours. Distortion of the features is due to muscle tone on the unaffected side, the affected side being expressionless. Recovery is usually complete within a few months although the condition is sometimes permanent.

Developmental abnormalities of the nervous system

Learning outcomes

After studying this section you should be able to:

- describe developmental abnormalities of the nervous system
- relate their effects to abnormal body function.

187

Spina bifida

This is a congenital malformation of the embryonic neural tube and spinal cord (Fig. 7.50). The vertebral (neural) arches are absent and the dura mater is abnormal, most commonly in the lumbosacral region. The causes are not known, although the condition is associated with dietary deficiency of folic acid at the time of conception. These neural tube defects may be of genetic origin or due to environmental factors, e.g. irradiation, or maternal infection (rubella) at a critical stage in development of the fetal vertebrae and spinal cord. The effects depend on the extent of the abnormality.

Occult spina bifida

The skin over the defect is intact and excessive growth of hair over the site may be the only sign of abnormality. This is sometimes associated with minor nerve defects that commonly affect the bladder.

Meningocele

The skin over the defect is very thin and may rupture after birth. There is dilatation of the subarachnoid space posteriorly. The spinal cord is correctly positioned.

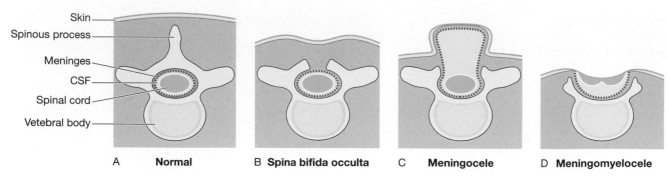

Skin
Spinous process
Meninges
CSF
Spinal cord
Vetebral body

A   **Normal**   B **Spina bifida occulta**   C   **Meningocele**   D   **Meningomyelocele**

Figure 7.50 Spina bifida.

Meningomyelocele

The meninges and spinal cord are grossly abnormal. The skin may be absent or rupture. In either case there is leakage of CSF, and the meninges may become infected. Serious nerve defects result in paraplegia and lack of sphincter control causing incontinence of urine and faeces. There may also be mental impairment.

Hydrocephalus (see p. 178)

Tumours of the nervous system

Learning outcome

After studying this section you should be able to:

- outline the effects of tumours of the nervous system.

Primary tumours of the nervous system usually arise from the neuroglia, meninges or blood vessels. Neurones are rarely involved because they do not normally multiply. Metastases of nervous tissue tumours are rare. Because of this, the rate of growth of a tumour is more important than the likelihood of spread outside the nervous system. In this context, 'benign' means slow growing and 'malignant' rapid growing. Early signs are typically headache, vomiting and *papilloedema* (swelling of the optic disc seen by ophthalmoscopy). Signs of raised ICP appear after the limits of compensation have been reached (see p. 177).

Within the confined space of the skull, haemorrhage within a tumour exacerbates the increased ICP caused by the tumour.

Slow-growing tumours

These allow time for adjustment to compensate for increasing intracranial pressure, so the tumour may be quite large before its effects are evident. Compensation involves gradual reduction in the volume of cerebrospinal fluid and circulating blood.

Rapidly growing tumours

These do not allow time for adjustment to compensate for the rapidly increasing ICP, so the effects quickly become apparent (Fig. 7.46C). Complications include:

- neurological impairment, depending on tumour site and size
- effects of increased ICP (p. 177)
- necrosis of the tumour, causing haemorrhage and oedema.

Specific tumours

Gliomas are usually astrocytomas, ranging from benign tumours to the highly malignant *glioblastoma multiforme*.

Meningiomas are usually benign, originating from arachnoid granulations.

Medulloblastomas are highly malignant neurone-cell tumours, occurring mainly in the cerebellum in children. They are believed to originate from primitive cells prior to differentiation into neurones and neuroglia.

Metastases in the brain

The most common primary sites that metastasise to the brain are the breast, lungs and bone marrow (leukaemias). The prognosis of this condition is poor and the effects depend on the site(s) and rate of growth of metastases. There are two forms:

- discrete multiple tumours, mainly in the cerebrum
- diffuse tumours in the arachnoid mater.

The special senses

8

The special senses of hearing, sight, smell and taste all have specialised sensory receptors (nerve endings) outside the brain. These are found in the ears, eyes, nose and mouth. The ear is also involved in the maintenance of balance. In the brain the incoming nerve impulses undergo complex processes of integration and coordination that result in perception of sensory information and a variety of responses inside and outside the body. Up to 80% of what we perceive comes from sensory stimuli.

Hearing and the ear

Learning outcomes

After studying this section you should be able to:

■ describe the structure of the outer, middle and inner parts of the ear

■ explain the physiology of hearing.

The ear is the organ of hearing. It is supplied by the 8th cranial nerve, i.e. the *cochlear part* of the *vestibulocochlear* nerve, which is stimulated by vibrations caused by sound waves.

With the exception of the auricle (pinna), the structures that form the ear are encased within the petrous portion of the temporal bone.

Structure

The ear is divided into three distinct parts (Fig. 8.1):

• outer ear
• middle ear (tympanic cavity)
• inner ear.

Outer ear

The outer ear consists of the auricle (pinna) and the external acoustic meatus (auditory canal).

The auricle (pinna)

The auricle is the expanded portion that projects from the side of the head. It is composed of fibroelastic cartilage covered with skin. It is deeply grooved and ridged; the most prominent outer ridge is the *helix*.

The *lobule* (earlobe) is the soft pliable part at the lower extremity, composed of fibrous and adipose tissue richly supplied with blood.

External acoustic meatus (auditory canal)

This is a slightly 'S'-shaped tube about 2.5 cm long extending from the auricle to the *tympanic membrane* (eardrum). The lateral third is cartilaginous and the remainder is a canal in the temporal bone. The meatus is lined with skin continuous with that of the auricle. There are numerous *ceruminous glands* and hair follicles, with associated *sebaceous glands*, in the skin of the lateral third. Ceruminous glands are modified sweat glands that secrete *cerumen* (earwax), a sticky material containing

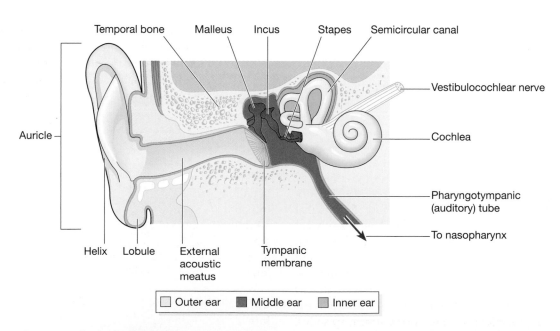

Figure 8.1 The parts of the ear.

lysozyme and immunoglobulins. Foreign materials, e.g. dust, insects and microbes, are prevented from reaching the tympanic membrane by wax, hairs and the curvature of the meatus. Movements of the temporomandibular joint during chewing and speaking 'massage' the cartilaginous meatus, moving the wax towards the exterior.

The tympanic membrane (eardrum) (Fig. 8.2) completely separates the external acoustic meatus from the middle ear. It is oval-shaped with the slightly broader edge upwards and is formed by three types of tissue: the outer covering of hairless skin, the middle layer of fibrous tissue and the inner lining of mucous membrane continuous with that of the middle ear.

Middle ear (tympanic cavity)

This is an irregular-shaped air-filled cavity within the petrous portion of the temporal bone. The cavity, its contents and the air sacs which open out of it are lined with either simple squamous or cuboidal epithelium.

The *lateral wall* of the middle ear is formed by the tympanic membrane.

The *roof and floor* are formed by the temporal bone.

The *posterior wall* is formed by the temporal bone with openings leading to the *mastoid antrum* through which air passes to the air cells within the mastoid process.

The *medial wall* is a thin layer of temporal bone in which there are two openings:

- oval window
- round window (see Fig. 8.6).

The oval window is occluded by part of a small bone called the *stapes* and the round window, by a fine sheet of fibrous tissue.

Air reaches the cavity through the *pharyngotympanic* (*auditory or Eustachian*) tube, which extends from the nasopharynx. It is about 4 cm long and is lined with ciliated columnar epithelium. The presence of air at atmospheric pressure on both sides of the tympanic membrane is maintained by the pharyngotympanic tube and enables the membrane to vibrate when sound waves strike it. The pharyngotympanic tube is normally closed but when there is unequal pressure across the tympanic membrane, e.g. at high altitude, it is opened by swallowing or yawning and the ears 'pop', equalising the pressure again.

Auditory ossicles (Fig. 8.3)

These are three very small bones that extend across the middle ear from the tympanic membrane to the oval window (Fig. 8.1). They form a series of movable joints with each other and with the medial wall of the cavity at the oval window. They are named according to their shapes.

The malleus. This is the lateral hammer-shaped bone. The handle is in contact with the tympanic membrane and the head forms a movable joint with the incus.

The incus. This is the middle anvil-shaped bone. Its body articulates with the malleus, the long process with the stapes, and it is stabilised by the short process, fixed by fibrous tissue to the posterior wall of the tympanic cavity.

191

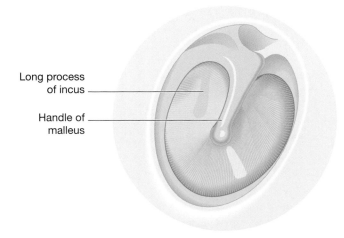

Figure 8.2 The tympanic membrane. Viewed through an auriscope showing the shadows cast by the malleus and the incus.

Long process of incus

Handle of malleus

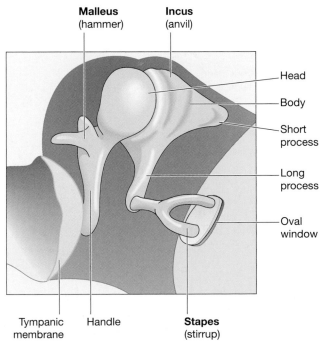

Malleus (hammer)

Incus (anvil)

Head

Body

Short process

Long process

Oval window

Tympanic membrane

Handle

Stapes (stirrup)

Figure 8.3 The auditory ossicles.

The stapes. This is the medial stirrup-shaped bone. Its head articulates with the incus and its footplate fits into the oval window.

The three ossicles are held in position by fine ligaments.

Inner ear (Fig. 8.4)

The inner (internal) ear or labyrinth (meaning 'maze') contains the organs of hearing and balance. It is described in two parts, the *bony labyrinth* and the *membranous labyrinth*.

Bony labyrinth

This is a cavity within the temporal bone lined with periosteum. It is larger than, and encloses, the membranous labyrinth of the same shape that fits into it, like a tube within a tube. Between the bony and membranous labyrinth there is a layer of watery fluid called *perilymph* and within the membranous labyrinth there is a similarly watery fluid, *endolymph*.

The bony labyrinth consists of:

- the vestibule
- the cochlea
- three semicircular canals.

The vestibule. This is the expanded part nearest the middle ear. It contains the oval and round windows in its lateral wall.

The cochlea. This resembles a snail's shell. It has a broad base where it is continuous with the vestibule

and a narrow apex, and it spirals round a central bony column.

The semicircular canals. These are three tubes arranged so that one is situated in each of the three planes of space. They are continuous with the vestibule.

Membranous labyrinth

This contains endolymph and lies within its bony counterpart. It comprises:

- the vestibule, which contains the *utricle* and *saccule*
- the cochlea
- three semicircular canals.

The cochlea

A cross-section of the cochlea (Fig. 8.5) contains three compartments:

- the scala vestibuli
- the scala media, or *cochlear duct*
- the scala tympani.

In cross-section the bony cochlea has two compartments containing perilymph: the scala vestibuli, which originates at the oval window, and the scala tympani, which ends at the round window. The two compartments are continuous with each other and Figure 8.6 shows the relationship between these structures. The cochlear duct is part of the membranous labyrinth and is triangular in shape. On the *basilar membrane*, or base of the triangle, there are *supporting cells* and specialised *cochlear hair cells* containing auditory receptors. These cells form the *spiral*

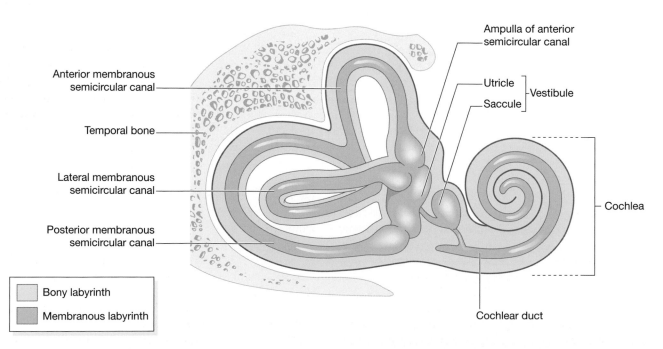

Anterior membranous semicircular canal

Temporal bone

Lateral membranous semicircular canal

Posterior membranous semicircular canal

Ampulla of anterior semicircular canal

Utricle
Saccule
Vestibule

Cochlea

Cochlear duct

Bony labyrinth

Membranous labyrinth

Figure 8.4 The inner ear. The membranous labyrinth within the bony labyrinth.

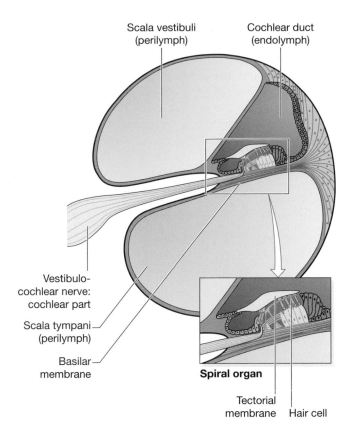

Figure 8.5 A cross-section of the cochlea showing the spiral organ (of Corti).

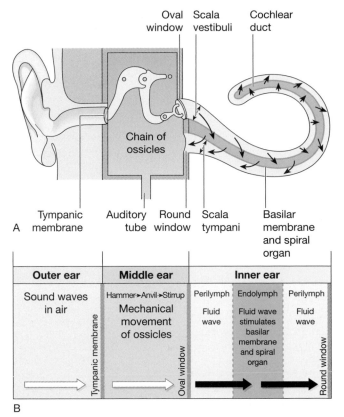

Figure 8.6 Passage of sound waves: A. The ear with cochlea uncoiled. **B.** Summary of transmission.

organ (of Corti), the sensory organ that responds to vibration by initiating nerve impulses that are then perceived as hearing by the brain. The *auditory receptors* are dendrites of efferent nerves that combine forming the cochlear (auditory) part of the vestibulocochlear nerve (8th cranial nerve), which passes through a foramen in the temporal bone to reach the hearing area in the temporal lobe of the cerebrum (see Fig. 7.16, p. 152).

Physiology of hearing

Every sound produces sound waves or vibrations in the air, which travel at about 332 metres per second. The auricle, because of its shape, collects and concentrates the waves and directs them along the external acoustic meatus causing the tympanic membrane to vibrate. Tympanic membrane vibrations are transmitted and amplified through the middle ear by movement of the ossicles (Fig. 8.6). At their medial end the footplate of the stapes rocks to and fro in the oval window, setting up fluid waves in the perilymph of the scala vestibuli. Some of the force of these waves is transmitted along the length of the scala vestibuli and scala tympani, but most of the pressure is transmitted into the cochlear duct. This causes a corresponding wave motion in the endolymph, resulting in vibration of the basilar membrane and stimulation of the auditory receptors in the hair cells of the spiral organ. The nerve impulses generated pass to the brain in the cochlear (auditory) portion of the vestibulocochlear nerve (8th cranial nerve). The fluid wave is finally expended into the middle ear by vibration of the membrane of the round window. The vestibulocochlear nerve transmits the impulses to the auditory nuclei in the medulla, where they synapse before they are conducted to the auditory area in the temporal lobe of the cerebrum (see Fig. 7.16, p. 152). Because some fibres cross over in the medulla and others remain on the same side, the left and right auditory areas of the cerebrum receive impulses from both ears.

Sound waves have the properties of *pitch* and *volume*, or intensity (Fig. 8.7). Pitch is determined by the frequency of the sound waves and is measured in Hertz (Hz). Sounds of different frequencies stimulate the basilar membrane (Fig. 8.6A) at different places along its length, allowing discrimination of pitch.

The volume depends on the magnitude of the sound waves and is measured in decibels (dB). The greater the

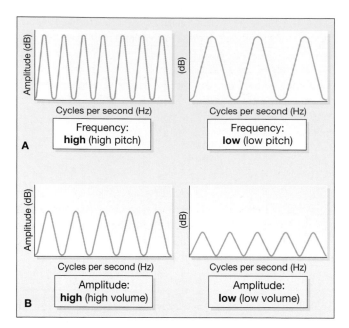

Figure 8.7 Behaviour of sound waves. A. Difference in frequency but of the same amplitude. **B.** Difference in amplitude but of the same frequency.

amplitude of the wave created in the endolymph, the greater is the stimulation of the auditory receptors in the hair cells in the spiral organ, enabling perception of volume. Very loud noise causes hearing loss, particularly when prolonged, because it damages the sensitive hair cells of the spiral organ.

Balance and the ear

Learning outcome

After studying this section you should be able to:

- describe the physiology of balance.

The semicircular canals and vestibule (Fig. 8.4)

The semicircular canals have no auditory function although they are closely associated with the cochlea. They provide information about the position of the head in space, contributing to maintenance of posture and balance.

There are three semicircular canals, one lying in each of the three planes of space. They are situated above, beside and behind the vestibule of the inner ear and open into it.

The semicircular canals, like the cochlea, are composed of an outer bony wall and inner membranous tubes or *ducts*. The membranous ducts contain endolymph and are separated from the bony wall by perilymph.

The utricle is a membranous sac which is part of the vestibule and the three membranous ducts open into it at their dilated ends, the *ampullae*. The *saccule* is a part of the vestibule and communicates with the utricle and the cochlea.

In the walls of the utricle, saccule and ampullae there are fine, specialised epithelial cells with minute projections, called *hair cells*. Amongst the hair cells there are receptors on sensory nerve endings, which combine forming the vestibular part of the vestibulocochlear nerve.

Physiology of balance

The semicircular canals and the vestibule (utricle and saccule) are concerned with balance. Any change of position of the head causes movement in the perilymph and endolymph, which bends the hair cells and stimulates the sensory receptors in the utricle, saccule and ampullae. The resultant nerve impulses are transmitted by the vestibular nerve, which joins the cochlear nerve to form the vestibulocochlear nerve. The vestibular branch passes first to the *vestibular nucleus*, then to the cerebellum.

The cerebellum also receives nerve impulses from the eyes and proprioceptors (sensory receptors) in the skeletal muscles and joints. Impulses from these three sources are coordinated and efferent nerve impulses pass to the cerebrum and to skeletal muscles. This results in awareness of body position, maintenance of upright posture and fixing of the eyes on the same point, independently of head movements.

Sight and the eye

Learning outcomes

After studying this section you should be able to:

- describe the gross structure of the eye
- describe the route taken by nerve impulses from the retina to the cerebrum
- explain how light entering the eye is focused on the retina
- state the functions of the extraocular eye muscles
- explain the functions of the accessory organs of the eye.

194

The eye is the organ of the sense of sight situated in the orbital cavity and it is supplied by the *optic nerve* (2nd cranial nerve).

It is almost spherical in shape and is about 2.5 cm in diameter. The space between the eye and the orbital cavity is occupied by adipose tissue. The bony walls of the orbit and the fat help to protect the eye from injury.

Structurally the two eyes are separate but, unlike the ear, some of their activities are coordinated so that they function as a pair. It is possible to see with only one eye, but three-dimensional vision is impaired when only one eye is used, especially in relation to the judgement of speed and distance.

Structure (Fig. 8.8)

There are three layers of tissue in the walls of the eye. They are:

- the outer fibrous layer: sclera and cornea
- the middle vascular layer or *uveal tract*: choroid, ciliary body and iris
- the inner nervous tissue layer: retina.

Structures inside the eyeball are the lens, aqueous fluid and vitreous body.

Sclera and cornea

The sclera, or white of the eye, forms the outermost layer of the posterior and lateral aspects of the eyeball and is continuous anteriorly with the transparent cornea. It consists of a firm fibrous membrane that maintains the shape of the eye and gives attachment to the *extrinsic muscles* of the eye (p. 201).

Anteriorly the sclera continues as a clear transparent epithelial membrane, the cornea. Light rays pass through the cornea to reach the retina. The cornea is convex anteriorly and is involved in refracting (bending) light rays to focus them on the retina.

Choroid (Figs 8.8 and 8.9)

The choroid lines the posterior five-sixths of the inner surface of the sclera. It is very rich in blood vessels and is deep chocolate brown in colour. Light enters the eye through the pupil, stimulates the sensory receptors in the retina and is then absorbed by the choroid.

Ciliary body

The ciliary body is the anterior continuation of the choroid consisting of *ciliary muscle* (smooth muscle fibres) and secretory epithelial cells. It gives attachment to the *suspensory ligament* which, at its other end, is attached to the capsule enclosing the lens. Contraction and relaxation of the ciliary muscle changes the thickness of the lens, which bends light rays entering the eye to focus them on the retina. The epithelial cells secrete *aqueous fluid* into the anterior segment of the eye, i.e. the space between the lens and the cornea (anterior and posterior chambers) (Fig. 8.8). The ciliary body is supplied by parasympathetic branches of the oculomotor nerve (3rd cranial nerve). Stimulation causes contraction of the ciliary muscle and accommodation of the eye (p. 200).

195

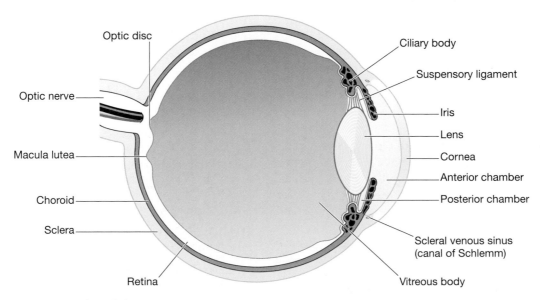

Figure 8.8 Section of the eye.

Optic disc

Optic nerve

Macula lutea

Choroid

Sclera

Retina

Ciliary body

Suspensory ligament

Iris

Lens

Cornea

Anterior chamber

Posterior chamber

Scleral venous sinus (canal of Schlemm)

Vitreous body

Iris

The iris is the visible coloured part of the eye and extends anteriorly from the ciliary body, lying behind the cornea and in front of the lens. It divides the *anterior segment* of the eye into anterior and posterior chambers which contain aqueous fluid secreted by the ciliary body. It is a circular body composed of pigment cells and two layers of smooth muscle fibres, one circular and the other radiating (Fig. 8.9). In the centre there is an aperture called the *pupil*.

The iris is supplied by parasympathetic and sympathetic nerves. Parasympathetic stimulation constricts the pupil and sympathetic stimulation dilates it (see Figs 7.42 and 7.43, pp. 171 and 172).

The colour of the iris is genetically determined and depends on the number of pigment cells present. Albinos have no pigment cells and people with blue eyes have fewer than those with brown eyes.

Lens (Fig. 8.10)

The lens is a highly elastic circular biconvex body, lying immediately behind the pupil. It consists of fibres enclosed within a capsule and it is suspended from the ciliary body by the suspensory ligament. Its thickness is controlled by the ciliary muscle through the suspensory ligament. When the ciliary muscle contracts, it moves forward, releasing its pull on the lens, increasing its thickness. The nearer is the object being viewed, the thicker the lens becomes to allow focusing.

The lens refracts light rays reflected by objects in front of the eye. It is the only structure in the eye that can vary

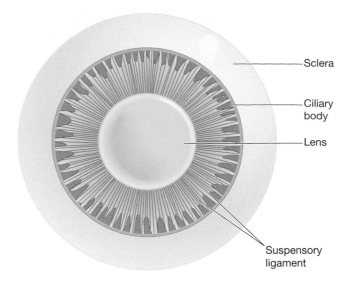

Figure 8.10 **The lens and suspensory ligament viewed from the front.** The iris has been removed.

its refractory power, which is achieved by changing its thickness.

Retina

The retina is the innermost layer of the wall of the eye (Fig. 8.8). It is an extremely delicate structure and is well adapted for stimulation by light rays. It is composed of several layers of nerve cell bodies and their axons, lying on a pigmented layer of epithelial cells which attach it to the choroid. The light-sensitive layer consists of sensory receptor cells: *rods* and *cones*.

The retina lines about three-quarters of the eyeball and is thickest at the back. It thins out anteriorly to end just behind the ciliary body. Near the centre of the posterior part is the *macula lutea*, or yellow spot (Figs 8.11 and 8.12). In the centre of the yellow spot is a little depression called the *fovea centralis*, consisting of only cones. Towards the anterior part of the retina there are fewer cones than rods (Fig. 8.11).

The rods and cones contain photosensitive pigments that convert light rays into nerve impulses.

About 0.5 cm to the nasal side of the macula lutea all the nerve fibres of the retina converge to form the optic nerve. The small area of retina where the optic nerve leaves the eye is the *optic disc* or *blind spot*. It has no light-sensitive cells.

Blood supply to the eye

The eye is supplied with arterial blood by the *ciliary arteries* and the *central retinal artery*. These are branches of the ophthalmic artery, one of the branches of the internal carotid artery.

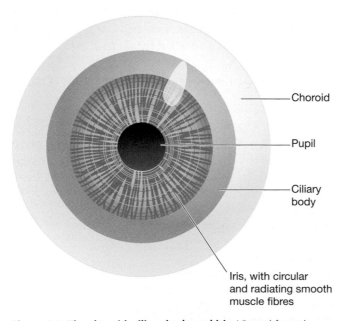

Choroid

Pupil

Ciliary body

Iris, with circular and radiating smooth muscle fibres

Figure 8.9 **The choroid, ciliary body and iris.** Viewed from the front.

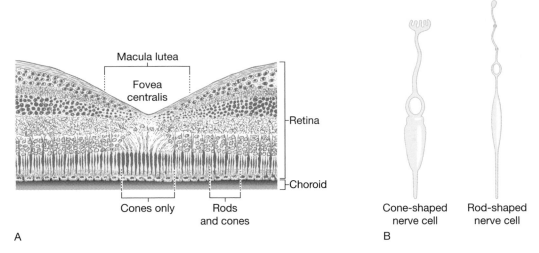

Figure 8.11 The retina. A. Magnified section. B. Light-sensitive nerve cells: rods and cones.

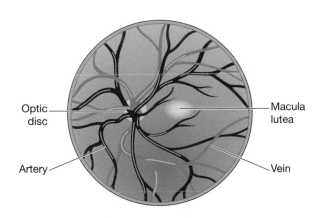

Figure 8.12 The retina as seen through the pupil with an ophthalmoscope.

Venous drainage is by a number of veins, including the *central retinal vein*, which eventually empty into a deep venous sinus.

The central retinal artery and vein are encased in the optic nerve, entering the eye at the optic disc.

Interior of the eye

The anterior segment of the eye, i.e. the space between the cornea and the lens, is incompletely divided into anterior and posterior chambers by the iris (Fig. 8.8). Both chambers contain a clear aqueous fluid secreted into the posterior chamber by ciliary glands. It circulates in front of the lens, through the pupil into the anterior chamber and returns to the venous circulation through the *scleral venous sinus* (canal of Schlemm) in the angle between the iris and cornea (Fig. 8.8). There is continuous production and drainage but the intraocular pressure remains

fairly constant between 1.3 and 2.6 kPa (10 to 20 mmHg). An increase in this pressure causes *glaucoma* (p. 208). Aqueous fluid supplies nutrients and removes wastes from the transparent structures in the front of the eye that have no blood supply, i.e. the cornea, lens and lens capsule.

Behind the lens and filling the posterior segment (cavity) of the eyeball is the *vitreous body*. This is a soft, colourless, transparent, jelly-like substance composed of 99% water, some salts and mucoprotein. It maintains sufficient intraocular pressure to support the retina against the choroid and prevent the walls of the eyeball from collapsing.

The eye keeps its shape because of the intraocular pressure exerted by the vitreous body and the aqueous fluid. It remains fairly constant throughout life.

Optic nerves (second cranial nerves)

(Fig. 8.13)

The fibres of the optic nerve originate in the retina and they converge to form the optic nerve about 0.5 cm to the nasal side of the macula lutea. The nerve pierces the choroid and sclera to pass backwards and medially through the orbital cavity. It then passes through the optic foramen of the sphenoid bone, backwards and medially to meet the nerve from the other eye at the *optic chiasma*.

Optic chiasma

This is situated immediately in front of and above the pituitary gland, which is in the hypophyseal fossa of the sphenoid bone (see Fig. 9.2, p. 213). In the optic chiasma the nerve fibres of the optic nerve from the nasal side of each retina cross over to the opposite side. The fibres

197

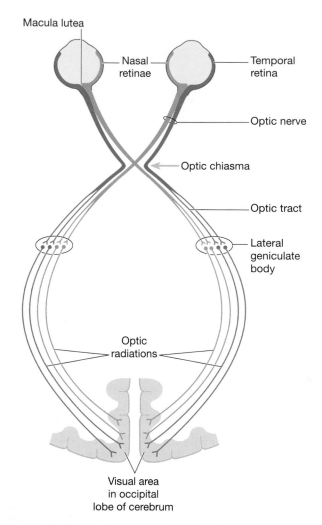

Figure 8.13 The optic nerves and their pathways.

and from the skeletal muscles and joints, they contribute to the maintenance of posture and balance.

Physiology of sight

Light waves travel at a speed of 300 000 kilometres (186 000 miles) per second. Light is reflected into the eyes by objects within the field of vision. White light is a combination of all the colours of the visual spectrum (rainbow), i.e. red, orange, yellow, green, blue, indigo and violet. This is demonstrated by passing white light through a glass prism which bends the rays of the different colours to a greater or lesser extent, depending on their wavelengths (Fig. 8.14). Red light has the longest wavelength and violet the shortest.

This range of colour is the *spectrum of visible light*. In a rainbow, white light from the sun is broken up by raindrops, which act as prisms and reflectors.

The electromagnetic spectrum

The electromagnetic spectrum is broad, but only a small part is visible to the human eye (Fig. 8.15). Beyond the long end are infrared waves (heat), microwaves and radio waves. Beyond the short end are ultraviolet (UV), X-rays and gamma rays. UV light is not normally visible because it is absorbed by a yellow pigment in the lens. Following removal of the lens (cataract extraction), UV light is visible and it has been suggested that long-term exposure may damage the retina.

A specific colour is perceived when only one wavelength is reflected by the object and all the others are absorbed, e.g. an object appears red when only the red wavelength is reflected. Objects appear white when all

from the temporal side do not cross but continue backwards on the same side. This crossing over provides both cerebral hemispheres with sensory input from each eye.

Optic tracts

These are the pathways of the optic nerves, posterior to the optic chiasma. Each tract consists of the nasal fibres from the retina of one eye and the temporal fibres from the retina of the other. The optic tracts pass backwards to synapse with nerve cells of the *lateral geniculate bodies* of the thalamus. From there the nerve fibres proceed backwards and medially as the *optic radiations* to terminate in the *visual area* of the cerebral cortex in the occipital lobes of the cerebrum (see Fig. 7.16, p. 152). Other neurones originating in the lateral geniculate bodies convey impulses from the eyes to the cerebellum where, together with impulses from the semicircular canals of the ears

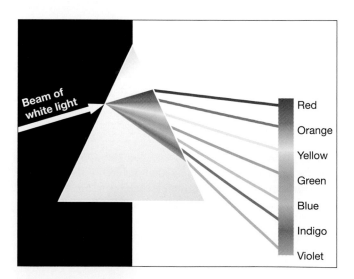

Figure 8.14 Refraction: white light broken into the colours of the visible spectrum when it passes through a prism.

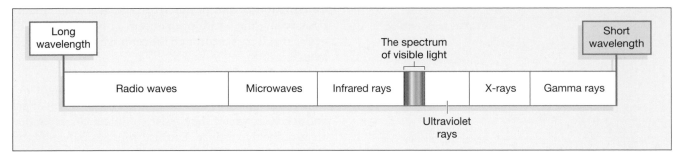

Figure 8.15 The electromagnetic spectrum.

wavelengths are reflected, and black when they are all absorbed.

In order to achieve clear vision, light reflected from objects within the visual field is focused on to the retina of each eye. The processes involved in producing a clear image are *refraction of the light rays*, changing the *size of the pupils* and *accommodation* (adjustment of the lens for near vision).

Although these may be considered as separate processes, effective vision is dependent upon their coordination.

Refraction of the light rays

When light rays pass from a medium of one density to a medium of a different density they are bent; for example, in the eye, the biconvex lens bends and focuses light rays (Fig. 8.16). This principle is used to focus light on the retina. Before reaching the retina, light rays pass successively through the conjunctiva, cornea, aqueous fluid, lens and vitreous body. They are all denser than air and, with the exception of the lens, they have a constant refractory power, similar to that of water.

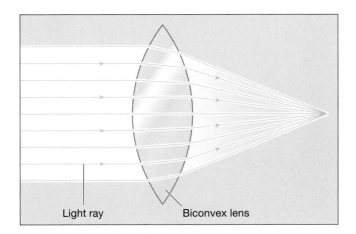

Figure 8.16 Refraction of light rays passing through a biconvex lens.

Abnormal refraction within the eye is corrected using biconvex or biconcave lenses, which are shown on page 210.

Lens

The lens is a biconvex elastic transparent body suspended behind the iris from the ciliary body by the suspensory ligament. It is the only structure in the eye that changes its refractive power. Light rays entering the eye need to be refracted to focus them on the retina. Light from distant objects needs least refraction and, as the object comes closer, the amount of refraction needed is increased. To increase the refractive power, the ciliary muscle contracts, releasing its pull on the suspensory ligament, and the anterior surface of the lens bulges forward, increasing its convexity. This focuses light rays from near objects on the retina. When the ciliary muscle relaxes it slips backwards, increasing its pull on the suspensory ligament, making the lens thinner (Fig. 8.17). This focuses light rays from distant objects on the retina.

Size of the pupils

Pupil size influences accommodation by controlling the amount of light entering the eye. In a bright light the pupils are constricted. In a dim light they are dilated.

If the pupils were dilated in a bright light, too much light would enter the eye and damage the sensitive retina. In a dim light, if the pupils were constricted, insufficient light would enter the eye to activate the photosensitive pigments in the rods and cones which stimulate the nerve endings in the retina.

The iris consists of one layer of circular and one of radiating smooth muscle fibres. Contraction of the circular fibres constricts the pupil, and contraction of the radiating fibres dilates it. The size of the pupil is controlled by the autonomic nervous system. Sympathetic stimulation dilates the pupils and parasympathetic stimulation causes constriction.

199

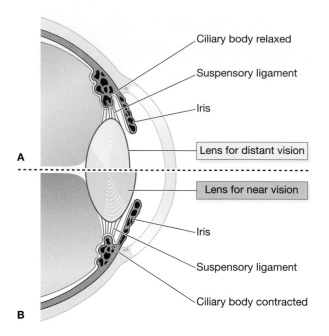

Figure 8.17 The shape of the lens. A. Distant vision. **B.** Near vision.

Accommodation

Close vision

In order to focus on near objects, i.e. within about 6 metres, accommodation is required and the eye must make the following adjustments:

- constriction of the pupils
- convergence
- changing the power of the lens.

Constriction of the pupils. This assists accommodation by reducing the width of the beam of light entering the eye so that it passes through the central curved part of the lens (Fig. 8.18).

Convergence (movement of the eyeballs). Light rays from nearby objects enter the two eyes at different angles and for clear vision they must stimulate corresponding areas of the two retinae. Extrinsic muscles move the eyes and to obtain a clear image they rotate the eyes so that they converge on the object viewed. This coordinated muscle activity is under autonomic control. When there is voluntary movement of the eyes both eyes move and convergence is maintained. The nearer an object is to the eyes the greater the eye rotation needed to achieve convergence, e.g. an individual focusing near the tip of his nose appears to be 'cross-eyed'. If convergence is not complete the eyes are focused on different objects or on different points of the same object. There are then two images sent to the brain and this leads to double vision, *diplopia*. If convergence is not possible, the brain tends to ignore the impulses received from the divergent eye (see Squint, p. 209).

Changing the power of the lens. Changes in the thickness of the lens are made to focus light on the retina. The amount of adjustment depends on the distance of the object from the eyes, i.e. the lens is thicker for near vision and at its thinnest when focusing on objects at more than 6 metres' distance (Fig. 8.17). Looking at near objects 'tires' the eyes more quickly, owing to the continuous use of the ciliary muscle.

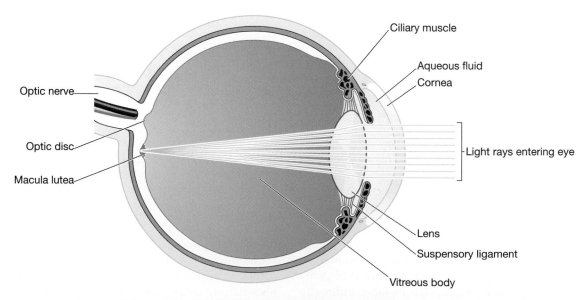

Figure 8.18 Section of the eye showing the focusing of light rays on the retina.

Distant vision

Objects more than 6 metres away from the eyes are focused on the retina without adjustment of the lens or convergence of the eyes.

Functions of the retina

The retina is the *photosensitive* part of the eye. The light-sensitive nerve cells are the rods and cones and their distribution in the retina is shown in Figure 8.11A. Light rays cause chemical changes in photosensitive pigments in these cells and they generate nerve impulses which are conducted to the occipital lobes of the cerebrum via the optic nerves (Fig. 8.13).

The *rods* are more sensitive than the cones. They are stimulated by low-intensity or dim light, e.g. by the dim light in a darkened room.

The *cones* are sensitive to bright light and colour. The different wavelengths of visible light stimulate photosensitive pigments in the cones, resulting in the perception of different colours. In bright light the light rays are focused on the macula lutea.

The rods are more numerous towards the periphery of the retina. *Visual purple (rhodopsin)* is a photosensitive pigment present only in the rods. It is bleached (degraded) by bright light and is quickly regenerated, provided an adequate supply of vitamin A is available.

Dark adaptation. When exposed to bright light, the rhodopsin within the sensitive rods is completely degraded. This is not significant until the individual moves into a darkened area where the light intensity is insufficient to stimulate the cones, and temporary visual impairment results whilst the rhodopsin is being regenerated within the rods, 'dark adaptation'. When regeneration of rhodopsin has occurred, normal sight returns.

It is easier to see a dim star in the sky at night if the head is turned slightly away from it because light of low intensity is then focused on an area of the retina where there is a greater concentration of rods. If looked at directly the light intensity of a dim star is not sufficient to stimulate the less sensitive cones in the area of the macula lutea. In dim evening light, different colours cannot be distinguished because the light intensity is insufficient to stimulate colour-sensitive pigments in cones.

Breakdown and regeneration of the visual pigments in cones is similar to that of rods.

Binocular vision (Fig. 8.19)

Binocular or stereoscopic vision enables three-dimensional views although each eye 'sees' a scene slightly differently. The visual fields overlap in the middle but the left eye sees more on the left than can be seen by the

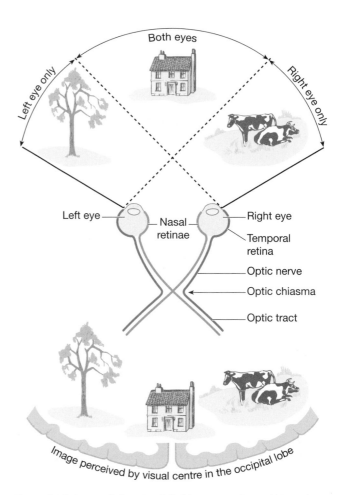

Figure 8.19 Parts of the visual field – monocular and binocular.

other eye and vice versa. The images from the two eyes are fused in the cerebrum so that only one image is perceived.

Binocular vision provides a much more accurate assessment of one object relative to another, e.g. its distance, depth, height and width. People with monocular vision may find it difficult, for example, to judge the speed and distance of an approaching vehicle.

Extraocular muscles of the eye

These include the muscles of the eyelids (p. 203) and those that move the eyeballs. The eyeball is moved by six *extrinsic muscles*, attached at one end to the eyeball and at the other to the walls of the orbital cavity. There are four *straight* (rectus) muscles and two *oblique* muscles (Fig. 8.20).

Moving the eyes to look in a particular direction is under voluntary control, but coordination of movement, needed for convergence and accommodation to near or distant vision, is under autonomic (involuntary) control.

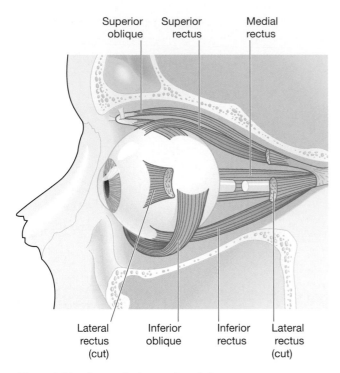

Superior oblique   Superior rectus   Medial rectus

Lateral rectus (cut)   Inferior oblique   Inferior rectus   Lateral rectus (cut)

Figure 8.20   The extrinsic muscles of the eye.

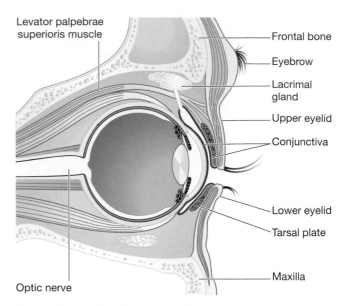

Levator palpebrae superioris muscle

Frontal bone

Eyebrow

Lacrimal gland

Upper eyelid

Conjunctiva

Lower eyelid

Tarsal plate

Maxilla

Optic nerve

Figure 8.21 Section of the eye and its accessory structures.

Movements of the eyes resulting from the action of these muscles are shown in Table 8.1.

Nerve supply to the muscles of the eye

Nerves shown in Table 8.1 supply the extrinsic muscles. The *oculomotor nerves* supply the *intrinsic eye muscles* of the iris and ciliary body.

Accessory organs of the eye

The eye is a delicate organ which is protected by several structures (Fig. 8.21):

- eyebrows
- eyelids and eyelashes
- lacrimal apparatus.

Eyebrows

These are two arched ridges of the supraorbital margins of the frontal bone. Numerous hairs (eyebrows) project obliquely from the surface of the skin. They protect the eyeball from sweat, dust and other foreign bodies.

Eyelids (palpebrae)

The eyelids are two movable folds of tissue situated above and below the front of each eye. On their free edges there are short curved hairs, the *eyelashes*. The layers of tissue forming the eyelids are:

Table 8.1 Extrinsic muscles of the eye: their actions and cranial nerve supply		
Name	**Action**	**Cranial nerve supply**
Medial rectus	Rotates eyeball inwards	Oculomotor nerve (3rd cranial nerve)
Lateral rectus	Rotates eyeball outwards	Abducent nerve (6th cranial nerve)
Superior rectus	Rotates eyeball upwards	Oculomotor nerve (3rd cranial nerve)
Inferior rectus	Rotates eyeball downwards	Oculomotor nerve (3rd cranial nerve)
Superior oblique	Rotates eyeball downwards and outwards	Trochlear nerve (4th cranial nerve)
Inferior oblique	Rotates eyeball upwards and outwards	Oculomotor nerve (3rd cranial nerve)

- a thin covering of skin
- a thin sheet of subcutaneous connective (loose areolar) tissue
- two muscles – the *orbicularis oculi* and *levator palpebrae superioris*
- a thin sheet of dense connective tissue, the *tarsal plate*, larger in the upper than in the lower eyelid, which supports the other structures
- a lining of *conjunctiva*.

Conjunctiva

This is a fine transparent membrane that lines the eyelids and the front of the eyeball (Fig. 8.21). Where it lines the eyelids it consists of highly vascular columnar epithelium. Corneal conjunctiva consists of avascular stratified epithelium, i.e. epithelium without blood vessels. When the eyelids are closed the conjunctiva becomes a closed sac. It protects the delicate cornea and the front of the eye. When eyedrops are administered they are placed in the lower conjunctival sac. The medial and lateral angles of the eye where the upper and lower lids come together are called respectively the *medial canthus* and the *lateral canthus*.

Eyelid margins

Along the edges of the lids there are numerous *sebaceous glands*, some with ducts opening into the hair follicles of the eyelashes and some on to the eyelid margins between the hairs. *Tarsal glands* (Meibomian glands) are modified sebaceous glands embedded in the tarsal plates with ducts that open on to the inside of the free margins of the eyelids. They secrete an oily material, spread over the conjunctiva by blinking, which delays evaporation of tears.

Functions

The eyelids and eyelashes protect the eye from injury:

- reflex closure of the lids occurs when the conjunctiva or eyelashes are touched, when an object comes close to the eye or when a bright light shines into the eye – this is called the *corneal reflex*
- blinking at about 3- to 7-second intervals spreads tears and oily secretions over the cornea, preventing drying.

When the orbicularis oculi contract, the eyes close. When the levator palpebrae contract, the eyelids open (see Fig. 16.54, p. 419).

Lacrimal apparatus (Fig. 8.22)

For each eye this consists of:

- 1 lacrimal gland and its ducts
- 2 lacrimal canaliculi

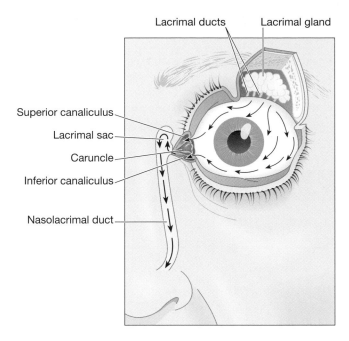

Figure 8.22 The lacrimal apparatus. Arrows show the direction of the flow of tears.

- 1 lacrimal sac
- 1 nasolacrimal duct.

The lacrimal glands are exocrine glands situated in recesses in the frontal bones on the lateral aspect of each eye just behind the supraorbital margin. Each gland is approximately the size and shape of an almond, and is composed of secretory epithelial cells. The glands secrete *tears* composed of water, mineral salts, antibodies, and *lysozyme*, a bactericidal enzyme.

The tears leave the lacrimal gland by several small ducts and pass over the front of the eye under the lids towards the medial canthus where they drain into the *two lacrimal canaliculi*; the opening of each is called the *punctum*. The two canaliculi lie one above the other, separated by a small red body, the *caruncle*. The tears then drain into the *lacrimal sac*, which is the upper expanded end of the *nasolacrimal duct*. This is a membranous canal approximately 2 cm long, extending from the lower part of the lacrimal sac to the nasal cavity, opening at the level of the inferior concha. Normally the rate of secretion of tears keeps pace with the rate of drainage. When a foreign body or other irritant enters the eye the secretion of tears is greatly increased and the conjunctival blood vessels dilate. Secretion of tears is also increased in emotional states, e.g. crying, laughing.

Functions

The fluid that fills the conjunctival sac consists of tears and the oily secretion of tarsal glands and is spread over

203

the cornea by blinking. The functions of this mixture of fluids include:

- washing away irritating materials, e.g. dust, grit
- the bacteriocidal enzyme lysozyme prevents microbial infection
- its oiliness delays evaporation and prevents drying of the conjunctiva.

Sense of smell

Learning outcome

After studying this section you should be able to:

■ describe the physiology of smell.

The sense of smell, or *olfaction*, originates in the nasal cavity, which also acts as a passageway for respiration (see Ch. 10).

Olfactory nerves (first cranial nerves)

These are the sensory nerves of smell. They originate as specialised olfactory nerve endings (*chemoreceptors*) in the mucous membrane of the roof of the nasal cavity above the superior nasal conchae (Fig. 8.23). On each side of the nasal septum nerve fibres pass through the cribriform plate of the ethmoid bone to the *olfactory bulb* where

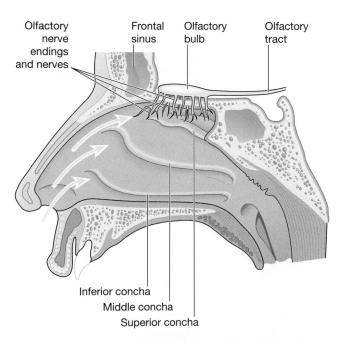

Figure 8.23 The olfactory structures.

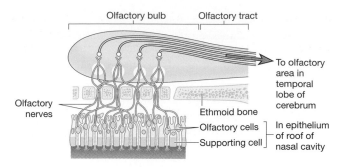

Figure 8.24 An enlarged section of the olfactory apparatus in the nose and on the inferior surface of the cerebrum.

interconnections and synapses occur (Fig. 8.24). From the bulb, bundles of nerve fibres form the *olfactory tract*, which passes backwards to the olfactory area in the temporal lobe of the cerebral cortex in each hemisphere where the impulses are interpreted and odour perceived (see Fig. 7.16, p. 152).

Physiology of smell

The human sense of smell is less acute than in other animals. Many animals secrete odorous chemicals called *pheromones* that play an important part in chemical communication in, for example, territorial behaviour, mating and the bonding of mothers and their newborn offspring. The role of pheromones in human communication is unknown.

All odorous materials give off volatile molecules, which are carried into the nose with the inhaled air and even very low concentrations, when dissolved in mucus, stimulate the olfactory chemoreceptors.

The air entering the nose is warmed, and convection currents carry eddies of inspired air to the roof of the nasal cavity. 'Sniffing' concentrates volatile molecules in the roof of the nose. This increases the number of olfactory receptors stimulated and thus the perception of the smell. The sense of smell may affect the appetite. If the odours are pleasant the appetite may improve and vice versa. When accompanied by the sight of food, an appetising smell increases salivation and stimulates the digestive system (see Ch. 12). The sense of smell may create long-lasting memories, especially for distinctive odours, e.g. hospital smells, favourite or least-liked foods.

Inflammation of the nasal mucosa prevents odorous substances from reaching the olfactory area of the nose, causing loss of the sense of smell (*anosmia*). The usual cause is a cold.

Adaptation. When an individual is continuously exposed to an odour, perception of the odour decreases and ceases within a few minutes. This loss of perception affects only that specific odour and adaptation probably occurs in both neurones within the central nervous system and the sensory receptors in the nasal cavity.

Sense of taste

Learning outcome

After studying this section you should be able to:

■ describe the physiology of taste.

The sense of taste, or *gustation*, is closely linked to the sense of smell and, like smell, also involves stimulation of chemoreceptors by dissolved chemicals.

Taste buds contain sensory receptors (chemoreceptors) that are found in the papillae of the tongue and widely distributed in the epithelia of the tongue, soft palate, pharynx and epiglottis. They consist of small sensory nerve endings of the glossopharyngeal, facial and vagus nerves (cranial nerves VII, IX and X). Some of the cells have hair-like microvilli on their free border, projecting towards tiny pores in the epithelium (Fig. 8.25). The sensory receptors are stimulated by chemicals that enter the pores dissolved in saliva. Nerve impulses are generated and conducted along the glossopharyngeal, facial and vagus nerves before synapsing in the medulla and thalamus. Their final destination is the *taste area* in the parietal lobe of the cerebral cortex where taste is perceived (see Fig. 7.16, p. 152).

Physiology of taste

Four fundamental sensations of taste have been described – sweet, sour, bitter and salt. This is probably an oversimplification because perception varies widely

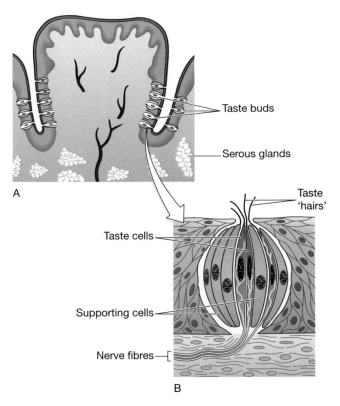

Figure 8.25 Structure of taste buds. A. A section of a papilla. B. A taste bud – greatly magnified.

and many 'tastes' cannot be easily classified. However, some tastes consistently stimulate taste buds in specific parts of the tongue (see Fig. 12.9, p. 288):

- sweet and salty, mainly at the tip
- sour, at the sides
- bitter, at the back.

The sense of taste triggers salivation and the secretion of gastric juice (see Ch. 12). It also has a protective function, e.g. when foul-tasting food is eaten, reflex gagging or vomiting may be induced.

The sense of taste is impaired when the mouth is dry, because substances can only be 'tasted' when in solution.

205

Disorders of the ear

Learning outcomes

After studying this section you should be able to:

■ compare and contrast the features of conductive and sensorineural hearing loss

■ describe the causes and effects of diseases of the ear.

Hearing loss

Hearing impairment can be classified in two main categories: *conductive* and *sensorineural*. Common causes are shown in Box 8.1. Hearing impairment can also be *mixed* when there is a combination of conductive and sensorineural hearing loss in one ear.

Conductive hearing impairment

This is due to reduced transmission of sound waves when an abnormality of the outer or middle ear impairs conduction of sound waves to the oval window.

Otosclerosis

This is a common cause of progressive conductive hearing loss in young adults that may affect one ear but is more commonly bilateral. It is usually hereditary, more common in females than males and often worsens during pregnancy. Abnormal bone develops around the footplate of the stapes fusing it to the oval window, reducing the ability to transmit sound waves across the tympanic cavity.

Box 8.1 Common causes of deafness

Conductive	Sensorineural
Impacted earwax or foreign body	Presbycusis
Acute otitis media	Noise pollution
Serous otitis media	Congenital
Chronic otitis media	Ménière's disease
Barotrauma	Ototoxic drugs, e.g.
Otosclerosis	aminoglycoside antibiotics,
External otitis	diuretics, chemotherapy
Injury of the tympanic membrane	Infections, e.g. mumps, herpes zoster, meningitis, syphilis

---

Sensorineural (perceptive) hearing impairment

This is the result of a disorder of the inner ear or the central nervous system, e.g. the cochlea, cochlear branch of the vestibular nerve or the auditory area of the cerebrum. The individual usually perceives noise but cannot discriminate between sounds.

Risk factors for congenital sensorineural hearing impairment include:

● family history
● exposure to intrauterine viruses, e.g. maternal rubella
● acute hypoxia at birth.

Presbycusis

This form of hearing impairment commonly accompanies the ageing process and is therefore common in older people. Degenerative changes in the sensory cells of the spiral organ (of Corti) result in sensorineural hearing loss. Perception of high-frequency sound is impaired first and later low-frequency sound may also be affected. The individual develops difficulty in discrimination, e.g. following a conversation, especially in the presence of background noise.

Ear infections

External otitis

Infection by *Staphylococcus aureus* is the usual cause of localised inflammation (boils) in the auditory canal. When more generalised, the inflammation may be caused by prolonged exposure to moisture, bacteria or fungi or by an allergic reaction to, e.g., dandruff, soaps, hair sprays, hair dyes.

Acute otitis media

This is inflammation of the middle ear cavity usually caused by upward spread of microbes from an upper respiratory tract infection via the auditory tube. It is very common in children and is accompanied by severe earache. Occasionally it spreads inwards from the outer ear through a perforation in the tympanic membrane.

Microbial infection leads to the accumulation of pus and the outward bulging of the tympanic membrane. Sometimes there is rupture of the tympanic membrane and purulent discharge from the ear (*otorrhoea*). The spread of infection may cause *mastoiditis* and *labyrinthitis*. As the petrous portion of the temporal bone is very thin the infection may spread through the bone and cause meningitis and brain abscess.

Serous otitis media

Also known as *'glue ear'*, or secretory otitis media, this is a collection of fluid (*effusion*) in the middle ear cavity. Causes include:

- obstruction of the auditory tube by, for example, pharyngeal swelling, enlarged adenoids or tumour
- barotrauma (usually caused by descent in an aeroplane when suffering from a cold)
- untreated acute otitis media.

In adults the individual suffers from hearing loss and (usually painless) blockage of the ear, whereas young children show delay in speech development and behavioural disorders due to hearing impairment. Air already present in the middle ear cavity is absorbed and a negative pressure develops. At first there is retraction of the tympanic membrane, then fluid is drawn into the low-pressure cavity from surrounding blood vessels. Conductive hearing loss occurs and there may or may not be secondary infection. This is a common cause of hearing impairment in children.

Chronic otitis media

In this condition there is permanent perforation of the tympanic membrane following acute otitis media (especially when recurrent, persistent or untreated) and mechanical or blast injuries. During the healing process stratified epithelium from the outer ear sometimes grows into the middle ear, forming a *cholesteatoma*. This is a collection of desquamated epithelial cells and purulent material. Continued development of cholesteatoma may lead to:

- destruction of the ossicles and conductive hearing loss
- erosion of the roof of the middle ear and meningitis
- spread of infection to the inner ear that may cause labyrinthitis (see below).

Ménière's disease

In this condition there is accumulation of endolymph causing distension and increased pressure within the membranous labyrinth with destruction of the sensory cells in the ampulla and cochlea. It is usually unilateral at first but both ears may be affected later. The cause is not known. Ménière's disease is associated with recurrent episodes of incapacitating dizziness (*vertigo*), nausea and vomiting, lasting for several hours. Periods of remission vary from days to months. During and between attacks there may be continuous ringing in the affected ear (*tinnitus*). Loss of hearing is experienced during episodes, and permanent hearing impairment may gradually develop over a period of years as the spiral organ (of Corti) is destroyed.

Labyrinthitis

This complication of middle ear infection may be caused by development of a fistula from a cholesteatoma (see above). It is accompanied by vertigo, nausea and vomiting, and nystagmus. In some cases the spiral organ is destroyed, causing sudden profound sensorineural hearing loss in the affected ear.

Motion sickness

Repetitive motion causes excessive stimulation of the semicircular canals and vestibular apparatus and results in nausea and vomiting in some people.

Disorders of the eye

Learning outcome

After studying this section you should be able to:

- describe the pathological changes and effects of diseases of the eye.

Inflammatory conditions

Stye (hordeolum)
This is an acute and painful bacterial infection of sebaceous or tarsal glands of the eyelid margin. A 'crop' of styes may occur due to localised spread to adjacent glands. Infection of tarsal glands may block their ducts, leading to cyst formation (*chalazion*), which may damage the cornea. The most common infecting organism is *Staphylococcus aureus*.

Blepharitis
This is chronic inflammation of the eyelid margins, usually caused by microbes or allergy, e.g. staphylococcal infection or seborrhoea (excessive sebaceous gland secretion). If ulceration occurs, healing by fibrosis may distort the eyelid margins, preventing complete closure of the eye. This may lead to drying of the eye, conjunctivitis and possibly corneal ulceration.

Conjunctivitis
Inflammation of the conjunctiva may be caused by irritants, such as smoke, dust, wind, cold or dry air, microbes

or antigens. Corneal ulceration (see below) is a rare complication.

Microbial infection. This is highly contagious and in adults is usually caused by strains of staphylococci, streptococci, pneumococci and haemophilus.

Neonatal conjunctivitis. This occurs within 28 days of birth and is commonly caused by *Neisseria gonorrhoea*, *Chlamydia trachomatis* or herpes simplex virus. It is usually acquired when microbes contaminate the baby's eyes during delivery. Infection may cause corneal ulceration (see below).

Allergic conjunctivitis. This may be a complication of hay fever, or be caused by a wide variety of airborne antigens, e.g. dust, pollen, fungus spores, animal dander, cosmetics, hair sprays, soaps. The condition sometimes becomes chronic.

Trachoma. This is a chronic inflammatory condition caused by *Chlamydia trachomatis* in which fibrous tissue forms in the conjunctiva and cornea, leading to eyelid deformity, and is a common cause of loss of sight in tropical countries. The microbes are spread by poor hygiene, e.g. communal use of contaminated washing water, cross-infection between mother and child, or contaminated towels and clothing.

Corneal ulcer

This is local necrosis of corneal tissue, usually associated with corneal infection (*keratitis*) following trauma (e.g. abrasion), or infection spread from the conjunctiva or eyelids. Common infecting microbes include staphylococci, pneumococci and herpes simplex viruses. Acute pain, *injection* (redness of the cornea), photophobia and lacrimation interfere with sight during the acute phase. In severe cases extensive ulceration or perforation and healing by fibrosis can cause opacity of the cornea requiring corneal transplantation.

Inflammation of the uveal tract (iris, ciliary body, choroid)

Anterior uveitis (iritis, iridocyclitis). Iridocyclitis (inflammation of iris and ciliary body) is the more common and it may be acute or chronic. The infection may have spread from the outer eye but in most cases the cause is unknown. There is usually moderate to severe pain, redness, blurring of vision, lacrimation and *photophobia* (intolerance of light). In severe cases adhesions form between the iris and lens capsule, preventing the circulation of aqueous fluid in the posterior and anterior chambers. This may cause the lens to bulge and block the scleral venous sinus (canal of Schlemm), raising intra-

ocular pressure causing *chronic closed-angle glaucoma* (see below). Acute infection usually resolves in several days or weeks while the chronic form may last for months or years.

Posterior uveitis (choroiditis, chorioretinitis). This affects the posterior segment of the eye and chorioretinitis is the more common condition. It may be caused by spread of infection from the anterior segment (front) of the eye or be secondary to a wide variety of systemic conditions, including rheumatoid arthritis, Reiter's syndrome, inflammatory bowel disease and brucellosis. Complications of uveitis include retinal detachment due to accumulation of inflammatory exudate, secondary glaucoma or cataract.

Glaucoma

This is a group of conditions in which there is increased intraocular pressure due to impaired drainage of aqueous fluid through the scleral venous sinus (canal of Schlemm) in the angle between the iris and cornea in the anterior chamber. Persistently raised intraocular pressure may damage the optic nerve by:

- mechanical compression
- compression of its blood supply causing ischaemia.

Damage to the optic nerve impairs vision, and the extent varies from some visual impairment to complete loss of sight.

Primary glaucomas

Chronic open-angle glaucoma. There is a gradual painless rise in intraocular pressure with progressive loss of vision. Peripheral vision is lost first but may not be noticed until only central (*tunnel*) vision remains. As the condition progresses, atrophy of the optic disc occurs leading to irreversible loss of vision. It is commonly bilateral and occurs mostly in people over 40 years of age. The cause is not known but there is a familial tendency.

Acute closed-angle glaucoma. This is most common in people over 40 years of age and usually affects one eye. During life the lens gradually increases in size, pushing the iris forward. In dim light when the pupil dilates, the lax iris bulges still further forward, and may come into contact with the cornea, blocking the scleral venous sinus (canal of Schlemm) suddenly raising the intraocular pressure. Sudden severe pain, photophobia, lacrimation and loss of vision accompany an acute attack. It may resolve spontaneously if the iris responds to bright light, constricting the pupil and releasing the pressure on the scleral venous sinus. After repeated attacks spontaneous recovery may be incomplete and vision is progressively impaired.

Chronic closed-angle glaucoma. The intraocular pressure rises gradually without symptoms. Peripheral vision deteriorates first followed by atrophy of the optic disc and loss of sight.

Congenital glaucoma. This abnormal development of the anterior chamber is often familial or due to maternal infection with rubella in early pregnancy.

Secondary glaucoma

The most common primary disorder is anterior uveitis with the formation of adhesions (see above). Other predisposing primary conditions include intraocular tumours, enlarged cataracts, central retinal vein occlusion, intraocular haemorrhage, and trauma to the eye.

Strabismus (squint, cross-eye)

This is the inability of the eyes to move together so that the same image falls on the corresponding parts of the retina in both eyes. Only one eye is directed at the observed object and the other diverges (is directed elsewhere). The result is that two images are sent to the brain, one from each eye, instead of one integrated image. It is caused by one-sided extrinsic muscle weakness or impairment of the cranial nerve (III, IV or VI) supply to the extrinsic muscles. In most cases the image from the squinting eye is suppressed by the brain, otherwise there is double vision (*diplopia*).

Presbyopia

Ageing changes affect the eye leading to loss of accommodation as the lens loses its elasticity and becomes firmer. This results in difficulty with reading after the age of 40 years as the individual needs to hold reading material at arm's length. Correction is achieved using convex lenses.

Cataract

This is opacity of the lens which may be age-related or congenital, bilateral or unilateral.

In *age-related cataract* there is gradual development of lens opacity that usually develops during older age as the result of exposure to a variety of predisposing factors including: UV light, X-rays, cigarette smoke, diabetes mellitus, ocular trauma, uveitis, systemic drug therapy, e.g. corticosteroids, chlorpromazine.

Congenital cataract may be due to genetic abnormality, e.g. Down's syndrome, or maternal infection in early pregnancy, e.g. rubella. Early treatment is required to prevent permanent loss of sight.

The extent of visual impairment depends on the location and extent of the opacity.

Keratomalacia

In this condition, lack of tears causes dryness of the cornea leading to corneal ulceration, usually with secondary infection. The lacrimal glands and conjunctiva may also be involved. It is associated with vitamin A deficiency and protein-energy malnutrition. There may be softening or even perforation of the cornea. Night blindness (ineffective adaptation to dim light) is usually an early sign of vitamin A deficiency.

Retinopathies

Vascular retinopathies

Occlusion of the central retinal artery or vein causes sudden painless unilateral loss of vision. *Arterial occlusion* is usually due to embolism from, e.g. atheromatous plaques, endocarditis. *Venous occlusion* is usually associated with increased intraocular pressure, e.g. glaucoma, diabetes mellitus, hypertension, increased blood viscosity. The retinal veins become distended and retinal haemorrhages occur.

Diabetic retinopathy

This occurs in Type I and Type II diabetes mellitus (p. 232) and is the commonest cause of blindness in adults aged between 30 and 65 years in developed countries. Changes in retinal blood vessels increase with the severity and duration of hyperglycaemia. Capillary microaneurysms develop and later there may be proliferation of blood vessels. Haemorrhages, fibrosis and secondary retinal detachment may occur, leading to retinal degeneration and loss of vision.

Retinopathy of prematurity

Previously known as retrolental fibroplasia, this condition affects premature babies. Known risk factors include: birth before 32 weeks' gestation, birth weight less than 1500 g, requirement for oxygen therapy, apnoea and sepsis. There is abnormal development of retinal blood vessels and formation of fibrovascular tissue in the vitreous body causing varying degrees of interference with light transmission. In severe cases there may also be haemorrhage in the vitreous body, retinal detachment and loss of vision.

Retinal detachment

This painless condition occurs when a tear or hole in the retina allows fluid to accumulate between the layers of retinal cells or between the retina and choroid. It is usually localised at first but as fluid collects the detachment spreads. There are spots before the eyes, flashing lights due to abnormal stimulation of sensory receptors, and progressive loss of vision, sometimes described as a 'shadow' or 'curtain'. In many cases the cause is unknown but it may be associated with trauma to the eye or head, tumours, haemorrhage, cataract surgery when the pressure in the eye is reduced or diabetic retinopathy.

Retinitis pigmentosa

This is an hereditary disease in which there is degeneration of the retina, mainly affecting the rods. Visual impairment, especially in dim light, usually becomes apparent in early childhood, leading to tunnel vision and eventually, loss of sight.

Tumours

Choroidal malignant melanoma

This is the most common ocular malignancy and it occurs between 40 and 70 years of age. Vision is not normally affected until the tumour causes retinal detachment or secondary glaucoma, usually when well advanced. The tumour spreads locally in the choroid, and blood-borne metastases develop mainly in the liver.

Retinoblastoma

This is a malignant tumour derived from embryonic retinal cells. A small number of cases are familial. It is usually evident before the age of 4 years and may be bilateral. The condition presents with a squint and enlargement of the eye. As the tumour grows visual impairment develops and the pupil looks pale. It spreads locally to the vitreous body and may grow along the optic nerve, invading the brain.

Refractive errors of the eye

Learning outcome

After studying this section you should be able to:

■ explain how corrective lenses overcome refractive errors of the eye.

In the *emetropic* or normal eye, light from near and distant objects is focused on the retina (Fig. 8.26A).

In *hypermetropia*, or farsightedness, a near image is focused behind the retina because the eyeball is too short (Fig. 8.26B). A *biconvex lens* corrects this (Fig. 8.26C). Distant objects are focused normally.

In *myopia*, or nearsightedness, the eyeball is too long and distant objects are focused in front of the retina (Fig. 8.26D). Correction is achieved using a *biconcave lens* (Fig. 8.26E). Near objects are seen in focus as the eye can accommodate normally.

Astigmatism results in blurred vision when there is abnormal curvature of part of the cornea or lens that prevents focusing on the retina. Correction requires cylindrical lenses. It may coexist with hypermetropia, myopia or presbycusis.

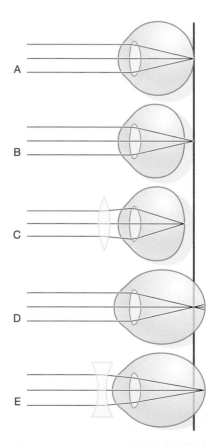

Figure 8.26 Common refractive errors of the eye and corrective lenses. A. Normal eye. B and C. Farsightedness. D and E. Nearsightedness.

The endocrine system

9

The endocrine system consists of glands widely separated from each other with no direct links (Fig. 9.1). Endocrine glands consist of groups of secretory cells surrounded by an extensive network of capillaries that facilitates diffusion of *hormones* (chemical messengers) from the secretory cells into the bloodstream. They are commonly referred to as the *ductless glands* because the hormones diffuse directly into the bloodstream. The hormone is then carried in the bloodstream to *target tissues* and *organs* that may be quite distant, where they influence cellular growth and metabolism.

Homeostasis of the internal environment is maintained partly by the autonomic nervous system and partly by the endocrine system. The autonomic nervous system is concerned with rapid changes, while hormones of the endocrine system are mainly involved in slower and more precise adjustments.

The endocrine system consists of a number of distinct glands and some tissues in other organs. Although the hypothalamus is classified as a part of the brain and not as an endocrine gland it controls the pituitary gland and has an indirect effect on many others. The endocrine glands are shown in Figure 9.1.

Box 9.1 **Examples of lipid-based and peptide hormones**	
Lipid-based hormones	Peptide hormones
Steroids e.g. glucocorticoids, mineralocorticoids	Adrenaline (epinephrine), noradrenaline (norepinephrine)
	Insulin
Thyroid hormones	Glucagon

The ovaries and the testes secrete hormones associated with the reproductive system after puberty. Their functions are described in Chapter 18.

When a hormone arrives at its target cell, it binds to a specific area, the *receptor*, where it acts as a switch influencing chemical or metabolic reactions inside the cell. The receptors for peptide hormones are situated on the cell membrane and those for lipid-based hormones are inside the cell. Examples are shown in Box 9.1.

The level of a hormone in the blood is variable and self-regulating within its normal range. A hormone is released in response to a specific stimulus and usually its action reverses or negates the stimulus through a *negative feedback mechanism* (see p. 5). This may be controlled either indirectly through the release of hormones by the hypothalamus and the anterior pituitary gland, e.g. steroid and thyroid hormones, or directly by blood levels of the stimulus, e.g. insulin and glucagon.

The effect of a *positive feedback mechanism* is amplification of the stimulus and increasing release of the hormone until a particular process is complete and the stimulus ceases, e.g. release of oxytocin during labour (p. 6).

In addition to the hormones that have the characteristics and actions outlined above there are also other hormones that do not travel to remote target organs but act locally, and these are considered briefly at the end of the chapter.

Pituitary gland and hypothalamus

Learning outcomes

After studying this section you should be able to:

- describe the structure of the hypothalamus and the pituitary gland
- explain the influence of the hypothalamus on the lobes of the pituitary gland
- outline the actions of the hormones secreted by the anterior and posterior lobes of the pituitary gland.

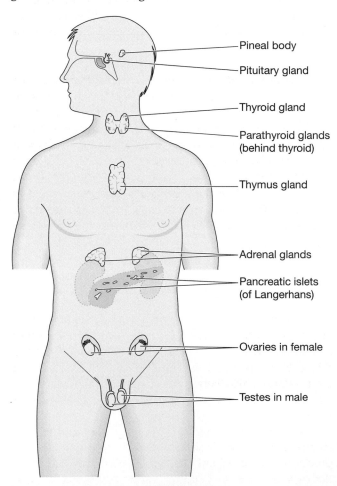

- Pineal body
- Pituitary gland
- Thyroid gland
- Parathyroid glands (behind thyroid)
- Thymus gland
- Adrenal glands
- Pancreatic islets (of Langerhans)
- Ovaries in female
- Testes in male

Figure 9.1 Positions of the endocrine glands.

The pituitary gland (hypophysis) and the hypothalamus act as a unit, regulating the activity of most of the other endocrine glands. The pituitary gland lies in the hypophyseal fossa of the sphenoid bone below the hypothalamus, to which it is attached by a *stalk* (Fig. 9.2). It is the size of a pea, weighs about 500 mg and consists of three distinct parts that originate from different types of cells. The *anterior pituitary* (adenohypophysis) is an upgrowth of glandular epithelium from the pharynx and the *posterior pituitary* (neurohypophysis) is a downgrowth of nervous tissue from the brain. There is a network of nerve fibres between the hypothalamus and the posterior pituitary. Between these lobes there is a thin strip of tissue called the *intermediate lobe* and its function in humans is not known.

Blood supply

Arterial blood. This is supplied by branches from the internal carotid artery. The anterior lobe is supplied indirectly by blood that has already passed through a capillary bed in the hypothalamus but the posterior lobe is supplied directly.

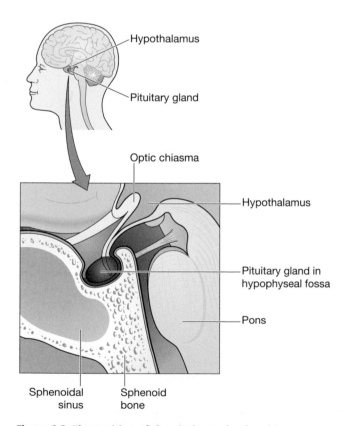

Figure 9.2 The position of the pituitary gland and its associated structures.

Hypothalamus

Pituitary gland

Optic chiasma

Hypothalamus

Pituitary gland in hypophyseal fossa

Pons

Sphenoidal sinus

Sphenoid bone

Venous drainage. This comes from both lobes, containing hormones, and leaves the gland in short veins that enter the venous sinuses between the layers of dura mater.

The influence of the hypothalamus on the pituitary gland

The influence of the hypothalamus on the release of hormones is different in the anterior and posterior lobes of the pituitary gland.

The anterior pituitary. This is supplied indirectly with arterial blood that has already passed through a capillary bed in the hypothalamus (Fig. 9.3A). This network of blood vessels forms part of the *pituitary portal system*, which transports blood from the hypothalamus to the anterior pituitary where it enters thin-walled vascular sinusoids and is in very close contact with the secretory cells. As well as providing oxygen and nutrients, this blood transports *releasing* and *inhibiting hormones* secreted by the *hypothalamus*. These hormones influence secretion and release of other hormones formed in the anterior pituitary. The releasing and inhibiting hormones that stimulate and inhibit secretion of specific anterior pituitary hormones are shown in Table 9.1.

The posterior pituitary. This is formed from nervous tissue and consists of nerve cells surrounded by supporting cells called *pituicytes*. These neurones have their cell bodies in the supraoptic and paraventricular nuclei of the hypothalamus and their axons form a bundle known as the *hypothalamohypophyseal tract* (Fig. 9.3A). Posterior pituitary hormones are synthesised in the nerve cell bodies, transported along the axons and then stored in vesicles within the axon terminals within the posterior pituitary (Fig. 9.3B). Their release by exocytosis is triggered by nerve impulses from the hypothalamus.

Anterior pituitary

Some of the hormones secreted by the anterior lobe (adenohypophysis) stimulate or inhibit secretion by other endocrine glands (target glands) while others have a direct effect on target tissues. Table 9.1 summarises the main relationships between the hormones of the hypothalamus, the anterior pituitary and target glands or tissues.

The release of an anterior pituitary hormone follows stimulation of the gland by a specific *releasing hormone* produced by the hypothalamus and carried to the gland through the pituitary portal system of blood vessels. The whole system is controlled by a *negative feedback*

213

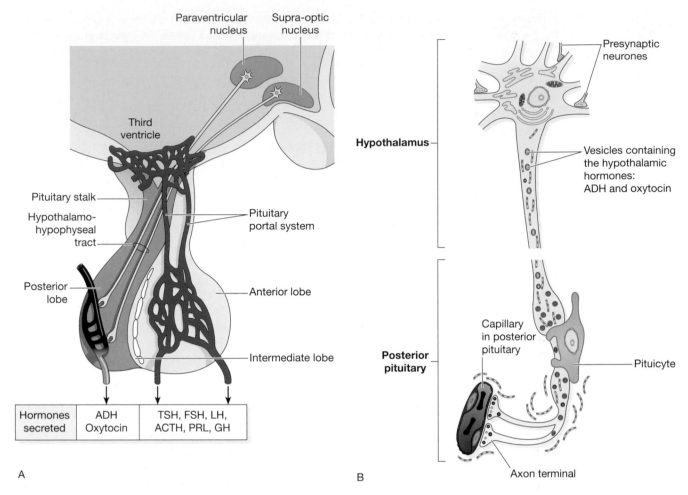

Figure 9.3 The pituitary gland. A. The lobes of the pituitary gland and their relationship with the hypothalamus. **B.** Synthesis and storage of antidiuretic hormone and oxytocin.

mechanism. That is, when there is a low level of a hormone in the blood supplying the hypothalamus it produces the appropriate releasing hormone that stimulates release of a *trophic hormone* by the anterior pituitary. This in turn stimulates the target gland to produce and release its hormone. As a result the blood level of that hormone rises and inhibits the secretion of releasing factor by the hypothalamus (Fig. 9.4).

Growth hormone (GH)

This is the most abundant hormone synthesised by the anterior pituitary. It stimulates growth and division of most body cells but especially those in the bones and skeletal muscles. Body growth in response to the secretion of GH is evident during childhood and adolescence, and thereafter secretion of GH maintains the mass of bones and skeletal muscles. It also regulates aspects of metabolism in many organs, e.g. liver, intestines and pancreas; stimulates protein synthesis; promotes break-

down of fats; and increases blood glucose levels (see Ch. 12).

Its release is stimulated by *growth hormone releasing hormone* (GHRH) and suppressed by *growth hormone release inhibiting hormone* (GHRIH) both of which are secreted by the hypothalamus. Secretion of GH is greater at night during sleep and is also stimulated by hypoglycaemia, exercise and anxiety. The daily amount secreted peaks in adolescence and then declines with age. Inhibition of GH secretion occurs by a negative feedback mechanism when the blood level rises and also when GHRIH (*somatostatin*) is released by the hypothalamus. GHRIH also suppresses secretion of TSH and gastrointestinal secretions, e.g. gastric juice, gastrin and cholecystokinin (see Ch. 12).

Thyroid stimulating hormone (TSH)

This hormone is synthesised by the anterior pituitary and its release is stimulated by TRH from the hypothalamus.

Table 9.1 Hormones of the hypothalamus, anterior pituitary and their target tissues

Hypothalamus	Anterior pituitary	Target gland or tissue
GHRH	GH	Most tissues
		Many organs
GHRIH	GH inhibition	Thyroid gland
	TSH inhibition	Pancreatic islets
		Most tissues
TRH	TSH	Thyroid gland
CRH	ACTH	Adrenal cortex
PRH	PRL	Breast
PIH	PRL inhibition	Breast
LHRH or	FSH	Ovaries and testes
GnRH	LH	Ovaries and testes

GHRH = growth hormone releasing hormone
GH   = growth hormone (somatotrophin)
GHRIH = growth hormone release inhibiting hormone (somatostatin)
TRH   = thyroid releasing hormone
TSH   = thyroid stimulating hormone
CRH   = corticotrophin releasing hormone
ACTH = adrenocorticotrophic hormone
PRH   = prolactin releasing hormone
PRL   = prolactin (lactogenic hormone)
PIH   = prolactin inhibiting hormone (dopamine)
LHRH = luteinising hormone releasing hormone
GnRH = gonadotrophin releasing hormone
FSH   = follicle stimulating hormone
LH   = luteinising hormone

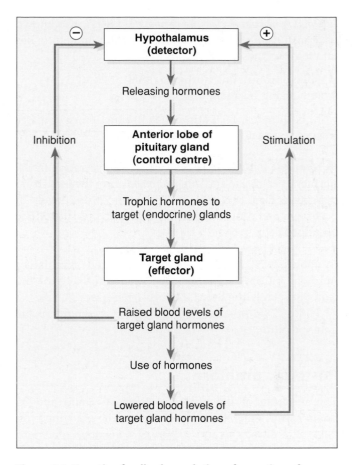

Figure 9.4 Negative feedback regulation of secretion of hormones by the anterior lobe of the pituitary gland.

215

It stimulates growth and activity of the thyroid gland, which secretes the hormones *thyroxine* (T_4) and *tri-iodothyronine* (T_3). Release is lowest in the early evening and highest during the night. Secretion is regulated by a negative feedback mechanism (Fig. 9.4). When the blood level of thyroid hormones is high, secretion of TSH is reduced, and vice versa.

Adrenocorticotrophic hormone (corticotrophin, ACTH)

Corticotrophin releasing hormone (CRH) from the hypothalamus promotes the synthesis and release of ACTH by the anterior pituitary. This increases the concentration of cholesterol and steroids within the adrenal cortex and the output of steroid hormones, especially *cortisol*.

ACTH levels are highest at about 8 a.m. and fall to their lowest about midnight, although high levels sometimes occur at midday and 6 p.m. This circadian rhythm is maintained throughout life. It is associated with the sleep pattern and adjustment to changes takes several days, following, e.g., changing work shifts, travelling to a different time zone (jet lag).

Secretion is also regulated by a negative feedback mechanism, being suppressed when the blood level of ACTH rises (Fig. 9.4). Other factors that stimulate secre-tion include hypoglycaemia, exercise and other stressors, e.g. emotional states and fever.

Prolactin

This hormone stimulates *lactation* (milk production) and has a direct effect on the breasts immediately after parturition (childbirth). The blood level of prolactin is stimulated by prolactin releasing hormone (PRH) released from the hypothalamus and it is lowered by prolactin inhibiting hormone (PIH, *dopamine*) and by an increased blood level of prolactin. After birth, suckling stimulates prolactin secretion and lactation. The resultant high blood level is a factor in reducing the incidence of conception during lactation.

Prolactin together with oestrogens, corticosteroids, insulin and thyroxine is involved in initiating and maintaining lactation. Prolactin secretion is related to sleep, i.e. it is raised during any period of sleep, night or day. Emotional stress increases production.

Gonadotrophins

After puberty two gonadotrophins (sex hormones) are secreted by the anterior pituitary in response to *luteinising hormone releasing hormone* (LHRH), also known as *gonadotrophin releasing hormone* (GnRH). In both males and females these are:

- follicle stimulating hormone (FSH)
- luteinising hormone (LH).

In both sexes. FSH stimulates production of gametes (ova or spermatozoa).

In females. LH and FSH are involved in secretion of the hormones *oestrogen* and *progesterone* during the menstrual cycle (see Figs 18.8 and 18.9, p. 448). As the levels of oestrogen and progesterone rise, secretion of LH and FSH is suppressed.

In males. LH, also called interstitial cell stimulating hormone (ICSH) stimulates the interstitial cells of the testes to secrete the hormone *testosterone* (see Ch. 18). Table 9.2 summarises the hormonal secretions of the anterior pituitary.

Posterior pituitary

The structure of the posterior pituitary gland and its relationship with the hypothalamus is explained on page 213. *Oxytocin* and *antidiuretic hormone* (ADH or vasopressin) are the hormones synthesised in the hypothalamus and then stored in the axon terminals within the posterior pituitary gland (Fig. 9.3B). These hormones act directly on non-endocrine tissue and their release from synaptic vesicles by exocytosis is stimulated by nerve impulses from the hypothalamus.

Oxytocin

Oxytocin stimulates two target tissues during and after childbirth (parturition): uterine smooth muscle and the muscle cells of the lactating breast.

During childbirth increasing amounts of oxytocin are released by the posterior pituitary into the bloodstream in response to increasing distension of sensory stretch receptors in the uterine cervix by the baby's head. Sensory impulses are generated and travel to the control centre in the hypothalamus, stimulating the posterior pituitary to release more oxytocin. In turn this stimulates more forceful uterine contractions and greater stretching of the uterine cervix as the baby's head is forced further downwards. This is an example of a *positive feedback mechanism* which stops soon after the baby is delivered when distension of the uterine cervix is greatly reduced (Fig. 9.5).

The process of milk ejection also involves a positive feedback mechanism. Suckling generates sensory impulses that are transmitted from the breast to the hypothalamus. The impulses trigger the release of oxytocin from the posterior pituitary and oxytocin stimulates contraction of the myoepithelial cells around the glandular cells and ducts of the lactating breast to contract, ejecting milk. Suckling also inhibits the release of *prolactin inhibiting hormone* (PIH), prolonging prolactin secretion and lactation. The role of this hormone in males and non-lactating females remains unclear.

Antidiuretic hormone (ADH) or vasopressin

The main effect of antidiuretic hormone is to reduce urine output (diuresis is the production of a large volume of

Table 9.2 Summary of the hormones secreted by the anterior pituitary gland and their functions

Hormone	Function
Growth hormone (GH)	Regulates metabolism, promotes tissue growth especially of bones and muscles
Thyroid stimulating hormone (TSH)	Stimulates growth and activity of thyroid gland and secretion of T_3 and T_4
Adrenocorticotrophic hormone (ACTH)	Stimulates the adrenal cortex to secrete glucocorticoids
Prolactin (PRL)	Stimulates milk production in the breasts
Follicle stimulating hormone (FSH)	Stimulates production of sperm in the testes, stimulates secretion of oestrogen by the ovaries, maturation of ovarian follicles, ovulation
Luteinising hormone (LH)	Stimulates secretion of testosterone by the testes, stimulates secretion of progesterone by the corpus luteum

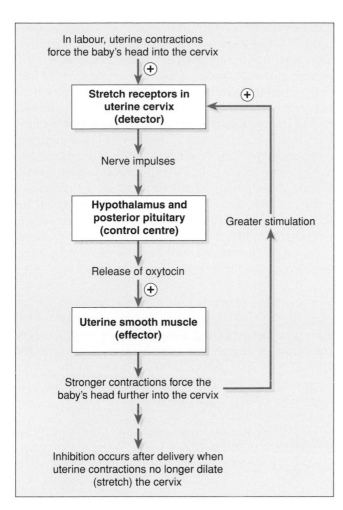

In labour, uterine contractions force the baby's head into the cervix

Stretch receptors in uterine cervix (detector)

Nerve impulses

Hypothalamus and posterior pituitary (control centre)

Greater stimulation

Release of oxytocin

Uterine smooth muscle (effector)

Stronger contractions force the baby's head further into the cervix

Inhibition occurs after delivery when uterine contractions no longer dilate (stretch) the cervix

Figure 9.5 Regulation of secretion of oxytocin through a positive feedback mechanism.

urine). ADH increases the permeability to water of the distal convoluted and collecting tubules of the nephrons of the kidneys (Ch. 13). As a result the reabsorption of water from the glomerular filtrate is increased. The amount of ADH secreted is influenced by the osmotic pressure of the blood circulating to the *osmoreceptors* in the hypothalamus.

As the osmotic pressure rises, the secretion of ADH increases as in, for example, dehydration and following haemorrhage. More water is therefore reabsorbed and the urine output is reduced. This means that the body retains more water and the rise in osmotic pressure is reversed. Conversely, when the osmotic pressure of the blood is low, for example after a large fluid intake, secretion of ADH is reduced, less water is reabsorbed and more urine is produced (Fig. 9.11).

At high concentrations, for example after severe blood loss, ADH causes smooth muscle contraction, especially vasoconstriction in the blood vessels of the skin and abdominal organs. This has a *pressor effect*, raising systemic blood pressure; the alternative name of this hormone, vasopressin, reflects this effect.

Thyroid gland (Fig. 9.6)

Learning outcomes

After studying this section you should be able to:

- describe the position of the thyroid gland and its related structures

- describe the microscopic structure of the thyroid gland

- outline the actions of the thyroid hormones

- explain how blood levels of the thyroid hormones T_3 and T_4 are regulated.

The thyroid gland is situated in the neck in front of the larynx and trachea at the level of the 5th, 6th and 7th cervical and 1st thoracic vertebrae. It is a highly vascular gland that weighs about 25 g and is surrounded by a fibrous capsule. It resembles a butterfly in shape,

217

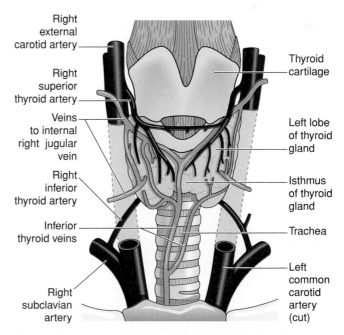

Right external carotid artery

Right superior thyroid artery

Veins to internal right jugular vein

Right inferior thyroid artery

Inferior thyroid veins

Right subclavian artery

Thyroid cartilage

Left lobe of thyroid gland

Isthmus of thyroid gland

Trachea

Left common carotid artery (cut)

Figure 9.6 The position of the thyroid gland and its associated structures. Anterior view.

consisting of two *lobes*, one on either side of the thyroid cartilage and upper cartilaginous rings of the trachea. The lobes are joined by a narrow *isthmus*, lying in front of the trachea.

The lobes are roughly cone shaped, about 5 cm long and 3 cm wide.

The *arterial blood supply* to the gland is through the superior and inferior thyroid arteries. The superior thyroid artery is a branch of the external carotid artery and the inferior thyroid artery is a branch of the subclavian artery.

The *venous return* is by the thyroid veins, which drain into the internal jugular veins.

Two parathyroid glands lie against the posterior surface of each lobe and are sometimes embedded in thyroid tissue. The recurrent laryngeal nerve passes upwards close to the lobes of the gland and on the right side it lies near the inferior thyroid artery (see Fig. 9.9).

The gland is composed of cuboidal epithelium that forms spherical follicles. These secrete and store *colloid*, a thick sticky protein material (Fig. 9.7). Between the follicles there are other cells found singly or in small groups: *parafollicular cells*, also called C-cells, which secrete the hormone *calcitonin*.

Thyroxine and tri-iodothyronine

Iodine is essential for the formation of the thyroid gland hormones, thyroxine (T_4) and tri-iodothyronine (T_3). The body's main sources of iodine are seafood, vegetables grown in iodine-rich soil and iodinated table salt in the diet. The thyroid gland selectively takes up iodine from the blood, a process called *iodine trapping*.

The thyroid hormones are synthesised as large precursor molecules called *thyroglobulin*, the major constituent of colloid. The release of T_3 and T_4 into the blood is regulated by *thyroid stimulating hormone* (TSH) from the anterior pituitary.

Secretion of TSH is stimulated by *thyroid releasing hormone* (TRH) from the hypothalamus and secretion of TRH is stimulated by exercise, stress, malnutrition, low plasma glucose and sleep. The level of secretion of TSH depends on the plasma levels of T_3 and T_4 because these hormones affect the sensitivity of the anterior pituitary to TRH. Through the negative feedback mechanism, increased levels of T_3 and T_4 decrease TSH secretion and vice versa (Fig. 9.8). When the supply of iodine is deficient, excess TSH is secreted and there is proliferation of thyroid gland cells and enlargement of the gland (see Goitre, p. 228). Secretion of T_3 and T_4 begins about the third month of fetal life and is increased at puberty and in women during the reproductive years, especially during pregnancy. Otherwise, it remains fairly constant throughout life.

218

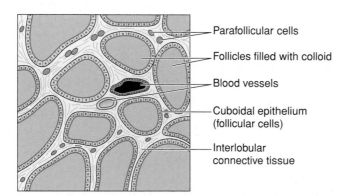

Figure 9.7 The microscopic structure of the thyroid gland.

Parafollicular cells

Follicles filled with colloid

Blood vessels

Cuboidal epithelium (follicular cells)

Interlobular connective tissue

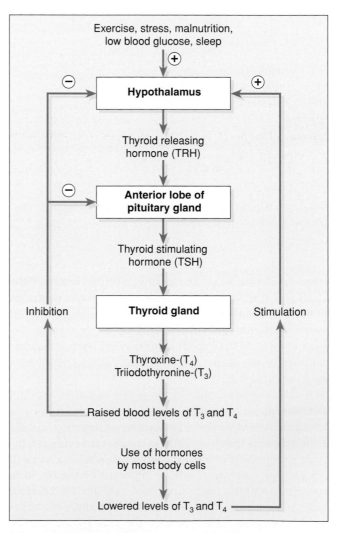

Figure 9.8 Negative feedback regulation of the secretion of thyroxine (T_4) and tri-iodothyronine (T_3).

Exercise, stress, malnutrition, low blood glucose, sleep

Hypothalamus

Thyroid releasing hormone (TRH)

Anterior lobe of pituitary gland

Thyroid stimulating hormone (TSH)

Inhibition   Thyroid gland   Stimulation

Thyroxine-(T_4) Triiodothyronine-(T_3)

Raised blood levels of T_3 and T_4

Use of hormones by most body cells

Lowered levels of T_3 and T_4

Table 9.3 Common effects of abnormal secretion of thyroid hormones

Hyperthyroidism: increased T_3 and T_4 secretion	Hypothyroidism: decreased T_3 and T_4 secretion
Increased basal metabolic rate	Decreased basal metabolic rate
Weight loss, good appetite	Weight gain, anorexia
Anxiety, physical restlessness, mental excitability	Depression, psychosis, mental slowness, lethargy
Hair loss	Dry skin, brittle hair
Tachycardia, palpitations, atrial fibrillation	Bradycardia
Warm sweaty skin, heat intolerance	Dry cold skin, prone to hypothermia
Diarrhoea	Constipation
Exophthalmos in Graves' disease	

Thyroid hormones enter the target cells and regulate the expression of genes in the nucleus, i.e. they increase or decrease the synthesis of some proteins including enzymes. They combine with specific receptor sites and enhance the effects of other hormones, e.g. adrenaline (epinephrine) and noradrenaline (norepinephrine).

T_3 and T_4 affect most cells of the body by:

- increasing the basal metabolic rate and heat production
- regulating metabolism of carbohydrates, proteins and fats.

T_3 and T_4 are essential for normal growth and development, especially of the skeleton and nervous system. Most other organs and systems are also influenced by thyroid hormones – physiological effects of T_3 and T_4 on the heart, skeletal muscles, skin, digestive and reproductive systems are more evident when there is underactivity or overactivity of the thyroid gland. These changes are listed in Table 9.3.

Calcitonin

This hormone is secreted by the parafollicular or C-cells in the thyroid gland (Fig. 9.7). It acts on bone and the kidneys to reduce the blood calcium (Ca^{2+}) level when it is raised. It reduces the reabsorption of calcium from bones and inhibits reabsorption of calcium by the renal tubules. Its effect is opposite to that of parathyroid hormone, the hormone secreted by the parathyroid glands. Release of calcitonin is stimulated by an increase in the blood calcium level.

This hormone is important during childhood when bones undergo considerable changes in size and shape.

219

Parathyroid glands

Learning outcomes

After studying this section you should be able to:

- describe the position and gross structure of the parathyroid glands

- outline the functions of parathyroid hormone and calcitonin

- explain how blood levels of parathyroid hormone and calcitonin are regulated.

There are four small parathyroid glands, two embedded in the posterior surface of each lobe of the thyroid gland (Fig. 9.9). They are surrounded by fine connective tissue capsules. The cells forming the glands are spherical in shape and are arranged in columns with channels containing blood between them.

Function

The parathyroid glands secrete *parathyroid hormone* (PTH, parathormone). Secretion is regulated by the blood level

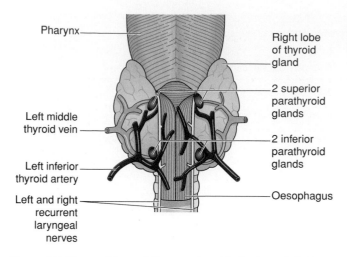

Pharynx

Right lobe of thyroid gland

2 superior parathyroid glands

Left middle thyroid vein

2 inferior parathyroid glands

Left inferior thyroid artery

Left and right recurrent laryngeal nerves

Oesophagus

Figure 9.9 The positions of the parathyroid glands and their related structures, viewed from behind.

of calcium. When this falls, secretion of PTH is increased and vice versa.

The main function of PTH is to increase the blood calcium level when it is low. This is achieved by indirectly increasing the amount of calcium absorbed from the small intestine and reabsorbed from the renal tubules. If these sources provide inadequate supplies then PTH stimulates osteoclasts (bone-destroying cells) and resorption of calcium from bones.

Parathormone and calcitonin from the thyroid gland act in a complementary manner to maintain blood calcium levels within the normal range. This is needed for:

- muscle contraction
- blood clotting
- nerve impulse transmission.

Adrenal (suprarenal) glands

Learning outcomes

After studying this section you should be able to:

- describe the structure of the adrenal glands

- describe the actions of each of the three groups of adrenocorticoid hormones

- explain how blood levels of glucocorticoids are regulated

- describe the actions of adrenaline (epinephrine) and noradrenaline (norepinephrine)

- outline how the adrenal glands respond to stress.

There are two adrenal glands, one situated on the upper pole of each kidney enclosed within the renal fascia. They are about 4 cm long and 3 cm thick.

The *arterial blood supply* to the glands is by branches from the abdominal aorta and renal arteries.

The *venous return* is by suprarenal veins. The right gland drains into the inferior vena cava and the left into the left renal vein.

The glands are composed of two parts which have different structures and functions. The outer part is the *cortex* and the inner part the *medulla*. The adrenal cortex is essential to life but the medulla is not.

Adrenal cortex

The adrenal cortex produces three groups of steroid hormones from cholesterol. They are collectively called *adrenocorticocoids* (corticosteroids, corticoids). They are:

- glucocorticoids
- mineralocorticoids
- sex hormones (androgens).

The hormones in each group have different characteristic actions but due to their structural similarity their actions may overlap.

Glucocorticoids

Cortisol (hydrocortisone), is the main glucocorticoid but small amounts of *corticosterone* and *cortisone* are also produced. They are essential for life, regulating metabolism and responses to stress. Secretion is controlled through a negative feedback system involving the hypothalamus and anterior pituitary. It is stimulated by ACTH from the anterior pituitary and by stress (Fig. 9.10). In non-stressful conditions, secretion has marked circadian variations. The highest level of hormones occurs between 4 a.m. and 8 a.m. and the lowest, between midnight and 3 a.m. When the sleeping and waking pattern is changed it takes several days for adjustment of the ACTH/cortisol secretion to take place (see p. 215).

Glucocorticoids have widespread metabolic effects and these include:

- *gluconeogenesis* (formation of new sugar from, for example, protein) and hyperglycaemia (raised blood glucose level)
- *lipolysis* (breakdown of triglycerides into fatty acids and glycerol for energy production)
- stimulating breakdown of protein, releasing amino acids, which can be used for synthesis of other proteins, e.g. enzymes, or for energy (ATP) production (p. 314)
- promoting absorption of sodium and water from renal tubules (a weak mineralocorticoid effect).

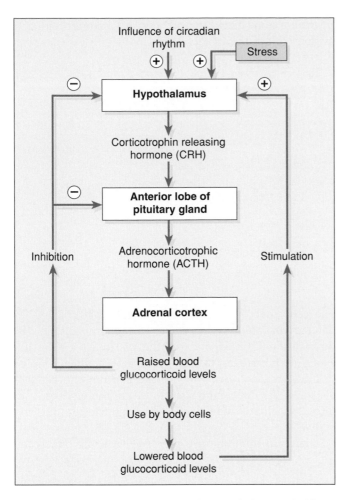

Figure 9.10 Negative feedback regulation of glucocorticoid secretion.

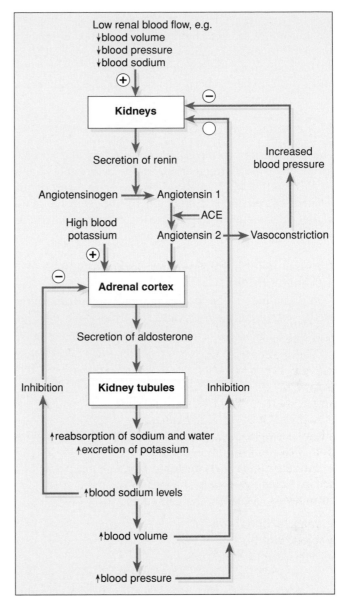

221

Figure 9.11 Negative feedback regulation of aldosterone secretion.

In pathological and pharmacological quantities glucocorticoids also have other effects including:

- anti-inflammatory actions
- suppression of immune responses
- delayed wound healing.

Mineralocorticoids (aldosterone)

Aldosterone is the main mineralocorticoid. Its functions are associated with the maintenance of water and electrolyte balance in the body. Through a negative feedback system it stimulates the reabsorption of sodium (Na^+) by the renal tubules and excretion of potassium (K^+) in the urine. Sodium reabsorption is also accompanied by retention of water and therefore aldosterone is involved in the regulation of blood volume and blood pressure too.

The blood potassium level regulates the amount of aldosterone produced by the adrenal cortex. When the blood potassium level rises, more aldosterone is secreted (Fig. 9.11). Low blood potassium has the opposite effect.

Angiotensin (see below) also stimulates the release of aldosterone.

Renin–angiotensin–aldosterone system. When renal blood flow is reduced or blood sodium levels fall, the enzyme *renin* is secreted by kidney cells. Renin converts the plasma protein *angiotensinogen*, produced by the liver, to *angiotensin 1*. Angiotensin converting enzyme (ACE), formed in small quantities in the lungs, proximal kidney tubules and other tissues converts angiotensin 1 to *angiotensin 2*, which stimulates secretion of aldosterone (Fig. 9.11). It also causes vasoconstriction and increases blood pressure.

Sex hormones

Sex hormones secreted by the adrenal cortex are mainly *androgens* (male sex hormones) and the amounts produced are insignificant compared with those secreted by the testes and ovaries in late puberty and adulthood (see Ch. 18).

Adrenal medulla

The medulla is completely surrounded by the adrenal cortex. It develops from nervous tissue in the embryo and is part of the sympathetic division of the autonomic nervous system. It is stimulated by its extensive sympathetic nerve supply to produce the hormones *adrenaline (epinephrine)* and *noradrenaline (norepinephrine)*.

Adrenaline (epinephrine) and noradrenaline (norepinephrine)

Noradrenaline is the postganglionic neurotransmitter of the sympathetic division of the autonomic nervous system (see Fig. 7.8, p. 147). Adrenaline and some noradrenaline are released into the blood from the adrenal medulla during stimulation of the sympathetic nervous system (see Fig. 7.42, p. 171). They are structurally very similar and this explains their similar effects. Together they potentiate the fight or flight response by:

- increasing heart rate
- increasing blood pressure
- diverting blood to essential organs including the heart, brain and skeletal muscles by dilating their blood vessels and constricting those of less essential organs, such as the skin
- increasing metabolic rate
- dilating the pupils.

Adrenaline has a greater effect on the heart and metabolic processes whereas noradrenaline has more influence on blood vessels.

Response to stress

When the body is under stress homeostasis is disturbed. To restore it and, in some cases, to maintain life there are immediate and, if necessary, longer-term responses. Stressors include exercise, fasting, fright, temperature changes, infection, disease and emotional disturbances/situations.

The *immediate response* is sometimes described as preparing for 'fight or flight'. This is mediated by the sympathetic part of the autonomic nervous system and the principal effects are shown in Figure 9.12.

In the *longer term*, ACTH from the anterior pituitary stimulates the release of glucocorticoids and mineralo-

corticoids from the adrenal cortex and a more prolonged response to stress occurs (Fig. 9.12).

Pancreatic islets

Learning outcomes

After studying this section you should be able to:

- list the hormones secreted by the endocrine pancreas
- describe the actions of insulin and glucagon
- explain how blood glucose levels are regulated.

The cells that make up the pancreatic islets (islets of Langerhans) are found in clusters irregularly distributed throughout the substance of the pancreas. Unlike the exocrine pancreas, which produces pancreatic juice (p. 304), there are no ducts leading from the clusters of islet cells. Pancreatic hormones are secreted directly into the bloodstream and circulate throughout the body.

There are three main types of cells in the pancreatic islets:

- α (alpha) cells, which secrete *glucagon*
- β (beta) cells, which secrete *insulin*
- δ (delta) cells, which secrete *somatostatin* (GHRIH, pp. 214 and 223).

The normal blood glucose level is between 3.5 and 8 mmol/litre (63 to 144 mg/100 ml). Blood glucose levels are controlled mainly by the opposing actions of insulin and glucagon:

- glucagon increases blood glucose levels
- insulin reduces blood glucose levels.

Insulin

Insulin is a polypeptide consisting of about 50 amino acids. The main function of insulin is to lower raised blood nutrient levels, especially glucose but also amino acids and fatty acids. When these nutrients, especially glucose, are in excess of immediate needs insulin promotes their storage by:

- acting on cell membranes and stimulating uptake and use of glucose by muscle and connective tissue cells
- increasing conversion of glucose to glycogen (glycogenesis), especially in the liver and skeletal muscles

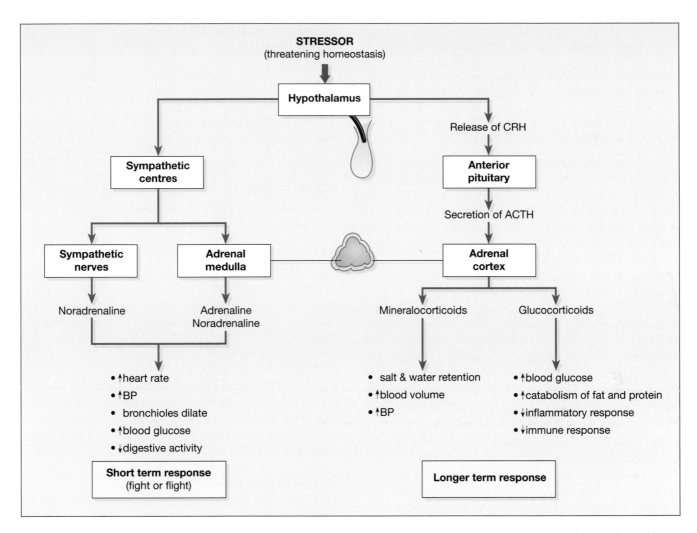

Figure 9.12 Responses to stressors that threaten homeostasis. CRH = corticotrophin releasing hormone. ACTH = adrenocorticotrophic hormone.

- accelerating uptake of amino acids by cells, and the synthesis of protein
- promoting synthesis of fatty acids and storage of fat in adipose tissue (lipogenesis)
- decreasing glycogenolysis (breakdown of glycogen, into glucose)
- preventing the breakdown of protein and fat, and *gluconeogenesis* (formation of new sugar from, e.g., protein).

Secretion of insulin is stimulated by increased blood glucose levels and to a lesser extent by parasympathetic stimulation, raised blood amino acid and fatty acid levels, and gastrointestinal hormones, e.g. gastrin, secretin and cholecystokinin. Secretion is decreased by sympathetic stimulation, glucagon, adrenaline, cortisol and somatostatin (GHRIH) secreted by the pancreatic islets.

Glucagon

The effects of glucagon increase blood glucose levels by stimulating:

- conversion of glycogen to glucose in the liver and skeletal muscles (glycogenolysis)
- gluconeogenesis.

Secretion of glucagon is stimulated by a low blood glucose level and exercise, and decreased by somatostatin and insulin.

Somatostatin (GHRIH)

The effect of this hormone, also produced by the hypothalamus, is to inhibit the secretion of both insulin and glucagon in addition to inhibiting the secretion of GH from the anterior pituitary.

Pineal gland or body

Learning outcomes

After studying this section you should be able to:

- state the position of the pineal gland
- outline the actions of melatonin.

The pineal gland is a small body attached to the roof of the third ventricle and is connected to it by a short stalk containing nerves, many of which terminate in the hypothalamus. The pineal gland is about 10 mm long, is reddish brown in colour and is surrounded by a capsule.

Melatonin

This is the hormone secreted by the pineal gland. Secretion is controlled by daylight and levels fluctuate during each 24-hour period, being highest at night and lowest around midday. Secretion is also influenced by the number of daylight hours, i.e. seasonal variations. Although its functions are not fully understood, melatonin is believed to be associated with:

- coordination of the circadian and diurnal rhythms of many tissues, possibly by influencing the hypothalamus
- inhibition of growth and development of the sex organs before puberty, possibly by preventing synthesis or release of gonadotrophins.

The gland tends to atrophy after puberty and may become calcified in later life.

Thymus gland

Learning outcomes

After studying this section you should be able to:

- state the position of the thymus gland
- outline the actions of thymosin.

The location and structure of the thymus gland are described on page 136.

Thymosin

This is the hormone secreted by the thymus gland and is required for the development of T-lymphocytes for cell-mediated immunity (Ch. 15).

Local hormones

Learning outcome

After studying this section you should be able to:

- name substances that act as local hormones.

A number of body tissues not normally described as endocrine glands secrete substances that act locally. Some of these are described below.

Histamine

This hormone is synthesised by mast cells in the tissues and basophils in blood. It is released as part of the inflammatory process, increasing capillary permeability and causing vasodilatation. It also causes contraction of smooth muscle of the bronchi and alimentary tract and stimulates the secretion of gastric juice.

Serotonin (5-hydroxytryptamine, 5-HT)

This is present in platelets, in the brain and in the intestinal wall. It causes intestinal secretion and contraction of smooth muscle and its role in haemostasis (blood clotting) is outlined in Chapter 4.

Prostaglandins (PGs)

These are lipid substances found in most tissues that act as local hormones and have wide-ranging physiological effects in:

- the inflammatory response
- potentiating pain
- fever
- regulating blood pressure
- blood clotting
- uterine contractions during labour.

Other chemically similar compounds include *leukotrienes* and *thromboxanes* e.g. thromboxane A_2, which is a potent aggregator of platelets. They are active substances found in only small amounts, as they are rapidly degraded.

Gastrointestinal hormones

Several local hormones, including gastrin, secretin and cholecystokinin (CCK), influence the secretion of digestive juices and their functions are explained in Chapter 12.

Endocrine disorders are commonly caused by *tumours* or *autoimmune diseases* and their effects are usually the result of:

- hypersecretion (overproduction) of hormones
- hyposecretion (underproduction) of hormones.

The effects of many of the conditions explained in this section can therefore be readily linked to the underlying abnormality.

Disorders of the anterior pituitary

Learning outcomes

After studying this section you should be able to:

- list the causes of diseases in this section
- explain the features of the diseases in this section.

Hypersecretion of anterior pituitary hormones

Gigantism and acromegaly

The most common cause is prolonged hypersecretion of growth hormone (GH), usually by a hormone-secreting pituitary tumour. The conditions are only occasionally due to excess growth hormone releasing hormone (GHRH) secreted by the hypothalamus. As the tumour increases in size, compression of nearby structures may lead to:

- hyposecretion of other pituitary hormones of both the anterior and posterior lobes
- damage to the optic nerves, causing visual disturbances.

Effects of excess GH
These include:

- excessive growth of bones
- enlargement of internal organs
- growth of excess connective tissue
- enlargement of the heart and a rise in blood pressure
- reduced glucose tolerance and a predisposition to diabetes mellitus.

Gigantism. This occurs in children when there is excess GH while epiphyseal cartilages of long bones are still growing, i.e. before ossification of bones is complete. It is

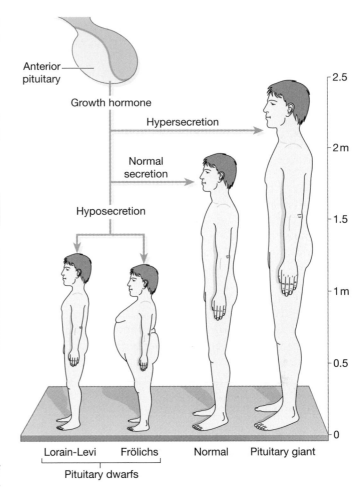

Figure 9.13 **Effects of normal and abnormal growth hormone secretion.**

evident mainly in the bones of the limbs, and affected individuals may grow to heights of 2.1 to 2.4 m, although body proportions remain normal (Fig. 9.13).

Acromegaly (meaning 'large extremities'). This occurs in adults when there is excess GH after ossification is complete. The bones become abnormally thick and there is thickening of the soft tissues. These changes are most noticeable as coarse facial features (especially excessive growth of the lower jaw), an enlarged tongue and excessively large hands and feet (Fig. 9.14).

Hyperprolactinaemia

This is caused by a hormone-secreting tumour. It causes *galactorrhoea* (inappropriate milk secretion), *amenorrhoea* (cessation of menstruation) and sterility in women and impotence in men.

225

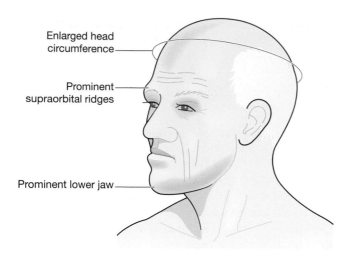

Enlarged head circumference

Prominent supraorbital ridges

Prominent lower jaw

Figure 9.14 Facial features in acromegaly.

Hyposecretion of anterior pituitary hormones

The number of hormones involved and the extent of hyposecretion varies. *Panhypopituitarism* is absence of all hormones. Causes of hyposecretion include:

- tumours of the hypothalamus or pituitary
- trauma, usually caused by fractured base of skull or surgery
- pressure caused by a tumour adjacent to the pituitary gland, e.g. glioma, meningioma
- infection, e.g. meningitis, encephalitis, syphilis
- ischaemic necrosis
- ionising radiation or cytotoxic drugs.

Ischaemic necrosis

Simmond's disease is hypofunction of the anterior pituitary gland. It only rarely affects the posterior lobe. The arrangement of the blood supply makes the gland unusually susceptible to a fall in systemic BP. Severe hypotensive shock may cause ischaemic necrosis of the gland. The effects include deficient stimulation of target glands and hypofunction of all or some of the thyroid, adrenal cortex and gonads. The outcome depends on the extent of pituitary necrosis and hormone deficiency. In severe cases, glucocorticoid deficiency may be life threatening or fatal. When this condition is associated with severe haemorrhage during or after childbirth it is known as *Sheehan's syndrome*, and in this situation the other effects are preceded by failure of lactation.

Pituitary dwarfism (Lorain–Lévi syndrome)

This is caused by severe deficiency of GH, and possibly of other hormones, in childhood. The individual is of small stature but is well proportioned and mental development is not affected. Puberty is delayed and there may be episodes of hypoglycaemia. The condition may be due to genetic abnormality or a tumour.

Fröhlich's syndrome

In this condition there is panhypopituitarism but the main features are associated with deficiency of GH, FSH and LH. In children the effects are diminished growth, lack of sexual development, obesity with female distribution of fat and learning disabilities. In a similar condition in adults, obesity and sterility are the main features. It may be the result of a tumour of the anterior pituitary and/or the hypothalamus but in most cases the cause is unknown.

Disorders of the posterior pituitary

Learning outcomes

After studying this section you should be able to:

- list the causes of diabetes insipidus
- relate the features of diabetes insipidus to abnormal secretion of antidiuretic hormone.

Diabetes insipidus

This is a relatively rare condition usually caused by hyposecretion of ADH due to damage to the hypothalamus by, e.g., trauma, tumour or encephalitis. Occasionally it occurs when the renal tubules do not respond to ADH. Water reabsorption by the renal tubules is impaired, leading to excretion of excessive amounts of dilute urine, often more than 10 litres daily, causing dehydration, extreme thirst and polydipsia. Water balance is disturbed unless fluid intake is greatly increased to compensate for excess losses.

Disorders of the thyroid gland

Learning outcome

After studying this section you should be able to:

- compare and contrast the effects of hyperthyroidism and hypothyroidism, relating them to the actions of T_3 and T_4.

These fall into three main categories:

- abnormal secretion of thyroid hormones (T_3 and T_4)
  - hyperthyroidism
  - hypothyroidism
- *goitre* – enlargements of the thyroid gland
- tumours.

Abnormal thyroid function may arise not only from thyroid disease but also from disorders of the pituitary or hypothalamus; in addition, insufficient dietary iodine causes deficiency in thyroid hormone production. The main effects are caused by an abnormally high or low basal metabolic rate.

Abnormal secretion of thyroid hormones

Hyperthyroidism

This syndrome, also known as *thyrotoxicosis*, arises as the body tissues are exposed to excessive levels of T_3 and T_4. The main effects are due to increased basal metabolic rate (see Table 9.3).

In older adults, cardiac failure is another common consequence as the ageing heart works harder to deliver more blood and nutrients to the hyperactive body cells. The main causes are:

- Graves' disease
- toxic nodular goitre
- toxic adenoma (a benign tumour, p. 228).

Graves' disease

Sometimes called *Graves' thyroiditis*, this condition accounts for 75% of cases of hyperthyroidism. It affects more women than men and may occur at any age, being most common between the ages of 30 and 50 years. It is an autoimmune disorder in which an antibody that mimics the effects of TSH is produced, causing:

- increased release of T_3 and T_4 and signs of hyperthyroidism (see Table 9.3)
- goitre (visible enlargement of the gland) as the antibody stimulates thyroid growth
- exophthalmos in many cases.

Exophthalmos. This is protrusion of the eyeballs due to the deposition of excess fat and fibrous tissue behind the eyes (Fig. 9.15); it is often present in Graves' disease. Effective treatment of hyperthyroidism does not completely reverse the exophthalmos although it may lessen after 2 to 3 years. In severe cases the eyelids become retracted and may not completely cover the eyes during blinking and sleep, leading to drying of the conjunctiva and predisposing to infection. It does not occur in other forms of hyperthyroidism.

Toxic nodular goitre

In this condition one or two nodules of a gland that is already affected by goitre (see Simple goitre, p. 228) become active and secrete excess T_3 and T_4 causing the effects of hyperthyroidism (Table 9.3). It is more common in women than men and after middle age. As this condition affects an older age group than Graves' disease, arrhythmias and cardiac failure are more common. Exophthalmos does not occur in this type of hyperthyroidism.

Hypothyroidism

This occurs when there is insufficient T_3 and T_4 secretion causing:

- congenital hypothyroidism in children
- myxoedema in adults.

Congenital hypothyroidism

Previously called cretinism, this is a profound deficiency or absence of thyroid hormones that becomes evident a few weeks or months after birth. Hypothyroidism is endemic in some parts of the world where the diet is severely deficient in iodine and contains insufficient for synthesis of T_3 and T_4. This results in profound impairment of growth and mental development. Unless treatment begins early in life, mental impairment remains and the individual typically has disproportionately short

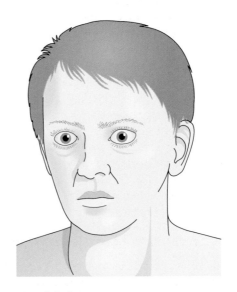

Figure 9.15 Exophthalmos.

limbs, a large protruding tongue, coarse dry skin, poor abdominal muscle tone and an umbilical hernia.

Myxoedema

This condition is prevalent in the elderly and is five times more common in females than males. Deficiency of T_3 and T_4 in adults results in an abnormally low metabolic rate and other effects shown in Table 9.3. There may be accumulation of polysaccharide substances in the subcutaneous tissues especially of the face. The commonest causes are:

- autoimmune thyroiditis
- severe iodine deficiency (see goitre)
- iatrogenic, e.g. antithyroid drugs, surgical removal of thyroid tissue, ionising radiation.

Autoimmune thyroiditis

The most common cause of acquired hypothyroidism is *Hashimoto's disease*. It is more common in women than men and, like Graves' disease, it is also an organ-specific autoimmune condition. Autoantibodies that react with thyroglobulin and thyroid gland cells develop and prevent synthesis and release of thyroid hormones causing hypothyroidism. Goitre is sometimes present.

Simple goitre

This is enlargement of the thyroid gland without signs of hyperthyroidism. It is caused by a relative lack of T_3 and T_4 and the low levels stimulate secretion of TSH resulting in hyperplasia of the thyroid gland (Fig. 9.16). Sometimes the extra thyroid tissue is able to maintain

normal hormone levels but if not, hypothyroidism develops. Causes are:

- persistent iodine deficiency. In some parts of the world where there is dietary iodine deficiency, this is a common condition known as *endemic goitre*
- genetic abnormality affecting synthesis of T_3 and T_4
- iatrogenic, e.g. antithyroid drugs, surgical removal of excess thyroid tissue.

The enlarged gland may cause pressure damage to adjacent tissues, especially if it lies in an abnormally low position, i.e. behind the sternum. The structures most commonly affected are the oesophagus, causing dysphagia; the trachea, causing dyspnoea; and the recurrent laryngeal nerve, causing hoarseness of voice.

Tumours of the thyroid gland

Benign tumours

Single adenomas are fairly common and may become cystic. Sometimes the adenoma secretes hormones and hyperthyroidism may develop. The tumours have a tendency to become malignant especially in the elderly.

Malignant tumours

These are rare and are usually well differentiated but are sometimes anaplastic (see p. 52).

Disorders of the parathyroid glands

> **Learning outcome**
>
> After studying this section you should be able to:
>
> ■ explain how the diseases in this section are related to abnormal secretion of parathyroid hormone.

Hyperparathyroidism

Excess secretion of parathyroid hormone (PTH), usually by benign tumours of a gland, causes reabsorption of calcium from bones, raising the blood calcium level (hypercalcaemia). The effects may be:

- polyuria and polydipsia
- formation of renal calculi

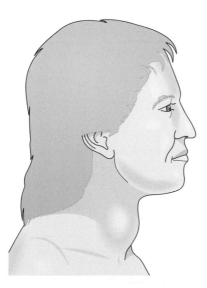

Figure 9.16 Enlarged thyroid gland in goitre.

228

- anorexia and constipation
- muscle weakness
- general fatigue.

Hypoparathyroidism

Parathyroid hormone (PTH) deficiency causes hypocalcaemia, i.e. an abnormally low level of calcium in the blood, and is much less common than hyperparathyroidism. There is reduced absorption of calcium from the small intestine and reabsorption from bones and glomerular filtrate. Low blood calcium causes:

- *tetany* (Fig. 9.17)
- psychiatric disturbances
- paraesthesia
- grand mal seizures
- in some cases development of cataract (opacity of the lens) and brittle nails.

The causes of hypoparathyroidism include: damage to or removal of the glands during thyroidectomy, ionising radiation, development of autoantibodies to PTH and parathyroid cells, and congenital abnormality of the glands.

Tetany

This is caused by hypocalcaemia, because it increases excitability of peripheral nerves. There are very strong painful spasms of skeletal muscles, causing characteristic bending inwards of the hands, forearms and feet (Fig. 9.17). In children there may be laryngeal spasm and seizures. Hypocalcaemia is associated with:

- hypoparathyroidism

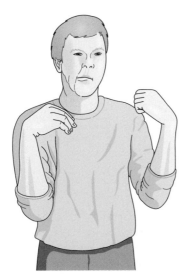

Figure 9.17 Characteristic positions adopted during tetanic spasms.

- deficiency of vitamin D or dietary deficiency of calcium
- chronic renal failure when there is excretion of excess calcium in the urine
- alkalosis; metabolic due to persistent vomiting, ingestion of excess alkali to alleviate gastric disturbances or respiratory due to hyperventilation
- acute pancreatitis.

Disorders of the adrenal cortex

Learning outcomes

After studying this section you should be able to:

- relate the features of Cushing's syndrome to the actions of adrenocorticoids
- relate the features of Addison's disease to the actions of adrenocorticoids.

Hypersecretion of glucocorticoids (Cushing's syndrome)

Cortisol is the main glucocorticoid hormone secreted by the adrenal cortex. Causes of hypersecretion include:

- hormone-secreting adrenal tumours, benign or malignant
- hypersecretion of adrenocorticotrophic hormone (ACTH) by the anterior pituitary
- abnormal secretion of ACTH by a non-pituitary tumour, e.g. bronchial carcinoma, pancreatic tumour, carcinoid tumours
- prolonged therapeutic use of ACTH or glucocorticoids, e.g. prednisolone, in high doses.

Hypersecretion of cortisol exaggerates its physiological effects (Fig. 9.18). These include:

- painful adiposity of the face (*moon face*), neck and abdomen
- excess protein breakdown, causing thinning of subcutaneous tissue and muscle wasting, especially of the limbs
- diminished protein synthesis
- suppression of growth hormone, causing arrest of growth in children
- osteoporosis, and kyphosis if vertebral bodies are involved
- pathological fractures because of calcium loss from bone

229

- excessive gluconeogenesis with hyperglycaemia and glycosuria
- atrophy of lymphoid tissue and depressed immune response
- susceptibility to infection due to reduced febrile response, depressed immune response and phagocytosis, impaired migration of phagocytes
- insomnia, excitability, euphoria, psychosis, depression
- hypertension due to salt and water retention
- menstrual disturbances
- formation of renal calculi
- peptic ulceration.

Hyposecretion of glucocorticoids

Inadequate secretion of cortisol causes diminished gluconeogenesis, low blood glucose, muscle weakness and pallor. It may be primary, i.e. due to disease of the adrenal cortex, or secondary due to deficiency of ACTH from the anterior pituitary. In primary deficiency there is also hyposecretion of aldosterone (see below) but in secondary deficiency, aldosterone secretion is not usually affected because aldosterone release is controlled by the renin–angiotensin–aldosterone system (p. 343).

Hypersecretion of mineralocorticoids

Excess aldosterone affects kidney function, causing:

- excessive reabsorption of sodium chloride and water, causing increased blood volume and hypertension
- excessive excretion of potassium, causing *hypokalaemia*, which leads to cardiac arrhythmia, alkalosis, syncope and muscle weakness.

Primary hyperaldosteronism (Conn's syndrome)

This is due to an excessive secretion of mineralocorticoids, independent of the renin–angiotensin–aldosterone

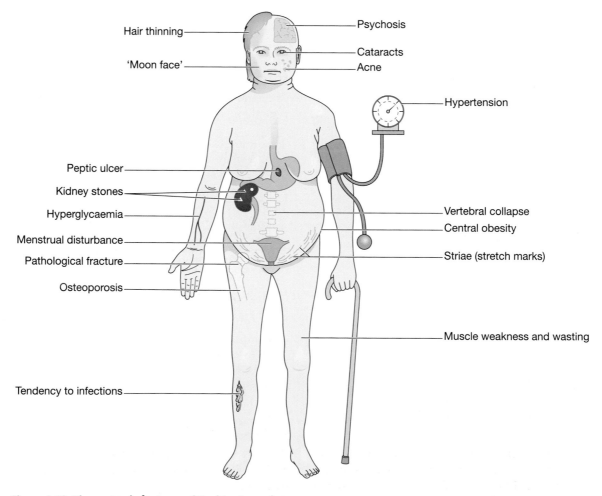

Hair thinning

'Moon face'

Psychosis

Cataracts

Acne

Hypertension

Peptic ulcer

Kidney stones

Hyperglycaemia

Menstrual disturbance

Pathological fracture

Osteoporosis

Vertebral collapse

Central obesity

Striae (stretch marks)

Muscle weakness and wasting

Tendency to infections

Figure 9.18 The systemic features of Cushing's syndrome.

system. It is usually caused by a tumour affecting only one adrenal gland.

Secondary hyperaldosteronism

This is caused by overstimulation of normal glands by the excessively high blood levels of renin and angiotensin that result from low renal perfusion or low blood sodium.

Hyposecretion of mineralocorticoids

Hypoaldosteronism results in failure of the kidneys to regulate sodium, potassium and water excretion, leading to:

- blood sodium deficiency (hyponatraemia) and potassium excess (hyperkalaemia)
- dehydration, low blood volume and low blood pressure.

There is usually hyposecretion of other cortical hormones, as in Addison's disease.

Chronic adrenocortical insufficiency (Addison's disease)

This is due to hyposecretion of glucocorticoid and mineralocorticoid hormones. The most common causes are development of autoantibodies to cortical cells, metastatic tumours and infections. Autoimmune disease of some other glands is associated with Addison's disease, e.g. thyrotoxicosis and hypoparathyroidism. The most important effects are:

- muscle weakness and wasting
- gastrointestinal disturbances, e.g. vomiting, diarrhoea, anorexia
- increased pigmentation of the skin, especially of exposed areas, due to excess ACTH and the related melanin-stimulating hormone secreted by the anterior pituitary
- listlessness and tiredness
- hypoglycaemia
- mental confusion
- menstrual disturbances and loss of body hair in women
- electrolyte imbalance, including hyponatraemia, low blood chloride levels and hyperkalaemia
- chronic dehydration, low blood volume and hypotension.

The adrenal glands have a considerable reserve of tissue and Addison's disease is not usually severely debilitating unless more than 90% of cortical tissue is destroyed, but this condition is fatal without treatment.

Acute adrenocortical insufficiency (Addisonian crisis)

This is characterised by sudden severe nausea, vomiting, diarrhoea, hypotension, electrolyte imbalance (hyponatraemia and hyperkalaemia) and, in severe cases, circulatory collapse. It is precipitated when an individual with chronic adrenocortical insufficiency is subjected to stress, e.g. an acute infection.

Disorders of the adrenal medulla

Learning outcome

After studying this section you should be able to:

- explain how the features of the diseases in this section are related to excessive secretion of adrenaline (epinephrine) and noradrenaline (norepinephrine).

Tumours

Hormone-secreting tumours are the main abnormality. The effects of excess adrenaline (epinephrine) and noradrenaline (norepinephrine) include:

- hypertension, often associated with arteriosclerosis and cerebral haemorrhage
- weight loss
- nervousness
- headache
- excessive sweating and alternate flushing and blanching
- hyperglycaemia and glycosuria.

Phaeochromocytoma

This is usually a *benign tumour*, occurring in one or both glands. The secretion of hormones may be at a steady high level or in intermittent bursts often precipitated by raised intra-abdominal pressure, e.g. coughing or defaecation.

Neuroblastoma

This is a rare and *malignant tumour*, occurring in infants and children under 15 years of age. Tumours that develop early tend to be highly malignant but in this condition there may be spontaneous regression.

231

Disorders of the pancreatic islets

Learning outcomes

After studying this section you should be able to:

■ compare and contrast the onset and features of types I and II diabetes mellitus

■ state the common causes of secondary diabetes

■ relate the signs and symptoms of diabetes mellitus to deficiency of insulin

■ explain how the causes and effects of the following conditions occur: diabetic ketoacidosis and hypoglycaemic coma

■ describe the long-term complications of diabetes mellitus.

Diabetes mellitus

This is due to deficiency or absence of insulin or, rarely, to impairment of insulin activity (insulin resistance) causing varying degrees of disruption of carbohydrate and fat metabolism. The incidence of type 1 and, especially, type 2 diabetes (see below) is increasing worldwide.

Type I, insulin-dependent diabetes mellitus (IDDM)

This occurs mainly in children and young adults and the onset is usually sudden. The deficiency or absence of insulin is due to the destruction of β-islet cells of the pancreas. The exact cause remains unknown although, in most people, there is evidence of an autoimmune mechanism involving autoantibodies that destroy the β-islet cells. Genetic predisposition and environmental factors, including viral infections, are also thought to be involved.

Type II, non-insulin-dependent diabetes mellitus (NIDDM)

This is the most common form of diabetes, accounting for about 90% of cases. The causes are multifactorial and predisposing factors include:

- obesity
- sedentary lifestyle

- increasing age: affecting middle-aged and older people
- genetic factors.

It often goes undetected until signs are found on routine investigation or a complication occurs. Insulin secretion may be below or above normal. Deficiency of glucose inside body cells may occur despite hyperglycaemia and a high insulin level. This may be due to insulin resistance, i.e. changes in cell membranes that block the insulin-assisted movement of glucose into cells.

Secondary diabetes

This may develop as a complication of:

- acute and chronic pancreatitis
- some drugs, e.g. corticosteroids, phenytoin, thiazide diuretics
- secondary to other endocrine disorders involving hypersecretion of e.g. growth hormone, thyroid hormones, cortisol, adrenaline (epinephrine).

Gestational diabetes

This develops during pregnancy and may disappear after delivery; however, diabetes often recurs in later life. Raised plasma glucose levels during pregnancy predispose to the birth of large birth weight and stillborn babies and deaths shortly after birth.

Effects of diabetes mellitus

Raised plasma glucose level

After eating a carbohydrate-rich meal the plasma glucose level remains high because:

- cells are unable to take up and use glucose from the bloodstream
- conversion of glucose to glycogen in the liver and muscles is diminished
- there is gluconeogenesis from protein, in response to deficiency of intracellular glucose.

Glycosuria and polyuria

The concentration of glucose in the glomerular filtrate is the same as in the blood and, although diabetes raises the renal threshold for glucose, it is not all reabsorbed by the tubules (p. 340). The remaining glucose in the filtrate raises its osmotic pressure, water reabsorption is reduced and the volume of urine produced is increased (polyuria). This causes electrolyte imbalance and excretion of urine of high specific gravity. Polyuria can lead to hypovolaemia, extreme thirst (polydipsia) and increased fluid intake.

Weight loss

In diabetes, cells fail to metabolise glucose in the normal manner, resulting in weight loss due to:

- gluconeogenesis from amino acids and body protein, causing muscle wasting, tissue breakdown and further increases blood glucose
- catabolism of body fat, releasing some of its energy and excess production of ketone bodies.

Ketosis and ketoacidosis

In the absence of insulin, to promote normal intracellular glucose metabolism, alternative energy sources must be used instead and increased breakdown of fat occurs (see Fig. 12.45, p. 315). This leads to excessive production of ketone bodies, which are weakly acidic. Normal buffering systems maintain pH balance so long as the levels of ketone bodies are not excessive. *Ketosis* (see p. 313) develops as ketone bodies accumulate. Excretion of ketones is via:

- the urine (ketonuria)
- the lungs giving the breath a characteristic smell of acetone or 'pear drops'.

When worsening ketosis swamps the compensatory buffer systems, control of acid/base balance is lost; the blood pH falls and *ketoacidosis* occurs. The consequences if untreated are:

- increasing acidosis ($\downarrow$ blood pH) due to accumulation of ketoacids
- increasing hyperglycaemia
- hyperventilation as the lungs excrete excess hydrogen ions as CO_2
- acidification of urine – the result of kidney buffering
- polyuria (see above)
- dehydration and hypovolaemia ($\downarrow$BP and $\uparrow$ pulse) – caused by polyuria
- disturbances of electrolyte balance accompanying fluid loss, hyponatraemia ($\downarrow$ plasma sodium) and hypokalaemia ($\downarrow$ plasma potassium)
- confusion, coma and death.

Acute complications of diabetes mellitus

Diabetic ketoacidosis

This mainly affects people with insulin-dependent diabetes. Ketoacidosis develops owing to increased insulin requirement or increased resistance to insulin due to some added stress, such as pregnancy, microbial infection, infarction, or cerebrovascular accident. The inadequate supply of insulin may also be due to failure by the patient to administer the prescribed dose or inadequate adjustment of the prescribed dose during times of increased need. In some cases severe and dangerous ketoacidosis may occur without loss of consciousness. The effects and consequences of diabetic ketoacidosis are outlined above.

Hypoglycaemic coma

This occurs in insulin-dependent diabetics when insulin administered is in excess of that needed to balance the food intake and expenditure of energy. Because neurones are more dependent on glucose for their energy needs than are other cells, glucose deprivation causes disturbed neurological function, leading to coma and, if prolonged, irreversible damage. Hypoglycaemia may be the result of:

- accidental overdose of insulin
- delay in eating after insulin administration
- gastrointestinal disturbances in which carbohydrate absorption is diminished, e.g., vomiting, diarrhoea
- increased metabolic rate in, e.g. unexpected exercise, acute febrile illness
- an insulin-secreting tumour, especially if it produces irregular bursts of secretion.

Common signs and symptoms of hypoglycaemia include drowsiness, confusion, speech difficulty, sweating, trembling and anxiety.

Long-term complications of diabetes mellitus

These increase with the severity and duration of hyperglycaemia and represent significant causes of morbidity in people with diabetes.

Cardiovascular disturbances

Diabetes mellitus is a significant risk factor for cardiovascular disorders. Changes in blood vessels (angiopathies) may still occur even when the disease is well controlled.

Diabetic macroangiopathy

The most common lesions are atheroma and calcification of the tunica media of the large arteries. In insulin-dependent diabetes these changes may occur at a relatively early age. The most common consequences are serious and often fatal:

- ischaemic heart disease, i.e. angina and myocardial infarction (p. 123)
- stroke (p. 180)
- peripheral vascular disease.

233

Diabetic microangiopathy

This affects small blood vessels and there is thickening of the epithelial basement membrane of arterioles, capillaries and, sometimes, venules. These changes may lead to:

- peripheral vascular disease, progressing to gangrene and 'diabetic foot'
- diabetic retinopathy (see p. 209)
- diabetic nephropathy (p. 349)
- peripheral neuropathy, especially when myelination is affected.

Infection

Diabetic people are highly susceptible to infection, especially by bacteria and fungi, possibly because phagocyte activity is depressed by insufficient intracellular glucose. Infection may cause:

- complications in areas affected by peripheral neuropathy and changes in blood vessels, e.g. in the feet when sensation and blood supply are impaired
- boils and carbuncles
- vaginal candidiasis (thrush)
- pyelonephritis (p. 350).

Renal failure

This is due to diabetic nephropathy (p. 349) and is a common cause of death in those with diabetes.

Blindness

Diabetic retinopathy (p. 209) is the commonest cause of blindness in adults between 30 and 65 years in developed countries. Diabetes also increases the risk of early development of cataracts (p. 209) and other visual disorders.

Intake of raw materials and elimination of waste

The respiratory system

The cells of the body need energy for all their metabolic activities. Most of this energy is derived from chemical reactions, which can only take place in the presence of oxygen (O_2). The main waste product of these reactions is carbon dioxide (CO_2). The respiratory system provides the route by which the supply of oxygen present in the atmospheric air enters the body, and it provides the route of excretion for carbon dioxide.

The condition of the atmospheric air entering the body varies considerably according to the external environment, e.g. it may be dry, cold and contain dust particles or it may be moist and hot. As the air breathed in moves through the air passages to reach the lungs, it is warmed or cooled to body temperature, moistened to become saturated with water vapour and 'cleaned' as particles of dust stick to the mucus which coats the lining membrane. Blood provides the transport system for these gases between the lungs and the cells of the body. Exchange of gases between the blood and the lungs is called *external respiration* and that between the blood and the cells *internal respiration*. The organs of the respiratory system are:

- nose
- pharynx
- larynx
- trachea
- two bronchi (one bronchus to each lung)
- bronchioles and smaller air passages
- two lungs and their coverings, the pleura

238

- muscles of breathing – the intercostal muscles and the diaphragm.

A general view of the organs of the respiratory system is given in Figure 10.1.

Nose and nasal cavity

Learning outcomes

After studying this section, you should be able to:

- describe the location of the nasal cavities
- relate the structure of the nasal cavities to their function in respiration
- outline the physiology of smell.

Position and structure

The nasal cavity is the main route of air entry, and consists of a large irregular cavity divided into two equal passages by a *septum*. The posterior bony part of the septum is formed by the perpendicular plate of the ethmoid bone and the vomer. Anteriorly, it consists of hyaline cartilage (Fig. 10.2).

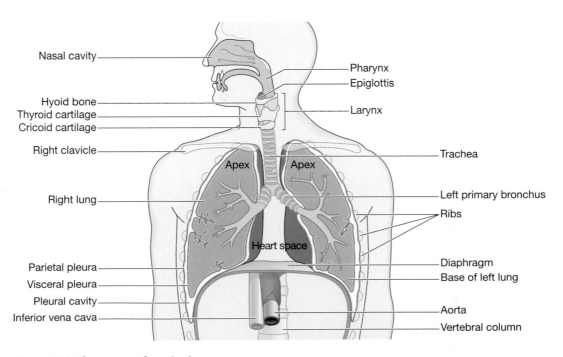

Figure 10.1 The organs of respiration.

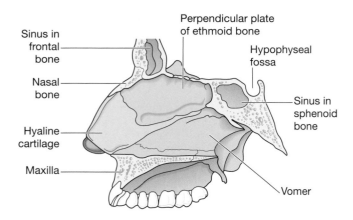

Figure 10.2 Structures forming the nasal septum.

The roof is formed by the cribriform plate of the ethmoid bone and the sphenoid bone, frontal bone and nasal bones.

The floor is formed by the roof of the mouth and consists of the hard palate in front and the soft palate behind. The hard palate is composed of the maxilla and palatine bones and the soft palate consists of involuntary muscle.

The medial wall is formed by the *septum*.

The lateral walls are formed by the maxilla, the ethmoid bone and the inferior conchae (Fig. 10.3).

The posterior wall is formed by the posterior wall of the pharynx.

Lining of the nose

The nose is lined with very vascular *ciliated columnar epithelium* (ciliated mucous membrane) which contains mucus-secreting goblet cells (p. 41). At the anterior nares this blends with the skin and posteriorly it extends into the nasal part of the pharynx.

Openings into the nasal cavity

The anterior nares, or nostrils, are the openings from the exterior into the nasal cavity. Nasal hairs are found here, coated in sticky mucus.

The posterior nares are the openings from the nasal cavity into the pharynx.

The paranasal sinuses are cavities in the bones of the face and the cranium, containing air. There are tiny openings between the paranasal sinuses and the nasal cavity. They are lined with mucous membrane, continuous with that of the nasal cavity. The main sinuses are:

- maxillary sinuses in the lateral walls
- frontal and sphenoidal sinuses in the roof (Fig. 10.3)
- ethmoidal sinuses in the upper part of the lateral walls.

The sinuses function in speech and also lighten the skull. *The nasolacrimal ducts* extend from the lateral walls of the nose to the conjunctival sacs of the eye (p. 203). They drain tears from the eyes.

Respiratory function of the nose

The nose is the first of the respiratory passages through which the inspired air passes. The function of the nose is to begin the process by which the air is warmed, moistened and filtered.

The projecting *conchae* (Figs 10.3 and 10.4) increase the surface area and cause turbulence, spreading inspired air

239

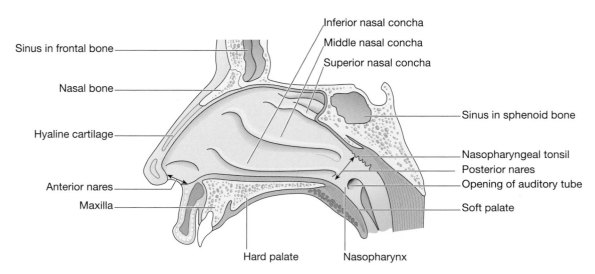

Figure 10.3 Lateral wall of right nasal cavity.

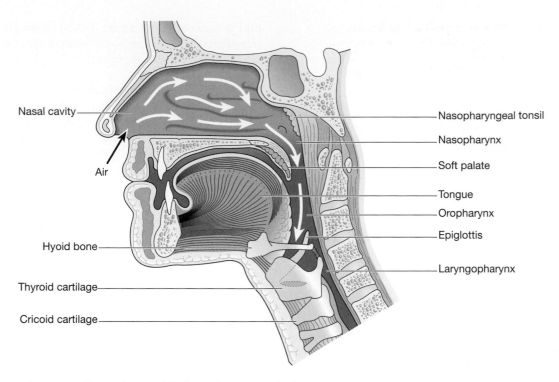

Figure 10.4 The pathway of air from the nose to the larynx.

over the whole nasal surface. The large surface area maximises warming, humidification and filtering.

Warming. This is due to the immense vascularity of the mucosa. This explains the large blood loss when a nosebleed (epistaxis) occurs.

Filtering and cleaning. This occurs as hairs at the anterior nares trap larger particles. Smaller particles such as dust and microbes settle and adhere to the mucus. Mucus protects the underlying epithelium from irritation and prevents drying. Synchronous beating of the cilia wafts the mucus towards the throat where it is swallowed or coughed up (expectorated).

Humidification. As air travels over the moist mucosa, it becomes saturated with water vapour. Irritation of the nasal mucosa results in *sneezing*, a reflex action that forcibly expels an irritant.

Olfactory function of the nose

The nose is the organ of the sense of smell. Nerve endings that detect smell are located in the roof of the nose in the area of the cribriform plate of the ethmoid bones and the superior conchae. These nerve endings are stimulated by airborne odours. The resultant nerve impulses are conveyed by the *olfactory nerves* to the brain where the sensation of smell is perceived (p. 204).

Pharynx

Learning outcomes

After studying this section, you should be able to:

- describe the location of the pharynx
- relate the structure of the pharynx to its function.

Position

The pharynx is a tube 12 to 14 cm long that extends from the base of the skull to the level of the 6th cervical vertebra. It lies behind the nose, mouth and larynx and is wider at its upper end.

Structures associated with the pharynx

Superiorly – the inferior surface of the base of the skull

Inferiorly – it is continuous with the oesophagus

240

Anteriorly – the wall is incomplete because of the openings into the nose, mouth and larynx

Posteriorly – areolar tissue, involuntary muscle and the bodies of the first six cervical vertebrae.

For descriptive purposes the pharynx is divided into three parts: *nasopharynx, oropharynx* and *laryngopharynx.*

The nasopharynx. The nasal part of the pharynx lies behind the nose above the level of the soft palate. On its lateral walls are the two openings of the *auditory tubes* (p. 190), one leading to each middle ear. On the posterior wall are the *pharyngeal tonsils* (adenoids), consisting of lymphoid tissue. They are most prominent in children up to approximately 7 years of age. Thereafter they gradually atrophy.

The oropharynx. The oral part of the pharynx lies behind the mouth, extending from below the level of the soft palate to the level of the upper part of the body of the 3rd cervical vertebra. The lateral walls of the pharynx blend with the soft palate to form two folds on each side. Between each pair of folds is a collection of lymphoid tissue called the *palatine tonsil.*

During swallowing, the nasal and oral parts are separated by the soft palate and the *uvula.*

The laryngopharynx. The laryngeal part of the pharynx extends from the oropharynx above and continues as the oesophagus below, i.e. from the level of the 3rd to the 6th cervical vertebrae.

Structure

The pharynx is composed of three layers of tissue:

Mucous membrane lining. The mucosa varies slightly in the different regions. In the nasopharynx it is continuous with the lining of the nose and consists of ciliated columnar epithelium; in the oropharynx and laryngopharynx it is formed by tougher stratified squamous epithelium, which is continuous with the lining of the mouth and oesophagus. This lining protects underlying tissues from the abrasive action of foodstuffs passing through prior to being swallowed.

Fibrous tissue. This forms the intermediate layer. It is thicker in the nasopharynx, where there is little muscle, and becomes thinner towards the lower end, where the muscle layer is thicker.

Smooth muscle. This consists of several involuntary constrictor muscles that play an important part in the mechanism of swallowing (deglutition, p. 293), which in the pharynx is not under voluntary control. The upper end of the oesophagus is closed by the lower constrictor muscle, except during swallowing.

Blood and nerve supply

Blood is supplied to the pharynx by several branches of the facial artery. The venous return is into the facial and internal jugular veins.

The nerve supply is from the pharyngeal plexus, formed by parasympathetic and sympathetic nerves. Parasympathetic supply is by the *vagus* and *glossopharyngeal* nerves. Sympathetic supply is by nerves from the *superior cervical ganglia* (p. 170).

Functions

Passageway for air and food. The pharynx is an organ involved in both the respiratory and the digestive systems: air passes through the nasal and oral sections, and food through the oral and laryngeal sections.

Warming and humidifying. By the same methods as in the nose, the air is further warmed and moistened as it passes through the pharynx.

Taste. There are olfactory nerve endings of the sense of taste in the epithelium of the oral and pharyngeal parts.

Hearing. The auditory tube, extending from the nasopharynx to each middle ear, allows air to enter the middle ear. Satisfactory hearing depends on the presence of air at atmospheric pressure on each side of the *tympanic membrane* (eardrum, p. 191).

Protection. The lymphatic tissue of the pharyngeal and laryngeal tonsils produces antibodies in response to antigens, e.g. microbes (Ch. 15). The tonsils are larger in children and tend to atrophy in adults.

Speech. The pharynx functions in speech; by acting as a resonating chamber for sound ascending from the larynx, it helps (together with the sinuses) to give the voice its individual characteristics.

241

Larynx

Learning outcomes

After studying this section, you should be able to:

■ describe the structure and function of the larynx

■ outline the physiology of speech generation.

Position

The larynx or 'voice box' extends from the root of the tongue and the hyoid bone to the trachea. It lies in front of the laryngopharynx at the level of the 3rd, 4th, 5th and 6th cervical vertebrae. Until puberty there is little difference in the size of the larynx between the sexes. Thereafter it grows larger in the male, which explains the prominence of the 'Adam's apple' and the generally deeper voice.

Structures associated with the larynx

Superiorly – the hyoid bone and the root of the tongue
Inferiorly – it is continuous with the trachea
Anteriorly – the muscles attached to the hyoid bone and the muscles of the neck
Posteriorly – the laryngopharynx and 3rd to 6th cervical vertebrae
Laterally – the lobes of the thyroid gland.

Structure

Cartilages

The larynx is composed of several irregularly shaped cartilages attached to each other by ligaments and membranes. The main cartilages are:

- 1 thyroid cartilage ⎫
- 1 cricoid cartilage ⎬ hyaline cartilage
- 2 arytenoid cartilages ⎭
- 1 epiglottis — elastic fibrocartilage.

The thyroid cartilage (Figs 10.5 and 10.6). This is the most prominent and consists of two flat pieces of hyaline cartilage, or *laminae*, fused anteriorly, forming the *laryngeal prominence* (Adam's apple). Immediately above the laryngeal prominence the laminae are separated, forming a V-shaped notch known as the *thyroid notch*. The thyroid cartilage is incomplete posteriorly, and the posterior border of each lamina is extended to form two processes called the *superior* and *inferior cornu*.

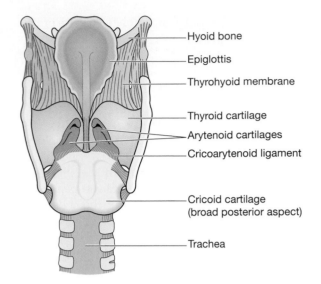

Figure 10.5 Larynx – viewed from behind.

Labels: Hyoid bone; Epiglottis; Thyrohyoid membrane; Thyroid cartilage; Arytenoid cartilages; Cricoarytenoid ligament; Cricoid cartilage (broad posterior aspect); Trachea

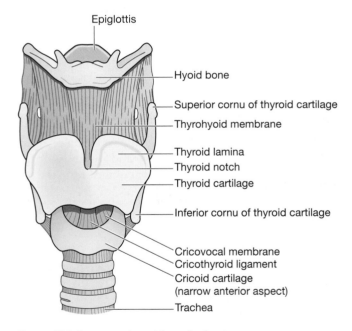

Figure 10.6 Larynx – viewed from the front.

Labels: Epiglottis; Hyoid bone; Superior cornu of thyroid cartilage; Thyrohyoid membrane; Thyroid lamina; Thyroid notch; Thyroid cartilage; Inferior cornu of thyroid cartilage; Cricovocal membrane; Cricothyroid ligament; Cricoid cartilage (narrow anterior aspect); Trachea

The upper part of the thyroid cartilage is lined with stratified squamous epithelium like the larynx, and the lower part with ciliated columnar epithelium like the trachea. There are many muscles attached to its outer surface.

The thyroid cartilage forms most of the anterior and lateral walls of the larynx.

The cricoid cartilage (Fig. 10.7). This lies below the thyroid cartilage and is also composed of hyaline cartilage. It is shaped like a signet ring, completely encircling

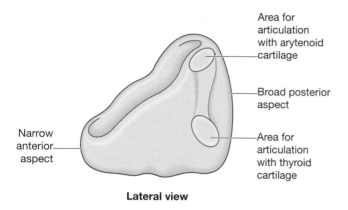

Area for
articulation
with arytenoid
cartilage

Broad posterior
aspect

Narrow
anterior
aspect

Area for
articulation
with thyroid
cartilage

Lateral view

Figure 10.7 The cricoid cartilage.

the larynx with the narrow part anteriorly and the broad part posteriorly. The broad posterior part articulates with the arytenoid cartilages and with the inferior cornu of the thyroid cartilage. It is lined with ciliated columnar epithelium and there are muscles and ligaments attached to its outer surface (Fig. 10.7). The lower border of the cricoid cartilage marks the end of the upper respiratory tract.

The arytenoid cartilages. These are two roughly pyramid-shaped hyaline cartilages situated on top of the broad part of the cricoid cartilage forming part of the posterior wall of the larynx (Fig. 10.8). They give attachment to the vocal cords and to muscles and are lined with ciliated columnar epithelium.

The epiglottis. This is a leaf-shaped fibroelastic cartilage attached to the inner surface of the anterior wall of the thyroid cartilage immediately below the thyroid notch (Fig. 10.4). It rises obliquely upwards behind the tongue and the body of the hyoid bone. It is covered with stratified squamous epithelium. If the larynx is likened to a box then the epiglottis acts as the lid; it closes off the larynx during swallowing, protecting the lungs from accidental inhalation of foreign objects.

Ligaments and membranes

There are several ligaments that attach the cartilages to each other and to the hyoid bone (Figs 10.5, 10.6 and 10.8).

Blood and nerve supply

Blood is supplied to the larynx by the superior and inferior laryngeal arteries and drained by the thyroid veins, which join the internal jugular vein.

The parasympathetic nerve supply is from the superior laryngeal and recurrent laryngeal nerves, which are branches of the vagus nerves. The sympathetic nerves are

from the superior cervical ganglia, one on each side. These provide the motor nerve supply to the muscles of the larynx and sensory fibres to the lining membrane.

Interior of the larynx

The *vocal cords* are two pale folds of mucous membrane with cord-like free edges, which extend from the inner wall of the thyroid prominence anteriorly to the arytenoid cartilages posteriorly (Fig. 10.8).

When the muscles controlling the vocal cords are relaxed, the vocal cords open and the passageway for air coming up through the larynx is clear; the vocal cords are said to be *abducted* (open, Fig. 10.9A). The pitch of the sound produced by vibrating the vocal cords in this position is low. When the muscles controlling the vocal cords contract, the vocal cords are stretched out tightly across the larynx (Fig. 10.9B), and are said to be *adducted* (closed). When the vocal cords are stretched to this extent, and are vibrated by air passing through from the lungs, the sound produced is high pitched. The pitch of the voice is therefore determined by the tension applied to the vocal cords by the appropriate sets of muscles. When not in use, the vocal cords are adducted. The space between the vocal cords is called the *glottis*.

243

Anterior

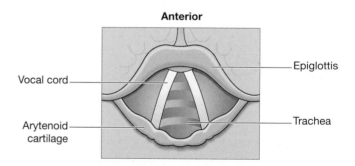

Vocal cord

Arytenoid
cartilage

Epiglottis

Trachea

Figure 10.8 Interior of the larynx viewed from above.

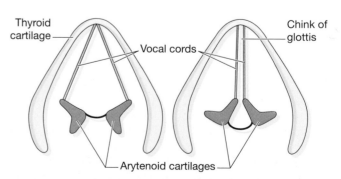

Thyroid
cartilage

Vocal cords

Chink of
glottis

Arytenoid cartilages

A   Vocal cords abducted   B   Vocal cords adducted

Figure 10.9 The extreme positions of the vocal cords.

Functions

Production of sound. Sound has the properties of *pitch, volume* and *resonance*.

- Pitch of the voice depends upon the *length* and *tightness* of the cords. At puberty, the male vocal cords begin to grow longer, hence the lower pitch of the adult male voice.
- Volume of the voice depends upon the *force* with which the cords vibrate. The greater the force of expired air, the more the cords vibrate and the louder the sound emitted.
- Resonance, or tone, is dependent upon the shape of the mouth, the position of the tongue and the lips, the facial muscles and the air in the paranasal sinuses.

Speech. This occurs during expiration when the sounds produced by the vocal cords are manipulated by the tongue, cheeks and lips.

Protection of the lower respiratory tract. During swallowing (deglutition) the larynx moves upwards, occluding the opening into it from the pharynx and the hinged epiglottis closes over the larynx. This ensures that food passes into the oesophagus and not into the lower respiratory passages.

Passageway for air. This is between the pharynx and trachea.

Humidifying, filtering and warming. These processes continue as inspired air travels through the larynx.

Trachea

Learning outcomes

After studying this section, you should be able to:

- describe the location of the trachea
- outline the structure of the trachea
- explain the functions of the trachea in respiration.

Position

The trachea or windpipe is a continuation of the larynx and extends downwards to about the level of the 5th thoracic vertebra where it divides (bifurcates) at the *carina* into the right and left primary bronchi, one bronchus going to each lung. It is approximately 10 to 11 cm long and lies mainly in the median plane in front of the oesophagus (Fig. 10.10).

Structures associated with the trachea
(Fig. 10.10)

Superiorly	– the larynx
Inferiorly	– the right and left bronchi
Anteriorly	– upper part: the isthmus of the thyroid gland lower part: the arch of the aorta and the sternum
Posteriorly	– the oesophagus separates the trachea from the vertebral column
Laterally	– the lungs and the lobes of the thyroid gland.

Structure

The trachea is composed of three layers of tissue, and held open by between 16 and 20 incomplete (C-shaped) rings of hyaline cartilage lying one above the other. The

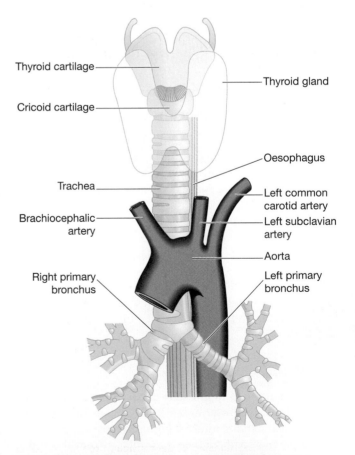

Figure 10.10 The trachea and some of its related structures.

rings are incomplete posteriorly. Connective tissue and involuntary muscle join the cartilages, and form the posterior wall where the rings are incomplete. The soft tissue posterior wall is in contact with the oesophagus (Fig. 10.11).

Three layers of tissue 'clothe' the cartilages of the trachea.

- The outer layer consists of fibrous and elastic tissue and encloses the cartilages.
- The middle layer consists of cartilages and bands of smooth muscle that wind round the trachea in a helical arrangement. There is some areolar tissue, containing blood and lymph vessels and autonomic nerves.
- The inner lining consists of ciliated columnar epithelium, containing mucus-secreting goblet cells (see Fig. 3.23, p. 41).

Blood and nerve supply, lymph drainage

The arterial blood supply is mainly by the inferior thyroid and bronchial arteries and the venous return is by the inferior thyroid veins into the brachiocephalic veins.

Parasympathetic nerve supply is by the recurrent laryngeal nerves and other branches of the vagi. Sympathetic supply is by nerves from the sympathetic ganglia. Parasympathetic stimulation constricts the trachea, and sympathetic stimulation dilates it.

Lymph from the respiratory passages drains through lymph nodes situated round the trachea and in the carina, the area where it divides into two bronchi.

Functions

Support and patency. The arrangement of cartilage and elastic tissue prevents kinking and obstruction of the airway as the head and neck move. The absence of cartilage posteriorly allows the trachea to dilate and constrict in response to nerve stimulation, and for indentation as the oesophagus distends during swallowing. The cartilages prevent collapse of the trachea when the internal pressure is less than intrathoracic pressure, i.e. at the end of forced expiration.

Mucociliary escalator. This is the synchronous and regular beating of the cilia of the mucous membrane lining that wafts mucus with adherent particles upwards towards the larynx where it is either swallowed or coughed up (Fig. 10.12).

Cough reflex. Nerve endings in the larynx, trachea and bronchi are sensitive to irritation, which generates nerve impulses conducted by the vagus nerves to the respiratory centre in the brain stem (p. 256). The reflex motor response is deep inspiration followed by closure of the glottis, i.e. closure of the vocal cords. The abdominal and respiratory muscles then contract and suddenly the air is released under pressure expelling mucus and/or foreign material from the mouth.

Warming, humidifying and filtering. These continue as in the nose, although air is normally saturated and at body temperature when it reaches the trachea.

245

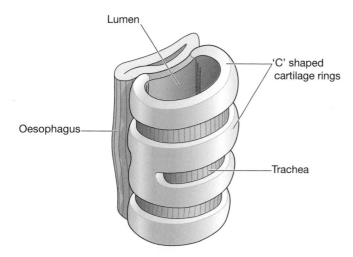

Figure 10.11 The relationship of the trachea to the oesophagus.

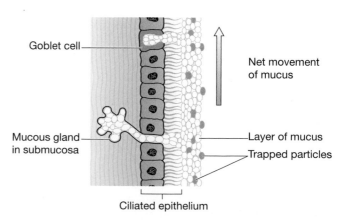

Figure 10.12 Microscopic view of ciliated mucus membrane.

Lungs

Learning outcomes

After studying this section, you should be able to:

- name the air passage of the bronchial tree in descending order of size
- describe the structure and changing functions of the different levels of airway
- describe the location and gross anatomy of the lungs
- identify the functions of the pleura
- describe the pulmonary blood supply.

Position and gross structure (Fig. 10.13)

There are two lungs, one lying on each side of the midline in the thoracic cavity. They are cone-shaped and have an *apex*, a *base, costal surface* and *medial surface.*

The apex. This is rounded and rises into the root of the neck, about 25 mm above the level of the middle third of the clavicle. It lies close to the first rib and the blood vessels and nerves in the root of the neck.

The base. This is concave and semilunar in shape, and lies on the thoracic surface of the diaphragm.

The costal surface. This surface is convex and lies against the costal cartilages, the ribs and the intercostal muscles.

The medial surface. This surface is concave and has a roughly triangular-shaped area, called the *hilum*, at the level of the 5th, 6th and 7th thoracic vertebrae. Structures forming the *root of the lung* enter and leave at the hilum. These include the primary bronchus, the pulmonary artery supplying the lung and the two pulmonary veins draining it, the bronchial artery and veins, and the lymphatic and nerve supply (Fig. 10.14).

The area between the lungs is the *mediastinum*. It is occupied by the heart, great vessels, trachea, right and left bronchi, oesophagus, lymph nodes, lymph vessels and nerves.

The right lung is divided into three distinct lobes: superior, middle and inferior. The left lung is smaller because the heart occupies space left of the midline. It is divided into only two lobes: superior and inferior.

Pleura and pleural cavity

The pleura consists of a closed sac of serous membrane (one for each lung) which contains a small amount of serous fluid. The lung is invaginated (pushed into) into this sac so that it forms two layers: one adheres to the lung and the other to the wall of the thoracic cavity (Figs 10.1 and 10.15).

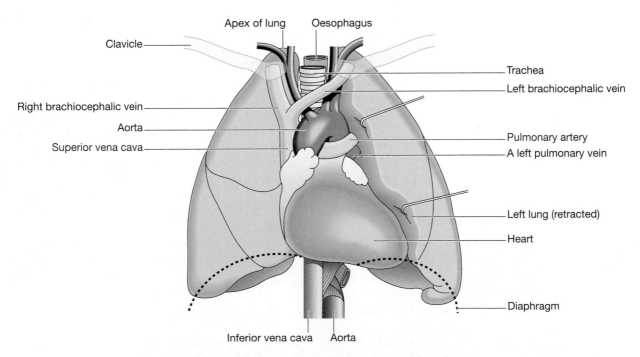

Figure 10.13 Organs associated with the lungs.

Labels: Clavicle, Apex of lung, Oesophagus, Trachea, Left brachiocephalic vein, Right brachiocephalic vein, Aorta, Superior vena cava, Pulmonary artery, A left pulmonary vein, Left lung (retracted), Heart, Diaphragm, Inferior vena cava, Aorta

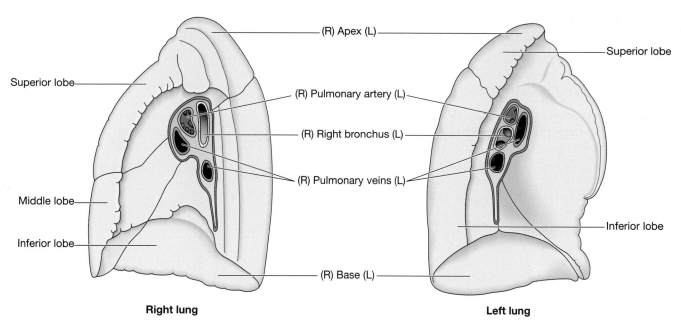

Right lung   **Left lung**

Figure 10.14 The lobes of the lungs and vessels/airways of each hilum – medial views.

247

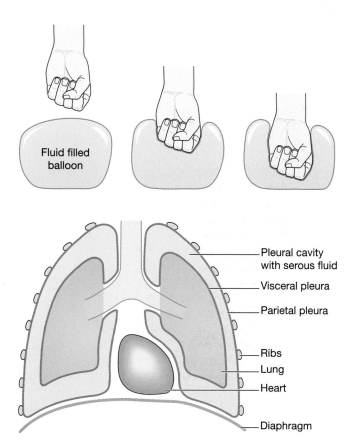

Figure 10.15 The relationship of the pleura to the lungs.

The visceral pleura. This is adherent to the lung, covering each lobe and passing into the fissures that separate them.

The parietal pleura. This is adherent to the inside of the chest wall and the thoracic surface of the diaphragm. It remains detached from the adjacent structures in the mediastinum and is continuous with the visceral pleura round the edges of the hilum.

The pleural cavity. This is only a potential space. In health, the two layers of pleura are separated by a thin film of serous fluid which allows them to glide over each other, preventing friction between them during breathing. The serous fluid is secreted by the epithelial cells of the membrane.

The two layers of pleura, with serous fluid between them, behave in the same way as two pieces of glass separated by a thin film of water. They glide over each other easily but can be pulled apart only with difficulty, because of the surface tension between the membranes and the fluid. If either layer of pleura is punctured, the underlying lung collapses owing to its inherent property of elastic recoil.

Interior of the lungs

The lungs are composed of the bronchi and smaller air passages, alveoli, connective tissue, blood vessels, lymph vessels and nerves, all embedded in an elastic connective tissue matrix. Each lobe is made up of a large number of *lobules*.

Pulmonary blood supply (Fig. 10.16)

The *pulmonary trunk* divides into the right and left pulmonary arteries, which transport deoxygenated blood to each lung. Within the lungs each pulmonary artery divides into many branches, which eventually end in a dense capillary network around the walls of the alveoli (see Fig. 10.18). The walls of the alveoli and the capillaries each consist of only one layer of flattened epithelial cells. The exchange of gases between air in the alveoli and blood in the capillaries takes place across these two very fine membranes (together called the *respiratory membrane*). The pulmonary capillaries join up, forming *two pulmonary veins* in each lung. They leave the lungs at the hilum and carry *oxygenated blood* to the left atrium of the heart. The innumerable blood capillaries and blood vessels in the lungs are supported by connective tissue.

The blood supply to the respiratory passages, lymphatic drainage and nerve supply is described later (p. 249).

Bronchi and bronchioles

The two primary bronchi are formed when the trachea divides, i.e. about the level of the 5th thoracic vertebra (Fig. 10.17).

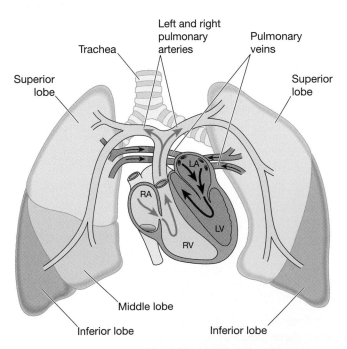

Figure 10.16 The flow of blood between heart and lungs.

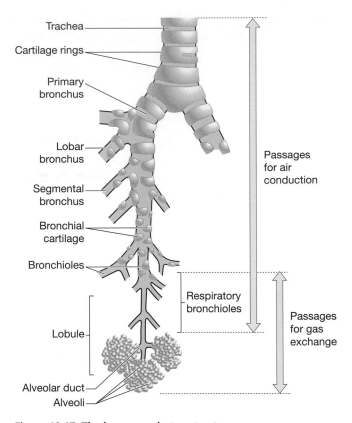

Figure 10.17 The lower respiratory tract.

The right bronchus. This is wider, shorter and more vertical than the left bronchus and is therefore more likely to become obstructed by an inhaled foreign body. It is approximately 2.5 cm long. After entering the right lung at the hilum it divides into three branches, one to each lobe. Each branch then subdivides into numerous smaller branches.

The left bronchus. This is about 5 cm long and is narrower than the right. After entering the lung at the hilum it divides into two branches, one to each lobe. Each branch then subdivides into progressively smaller tubes within the lung substance.

Structure

The bronchi are composed of the same tissues as the trachea, and are lined with ciliated columnar epithelium. The bronchi progressively subdivide into *bronchioles* (Fig. 10.17), *terminal bronchioles, respiratory bronchioles, alveolar ducts* and finally, *alveoli*. Towards the distal end of the bronchi the cartilages become irregular in shape and are absent at bronchiolar level. In the absence of cartilage the smooth muscle in the walls of the bronchioles becomes thicker and is responsive to autonomic nerve stimulation and irritation. Ciliated columnar mucous membrane changes gradually to non-ciliated cuboidal-shaped cells in the distal bronchioles. The wider passages are called *conducting airways* because their function is to bring air into the lungs, and their walls are too thick to permit gas exchange.

Blood and nerve supply, lymph drainage

The arterial supply to the walls of the bronchi and smaller air passages is through branches of the right and left bronchial arteries and the venous return is mainly through the bronchial veins. On the right side they empty into the azygos vein and on the left into the superior intercostal vein (see Figs 5.41 and 5.42, p. 102).

The vagus nerves (parasympathetic) stimulate contraction of smooth muscle in the bronchial tree, causing bronchoconstriction, and sympathetic stimulation causes bronchodilatation (see Ch. 7).

Lymph is drained from the walls of the air passages in a network of lymph vessels. It passes through lymph nodes situated around the trachea and bronchial tree then into the thoracic duct on the left side and right lymphatic duct on the other.

Functions

Control of air entry. The diameter of the respiratory passages is altered by contraction or relaxation of the involuntary muscles in their walls, thus regulating the volume of air entering the lungs. These changes are controlled by the autonomic nerve supply: parasympathetic stimulation causes constriction and sympathetic stimulation causes dilatation (p. 171).

The following functions continue as in the upper airways:

- warming and humidifying
- support and patency
- removal of particulate matter
- cough reflex.

Respiratory bronchioles and alveoli

Structure

Within each lobe, the lung tissue is further divided by fine sheets of connective tissue into *lobules*. Each lobule is supplied with air by a terminal bronchiole, which further subdivides into respiratory bronchioles, alveolar ducts and large numbers of alveoli (air sacs). There are about 150 million alveoli in the adult lung. It is in these structures that the process of gas exchange occurs. As airways progressively divide and become smaller and smaller, their walls gradually become thinner until muscle and connective tissue disappear, leaving a single layer of simple squamous epithelial cells in the alveolar ducts and alveoli. These distal respiratory passages are supported by a loose network of elastic connective tissue in which macrophages, fibroblasts, nerves and blood and lymph vessels are embedded. The alveoli are surrounded by a dense network of capillaries (Fig. 10.18). Exchange of gases in the lung (external respiration) takes place across a membrane made up of the alveolar wall and the capillary wall fused firmly together. This is called the *respiratory membrane*.

249

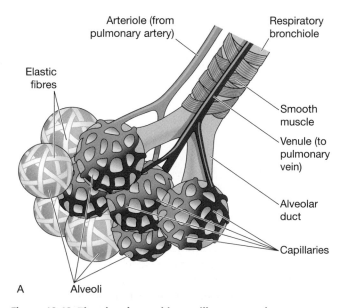

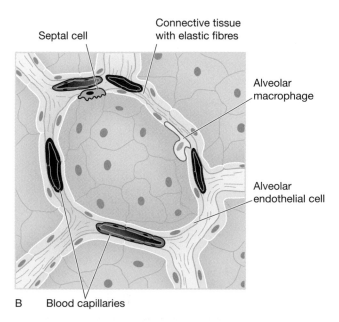

Figure 10.18 The alveolus and its capillary network.

Lying between the squamous cells are *septal* cells that secrete *surfactant*, a phospholipid fluid which prevents the alveoli from drying out. In addition, surfactant reduces surface tension and prevents alveolar walls collapsing during expiration. Secretion of surfactant into the distal air passages and alveoli begins about the 35th week of fetal life. Its presence in newborn babies facilitates expansion of the lungs and the establishment of respiration. It may not be present in sufficient amounts in the immature lungs of premature babies, causing serious breathing problems.

Nerve supply to bronchioles

Parasympathetic fibres from the vagus nerve cause bronchoconstriction. The absence of supporting cartilage means that small airways may be completely closed off by constriction of their smooth muscle. Sympathetic stimulation relaxes bronchiolar smooth muscle.

Functions

External respiration. (See p. 254.)

Defence against microbes. At this level, ciliated epithelium, goblet cells and mucus are no longer present, because their presence would impede gas exchange and encourage infection. By the time inspired air reaches the alveoli, it is usually clean. Defence relies on protective cells present within the lung tissue. These include lymphocytes and plasma cells, which produce antibodies in the presence of antigens, and macrophages and polymorphonuclear lymphocytes, which are phagocytic. These cells are most active in the distal air passages where ciliated epithelium has been replaced by flattened cells.

Warming and humidifying. These continue as in the upper airways. Inhalation of dry or inadequately humidified air over a period of time causes irritation of the mucosa and encourages infection.

Respiration

Learning outcomes

After studying this section, you should be able to:

- describe the actions of the main muscles involved in breathing
- compare and contrast the mechanical events occurring in inspiration and expiration
- define the terms compliance, elasticity and airflow resistance
- describe the principal lung volumes and capacities
- compare the processes of internal and external respiration, using the concept of diffusion of gases
- describe O_2 and CO_2 transport in the blood
- explain the main mechanisms by which respiration is controlled.

The term respiration means the exchange of gases between body cells and the environment. This involves two main processes:

Breathing (pulmonary ventilation). This is movement of air into and out of the lungs.

Exchange of gases. This takes place:

- in the lungs: *external respiration*
- in the tissues: *internal respiration*.

Each of these will be considered later in this section.

Breathing

Breathing supplies oxygen to the alveoli, and eliminates carbon dioxide.

Muscles of breathing

Expansion of the chest during inspiration occurs as a result of muscular activity, partly voluntary and partly involuntary. The main muscles used in normal quiet breathing are the *intercostal muscles* and the *diaphragm*. During difficult or deep breathing they are assisted by muscles of the neck, shoulders and abdomen.

Intercostal muscles
There are 11 pairs of intercostal muscles that occupy the spaces between the 12 pairs of ribs. They are arranged in

two layers, the external and internal intercostal muscles (Fig. 10.19).

The external intercostal muscle fibres. These extend downwards and forwards from the lower border of the rib above to the upper border of the rib below.

The internal intercostal muscle fibres. These extend downwards and backwards from the lower border of the rib above to the upper border of the rib below, crossing the external intercostal muscle fibres at right angles.

The first rib is fixed. Therefore, when the intercostal muscles contract they pull all the other ribs towards the first rib. Because of the shape and sizes of the ribs they move outwards when pulled upwards, enlarging the thoracic cavity. The intercostal muscles are stimulated to contract by the *intercostal nerves*.

Diaphragm

The diaphragm is a dome-shaped muscular structure separating the thoracic and abdominal cavities. It forms the floor of the thoracic cavity and the roof of the abdominal cavity and consists of a central tendon from which muscle fibres radiate to be attached to the lower ribs and sternum and to the vertebral column by two crura. When the muscle of the diaphragm is relaxed, the central tendon is at the level of the 8th thoracic vertebra (Fig. 10.20). When it contracts, its muscle fibres shorten and the central tendon is pulled downwards to the level of the 9th thoracic vertebra, enlarging the thoracic cavity in length. This decreases pressure in the thoracic cavity and increases it in the abdominal and pelvic cavities. The diaphragm is supplied by the *phrenic nerves*.

The intercostal muscles and the diaphragm contract simultaneously, enlarging the thoracic cavity in all direc-

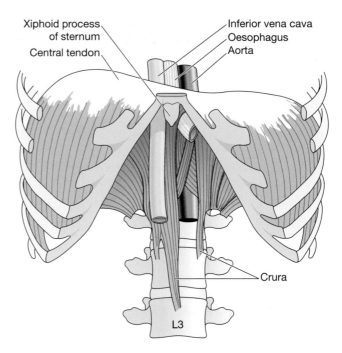

Figure 10.20 The diaphragm.

tions, that is from back to front, side to side and top to bottom (Fig. 10.21).

Cycle of breathing

The average respiratory rate is 12 to 15 breaths per minute. Each breath consists of three phases:

- inspiration
- expiration
- pause.

As described previously, the visceral pleura is adherent to the lungs and the parietal pleura to the inner wall of the thorax and to the diaphragm. Between them is a thin film of serous fluid (p. 247).

Inspiration

When the capacity of the thoracic cavity is increased by simultaneous contraction of the intercostal muscles and the diaphragm, the parietal pleura moves with the walls of the thorax and the diaphragm. This reduces the pressure in the pleural cavity to a level considerably lower than atmospheric pressure. The visceral pleura follows the parietal pleura, pulling the lung with it. This expands the lungs and the pressure within the alveoli and in the air passages falls, drawing air into the lungs in an attempt to equalise the atmospheric and alveolar air pressures.

The process of inspiration is *active*, as it needs energy for muscle contraction. The negative pressure created in the thoracic cavity aids venous return to the heart and is known as the *respiratory pump*.

At rest, inspiration lasts about 2 seconds.

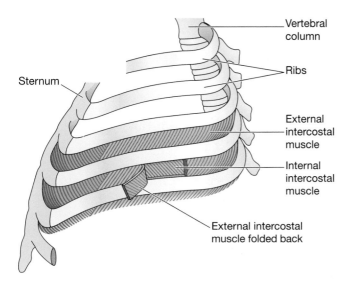

Figure 10.19 The intercostal muscles and the bones of the thorax.

251

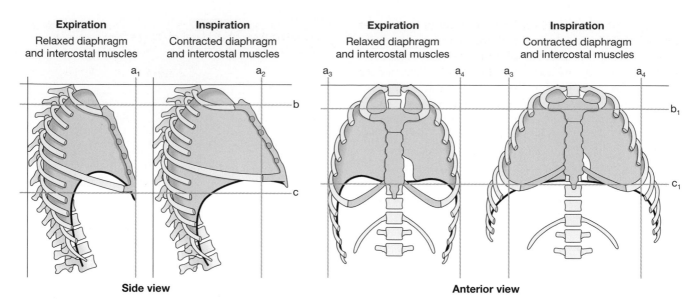

Figure 10.21 The changes in capacity of the thoracic cavity and the lungs during breathing.

Expiration

Relaxation of the intercostal muscles and the diaphragm results in downward and inward movement of the rib cage (Fig. 10.21) and elastic recoil of the lungs. As this occurs, pressure inside the lungs exceeds that in the atmosphere and so air is expelled from the respiratory tract. The lungs still contain some air, and are prevented from complete collapse by the intact pleura. This process is *passive* as it does not require the expenditure of energy.

At rest, expiration lasts about 3 seconds, and after expiration there is a pause before the next cycle begins.

Physiological variables affecting breathing

Elasticity. Elasticity is the term used to describe the ability of the lung to return to its normal shape after each breath. Loss of elasticity of the connective tissue in the lungs necessitates forced expiration and increased effort on inspiration.

Compliance. This is a measure of the distensibility of the lungs, i.e. the effort required to inflate the alveoli. The healthy lung is very compliant, and inflates with very little effort. When compliance is low the effort needed to inflate the lungs is greater than normal, e.g. in some diseases where elasticity is reduced or when insufficient surfactant is present. It should be noted that compliance and elasticity are opposing forces.

Airway resistance. When this is increased, e.g. in bronchoconstriction, more respiratory effort is required to inflate the lungs.

Lung volumes and capacities (Fig. 10.22)

In normal quiet breathing there are about 15 complete respiratory cycles per minute. The lungs and the air passages are never empty and, as the exchange of gases takes place only across the walls of the alveolar ducts and alveoli, the remaining capacity of the respiratory passages is called the *anatomical dead space* (about 150 ml).

Tidal volume (TV). This is the amount of air passing into and out of the lungs during each cycle of breathing (about 500 ml at rest).

Inspiratory reserve volume (IRV). This is the extra volume of air that can be inhaled into the lungs during maximal inspiration, i.e. over and above normal TV.

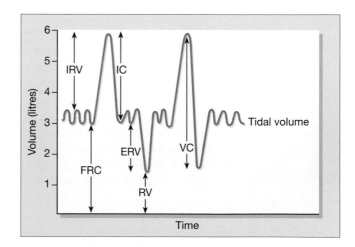

Figure 10.22 Lung volumes and capacities. IRV: inspiratory reserve volume; IC: inspiratory capacity; FRC: functional residual capacity; ERV: expiratory reserve volume; RV: residual volume; VC: vital capacity.

252

Inspiratory capacity (IC). This is the amount of air that can be inspired with maximum effort. It consists of the tidal volume (500 ml) plus the inspiratory reserve volume.

Functional residual capacity (FRC). This is the amount of air remaining in the air passages and alveoli at the end of quiet expiration. Tidal air mixes with this air, causing relatively small changes in the composition of alveolar air. As blood flows continuously through the pulmonary capillaries, this means that exchange of gases is not interrupted between breaths, preventing moment-to-moment changes in the concentration of blood gases. The functional residual volume also prevents collapse of the alveoli on expiration.

Expiratory reserve volume (ERV). This is the largest volume of air which can be expelled from the lungs during maximal expiration.

Residual volume (RV). This cannot be directly measured but is the volume of air remaining in the lungs after forced expiration.

Vital capacity (VC). This is the maximum volume of air which can be moved into and out of the lungs:

VC = Tidal volume + IRV + ERV

Alveolar ventilation. This is the volume of air that moves into and out of the alveoli per minute. It is equal to the tidal volume minus the anatomical dead space, multiplied by the respiratory rate:

Alveolar ventilation = (TV – anatomical dead space)
× respiratory rate
= (500 – 150) ml × 15 per minute
= 5.25 litres per minute

Lung function tests are carried out to determine respiratory function and are based on the parameters outlined above. Results of these tests can help in diagnosis and monitoring of respiratory disorders.

Exchange of gases

Although breathing involves the alternating processes of inspiration and expiration, gas exchange at the respiratory membrane and in the tissues is a continuous and ongoing process. Diffusion of oxygen and carbon dioxide depends on pressure differences, e.g. between atmospheric air and the blood, or blood and the tissues.

Composition of air

Atmospheric pressure at sea level is 101.3 kilopascals (kPa) or 760 mmHg. With increasing height above sea level, atmospheric pressure is progressively reduced and at 5500 m, about two-thirds the height of Mount Everest (8850 m), it is about half that at sea level. Under water,

Table 10.1 The composition of inspired and expired air

	Inspired air %	Expired air %
Oxygen	21	16
Carbon dioxide	0.04	4
Nitrogen and rare gases	78	78
Water vapour	Variable	Saturated

pressure increases by approximately 1 atmosphere per 10 m below sea level.

Air is a mixture of gases: nitrogen, oxygen, carbon dioxide, water vapour and small quantities of inert gases. The percentage of each is listed in Table 10.1. Each gas in the mixture exerts a part of the total pressure proportional to its concentration, i.e. the *partial pressure* (Table 10.2). This is denoted as, e.g. PO_2, PCO_2.

Alveolar air

The composition of alveolar air remains fairly constant and is different from atmospheric air. It is saturated with water vapour and contains more carbon dioxide, and less oxygen. Saturation with water vapour provides 6.3 kPa (47 mmHg) thus reducing the partial pressure of all the other gases present. Gaseous exchange between the alveoli and the bloodstream (*external respiration*) is a continuous process, as the alveoli are never empty, so it is independent of the respiratory cycle. During each inspiration only some of the alveolar gases are exchanged.

Expired air

This is a mixture of alveolar air and atmospheric air in the dead space (Table 10.1).

253

Table 10.2 Partial pressures of gases

Gas	Alveolar air		Deoxygenated blood		Oxygenated blood	
	kPa	mmHg	kPa	mmHg	kPa	mmHg
Oxygen	13.3	100	5.3	40	13.3	100
Carbon dioxide	5.3	40	5.8	44	5.3	40
Nitrogen and other inert gases	76.4	573	76.4	573	76.4	573
Water vapour	6.3	47				
	101.3	760				

Diffusion of gases

Exchange of gases occurs when a difference in partial pressure exists across a semipermeable membrane. Gases move by diffusion from the higher concentration to the lower until equilibrium is established (p. 26). Atmospheric nitrogen is not used by the body so its partial pressure remains unchanged and is the same in inspired and expired air, alveolar air and in the blood.

External respiration

This is exchange of gases by diffusion between the alveoli and the blood in the alveolar capillaries, across the respiratory membrane. Each alveolar wall is one cell thick and is surrounded by a network of tiny capillaries (the walls of which are also only one cell thick). The total area of respiratory membrane for gas exchange in the lungs is about equivalent to the area of a tennis court. Venous blood arriving at the lungs has travelled from all the tissues of the body, and contains high levels of CO_2 and low levels of O_2. Carbon dioxide diffuses from venous blood down its concentration gradient into the alveoli until equilibrium with alveolar air is reached. By the same process, oxygen diffuses from the alveoli into the blood. The slow flow of blood through the capillaries increases the time available for gas exchange to occur. When blood leaves the alveolar capillaries, the oxygen and carbon dioxide concentrations are in equilibrium with those of alveolar air (Fig. 10.23A).

Internal respiration

This is exchange of gases by diffusion between blood in the capillaries and the body cells. Gaseous exchange does not occur across the walls of the arteries carrying blood from the heart to the tissues, because their walls are too thick. PO_2 of blood arriving at the capillary bed is therefore the same as blood leaving the lungs. Blood arriving at the tissues has been cleansed of its CO_2 and saturated with O_2 during its passage through the lungs, and therefore has a higher PO_2 and a lower PCO_2 than the tissues. This creates concentration gradients between capillary blood and the tissues, and gaseous exchange therefore occurs (Fig. 10.23B). O_2 diffuses from the bloodstream through the capillary wall into the tissues. CO_2 diffuses from the cells into the extracellular fluid, then into the bloodstream towards the venous end of the capillary.

Figure 10.24 summarises the processes of internal and external respiration.

Transport of gases in the bloodstream

Transport of blood oxygen and carbon dioxide is essential for internal respiration to occur.

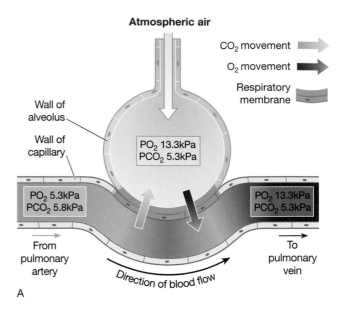

A

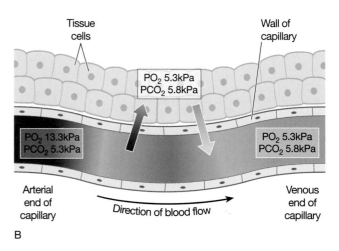

B

Figure 10.23 A: External respiration. B: internal respiration.

Oxygen

Oxygen is carried in the blood in:

- chemical combination with haemoglobin (see Fig. 4.5, p. 61) as *oxyhaemoglobin* (98.5%)
- solution in plasma water (1.5%).

Oxyhaemoglobin is an unstable compound that under certain conditions readily dissociates releasing oxygen. Factors that increase dissociation include low O_2 levels, low pH and raised temperature (see Ch. 4). In active tissues there is increased production of carbon dioxide and heat, which leads to increased release of oxygen. In this way oxygen is available to tissues in greatest need. When oxygen leaves the erythrocyte, the deoxygenated haemoglobin turns purplish in colour.

254

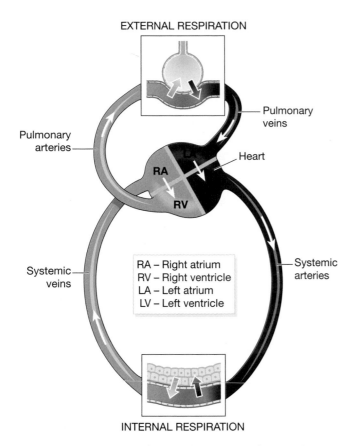

EXTERNAL RESPIRATION

Pulmonary veins

Pulmonary arteries

Heart

RA

RV

Systemic veins

RA – Right atrium
RV – Right ventricle
LA – Left atrium
LV – Left ventricle

Systemic arteries

INTERNAL RESPIRATION

Figure 10.24 Summary of external and internal respiration.

Carbon dioxide

Carbon dioxide is one of the waste products of metabolism. It is excreted by the lungs and is transported by three mechanisms:

- as bicarbonate ions (HCO_3^-) in the plasma (70%)
- some is carried in erythrocytes, loosely combined with haemoglobin as *carbaminohaemoglobin* (23%).
- some is dissolved in the plasma (7%).

Control of respiration

Control of respiration is normally involuntary. Voluntary control is exerted during activities such as speaking and singing but is overridden if blood CO_2 rises (hypercapnia).

The respiratory centre

This is formed by groups of nerves in the medulla, the *respiratory rhythmicity centre,* which control the respiratory pattern, i.e. the rate and depth of breathing (Fig. 10.25). Regular discharge of *inspiratory neurones* within this centre set the rate and depth of breathing. Activity of the respiratory rhythmicity centre is adjusted by nerves in the pons (the *pneumotaxic centre* and the *apneustic centre),* in response to input from other parts of the brain.

255

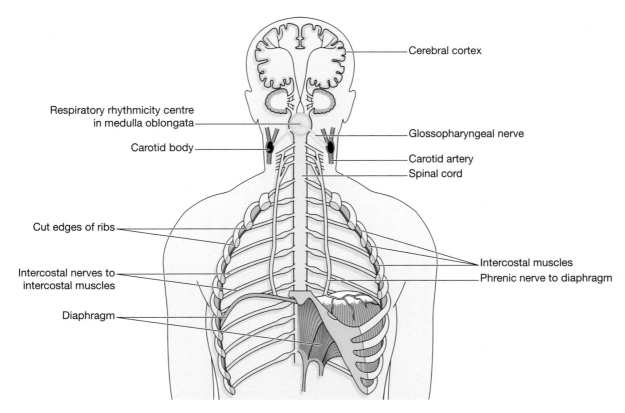

Cerebral cortex

Respiratory rhythmicity centre in medulla oblongata

Glossopharyngeal nerve

Carotid body

Carotid artery

Spinal cord

Cut edges of ribs

Intercostal muscles

Phrenic nerve to diaphragm

Intercostal nerves to intercostal muscles

Diaphragm

Figure 10.25 Some of the structures involved in control of respiration.

Motor impulses leaving the respiratory centre pass in the *phrenic* and *intercostal nerves* to the diaphragm and intercostal muscles respectively.

Chemoreceptors

These are receptors that respond to changes in the partial pressures of oxygen and carbon dioxide in the blood and cerebrospinal fluid. They are located centrally and peripherally.

Central chemoreceptors. These are located on the surface of the medulla oblongata and are bathed in cerebrospinal fluid. When arterial PCO_2 rises (hypercapnia), even slightly, the central chemoreceptors respond by stimulating the respiratory centre, increasing ventilation of the lungs and reducing arterial PCO_2. The sensitivity of the central chemoreceptors to raised arterial PCO_2 is the most important factor in controlling normal blood gas levels. A small reduction in PO_2 (hypoxaemia) has the same, but less pronounced effect, but a substantial reduction depresses breathing.

Peripheral chemoreceptors. These are situated in the arch of the aorta and in the carotid bodies (Fig. 10.25). They are more sensitive to small rises in arterial PCO_2 than to small decreases in arterial PO_2 levels. Nerve impulses, generated in the peripheral chemoreceptors, are conveyed by the *glossopharyngeal* and *vagus nerves* to the medulla and stimulate the respiratory centre. The rate and depth of breathing are then increased. An increase in blood acidity (decreased pH or raised $[H^+]$) stimulates the peripheral chemoreceptors, resulting in increased ventilation, increased CO_2 excretion and increased blood pH.

Other factors that influence respiration

Breathing may be modified by the higher centres in the brain by:

- speech, singing
- emotional displays, e.g. crying, laughing, fear
- drugs, e.g. sedatives, alcohol
- sleep.

Temperature influences breathing. In fever, respiration is increased due to increased metabolic rate, while in hypothermia it is depressed, as is metabolism. Temporary changes in respiration occur in swallowing, sneezing and coughing.

The *Hering–Breuer reflex* prevents overinflation of the lungs. Stretch receptors in the thoracic wall generate inhibitory nerve impulses when the lungs have inflated. They travel via the vagus nerves to the respiratory centre.

Usually, quiet breathing is adequate to maintain normal arterial PO_2 and PCO_2 levels; however, on strenuous exercise, both the rate and depth of breathing increase, increasing oxygen uptake and carbon dioxide excretion in order to meet increased needs. When intense respiratory effort is required, the *accessory muscles of respiration* are used. The most important is the *sternocleidomastoid* (see Fig. 16.54, p. 419). Contraction of these muscles in addition to the diaphragm and intercostal muscles ensures the maximum increase in the capacity of the thoracic cavity.

Effective control of respiration enables the body to regulate blood gas levels over a wide range of physiological, environmental and pathological conditions.

Disorders of the upper respiratory tract

Learning outcomes

After studying this section, you should be able to:

■ describe the main inflammatory and infectious disorders of the upper respiratory tract

■ outline the main tumours of the upper respiratory tract.

Infectious and inflammatory disorders

Inflammation of the upper respiratory tract can be caused by inhaling irritants, but is commonly due to infection. Such infections are usually caused by viruses that lower the resistance of the respiratory tract to other infections. This allows bacteria to invade the tissues. Such infections are a threat to life only if they spread to the lungs or other organs, or if inflammatory swelling and exudate block the airway.

Pathogens are usually spread by droplet infection, in dust or by contaminated equipment and dressings. If not completely resolved, acute infection may become chronic.

Viral infections cause acute inflammation of mucous membrane, leading to tissue congestion and profuse exudate of watery fluid. Secondary infection by bacteria usually results in purulent discharge.

Viral infections commonly cause severe illness and sometimes death in infants, young children and the elderly.

Common cold and influenza

The common cold (coryza) is usually caused by the rhinoviruses and is a highly infectious, normally mild illness characterised mainly by a runny nose (rhinorrhoea), sneezing, sore throat and sometimes slight fever. Normally a cold runs its course over a few days. Influenza is caused by a different group of viruses and produces far more severe symptoms than a cold, including very high temperatures and muscle pains; complete recovery can take weeks and secondary bacterial infections are more common than with a simple cold. In adults, most strains of influenza are incapacitating but rarely fatal unless infection spreads to the lungs.

Sinusitis

This is usually caused by spread of microbes from the nose and pharynx to the mucous membrane lining the paranasal sinuses. The primary viral infection is usually followed by bacterial infection. The congested mucosa may block the openings between the nose and the sinuses, preventing drainage of mucopurulent discharge. Symptoms include facial pain and headache. If there are repeated attacks or if recovery is not complete, the infection may become chronic.

Tonsillitis

Viruses and *Streptococcus pyogenes* are common causes of inflammation of the palatine tonsils, palatine arches and walls of the pharynx. Severe infection may lead to suppuration and abscess formation (*quinsy*). Occasionally the infection spreads into the neck causing cellulitis. Following acute tonsillitis, swelling subsides and the tonsil returns to normal but repeated infection may lead to chronic inflammation, fibrosis and permanent enlargement. Endotoxins from tonsillitis caused by *Streptococcus pyogenes* are associated with the development of rheumatic fever (p. 428) and glomerulonephritis (p. 348).

The nasopharyngeal tonsils lie on the upper wall of the nasopharynx (see Fig. 10.3) and, when inflamed, are better known as the *adenoids*. Temporary enlargement is a protective reaction to infection of the nasal and pharyngeal mucosa. The tissue returns to normal after the infection has subsided, but repeated infections can leave them enlarged and fibrotic. This can cause airway obstruction that can be a problem, especially in children.

Pharyngitis

This usually accompanies common colds and tonsillitis. Viruses, with superimposed bacterial infection, cause acute inflammation of the mucous membrane of the pharynx, nose and sinuses.

Laryngitis and tracheitis

The larynx and trachea are subject to the same viral and bacterial infections as the nose and pharynx. The infection may become chronic, especially in tobacco smokers and people who live or work in a polluted atmosphere.

Laryngotracheobronchitis (*croup* in children) is a rare but serious complication of upper respiratory tract infections. The airway is obstructed by marked swelling around the larynx and epiglottis, accompanied by wheeze and breathlessness (dyspnoea).

Diphtheria

This is a bacterial infection of the pharynx, caused by *Corynebacterium diphtheriae*, which may extend to the nasopharynx and trachea. A thick fibrous membrane forms over the area and may obstruct the airway. Powerful exotoxins may severely damage cardiac and skeletal muscle, the liver, kidneys and adrenal glands. Where immunisation is widespread, diphtheria is rare.

Hay fever (allergic rhinitis)

In this condition, *atopic* ('immediate') hypersensitivity (p. 379) develops to foreign proteins (antigens), e.g. pollen, mites in pillow feathers, animal dander. The acute inflammation of nasal mucosa and conjunctiva causes *rhinorrhoea* (excessive watery exudate from the nose), redness of the eyes and excessive secretion of tears. Atopic hypersensitivity tends to run in families, but no genetic factor has yet been identified. Other forms of atopic hypersensitivity include:

- childhood onset asthma (see below)
- eczema (p. 365) in infants and young children
- food allergies.

Tumours

Benign (haemangiomata)

These occur in the nasal septum. They consist of abnormal proliferations of blood vessels interspersed with collagen fibres of irregular size and arrangement. The blood vessels tend to rupture and cause persistent bleeding (epistaxis).

Malignant

Carcinoma of the nose, sinuses, nasopharynx and larynx is relatively rare.

Diseases of the bronchi

Learning outcomes

After studying this section, you should be able to:

- compare the causes and pathology of chronic and acute bronchitis

- discuss the causes and disordered physiology of asthma

- explain the main physiological abnormality in bronchiectasis.

Acute bronchitis

This is usually a secondary bacterial infection of the bronchi. It is usually preceded by a common cold or influenza and it may also complicate measles and whooping cough in children. The viruses depress normal defence mechanisms, allowing pathogenic bacteria already present in the respiratory tract to multiply. Downward spread of infection may lead to bronchiolitis. Bronchopneumonia may develop, especially in children and in debilitated or elderly adults.

Chronic bronchitis

Chronic bronchitis is defined clinically when an individual has had a cough with sputum for 3 months in 2 successive years. It is a progressive inflammatory disease resulting from prolonged irritation of the bronchial epithelium, often worsened by damp or cold conditions. One or more of the following predisposing factors are usually present:

- cigarette smoking
- acute bronchitis commonly caused by *Haemophilus influenzae* or *Streptococcus pneumoniae*
- atmospheric pollutants, e.g. motor vehicle exhaust fumes, industrial chemicals, sulphur dioxide, urban fog
- previous episodes of acute bronchitis.

It develops mostly in middle-aged men who are chronic heavy smokers and may have a familial predisposition. Acute exacerbations are common, and often associated with infection. The changes occurring in the bronchi include:

Increased size and number of mucus glands. The increased volume of mucus may block small airways, and overwhelm the ciliary escalator, leading to reduced clearance, a persistent cough and infection.

Oedema and other inflammatory changes. These cause swelling of the airway wall, narrowing the passageway and reducing airflow.

Reduction in number and function of ciliated cells. As ciliary efficiency is reduced, the problem of mucus accumulation is worsened, further increasing the risk of infection.

Fibrosis of the airways. Inflammatory changes lead to fibrosis and stiffening of airway walls, further reducing airflow.

Breathlessness (dyspnoea). This is worse with physical exertion and increases the work of breathing.

Ventilation of the lungs becomes severely impaired, causing breathlessness, leading to hypoxia, pulmonary hypertension and right-sided heart failure. As respiratory failure develops, arterial blood PO_2 is reduced (*hypoxaemia*) and is accompanied by a rise in arterial blood PCO_2 (*hypercapnia*). When the condition becomes more severe, the respiratory centre in the medulla responds to hypoxaemia rather than to hypercapnia. In the later stages, the inflammatory changes begin to affect the smallest bronchioles and the alveoli themselves, and emphysema develops (p. 260). The term *chronic obstructive pulmonary disease* (COPD) is sometimes used to describe this situation.

Asthma

Asthma is an inflammatory disease of the airways associated with episodes of reversible over-reactivity of the airway smooth muscle. The mucous membrane and muscle layers of the bronchi become thickened and the mucous glands enlarge, reducing airflow in the lower respiratory tract. During an asthmatic attack, spasmodic contraction of bronchial muscle (*bronchospasm*) constricts the airway and there is excessive secretion of thick sticky mucus, which further narrows the airway. Inspiration is normal but only partial expiration is achieved, so the lungs become hyperinflated and there is severe dyspnoea and wheezing. The duration of attacks usually varies from a few minutes to hours (*status asthmaticus*). In severe acute attacks the bronchi may be obstructed by mucus plugs, leading to acute respiratory failure, hypoxia and possibly death.

Non-specific factors that may precipitate asthma attacks include:

- cold air
- cigarette smoking
- air pollution
- upper respiratory tract infection
- emotional stress
- strenuous exercise.

There are two clinical categories of asthma, which generally give rise to identical symptoms and are treated in the same way. Important differences include typical age of onset and the contribution of an element of allergy. Asthma, whatever the aetiology, can usually be well controlled with inhaled anti-inflammatory and bronchodilator agents, enabling people to live a normal life.

Atopic (childhood onset, extrinsic) asthma

This occurs in children and young adults who have atopic (Type 1) hypersensitivity (p. 380) to foreign

protein, e.g. pollen, dust containing mites from carpets, feather pillows, animal dander, fungi. A history of infantile eczema or food allergies is common and there are often close family members with a history of allergy.

The same disease process occurs as in hay fever. Antigens (allergens) are inhaled and absorbed by the bronchial mucosa. This stimulates the production of IgE antibodies that bind to the surface of mast cells and basophils round the bronchial blood vessels. When the allergen is encountered again, the antigen/antibody reaction results in the release of histamine and other related substances that stimulate mucus secretion and muscle contraction that narrows the airways. Attacks tend to become less frequent and less severe with age.

Non-atopic (adult onset, intrinsic) asthma

This type occurs later in adult life and there is no history of childhood allergic reactions. It is often associated with chronic inflammation of the upper respiratory tract, e.g. chronic bronchitis, nasal polyps. Other trigger factors include exercise and occupational exposure, e.g. inhaled paint fumes. Aspirin triggers an asthmatic reaction in some people. Attacks tend to increase in severity over time and lung damage may be irreversible. Eventually, impaired lung ventilation leads to hypoxia, pulmonary hypertension and right-sided heart failure.

Bronchiectasis

This is permanent abnormal dilatation of bronchi and bronchioles. It is associated with chronic bacterial infection, and in some cases there is a history of childhood bronchiolitis and bronchopneumonia, cystic fibrosis, or bronchial tumour. The bronchi become obstructed by mucus, pus and inflammatory exudate and the alveoli distal to the blockage collapse as trapped air is absorbed. Interstitial elastic tissue degenerates and is replaced by fibrous adhesions that attach the bronchi to the parietal pleura. The pressure of inspired air in these damaged bronchi leads to dilatation proximal to the blockage. The persistent severe coughing to remove copious purulent sputum causes intermittent increases in pressure in the blocked bronchi, leading to further dilatation.

The lower lobe of the lung is usually affected. Suppuration is common. If a blood vessel is eroded, haemoptysis may occur, or pyaemia, leading to abscess formation elsewhere in the body, commonly the brain. Progressive fibrosis of the lung leads to hypoxia, pulmonary hypertension and right-sided heart failure.

Disorders of the lungs

Learning outcomes

After studying this section, you should be able to:

- discuss the pathologies of the main forms of emphysema

- describe the causes and effects of lung infection, including pneumonia, abscess and tuberculosis

- describe the main occupational lung diseases

- outline the main causes and consequences of chemically-induced lung disease

- describe the main causes and consequences of lung cancer

- discuss the causes and effects of collapse of all or part of a lung.

Emphysema (Fig. 10.26)

Pulmonary emphysema

In this form of the disease there is irreversible distension of the respiratory bronchioles, alveolar ducts and alveoli reducing the surface area for the exchange of gases. There are two main types and both are usually present.

Predisposing factors include:

- cigarette smoking, believed to promote the release of proteolytic enzymes from mast cells and basophils in the lungs
- acute inflammation of bronchi and alveoli

- increased pressure caused by coughing, stretching the already damaged structures
- congenital deficiency of an antiproteolytic enzyme, α_1-antitrypsin, leading to destruction of supporting elastic tissue in the lungs.

Panacinar emphysema

The walls between adjacent alveoli break down, the alveolar ducts dilate and interstitial elastic tissue is lost. The lungs become distended and their capacity is increased. Because the volume of air in each breath remains unchanged, it constitutes a smaller proportion of the total volume of air in the distended alveoli, reducing the partial pressure of oxygen. The consequence of this is reduction of the concentration gradient of O_2 across the alveolar membrane, therefore decreasing diffusion of O_2 into the blood. Merging of alveoli reduces the surface area for exchange of gases. Normal arterial blood O_2 and CO_2 levels are maintained at rest by hyperventilation, but as the disease progresses the combined effect of these changes may lead to hypoxia, pulmonary hypertension and eventually right-sided heart failure.

Centrilobular emphysema

In this form there is irreversible dilatation of the respiratory bronchioles in the centre of lobules. When inspired air reaches the dilated area the pressure falls, leading to a reduction in alveolar air pressure, reduced ventilation efficiency and reduced partial pressure of oxygen. As the disease progresses the resultant hypoxia leads to pulmonary hypertension and right-sided heart failure.

Interstitial emphysema

Interstitial emphysema means the presence of air in the thoracic interstitial tissues, and this may happen in one of the following ways:

- from the outside by injury, e.g. fractured rib, stab wound
- from the inside when an alveolus ruptures through the pleura, e.g. during an asthmatic attack, in bronchiolitis, coughing as in whooping cough.

The air in the tissues usually tracks upwards to the soft tissues of the neck where it is gradually absorbed, causing no damage. A large quantity in the mediastinum may limit heart movement.

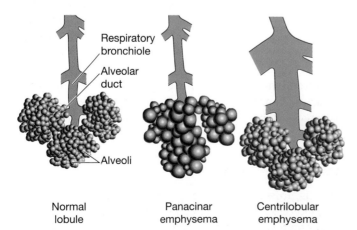

| Normal lobule | Panacinar emphysema | Centrilobular emphysema |

Figure 10.26 Emphysema.

Pneumonia (Fig. 10.27)

Pneumonia means infection of the alveoli. This occurs when protective processes fail to prevent inhaled or

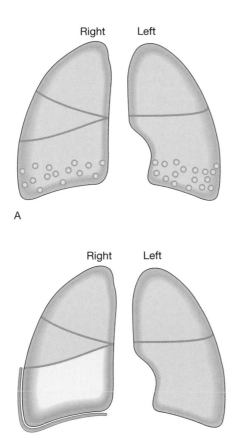

Right   Left

A

Right   Left

B

Figure 10.27 Distribution of infected tissue in:
A. Bronchopneumonia. B. Lobar pneumonia.

blood-borne microbes reaching and colonising the lungs. The following are some predisposing factors.

Impaired coughing. Coughing is an effective cleaning mechanism, but if it is impaired by e.g. unconsciousness, damage to respiratory muscles or the nerves supplying them, or painful coughing, then respiratory secretions may accumulate and become infected.

Damage to the epithelial lining of the tract. Ciliary action may be impaired or the epithelium destroyed by e.g. tobacco smoking, inhaling noxious gases, infection.

Impaired alveolar phagocytosis. Depressed macrophage activity may be caused by tobacco smoking, alcohol, anoxia, oxygen toxicity.

Other factors. These include:

- extremes of age
- leukopenia
- chronic disease, e.g. cardiac failure, cancer, chronic renal failure

- impaired immune response caused by e.g. ionising radiation, corticosteroid drugs
- unusually virulent infections
- hypothermia.

Pathogens associated with pneumonia

Streptococcus pneumoniae. This is the commonest causative organism in pneumonia, particularly lobar pneumonia.

Mycoplasma. This is the second commonest causative organism, and affects mainly children and young adults.

Staphylococcus aureus. Infection is usually preceded by influenza, measles, whooping cough or chronic lung disease. It is most common in hospitalised patients, but is increasingly seen in intravenous drug users.

Haemophilus influenzae. This may cause pneumonia following COPD exacerbations.

Klebsiella pneumoniae. This commensal is sometimes present in the upper respiratory tract, especially where there is advanced dental caries. It causes pneumonia in elderly people who have chronic disease, e.g. diabetes, alcoholism.

Legionella pneumonophilae. These microbes are widely distributed in water tanks, shower heads and air conditioning systems, and are therefore commonly found in institutions such as hospitals and hotels. They cause a severe form of pneumonia (*Legionnaires' disease*), complicated by gastrointestinal disturbances, headache, mental confusion and renal failure.

Pseudomonas pyocyanea. This organism causes a type of pneumonia acquired by cross-infection in hospitals, especially in patients with mechanically assisted ventilation or tracheostomy. It is resistant to many antibacterial agents and multiplies at room temperature in, e.g., water, soap solution, eye drops, ointments, weak antiseptics.

Other organisms. Some viruses, protozoa and fungi may cause pneumonia in people whose general resistance is lowered or whose immune systems are depressed by, e.g. HIV, immunosuppressant drugs.

Lobar pneumonia

This is infection of one or more lobes, usually by *Streptococcus pneumoniae*, leading to production of watery inflammatory exudate in the alveoli. This accumulates and fills the lobule which then overflows into and infects

261

adjacent lobules. It is of sudden onset and pleuritic pain accompanies inflammation of the visceral pleura. If not treated by antibacterial drugs the disease goes through a series of stages followed by resolution and reinflation of the lobes in 2 to 3 weeks. This form of pneumonia is most common in previously healthy young adults.

Bronchopneumonia

Infection spreads from the bronchi to terminal bronchioles and alveoli. As these become inflamed, fibrous exudate accumulates and there is an influx of leukocytes. Small foci of consolidation develop. There is frequently incomplete resolution with fibrosis. Bronchiectasis is a common complication leading to further acute attacks, lung fibrosis and progressive destruction of lung substance. Bronchopneumonia occurs most commonly in infancy and old age, and death is fairly common, especially when the condition complicates debilitating diseases. Predisposing factors include:

- debility due to, e.g., cancer, uraemia, cerebral haemorrhage, congestive heart failure, malnutrition, hypothermia
- chronic bronchitis
- bronchiectasis
- cystic fibrosis
- general anaesthetics, which depress respiratory and ciliary activity
- acute viral infections
- inhalation of gastric contents (*aspiration pneumonia*) in e.g. unconsciousness, very deep sleep, following excessive alcohol consumption, drug overdose
- inhalation of infected material from the paranasal sinuses or upper respiratory tract.

Lung abscess

This is localised suppuration and necrosis within the lung substance.

Sources of infection

- Inhalation of respiratory secretions or gastric contents (aspiration pneumonia, see above)
- Inadequately treated pneumonia
- Septic emboli, usually from thrombophlebitis or right-sided endocarditis
- Traumatic penetration of the lung, e.g. rib fracture, stab or gunshot wound, or during surgery, allowing pathogens to enter the lung
- Local spread of infection, e.g. from the pleural cavity, oesophagus, spine or a subphrenic abscess.

Outcomes

Recovery from lung abscess may either be complete or lead to complications, e.g.:

- chronic suppuration
- septic emboli may spread to other parts of the body, e.g. the brain, causing cerebral abscess or meningitis
- subpleural abscesses may spread and cause empyema and possibly bronchopleural fistula formation
- erosion of a pulmonary blood vessel, leading to haemorrhage.

Tuberculosis (TB)

This infection is caused by one of two similar forms of mycobacteria, the main one being *Mycobacterium tuberculosis*. Humans are the main host. The microbes cause pulmonary tuberculosis and are spread either by droplet infection from an individual with active tuberculosis, or in dust contaminated by infected sputum. Less commonly in developed countries because of pasteurisation of milk, TB can be caused by *Mycobacterium bovis*, from cows.

Phases of pulmonary tuberculosis

Primary tuberculosis

When microbes are inhaled they colonise a lung bronchiole, usually towards the apex of the lung. There may be no evidence of clinical disease during the initial stage of non-specific inflammation. Later, cell-mediated T-lymphocytes respond to the microbes (antigens) and the individual becomes *sensitised*. Macrophages surround the microbes at the site of infection, forming *Ghon foci* (tubercles). These walled-off tubercles shelter microbes from normal body defences. Some macrophages containing live microbes are spread in lymph and infect hilar lymph nodes. *Primary complexes* are formed, consisting of Ghon foci plus infected hilar lymph nodes. Necrosis (caseation) may reduce the core of foci to a cheese-like substance consisting of dead macrophages, dead lung tissue and live and dead microbes. Primary tuberculosis is usually asymptomatic. There are various outcomes.

- The disease may be permanently arrested, the foci becoming fibrosed and calcified.
- Microbes may survive in the foci and become the source of *secondary infection* months or years later.
- The disease may spread:
  - throughout the lung, forming multiple small foci; to the respiratory passages, causing bronchopneumonia or bronchiectasis; to the pleura, with or without effusion

– to other parts of the body via lymph and blood leading to widespread infection and the development of numerous small foci throughout the body (*miliary tuberculosis*).

Weight loss and malaise develop insidiously, and night sweats are common. Chronic cough, with or without blood in the sputum (haemoptysis) may be present.

Secondary (postprimary) tuberculosis

This occurs only in people carrying a primary lesion, usually in the apex of one or both lungs. It may be caused by a new infection or by reactivation of infection by microbes surviving within Ghon foci, often following reduction of immunity by age or illness. As sensitisation has already occurred, T-lymphocytes stimulate an immediate immune reaction. The subsequent course of the disease is variable. The infection may remain localised in the lung, with complete healing or persistence of live bacteria with their sealed pockets of infection. Progressive destruction of lung tissue leads to cavitation, pleurisy, pleural effusions and empyema (pus in the pleural space). Blood-borne spread may lead to infection of other tissues, e.g. bone and brain. Widely disseminated TB is always fatal unless effectively treated.

Occupational lung disease

This group of lung diseases is caused by inhaling atmospheric pollutants at work. Recognition of the damaging effects of these substances has led to legislation that limits workers' exposure to them. To cause disease, particles must be so small that they are carried in inspired air to the level of the respiratory bronchioles and alveoli, where they can only be cleared by phagocytosis. Larger particles are trapped by mucus higher up the respiratory tract and expelled by ciliary action and coughing. Other contributory factors include:

- high concentration of pollutants in the air
- long exposure to pollutants
- reduced numbers of macrophages and inefficient phagocytosis
- cigarette smoking.

Pneumoconiosis

The term pneumoconiosis describes the effects of coal dust in the lung. It occurs in two forms.

Simple pneumoconiosis

Particles of coal dust lodge mainly in the upper two-thirds of the lungs, and are ingested by macrophages inside the alveoli. Some macrophages remain in the alveoli and others migrate into surrounding tissues and adhere to the outside of the alveolar walls, respiratory bronchioles, blood vessels and the visceral pleura. Macrophages are unable to digest inorganic particles, but their activation leads to an inflammatory response that can cause fibrosis in the lung tissue. Fibrosis is progressive during exposure to coal dust but tends to stop when exposure stops. Early in the disease there may be few clinical signs unless emphysema develops or there is concurrent chronic bronchitis.

Pneumoconiosis with progressive massive fibrosis

This develops in a small number of cases, sometimes after the worker is no longer exposed to coal dust. Masses of fibrous tissue develop and progressively encroach on the blood vessels and bronchioles. Large parts of the lung are destroyed and emphysema is extensive, leading to pulmonary oedema, pulmonary hypertension and right-sided cardiac failure. The reasons for the severity of the disease are not clear. One factor may be hypersensitivity to antigens released by the large number of dead macrophages. About 40% of patients have tuberculosis.

Silicosis

This may be caused by long-term exposure to dust containing silicon compounds. High-risk industries are:

- quarrying: granite, slate, sandstone
- mining: hard coal, gold, tin, copper
- stone masonry and sand blasting
- glass and pottery work.

Inhaled silica particles accumulate in the alveoli. The particles are ingested by macrophages, and are actively toxic to these cells. The inflammatory reaction triggered when the macrophages die causes significant fibrosis.

Silicosis appears to predispose to the development of tuberculosis, which rapidly progresses to tubercular bronchopneumonia and possibly military TB. Gradual destruction of lung tissue leads to progressive reduction in pulmonary function, pulmonary hypertension and right-sided heart failure.

Asbestosis

Asbestosis, caused by inhaling asbestos fibres, usually develops after 10 to 20 years' exposure, but sometimes after only 2 years. Asbestos miners and workers involved in making and using some products containing asbestos are at risk. There are different types of asbestos, but blue asbestos is associated with the most serious disease.

263

In spite of their large size, asbestos particles penetrate to the level of respiratory bronchioles and alveoli. Macrophages accumulate in the alveoli and ingest shorter fibres. The larger fibres form *asbestos bodies*, consisting of fibres surrounded by macrophages, protein material and iron deposits. Their presence in sputum indicates exposure to asbestos but not necessarily asbestosis. The macrophages that have engulfed fibres migrate out of the alveoli and accumulate around respiratory bronchioles and blood vessels, stimulating the formation of fibrous tissue. Lung tissue is progressively destroyed, with the development of dyspnoea, chronic hypoxia, pulmonary hypertension and right-sided cardiac failure. The link between inhaled asbestos and fibrosis is not clear. It may be that asbestos stimulates the macrophages to secrete enzymes that promote fibrosis or that it stimulates an immune reaction causing fibrosis. Asbestos is linked to the development of mesothelioma (p. 265).

Byssinosis

This is caused by the inhalation of fibres of cotton, flax and hemp over several years. The fibres cause bronchial irritation and possibly the release of histamine-like substances. At first, breathless attacks similar to asthma occur only when the individual is at work. Later, they become more persistent and chronic bronchitis and emphysema may develop, leading to chronic hypoxia, pulmonary hypertension and right-sided heart failure.

Extrinsic allergic alveolitis

This group of conditions is caused by inhaling materials contaminated by moulds and fungi, e.g. those in Table 10.3. The contaminants act as antigens causing antigen/antibody reactions in the walls of the alveoli. There is excess fluid exudate and the accumulation of platelets, lymphocytes and plasma cells. The alveolar walls become thick and there is progressive fibrosis, leading to pulmonary hypertension and right-sided heart failure.

Table 10.3 Conditions caused by inhaled contaminants

Disease	Contaminant
Farmer's lung	Mouldy hay
Bagassosis	Mouldy sugar waste
Bird handler's lung	Moulds in bird droppings
Malt worker's lung	Mouldy barley

Chemically induced lung diseases

Paraquat

Within hours of ingestion of this weedkiller, it is blood-borne to the lungs and begins to cause irreversible damage. The alveolar membrane becomes swollen, pulmonary oedema develops and alveolar epithelium is destroyed. The kidneys are also damaged and death may be due to combined respiratory and renal failure or cardiac failure.

Cytotoxic drugs

Busulfan, bleomycin, methotrexate and other drugs used in cancer treatment may cause inflammation that heals by fibrosis of interstitial tissue in the lungs and is followed by alveolar fibrosis.

Oxygen toxicity

The lungs may be damaged by a high concentration of oxygen administered for several days, e.g. in intensive care units, to premature babies in incubators. The mechanisms involved are unknown but effects include:

- progressive decrease in lung compliance
- pulmonary oedema
- fibrosis of lung tissue
- breakdown of capillary walls.

In severe cases pneumonia may develop, followed by pulmonary hypertension and right-sided heart failure.

Retinopathy of prematurity. This affects premature babies requiring high-concentration oxygen therapy. The oxygen may stimulate immature retinal blood vessels to constrict causing fibrosis, retinal detachment and blindness (p. 209).

Lung tumours

Bronchial carcinoma

Primary bronchial carcinoma is a very common malignancy. The vast majority (up to 90%) of cases occur in smokers or those who inhale other people's smoke (passive smokers). Because it is seldom detected before spreading, the prognosis is usually very poor.

The tumour usually develops in a main bronchus, forming a large friable mass which projects into the lumen, sometimes causing obstruction. Mucus then collects and predisposes to development of infection. As the tumour grows it may erode a blood vessel, causing haemoptysis.

264

Spread of bronchial cancer

This does not follow any particular pattern or sequence. Spread is by infiltration of local tissues and the transport of tumour fragments in blood and lymph. If blood or lymph vessels are eroded, fragments may spread while the tumour is quite small. A metastatic tumour may, therefore, cause symptoms before the primary in the lung has been detected.

Local spread. This may be within the lung, to the other lung or to mediastinal structures, e.g. blood vessels, nerves, oesophagus.

Lymphatic spread. Tumour fragments spread along lymph vessels to successive lymph nodes in which they may cause metastatic tumours. Fragments may enter lymph draining from a tumour or gain access to a larger vessel if its walls have been eroded by a growing tumour.

Blood spread. Tumour cells can enter the blood if a blood vessel is eroded by a growing tumour. The most common sites of blood-borne metastases are the liver, brain, adrenal glands, bones and kidneys.

Pleural mesothelioma

The majority of cases of this malignant tumour of the pleura are linked with previous exposure to asbestos dust, e.g. asbestos workers and people living near asbestos mines and factories. Smoking multiplies the risk of mesothelioma development several fold in people exposed to asbestos. Mesothelioma may develop after widely varying duration of asbestos exposure, from 3 months to 60 years, and is usually associated with crocidolite fibres (blue asbestos). The tumour involves both layers of pleura and as it grows it obliterates the pleural cavity, compressing the lung. Lymph and blood-spread metastases are commonly found in the hilar and mesenteric lymph nodes, the other lung, liver, thyroid and adrenal glands, bone, skeletal muscle and the brain.

Lung collapse (Fig. 10.28)

The clinical effects of collapse of all or part of a lung depend on how much of the lung is affected. Fairly large sections of a single lung can be out of action without obvious symptoms. The term *atelectasis* is often used to describe lung collapse. There are four main causes of this condition:

- obstruction of an airway (absorption collapse)
- impaired surfactant function
- pressure collapse
- alveolar hypoventilation.

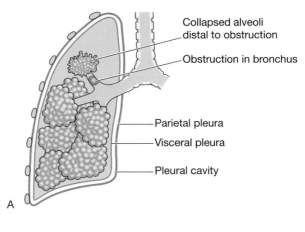

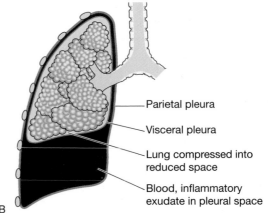

Figure 10.28 Collapse of a lung: A. Absorption collapse. B. Pressure collapse.

Obstruction of an airway (absorption collapse)

The amount of lung affected depends on the size of the obstructed air passage. Distal to the obstruction air is trapped and absorbed, the lung collapses and secretions collect. These may become infected, causing abscess formation. Short-term obstruction is usually followed by reinflation of the lung without lasting ill-effects. Prolonged obstruction leads to progressive fibrosis and permanent collapse. Sudden obstruction may be due to inhalation of a foreign body or a mucus plug formed during an asthmatic attack or in chronic bronchitis. Gradual obstruction may be due to a bronchial tumour or pressure on a bronchus by e.g., enlarged mediastinal lymph nodes, aortic aneurysm.

Impaired surfactant function

Premature babies, born before the 34th week, may be unable to expand their lungs by their own respiratory effort because their lungs are too immature to produce

265

surfactant (p. 250). Surfactant coats the inner surface of each alveolus and reduces surface tension, allowing alveolar expansion during inspiration. These babies may need to be mechanically ventilated until their lungs begin to produce surfactant. This is called *respiratory distress syndrome*.

In the condition called *adult respiratory distress syndrome* (ARDS), dilution of surfactant by fluid collecting in the alveoli (pulmonary oedema) causes surfactant efficiency to be reduced and atelectasis follows. These patients are nearly always gravely ill already, and collapse of substantial areas of lung contributes to the mortality rate of around 50%.

Pressure collapse

When air or fluid enters the pleural cavity the negative pressure becomes positive, preventing lung expansion. Fluids settle in the lung bases, whereas collections of air are usually found towards the lung apex (Fig. 10. 28B). The collapse usually affects only one lung and may be partial or complete. There is no obstruction of the airway.

Pneumothorax

In this condition there is air in the pleural cavity. It may occur spontaneously or be the result of trauma.

Tension pneumothorax. This occurs as a complication when a flap or one-way valve develops between the lungs and the pleural cavity. Air enters the pleural cavity during inspiration but cannot escape on expiration and steadily, but sometimes rapidly, accumulates. This causes shift of the mediastinum and compression of the other lung, resulting in severe respiratory distress that is often fatal unless promptly treated.

Spontaneous pneumothorax. This may be either primary or secondary. *Primary spontaneous pneumothorax* is of unknown cause and occurs in fit and healthy people, usually males between 20 and 40 years. *Secondary spontaneous pneumothorax* occurs when air enters the pleural cavity after the visceral pleura ruptures due to lung disease, e.g. emphysema, asthma, pulmonary tuberculosis, bronchial cancer.

Traumatic pneumothorax. This is due to a penetrating injury, e.g. compound fracture of rib, stab or gunshot wound, surgery.

Haemothorax

This is blood in the pleural cavity. It may be caused by:

- penetrating chest injury involving blood vessels

- ruptured aortic aneurysm
- erosion of a blood vessel by a malignant tumour.

Pleural effusion

This is excess fluid in the pleural cavity that may be caused by:

- increased hydrostatic pressure, e.g. heart failure, increased blood volume
- increased capillary permeability due to local inflammation, e.g. lobar pneumonia, pulmonary tuberculosis, bronchial cancer, mesothelioma
- decreased plasma osmotic pressure, e.g. nephrotic syndrome (p. 349), liver cirrhosis (p. 331)
- impaired lymphatic drainage, e.g. malignant tumour involving the pleura.

Following haemothorax and pleural effusion, fibrous adhesions which limit reinflation may form between the layers of pleura.

Alveolar hypoventilation

In the normal individual breathing quietly at rest there are always some collapsed lobules within the lungs because of the low tidal volume. These lobules will re-expand without difficulty at the next deep inspiration. Another common cause of hypoventilation collapse occurs postoperatively, particularly after chest and upper abdominal surgery, when pain restricts thoracic expansion. Postoperative collapse (atelectasis) predisposes to chest infections, because mucus collects in the under-ventilated airways and is not coughed up.

Cystic fibrosis (mucoviscidosis)

This is one of the most common genetic diseases, affecting 1 in 2500 babies. It is estimated that almost 5% of people carry the abnormal recessive gene which must be present in both parents to cause the disease.

The secretions of all exocrine glands have abnormally high viscosity, but the most severely affected are those of the lungs, pancreas, intestines, biliary tract, and the reproductive system in the male. Sweat glands secrete abnormally large amounts of salt during excessive sweating. In the pancreas, highly viscous mucus is secreted by the walls of the ducts and causes obstruction, parenchymal cell damage, the formation of cysts and defective enzyme secretion. In the newborn, intestinal obstruction may be caused by a plug of meconium and viscid mucus, leading to perforation and meconium peritonitis which is often fatal. In less acute cases there may be impairment of protein and fat digestion resulting in malabsorption, steatorrhoea and failure to thrive in infants. In older children:

- digestion of food and absorption of nutrients is impaired
- there may be obstruction of bile ducts in the liver, causing cirrhosis

- bronchitis, bronchiectasis and pneumonia may develop.

The life span of affected individuals is around 40 years; the main treatments offered are aimed at controlling pulmonary infection. Chronic lung and heart disease are common complications.

Introduction to nutrition

Before discussing the digestive system it is necessary to have an understanding of the nutritional needs of the body, i.e. the dietary constituents and their functions.

A *nutrient* is any substance that is digested, absorbed and used to promote body function. These substances are:

- carbohydrates
- proteins
- fats
- vitamins
- mineral salts
- water.

Many foods contain a number of nutrients, e.g. potatoes and bread are mainly carbohydrate, but both contain protein and some vitamins. Foods are described as carbohydrate or protein because they contain a higher proportion of one or the other. *Fibre*, more correctly known as *non-starch polysaccharide* (NSP), consists of indigestible material. It is not a nutrient, as it is not digested or absorbed, but it has many beneficial effects on the digestive tract.

The *diet* is the selection of foods eaten by an individual. A *balanced* diet is essential for health. It provides the appropriate amounts of all nutrients in the correct proportions to meet body requirements. An *essential nutrient* is a substance that cannot be made by the body and must therefore be included in the diet.

> **Box 11.1 Body mass index**
>
> **Calculation**
>
> $$\text{Body mass index (BMI)} = \frac{\text{Weight (kg)}}{\text{Height (m}^2)}$$
>
> **Interpretation of BMI**
>
> | | |
> |---|---|
> | < 16 | Severely underweight |
> | 16–19 | Underweight |
> | 20–25 | Normal range |
> | 26–30 | Overweight |
> | 31–40 | Obese |
> | > 41 | Severely obese |

The balanced diet

> ### Learning outcomes
>
> After studying this section, you should be able to:
>
> - list the constituent food groups of a balanced diet
>
> - calculate body mass index from an individual's weight and height.

A balanced diet contains all nutrients required for health in appropriate proportions, and is normally achieved by eating a variety of foods. If any nutrient is eaten in excess, or is deficient, health may be adversely affected. For example, a high-energy diet can lead to obesity, and an iron-deficient one to anaemia.

A balanced diet is important in maintaining a healthy body weight and can be assessed by calculating *body mass index* (BMI) (Box 11.1).

Eating a balanced diet requires a certain amount of knowledge and planning. An important dietary consideration is the amount of energy required. This should meet individual requirements. Daily energy requirements depend on several factors including basal metabolic rate (p. 311), age, gender and activity levels. Dietary carbohydrates, fats and proteins are the principal energy sources and fat is the most concentrated form. Dietary energy is correctly expressed in joules or kilojoules (kJ) although the older terms calories and kilocalories (kcal or Cal) are also still widely used in the UK.

Recommendations for daily food intake sort foods of similar origins and nutritional values into food groups, and advise that a certain number of servings from each group be eaten daily (Fig. 11.1). If this plan is followed, the resulting dietary intake is likely to be well balanced.

The five main food groups are:

- bread, rice, cereal and pasta
- fruit and vegetables
- meat and fish
- dairy products, e.g. milk and cheese
- fats, oils and sweets.

Bread, rice, cereal and pasta

Most (50–60%) of the daily energy requirements should come from these sources. In practice this means eating 6–11 servings from this food group every day. These foods contain large amounts of complex carbohydrates, which provide sustained energy release, as well as fibre.

> one serving = one slice of bread, one small bread roll, two large crackers, 25 g cereal

Fruit and vegetables

It is recommended that at least five portions should be eaten daily. Fruit and vegetables are high in vitamins, minerals and fibre, and (provided they have not been, for example, fried) are low in fat.

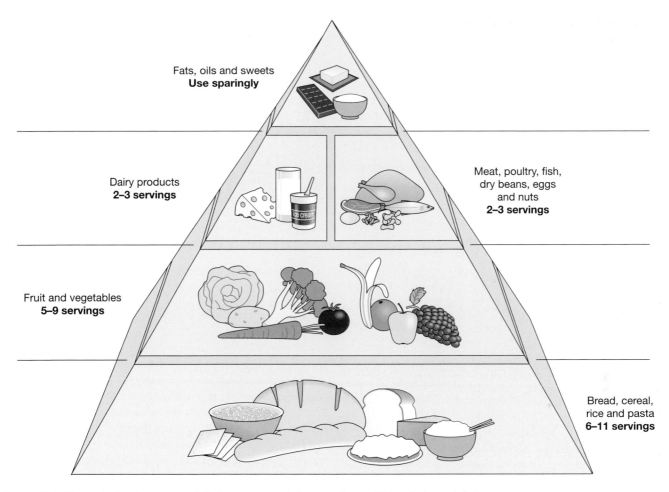

Figure 11.1 **The main food groups and their recommended proportions within a balanced diet.**

one serving = a medium apple, orange or banana; 100 g cooked/raw vegetables or tinned/fresh/cooked fruit; one wedge of melon; 125 ml fruit or vegetable juice

Meat, fish and alternatives

Current dietary habits in developed countries mean that too much of the daily energy requirements are met from this group of foods (which includes eggs and nuts) and from high-fat foods. Although these foods are high in protein, and some vitamins and minerals, only 2–3 servings daily are recommended because they have a high fat content.

one serving = one egg, 30 g peanut butter, 80 g lean cooked meat

Dairy products

This group includes milk, cheese and yoghurt, and is high in calcium and vitamins. 2–3 servings per day are recommended. Dairy foods are often high in fat.

1 serving = 250 ml milk or yoghurt; 50 g cheese

Fats, oils and sweets

These high-energy foods contain little other nutritional value and should be used sparingly, if at all.

Certain groups of people may require a diet different from the principles outlined above. For example, pregnant and lactating women have higher energy requirements to support the growing baby and milk production. Menstruating women need more iron in their diet than non-menstruating women to compensate for blood loss during menstruation. Babies and growing children have higher energy requirements than adults because they have higher growth and metabolic rates. In some gastrointestinal disorders there is intolerance of certain foods, which restricts that person's dietary choices, e.g. coeliac disease (p. 328).

Digestion, absorption and use of nutrients are explained in Chapter 12. Structures and chemistry of carbohydrates, proteins and fats are described in Chapter 2.

Carbohydrates

Learning outcomes

After studying this section, you should be able to:

- describe the main mono-, di- and polysaccharides
- list the nutritional function of digestible carbohydrates.

These are found in a wide variety of foods, e.g. sugar, jam, cereals, bread, biscuits, pasta, convenience foods, fruit and vegetables. They consist of carbon, hydrogen and oxygen, the hydrogen and oxygen being in the same proportion as in water. Carbohydrates are classified according to the complexity of the chemical substances from which they are formed.

Monosaccharides

Carbohydrates are digested in the alimentary canal and absorbed as monosaccharides. Examples include glucose (see Fig. 2.7, p. 23), fructose and galactose. These are, chemically, the simplest form in which a carbohydrate can exist.

Disaccharides

These consist of two monosaccharide molecules chemically combined, e.g. sucrose (see Fig. 2.7), maltose and lactose. When split into their constituent monosaccharides, energy is released for metabolic work.

Polysaccharides

These consist of complex molecules made up of large numbers of monosaccharide molecules in chemical combination, e.g. starches, glycogen, cellulose and dextrins. The monosaccharide constituents of digestible polysaccharides are used in metabolic processes.

Not all polysaccharides can be digested by humans; e.g. cellulose and other substances present in vegetables, fruit and some cereals pass through the alimentary canal almost unchanged (see NSP, p. 278).

Functions of digestible carbohydrates

These include:

- provision of rapidly available energy and heat, glucose is the main fuel molecule for energy production (p. 311)
- 'protein sparing'; i.e. when there is an adequate supply of carbohydrate in the diet, protein does not need to be used to provide energy and heat

- provision of a store of energy when carbohydrate is eaten in excess of the body's needs as it is converted to:
    - glycogen – as a short-term energy store in the liver and skeletal muscles (see p. 312)
    - fat and deposited in the fat depots, e.g. under the skin.

Proteins or nitrogenous foods

Learning outcomes

After studying this section, you should be able to:

- list the sources of animal and vegetarian protein
- list the nutritional functions of dietary proteins.

Proteins are broken down into their constituent amino acids by digestion and it is in this form that they are absorbed through the intestinal wall. Dietary protein is the main source of nitrogen used in the body. If it is absent, or deficient, in the diet the body goes into *negative nitrogen balance*. This is because amino acids are constantly being used to form enzymes, hormones and cell proteins and the turnover of cells is accompanied by the formation of nitrogenous waste materials that are excreted by the kidneys.

Amino acids (see Fig. 2.8)

These are composed of the elements carbon, hydrogen, oxygen and nitrogen. Some contain minerals such as iron, copper, zinc, iodine, sulphur and phosphate. They are divided into two categories: *essential* and *non-essential*.

Essential amino acids cannot be synthesised in the body, therefore they must be included in the diet. *Non-essential amino acids* are those that can be synthesised in the body. The essential and non-essential amino acids are shown in Box 11.2.

The nutritional value of a protein depends on the amino acids of which it is composed.

Complete proteins

This term is given to protein foods which contain all the essential amino acids in the proportions required to maintain health. They are derived almost entirely from animal sources and include meat, fish, milk, eggs, soya beans and milk products (excluding butter).

Box 11.2 Essential and non-essential amino acids	
Essential amino acids	**Non-essential amino acids**
Histidine	Alanine
Isoleucine	Arginine
Leucine	Asparagine
Lysine	Aspartic acid
Methionine	Cysteine
Phenylalanine	Cystine
Threonine	Glutamic acid
Tryptophan	Glutamine
Valine	Glycine
	Hydroxyproline
	Proline
	Serine
	Tyrosine

Protein quality

The nutritional value of a protein (its *quality*) is measured by how well it meets the nutritional needs of the body. High-quality protein is usually of animal origin, easily digested and contains all essential amino acids in the proportions required by the body. A balanced diet, containing all the amino acids required, may also be achieved by eating a range of foods containing low-quality proteins, provided that deficiencies in amino acid content of any one of the constituent proteins of the diet is supplied by another. A balanced vegetarian diet, which consists primarily of lower-quality protein, e.g. vegetables, cereals and pulses, is based on this principle.

Functions of proteins

Amino acids are used for:

- growth and repair of body cells and tissues
- synthesis of enzymes, plasma proteins, antibodies (immunoglobulins) and some hormones
- provision of energy. Normally a secondary function, this becomes important only when there is not enough carbohydrate in the diet and fat stores are depleted.

When protein is eaten in excess of the body's needs, the nitrogenous part is detached, i.e. it is deaminated, and excreted by the kidneys. The remainder is converted to fat for storage in the fat depots, e.g. in the fat cells of adipose tissue (p. 37).

Fats

Learning outcomes

After studying this section, you should be able to:

- outline the main sources of dietary fat
- list the functions of fats in the body.

Fats (see Fig. 2.9, p. 24) consist of carbon, hydrogen and oxygen, but they differ from carbohydrates in that the hydrogen and oxygen are not in the same proportions as in water. Fats are divided into two groups, *saturated* and *unsaturated*.

Saturated or *animal fat*, containing mainly saturated fatty acids and glycerol, is found in milk, cheese, butter, eggs, meat and oily fish such as herring, cod and halibut. All animal sources of protein contain some saturated fat.

Cholesterol is synthesised in the body and is also obtained in the diet from full fat dairy products, fatty meat and egg yolk.

Unsaturated or *vegetable fat*, containing mainly unsaturated fatty acids and glycerol, is found in some margarine and in most vegetable oils.

Linoleic, linolenic and arachidonic acids are polyunsaturated fatty acids that are essential in the diet because they cannot be synthesised in the body. They are needed for plasma membrane phospholipids and synthesis of prostaglandins, thromboxanes and leukotrienes (p. 224).

Functions of fats

These include:

- provision of the most concentrated source of chemical energy and heat
- support of certain body organs, e.g. the kidneys, the eyes
- transport and storage of the fat-soluble vitamins: A, D, E, K
- constituent of nerve sheaths and of sebum, the secretion of sebaceous glands in the skin
- formation of cholesterol and steroid hormones
- storage of energy as fat in adipose tissue under the skin and in the mesentery, especially when eaten in excess of requirements
- insulation – as a subcutaneous layer it reduces heat loss through the skin
- satiety value – when gastric contents (chyme) containing fat enter the duodenum, the emptying time of the stomach is prolonged, postponing the return of hunger.

273

Vitamins

Vitamins are chemical compounds, required in very small quantities, which are essential for normal metabolism and health. They are found widely distributed in food and are divided into two main groups:

• fat-soluble vitamins: A, D, E and K
• water-soluble vitamins: B complex, C.

Fat-soluble vitamins

Vitamin A (retinol)

This vitamin is found in such foods as cream, egg yolk, liver, fish oil, milk, cheese and butter. It is absent from vegetable fats and oils but is added to margarine during manufacture. It can be formed in the body from certain carotenes, the main dietary sources of which are green vegetables, fruit and carrots. Vitamin A and carotene are absorbed from the small intestine only if fat absorption is normal. Although some is synthesised in the body the daily dietary requirement is 600 to 700 µg. The main roles of vitamin A in the body are:

• generation of the light-sensitive pigment rhodopsin (visual purple) in the retina of the eye
• cell growth and differentiation; this is especially important in fast-growing cells, such as the epithelial cells covering both internal and external body surfaces
• promotion of immunity and defence against infection
• promotion of growth, e.g. in bones.

The first sign of vitamin A deficiency is night blindness due to defective retinal pigment. Other consequences include xerophthalmia, which is drying and thickening of the conjunctiva and, ultimately, ulceration and destruction of the conjunctiva. This is a common cause of blindness in developing countries. Atrophy and keratinisation of other epithelial tissues leads to increased incidence of infections of the ear, and the respiratory, genitourinary and alimentary tracts. Immunity is compromised and bone development may be abnormal and delayed.

Vitamin D

Vitamin D is found mainly in animal fats such as eggs, butter, cheese, fish liver oils. Humans and other animals can synthesise vitamin D by the action of the ultraviolet rays of the sun on a form of cholesterol (7-dehydrocholesterol) in the skin (see p. 362).

Vitamin D regulates calcium and phosphate metabolism by increasing their absorption in the gut and stimulating their retention by the kidneys. It therefore promotes the calcification of bones and teeth.

Deficiency causes *rickets* in children and *osteomalacia* in adults (p. 426), due to deficient absorption and use of calcium and phosphate. The daily requirement is 10 µg and stores in fat and muscle are such that deficiency may not be apparent for several years.

Vitamin E

This is a group of eight substances called *tocopherols*. They are found in nuts, egg yolk, wheat germ, whole cereal, milk and butter.

Vitamin E is an antioxidant, which means that it protects body constituents such as membrane lipids from being destroyed in oxidative reactions. Deficiency is rare, because of the widespread occurrence of this vitamin in foods, and is usually seen only in premature babies and in conditions associated with impaired fat absorption, e.g. cystic fibrosis. Haemolytic anaemia occurs, as abnormal red blood cell membranes rupture. White blood cells can likewise be affected, and vitamin E supplements boost immune function. Neurological abnormalities such as ataxia and visual disturbances may occur if the deficiency is severe. Recently, vitamin E has been shown to protect against coronary heart disease. Recommended daily intake is 10 mg for men and 8 mg for women, but this should be increased in high-fat diets.

Vitamin K

The sources of vitamin K are liver, some vegetable oils and leafy green vegetables. It is synthesised in the large intestine by microbes and significant amounts are absorbed. Absorption is dependent upon the presence of bile salts in the small intestine. The normal daily requirement is 1 µg/kg body weight and only a small amount is stored in the liver.

Vitamin K is required by the liver for the production of prothrombin and factors VII, IX and X, all essential for the clotting of blood (p. 66). Deficiency therefore prevents normal blood coagulation. It may occur in adults when there is obstruction to the flow of bile, severe liver damage and in malabsorption conditions, such as *coeliac disease*. Newborn infants may be given vitamin K because their intestines are sterile and require several weeks to become colonised with vitamin K-producing bacteria.

Water-soluble vitamins

Vitamin B complex

This is a group of water-soluble vitamins that promote activity of enzymes involved in the chemical breakdown (catabolism) of nutrients to release energy.

Vitamin B$_1$ (thiamine). This vitamin is present in nuts, yeast, egg yolk, liver, legumes, meat and the germ of cereals. It is rapidly destroyed by heat. The daily requirement is 0.8 to 1 mg and the body stores only about 30 mg. Thiamine is essential for the complete aerobic release of energy from carbohydrate. When it is absent there is accumulation of lactic and pyruvic acids, which may lead to accumulation of tissue fluid (oedema) and heart failure. Thiamine is also important for nervous system function because of the dependency of these tissues on glucose for fuel.

Deficiency causes *beriberi*, which occurs mainly in countries where polished rice is the chief constituent of the diet. In beriberi there is:

- severe muscle wasting
- delayed growth in children
- polyneuritis, causing degeneration of motor, sensory and some autonomic nerves
- susceptibility to infections.

If untreated, death occurs owing to cardiac failure or severe microbial infection.

The main cause of thiamine deficiency in developed countries is alcoholism, where the diet is usually poor. Neurological symptoms, which are usually irreversible, include memory loss, ataxia and visual disturbances.

Vitamin B$_2$ (riboflavine). Riboflavine is found in yeast, green vegetables, milk, liver, eggs, cheese and fish roe. The daily requirement is 1.1 to 1.3 mg; only small amounts are stored in the body and it is destroyed by light and alkalis. It is concerned with carbohydrate and protein metabolism, especially in the eyes and skin. Deficiency leads to cracking of the skin, commonly around the mouth (angular stomatitis), and inflammation of the tongue (glossitis).

Folate (folic acid). This is found in liver, kidney, fresh leafy green vegetables and yeast. It is synthesised by bacteria in the large intestine, and significant amounts derived from this source are believed to be absorbed. It is destroyed by heat and moisture. The daily requirement is 200 µg, and, as only a small amount is stored in the body, deficiency is evident within a short time. It is essential for DNA synthesis, and when lacking mitosis (cell division) is impaired. This manifests particularly in rapidly dividing tissues such as blood, and folate deficiency therefore leads to a type of megaloblastic anaemia (p. 69), which is reversible with folate supplements. Deficiency at conception and during early pregnancy is linked to an increased incidence of spina bifida (p. 187).

Niacin (nicotinic acid equivalent). This is found in liver, cheese, yeast, whole cereals, eggs, fish and nuts; in addition, the body can synthesise it from the amino acid tryptophan. It is associated with energy-releasing reactions in cells. In fat metabolism it inhibits the production of cholesterol and assists in fat breakdown. Deficiency occurs mainly in areas where maize is the chief constituent of the diet because niacin in maize is in an unusable form. The daily requirement is 12 to 17 mg and it is fairly stable.

Pellagra develops within 6 to 8 weeks of severe deficiency. It is characterised by:

- dermatitis – redness of the skin in parts exposed to light, especially the neck
- anorexia, nausea, dysphagia and inflammation of the oral mucosa
- delirium, mental disturbance and dementia.

Vitamin B$_6$ (pyridoxine). This stable vitamin is found in egg yolk, peas, beans, soya beans, yeast, meat and liver. The daily requirement is about 1.2 to 1.4 mg and dietary deficiency is rare, although certain drugs, e.g. alcohol and antituberculous drugs, antagonise the vitamin and can induce deficiency states. It is associated with amino acid metabolism, including the synthesis of non-essential amino acids and molecules such as haem and nucleic acids.

Vitamin B$_{12}$ (cobalamin). Vitamin B$_{12}$ consists of a number of *cobalamin compounds* (containing cobalt). It is found in liver, meat, eggs, milk and fermented liquors, and is destroyed by heat. The normal daily requirement is 1.5 µg.

Like folic acid, vitamin B$_{12}$ is essential for DNA synthesis, and deficiency also leads to a megaloblastic anaemia, which is correctable with supplements. However, vitamin B$_{12}$ is also required for formation and maintenance of myelin, the fatty substance that surrounds and protects some nerves. Deficiency accordingly causes irreversible damage such as peripheral neuropathy and/or subacute spinal cord degeneration. The presence of intrinsic factor in the stomach is essential for vitamin B$_{12}$ absorption, and deficiency is usually associated with insufficient intrinsic factor.

Pantothenic acid. This is found in many foods and is associated with amino acid metabolism. The daily safe intake is 3 to 7 mg and no deficiency diseases have been identified. It is destroyed by excessive heat and freezing.

Biotin. This is found in yeast, egg yolk, liver, kidney and tomatoes and is synthesised by microbes in the intestine. It is associated with the metabolism of carbohydrates. The daily safe intake is 10 to 20 µg, deficiency is rare and it is a stable compound.

Vitamin C (ascorbic acid)

This is found in fresh fruit, especially blackcurrants, oranges, grapefruit and lemons, and also in rosehips and green vegetables. The vitamin is very water soluble and is easily destroyed by heat, ageing, chopping, salting and drying. These processes may predispose to the development of *scurvy* (deficiency). The daily requirement is 40 mg and after 2 to 3 months deficiency becomes apparent.

Vitamin C is associated with protein metabolism, especially the laying down of collagen fibres in connective tissue. Vitamin C, like vitamin E, acts as an antioxidant, protecting body molecules from damaging oxidative reactions. When scurvy occurs, collagen production is affected, leading to fragility of blood vessels, delayed wound healing and poor bone repair. Gums become swollen and spongy and the teeth loosen in their sockets.

Summary of the vitamins

Tables 11.1 and 11.2 summarise the vitamins: their chemical names, sources, functions and deficiency diseases.

Mineral salts

Learning outcomes

After studying this section, you should be able to:

- list the commonest mineral salts required by the body
- describe their functions.

Mineral salts (inorganic compounds) are necessary within the body for all body processes, usually in only small quantities.

Calcium

This is found in milk, cheese, eggs, green vegetables and some fish. An adequate supply should be obtained from a normal, well-balanced diet, although requirements are higher in pregnant women and growing children. 99% of body calcium is found in the bones, where it is an essential structural component. Calcium is also involved in coagulation of blood and muscle contraction.

Phosphate

Sources of phosphate include cheese, oatmeal, liver and kidney. If there is sufficient calcium in the diet it is unlikely that there will be phosphate deficiency.

276

Table 11.1 Summary – fat-soluble vitamins (DoH 1991)

Vitamin	Chemical name	Source	Functions	Effects of deficiency
A	Retinol (carotene provitamin in plants)	Milk, butter, cheese, egg yolk, fish, liver oils, green and yellow vegetables	Maintains healthy epithelial tissues and cornea. Formation of rhodopsin (visual purple)	Keratinisation Xerophthalmia Stunted growth Night blindness
D	Calciferol	Fish, liver, oils, milk, cheese, egg yolk, irradiated 7-dehydrocholesterol in human skin	Facilitates the absorption and use of calcium and phosphate in the maintenance of healthy bones and teeth	Rickets (children) Osteomalacia (adults)
E	Tocopherols	Egg yolk, milk, butter, green vegetables, nuts	Antioxidant Promotes immune function	Anaemia Ataxia Visual disturbances
K	Phylloquinone	Leafy vegetables, fish, liver, fruit	Formation of prothrombin and factors VII, IX and X in the liver	Slow blood clotting Haemorrhages in the newborn

Bile is necessary for the absorption of these vitamins. Mineral oils interfere with absorption.

Table 11.2 Summary – water-soluble vitamins (DoH 1991)

Vitamin	Chemical name	Source	Functions	Effects of deficiency
B$_1$	Thiamine	Yeast, liver, germ of cereals, nuts, pulses, rice polishings, egg yolk, liver, legumes	Metabolism of carbohydrates and nutrition of nerve cells	General fatigue and loss of muscle tone Ultimately leads to beriberi Stunted growth
B$_2$	Riboflavine	Liver, yeast, milk, eggs, green vegetables, kidney, fish roe	Carbohydrate and protein metabolism Healthy skin	Angular stomatitis Dermatitis
B$_6$	Pyridoxine	Meat, liver, vegetables, bran of cereals, egg yolk, beans	Protein metabolism	Very rare
B$_{12}$	Cobalamin	Liver, milk, moulds, fermenting liquors, egg	DNA synthesis	Megaloblastic anaemia Degeneration of nerve fibres of the spinal cord
B	Folate (folic acid)	Dark green vegetables, liver, kidney, eggs Synthesised in colon	DNA synthesis Normal development of spinal cord in early pregnancy	Anaemia Increased incidence of spina bifida
B	Niacin	Yeast, offal, fish, pulses, wholemeal cereals Synthesised in the body from tryptophan	Necessary for cell respiration Inhibits production of cholesterol	Prolonged deficiency causes pellagra, i.e. dermatitis, diarrhoea, dementia
B	Pantothenic acid	Liver, yeast, egg yolk, fresh vegetables	Associated with amino acid metabolism	Unknown
B	Biotin	Yeasts, liver, kidney, pulses, nuts	Carbohydrates and fat metabolism	Dermatitis Hypercholesterolaemia
C	Ascorbic acid	Citrus fruits, currants, berries, green vegetables, potatoes, liver and glandular tissue in animals	Formation of collagen Maturation of RBCs Antioxidant	Multiple haemorrhages Slow wound healing Anaemia Gross deficiency causes scurvy

It is associated with calcium and vitamin D in the hardening of bones and teeth; 85% of body phosphate is found in these sites. Phosphates are an essential part of nucleic acids (DNA and RNA, see p. 433) and energy storage molecules inside cells as adenosine triphosphate (ATP, Fig. 2.10, p. 25).

Sodium

Sodium is found in most foods, especially fish, meat, eggs, milk, most processed foods and also added during cooking or as table salt. Intake of sodium chloride usually exceeds requirements and excess is excreted in the urine.

It is the most commonly occurring *extracellular cation* and is associated with:

- muscle contraction
- transmission of nerve impulses along axons
- maintenance of electrolyte balance in the body.

Potassium

This substance is found widely distributed in all foods, especially fruit and vegetables and intake usually exceeds potassium requirements.

It is the most commonly occurring *intracellular cation* and is involved in many chemical activities inside cells including:

- muscle contraction
- transmission of nerve impulses
- maintenance of electrolyte balance in the body.

Iron

Iron, as a soluble compound, is found in liver, kidney, beef, egg yolk, wholemeal bread and green vegetables. In normal adults about 1 mg of iron is lost from the body daily. The normal daily diet contains more, i.e. 9 to 15 mg, but only 5–15% of intake is absorbed. Iron is essential for the formation of haemoglobin in red blood cells. It is also necessary for oxidation of carbohydrates and the synthesis of some hormones and neurotransmitters.

Iron deficiency is a relatively common condition, and causes anaemia (p. 68) if iron stores become sufficiently depleted. Menstruating and pregnant women have increased iron requirements, as do young people experiencing growth spurts. Iron deficiency anaemia may also occur in chronic bleeding, e.g. peptic ulcer disease.

Iodine

Iodine is found in salt-water fish and in vegetables grown in soil containing iodine. In some parts of the world where iodine is deficient in soil, very small quantities are added to table salt to prevent goitre (p. 228). Daily iodine requirement depends upon metabolic rate. Some people have a higher normal metabolic rate than others and their iodine requirements are greater.

It is essential for the formation of *thyroxine* and *tri-iodothyronine*, two hormones secreted by the thyroid gland (p. 28).

Non-starch polysaccharide (NSP)

Learning outcome

After studying this section, you should be able to:

■ describe the sources and functions of non-starch polysaccharide.

Non-starch polysaccharide (NSP) is the correct term for dietary fibre although the latter term continues to be more commonly used in the UK. It is the indigestible part of the diet and consists of bran, cellulose and other polysaccharides. It is widely distributed in wholemeal flour, the husks of cereals and in fruit and vegetables. Dietary fibre is partly digested by microbes in the large intestine with gas (flatus) formation. The daily requirement is at least 20 g.

Functions of NSP (dietary fibre)

Dietary fibre:

- provides bulk to the diet and helps to satisfy the appetite
- stimulates peristalsis (see p. 285)

- attracts water, increasing bulk and softness of faeces
- increases frequency of defaecation, preventing constipation
- prevents some gastrointestinal disorders, e.g. colorectal cancer and diverticular disease (p. 325).

Water

Learning outcomes

After studying this section, you should be able to:

■ explain the distribution of water within the body

■ describe the functions of water within the body.

Water makes up about 60% of the body weight in men and about 55% in women.

A man weighing 70 kg contains about 40 litres of water, 28 of which are intracellular and 12 extracellular. Extracellular water consists of 2 to 3 litres in plasma and the remainder, interstitial fluid (see Fig. 2.14, p. 27).

A large amount of water is lost each day in urine, sweat and faeces. This is normally balanced by intake in food and fluids, to satisfy thirst. Dehydration, with serious consequences, may occur if intake does not balance loss.

Functions of water

These include:

- provision of the moist internal environment required by all living cells in the body, i.e. all the cells except the superficial layers of the skin, the nails, the hair and outer hard layer of the teeth
- participation in all the chemical reactions that occur inside and outside the body cells
- moistening of food (see saliva, p. 291)
- regulation of body temperature – as a constituent of sweat, which is secreted onto the skin, it evaporates, cooling the body surface
- a major constituent of blood and tissue fluid, it transports some substances in solution and some in suspension round the body
- dilution of waste products and poisonous substances in the body
- providing the medium for the excretion of waste products, e.g. urine and faeces.

Disorders of nutrition

Learning outcome

After studying this section, you should be able to:

■ describe the main consequences of malnutrition, malabsorption and obesity.

The importance of nutrition is increasingly recognised as essential for health, and illness often alters nutritional requirements.

Malnutrition

This may be due to:

- protein-energy malnutrition (PEM)
- vitamin deficiencies (Tables 11.1 and 11.2)
- both PEM and vitamin deficiencies.

The degree of malnutrition can be assessed from measurement of body mass index (Box 11.3).

Protein-energy malnutrition (Fig. 11.2)

This is the result of inadequate intake of protein, carbohydrate and fat. It occurs during periods of starvation and when dietary intake is inadequate to meet increased requirements, e.g. trauma, fever and illness. Infants and young children are especially susceptible as they need sufficient nutrients to grow and develop normally. If dietary intake is inadequate, it is not uncommon for vitamin deficiency to develop at the same time. Poor nutrition (malnutrition) reduces the ability to combat other illness and infection.

Kwashiorkor

This is mainly caused by protein deficiency, and occurs in infants and children in some developing countries and when there has been serious drought and crop failure. Reduced plasma proteins lead to ascites and oedema

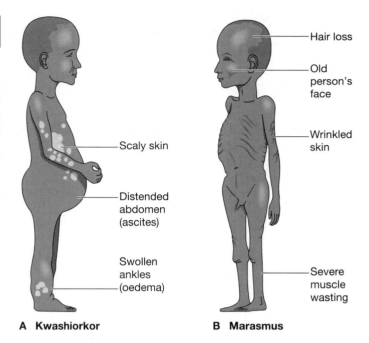

A Kwashiorkor   **B Marasmus**

Figure 11.2 Features of protein-energy malnutrition.

(p. 120) in the lower limbs that masks emaciation. There is severe liver damage. Growth stops and there is loss of weight and loss of pigmentation of skin and hair accompanied by listlessness, apathy and irritability.

Marasmus

This is caused by deficiency of both protein and carbohydrate. It is characterised by severe emaciation due to breakdown (catabolism) of muscle and fat. Growth is retarded, the skin becomes wrinkled due to absence of subcutaneous fat and hair is lost.

Malabsorption

The causes of malabsorption vary widely, from short-term problems such as gastrointestinal infections to chronic conditions such as cystic fibrosis (p. 266). Malabsorption may be specific for one nutrient, e.g. vitamin B_{12} in pernicious anaemia (p. 69), or it may apply across a spectrum of nutrients, e.g. in tropical sprue (p. 328).

Obesity

In developed countries, this is a very common nutritional disorder in which there is accumulation of excess body fat. Clinically, obesity is present when body mass index exceeds 31 (see Box 11.1). It occurs when energy intake exceeds energy expenditure, e.g. in inactive individuals who exceed daily energy requirements.

279

Box 11.3 Body mass index in malnutrition	
> 20	Normal
18.5–20	Marginal
17–18.5	Mild malnutrition
16–17	Moderate malnutrition
< 16	Severe malnutrition

Obesity predisposes to:

- gallstones (p. 333)
- cardiovascular diseases, e.g. ischaemic heart disease (p. 123), hypertension (p. 128)
- hernias (p. 326)
- varicose veins (p. 119)
- osteoarthritis (p. 429)

- type II (non-insulin-dependent) diabetes mellitus (p. 232)
- increased incidence of postoperative complications.

Phenylketonuria

See page 439.

The digestive system

12

The digestive system is the collective name used to describe the *alimentary canal,* some *accessory organs* and a variety of *digestive processes* that take place at different levels in the canal to prepare food eaten in the diet for absorption. The alimentary canal begins at the mouth, passes through the thorax, abdomen and pelvis and ends at the anus (Fig. 12.1). It has a general structure which is modified at different levels to provide for the processes occurring at each level (Fig. 12.2). The digestive processes gradually break down the foods eaten until they are in a form suitable for absorption. For example, meat, even when cooked, is chemically too complex to be absorbed from the alimentary canal. It therefore goes through a series of changes that release its constituent nutrients: amino acids, mineral salts, fat and vitamins. Chemical substances or *enzymes* (p. 25) that effect these changes are secreted into the canal by specialised glands, some of which are in the walls of the canal and some outside the canal, but with ducts leading into it.

After absorption, nutrients are used to synthesise body constituents. They provide the raw materials for the man-ufacture of new cells, hormones and enzymes, and the energy needed for these and other processes and for the disposal of waste materials.

The activities in the digestive system can be grouped under five main headings.

Ingestion. This is the taking of food into the alimentary tract, i.e. eating and drinking.

Propulsion. This mixes and moves the contents along the alimentary tract.

Digestion. This consists of:

- *mechanical breakdown* of food by, e.g. mastication (chewing)
- *chemical digestion* of food into small molecules by enzymes present in secretions produced by glands and accessory organs of the digestive system.

Absorption. This is the process by which digested food substances pass through the walls of some organs of the

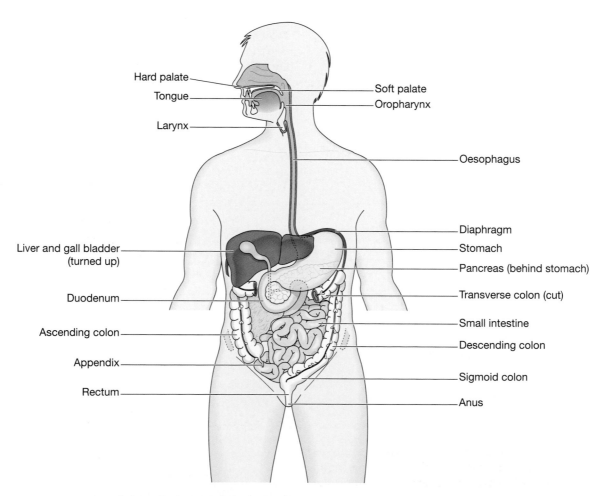

Figure 12.1 The digestive system.

alimentary canal into the blood and lymph capillaries for circulation and use by body cells.

Elimination. Food substances that have been eaten but cannot be digested and absorbed are excreted from the alimentary canal as *faeces* by the process of *defaecation*.

Organs of the digestive system

(Fig. 12.1)

Learning outcomes

After studying this section, you should be able to:

■ list the main organs of the alimentary tract

■ list the accessory organs of digestion.

Alimentary tract

Also known as the gastrointestinal (GI) tract, this is a long tube through which food passes. It commences at the mouth and terminates at the anus, and the various parts are given separate names, although structurally they are remarkably similar. The parts are:

● mouth
● pharynx
● oesophagus
● small intestine
● stomach
● large intestine
● rectum and anal canal.

Accessory organs

Various secretions are poured into the alimentary tract, some by glands in the lining membrane of the organs, e.g. gastric juice secreted by glands in the lining of the stomach, and some by glands situated outside the tract. The latter are the accessory organs of digestion and their secretions pass through ducts to enter the tract. They consist of:

● 3 pairs of salivary glands
● the pancreas
● the liver and biliary tract.

The organs and glands are linked physiologically as well as anatomically in that digestion and absorption occur in stages, each stage being dependent upon the previous stage or stages.

Basic structure of the alimentary canal (Fig. 12.2)

Learning outcomes

After studying this section, you should be able to:

■ describe the distribution of the peritoneum

■ explain the function of smooth muscle in the walls of the alimentary canal

■ discuss the structures of the alimentary mucosa

■ outline the nerve supply of the alimentary canal.

The layers of the walls of the alimentary canal follow a consistent pattern from the oesophagus onwards. This basic structure does not apply so obviously to the mouth and the pharynx, which are considered later in the chapter.

In the organs from the oesophagus onwards, modifications of structure are found which are associated with special functions. The basic structure is described here and any modifications in structure and function are described in the appropriate section.

283

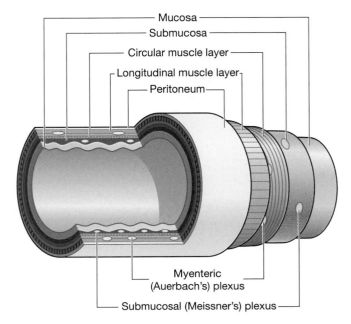

Figure 12.2 General structure of the alimentary canal.

The walls of the alimentary tract are formed by four layers of tissue:

- adventitia or serosa – outer covering
- muscle layer
- submucosa
- mucosa – lining.

Adventitia or serosa

This is the outermost layer. In the thorax it consists of *loose fibrous tissue* and in the abdomen the organs are covered by a serous membrane (serosa) called *peritoneum*.

Peritoneum

The peritoneum is the largest serous membrane of the body (Fig. 12.3A). It consists of a closed sac, containing a small amount of serous fluid, within the abdominal cavity. It is richly supplied with blood and lymph vessels, and contains many lymph nodes. It provides a physical barrier to local spread of infection, and can isolate an infective focus such as appendicitis, preventing involvement of other abdominal structures. It has two layers:

- the *parietal layer*, which lines the abdominal wall
- the *visceral layer*, which covers the organs (viscera) within the abdominal and pelvic cavities.

The arrangement of the peritoneum is such that the organs are invaginated into the closed sac from below, behind and above so that they are at least partly covered by the visceral layer, and attached securely within the abdominal cavity. This means that:

- pelvic organs are covered only on their superior surface
- the stomach and intestines, deeply invaginated from behind, are almost completely surrounded by peritoneum and have a double fold (the *mesentery*) that attaches them to the posterior abdominal wall. The fold of peritoneum enclosing the stomach extends beyond the greater curvature of the stomach, and hangs down in front of the abdominal organs like an apron (Fig. 12.3B). This is the *greater omentum*, and it stores fat, which provides both insulation and a long-term energy store
- the pancreas, spleen, kidneys and adrenal glands are invaginated from behind but only their anterior surfaces are covered and are therefore *retroperitoneal*
- the liver is invaginated from above and is almost completely covered by peritoneum, which attaches it to the inferior surface of the diaphragm
- the main blood vessels and nerves pass close to the posterior abdominal wall and send branches to the organs between folds of peritoneum.

284

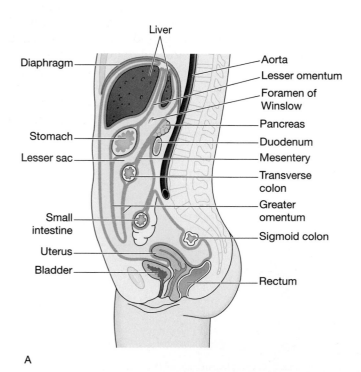

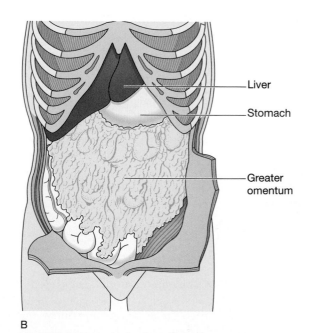

A

B

Figure 12.3 A. The peritoneal cavity (gold), the abdominal organs of the digestive system and the pelvic organs. **B.** The greater omentum.

The parietal peritoneum lines the anterior abdominal wall.

The two layers of peritoneum are actually in contact, and friction between them is prevented by the presence of serous fluid secreted by the peritoneal cells, thus the *peritoneal cavity* is only a *potential cavity*. A similar arrangement is seen with the membranes covering the lungs, the pleura (p. 246). In the male, the peritoneal cavity is completely closed but in the female the uterine tubes open into it and the ovaries are the only structures inside (Ch. 18).

Muscle layer

With some exceptions this consists of two layers of *smooth (involuntary)* muscle. The muscle fibres of the outer layer are arranged longitudinally, and those of the inner layer encircle the wall of the tube. Between these two muscle layers are blood vessels, lymph vessels and a plexus (network) of sympathetic and parasympathetic nerves, called the *myenteric* or *Auerbach's plexus* (Fig. 12.2). These nerves supply the adjacent smooth muscle and blood vessels.

Contraction and relaxation of these muscle layers occurs in waves, which push the contents of the tract onwards. This type of contraction of smooth muscle is called *peristalsis* (Fig. 12.4). Muscle contraction also mixes food with the digestive juices. Onward movement of the contents of the tract is controlled at various points by *sphincters*, which are thickened rings of circular muscle. Contraction of sphincters regulates forward movement. They also act as valves, preventing backflow in the tract. This control allows time for digestion and absorption to take place.

Submucosa

This layer consists of loose connective tissue collagen and some elastic fibres. Within it are plexuses of blood vessels and nerves, lymph vessels and varying amounts of lymphoid tissue. The blood vessels are arterioles, venules and capillaries. The nerve plexus is the *submucosal* or *Meissner's plexus* (Fig. 12.2), containing sympathetic and parasympathetic nerves that supply the mucosal lining.

Mucosa

This consists of three layers of tissue:

- *mucous membrane* formed by columnar epithelium is the innermost layer, and has three main functions: *protection, secretion* and *absorption*
- *lamina propria* consisting of loose connective tissue, which supports the blood vessels that nourish the inner epithelial layer, and varying amounts of lymphoid tissue that has a protective function
- *muscularis mucosa*, a thin outer layer of smooth muscle that provides involutions of the mucosa layer, e.g. gastric glands, villi.

Mucous membrane

In parts of the tract that are subject to great wear and tear or mechanical injury, this layer consists of *stratified squamous epithelium* with mucus-secreting glands just below the surface. In areas where the food is already soft and moist and where secretion of digestive juices and absorption occur, the mucous membrane consists of *columnar epithelial cells* interspersed with mucus-secreting goblet cells (Fig. 12.5). Mucus lubricates the walls of the tract and protects them from digestive enzymes. Below the surface in the regions lined with columnar epithelium are collections of specialised cells, or glands, which release their secretions into the lumen of the tract. The secretions include:

- *saliva* from the salivary glands
- *gastric juice* from the gastric glands

285

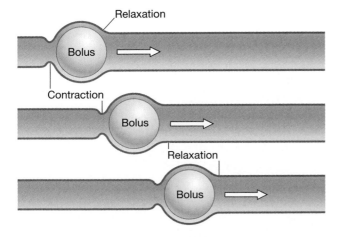

Figure 12.4 Movement of a bolus by peristalsis.

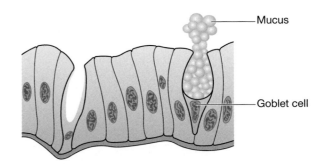

Figure 12.5 Columnar epithelium with goblet cells.

- *intestinal juice* from the intestinal glands
- *pancreatic juice* from the pancreas
- *bile* from the liver.

These are *digestive juices* and most contain enzymes that chemically break down food. Under the epithelial lining are varying amounts of lymphoid tissue.

Nerve supply

The alimentary tract and its related accessory organs are supplied by nerves from both divisions of the autonomic nervous system, i.e. parasympathetic and sympathetic parts (Fig. 12.6). Their actions are antagonistic and one has a greater influence than the other, according to body needs, at any particular time. When digestion is required, this is normally the parasympathetic nervous system.

The parasympathetic supply. One pair of cranial nerves, the *vagus nerves*, provides this supply to most of the alimentary tract and the accessory organs. Sacral nerves supply the most distal part of the tract. The effects of parasympathetic stimulation are:

- increased muscular activity, especially peristalsis, through activity of the myenteric plexus
- increased glandular secretion, through activity of the submucosal plexus (Fig. 12.2).

The sympathetic supply. This is provided by numerous nerves that emerge from the spinal cord in the thoracic and lumbar regions. These form plexuses in the thorax, abdomen and pelvis, from which nerves pass to the organs of the alimentary tract. The effects of sympathetic stimulation are to:

- decrease muscular activity, especially peristalsis, because there is less stimulation of the myenteric plexus
- decrease glandular secretion, as stimulation of the submucosal plexus is reduced.

286

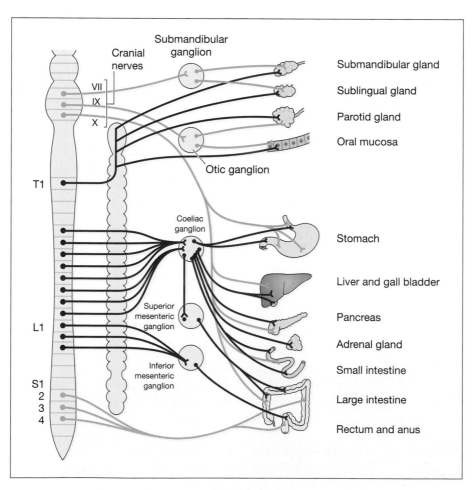

Figure 12.6 Autonomic nerve supply to the digestive system. Parasympathetic – blue; sympathetic – red.

Mouth (Fig. 12.7)

Learning outcomes

After studying this section, you should be able to:

- list the principal structures associated with the mouth

- describe the structure of the mouth

- describe the structure and function of the tongue

- describe the structure and function of the teeth

- outline the arrangement of normal primary and secondary dentition.

The mouth or oral cavity is bounded by muscles and bones:

Anteriorly – by the lips
Posteriorly – it is continuous with the oropharynx
Laterally – by the muscles of the cheeks
Superiorly – by the bony hard palate and muscular soft palate
Inferiorly – by the muscular tongue and the soft tissues of the floor of the mouth.

The oral cavity is lined throughout with *mucous membrane*, consisting of stratified squamous epithelium containing small mucus-secreting glands.

The part of the mouth between the gums and the cheeks is the *vestibule* and the remainder of the cavity is the *oral cavity*. The mucous membrane lining of the cheeks and the lips is reflected onto the gums or

alveolar ridges and is continuous with the skin of the face.

The *palate* forms the roof of the mouth and is divided into the anterior *hard palate* and the posterior *soft palate* (Fig. 12.1). The hard palate is formed by the maxilla and the palatine bones. The soft palate is muscular, curves downwards from the posterior end of the hard palate and blends with the walls of the pharynx at the sides.

The *uvula* is a curved fold of muscle covered with mucous membrane, hanging down from the middle of the free border of the soft palate. Originating from the upper end of the uvula are four folds of mucous membrane, two passing downwards at each side to form membranous arches. The posterior folds, one on each side, are the *palatopharyngeal arches* and the two anterior folds are the *palatoglossal arches*. On each side, between the arches, is a collection of lymphoid tissue called the *palatine tonsil*.

Tongue

The tongue is a voluntary muscular structure that occupies the floor of the mouth. It is attached by its base to the *hyoid bone* (see Fig. 10.4, p. 240) and by a fold of its mucous membrane covering, called the *frenulum*, to the floor of the mouth (Fig. 12.8). The superior surface consists of stratified squamous epithelium, with numerous *papillae* (little projections). These contain sensory receptors (specialised nerve endings) for the sense of taste in the *taste buds* (see Fig. 8.25, p. 205). There are three varieties of papillae (Fig. 12.9).

Vallate papillae, usually between 8 and 12 altogether, are arranged in an inverted V shape towards the base of the tongue. These are the largest of the papillae and are the most easily seen.

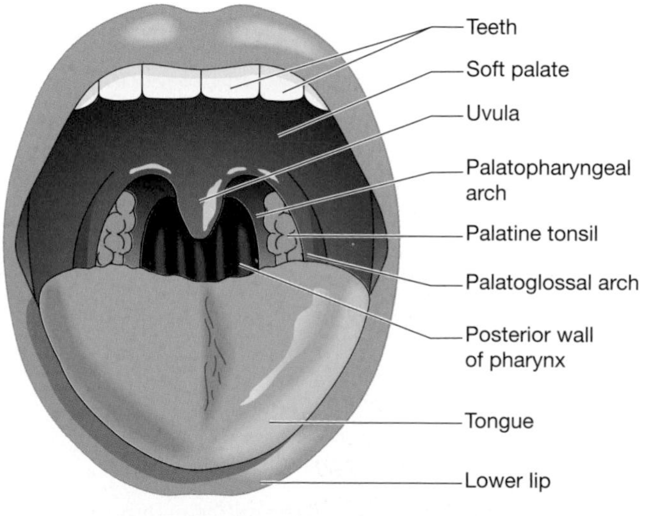

287

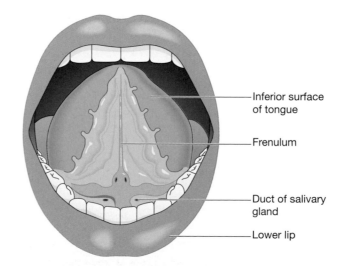

Teeth
Soft palate
Uvula
Palatopharyngeal arch
Palatine tonsil
Palatoglossal arch
Posterior wall of pharynx
Tongue
Lower lip

Inferior surface of tongue
Frenulum
Duct of salivary gland
Lower lip

Figure 12.7 Structures seen in the widely open mouth.

Figure 12.8 The inferior surface of the tongue.

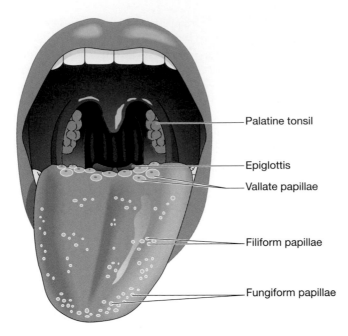

Figure 12.9 **Locations of the papillae of the tongue and related structures.**

Fungiform papillae are situated mainly at the tip and the edges of the tongue and are more numerous than the vallate papillae.

Filiform papillae are the smallest of the three types. They are most numerous on the surface of the anterior two-thirds of the tongue.

Blood supply

The main arterial blood supply to the tongue is by the *lingual branch* of the *external carotid artery*. Venous drainage is by the *lingual vein*, which joins the *internal jugular vein*.

Nerve supply

The nerves involved are:

- the *hypoglossal nerves* (12th cranial nerves), which supply the voluntary muscle
- the *lingual branch of the mandibular nerves*, the nerves of somatic (ordinary) sensation, i.e. pain, temperature and touch
- the *facial* and *glossopharyngeal nerves* (7th and 9th cranial nerves), the nerves of taste.

Functions of the tongue

The tongue plays an important part in:

- mastication (chewing)
- deglutition (swallowing)

- speech (p. 244)
- taste (p. 205).

Nerve endings of the sense of taste are present in the papillae and widely distributed in the epithelium of the tongue, soft palate, pharynx and epiglottis.

Teeth

The teeth are embedded in the alveoli or sockets of the alveolar ridges of the mandible and the maxilla (Fig. 12.10). Babies are born with two sets, or *dentitions*, the *temporary* or *deciduous teeth* and the *permanent teeth* (Figs 12.11 and 12.12). At birth the teeth of both dentitions are present, in immature form, in the mandible and maxilla.

There are 20 temporary teeth, 10 in each jaw. They begin to erupt when the child is about 6 months old, and should all be present by 24 months (Table 12.1).

The permanent teeth begin to replace the deciduous teeth in the 6th year of age and this dentition, consisting of 32 teeth, is usually complete by the 24th year.

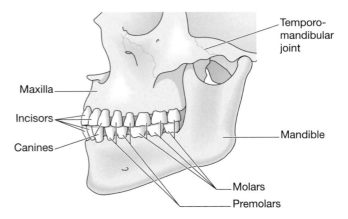

Figure 12.10 **The permanent teeth and the jaw bones.**

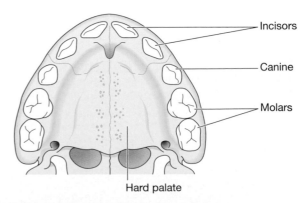

Figure 12.11 **The roof of the mouth and the deciduous teeth –** viewed from below.

288

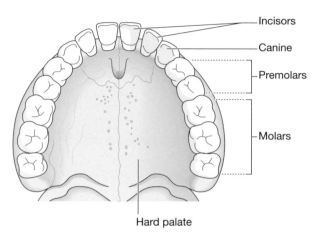

Figure 12.12 **The roof of the mouth and the permanent teeth –** viewed from below.

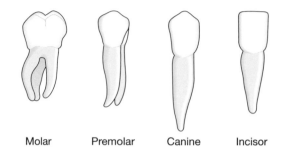

Figure 12.13 **The shapes of the permanent teeth.**

Functions of the teeth

The *incisor* and *canine* teeth are the cutting teeth and are used for biting off pieces of food, whereas the *premolar* and *molar* teeth, with broad, flat surfaces, are used for grinding or chewing food (Fig. 12.13).

Structure of a tooth (Fig. 12.14)

Although the shapes of the different teeth vary, the structure is the same and consists of:

- *the crown* – the part that protrudes from the gum
- *the root* – the part embedded in the bone
- *the neck* – the slightly narrowed region where the crown merges with the root.

In the centre of the tooth is the *pulp cavity* containing blood vessels, lymph vessels and nerves, and surrounding this is a hard ivory-like substance called *dentine*. Outside the dentine of the crown is a thin layer of very hard substance, the *enamel*. The root of the tooth, on the other hand, is covered with a substance resembling bone,

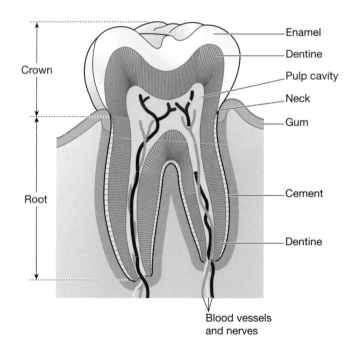

Figure 12.14 **A section of a tooth.**

289

Table 12.1 Deciduous and permanent dentitions								
Jaw	Molars	Premolars	Canine	Incisors	Incisors	Canine	Premolars	Molars
Deciduous teeth								
Upper	2	–	1	2	2	1	–	2
Lower	2	–	1	2	2	1	–	2
Permanent teeth								
Upper	3	2	1	2	2	1	2	3
Lower	3	2	1	2	2	1	2	3

called *cement*, which secures the tooth in its socket. Blood vessels and nerves pass to the tooth through a small foramen at the apex of each root.

Blood supply

Most of the arterial blood supply to the teeth is by branches of the *maxillary arteries*. The venous drainage is by a number of veins which empty into the *internal jugular veins*.

Nerve supply

The nerve supply to the upper teeth is by branches of the *maxillary nerves* and to the lower teeth by branches of the *mandibular nerves*. These are both branches of the *trigeminal nerves* (5th cranial nerves) (see p. 168).

Salivary glands (Fig. 12.15)

Learning outcomes

After studying this section, you should be able to:

■ describe the structure and the function of the principal salivary glands

■ explain the role of saliva in digestion.

Salivary glands release their secretions into ducts that lead to the mouth. There are three main pairs: the parotid glands, the submandibular glands and the sublingual glands. There are also numerous smaller salivary glands scattered around the mouth.

Parotid glands

These are situated one on each side of the face just below the external acoustic meatus (see Fig. 8.1, p. 190). Each gland has a *parotid duct* opening into the mouth at the level of the second upper molar tooth.

Submandibular glands

These lie one on each side of the face under the angle of the jaw. The two *submandibular ducts* open on the floor of the mouth, one on each side of the frenulum of the tongue.

Sublingual glands

These glands lie under the mucous membrane of the floor of the mouth in front of the submandibular glands. They have numerous small ducts that open into the floor of the mouth.

Structure of the salivary glands

The glands are all surrounded by a *fibrous capsule*. They consist of a number of *lobules* made up of small acini lined with *secretory cells* (Fig. 12.15B). The secretions are poured

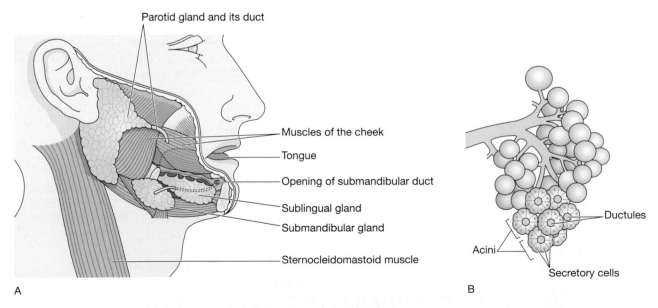

Figure 12.15 A. The position of the salivary glands. **B.** Enlargement of part of a gland.

into ductules that join up to form larger ducts leading into the mouth.

Blood supply

Arterial supply is by various branches from the external carotid arteries and venous drainage is into the external jugular veins.

Composition of saliva

Saliva is the combined secretions from the salivary glands and the small mucus-secreting glands of the oral mucosa. About 1.5 litres of saliva is produced daily and it consists of:

- water
- mineral salts
- an enzyme: salivary amylase
- mucus
- lysozyme
- immunoglobulins
- blood-clotting factors.

Secretion of saliva

Secretion of saliva is under autonomic nerve control. Parasympathetic stimulation causes vasodilatation and profuse secretion of watery saliva with a relatively low content of enzymes and other organic substances. Sympathetic stimulation causes vasoconstriction and secretion of small amounts of saliva rich in organic material, especially from the submandibular glands. Reflex secretion occurs when there is food in the mouth and the reflex can easily become *conditioned* so that the sight, smell and even the thought of food stimulates the flow of saliva.

Functions of saliva

Chemical digestion of polysaccharides. Saliva contains the enzyme *amylase* that begins the breakdown of complex sugars, including starches, reducing them to the disaccharide maltose. The optimum pH for the action of salivary amylase is 6.8 (slightly acid). Salivary pH ranges from 5.8 to 7.4 depending on the rate of flow; the higher the flow rate, the higher is the pH. Enzyme action continues during swallowing until terminated by the strongly acidic pH (1.5 to 1.8) of the gastric juices, which degrades the amylase.

Lubrication of food. Dry food entering the mouth is moistened and lubricated by saliva before it can be made into a bolus ready for swallowing.

Cleaning and lubricating. An adequate flow of saliva is necessary to clean the mouth, and to keep it soft, moist and pliable. It helps to prevent damage to the mucous membrane by rough or abrasive food.

Non-specific defence. Lysozyme, immunoglobulins and clotting factors combat invading microbes.

Taste. The taste buds are stimulated only by chemical substances in solution and therefore dry foods only stimulate the sense of taste after thorough mixing with saliva. The senses of taste and smell are closely linked and involved in the enjoyment, or otherwise, of food.

Pharynx

Learning outcome

After studying this section, you should be able to:

- describe the structure of the pharynx.

The pharynx is divided for descriptive purpose into three parts, the nasopharynx, oropharynx and laryngopharynx (see p. 240). The nasopharynx is important in respiration. The oropharynx and laryngopharynx are passages common to both the respiratory and the digestive systems. Food passes from the oral cavity into the pharynx then to the oesophagus below, with which it is continuous. The walls of the pharynx consist of three layers of tissue.

The lining membrane (mucosa) is stratified squamous epithelium, continuous with the lining of the mouth at one end and the oesophagus at the other.

The middle layer consists of fibrous tissue which becomes thinner towards the lower end and contains blood and lymph vessels and nerves.

The outer layer consists of a number of involuntary muscles that are involved in swallowing. When food reaches the pharynx swallowing is no longer under voluntary control.

Blood supply

The blood supply to the pharynx is by several branches of the facial arteries. Venous drainage is into the facial veins and the internal jugular veins.

Nerve supply

This is from the pharyngeal plexus and consists of parasympathetic and sympathetic nerves. Parasympathetic supply is mainly by the glossopharyngeal and vagus nerves and sympathetic from the cervical ganglia.

Oesophagus (Fig. 12.16)

Learning outcomes

After studying this section, you should be able to:

■ describe the location of the oesophagus

■ outline the structure of the oesophagus

■ explain the mechanisms involved in swallowing, and the route taken by a bolus.

The oesophagus is about 25 cm long and about 2 cm in diameter and lies in the median plane in the thorax in front of the vertebral column behind the trachea and the heart. It is continuous with the pharynx above and just below the diaphragm it joins the stomach. It passes between muscle fibres of the diaphragm behind the central tendon at the level of the 10th thoracic vertebra.

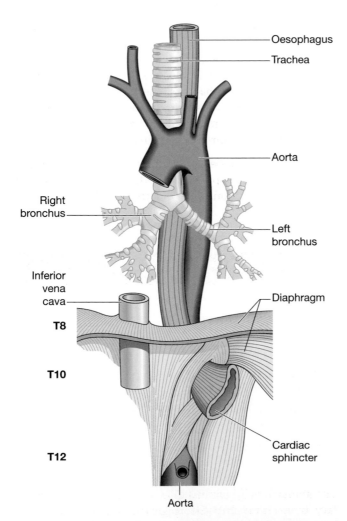

Figure 12.16 The oesophagus and some related structures.

Immediately the oesophagus has passed through the diaphragm it curves upwards before opening into the stomach. This sharp angle is believed to be one of the factors that prevents the regurgitation (backflow) of gastric contents into the oesophagus. The upper and lower ends of the oesophagus are closed by sphincters. The upper *cricopharyngeal* or *upper oesophageal sphincter* prevents air passing into the oesophagus during inspiration and the aspiration of oesophageal contents. The *cardiac* or *lower oesophageal sphincter* prevents the reflux of acid gastric contents into the oesophagus. There is no thickening of the circular muscle in this area and this sphincter is therefore 'physiological', i.e. this region can act as a sphincter without the presence of the anatomical features. When intra-abdominal pressure is raised, e.g. during inspiration and defaecation, the tone of the lower oesophageal sphincter increases. There is an added pinching effect by the contracting muscle fibres of the diaphragm.

Structure

There are four layers of tissue as shown in Figure 12.2. As the oesophagus is almost entirely in the thorax the outer covering, the adventitia, consists of *elastic fibrous tissue* that attaches the oesophagus to the surrounding structures. The proximal third is lined by stratified squamous epithelium and the distal third by columnar epithelium. The middle third is lined by a mixture of the two.

Blood supply

Arterial. The thoracic region is supplied mainly by the paired oesophageal arteries, branches from the thoracic aorta. The abdominal region is supplied by branches from the inferior phrenic arteries and the left gastric branch of the coeliac artery.

Venous drainage. From the thoracic region venous drainage is into the azygos and hemiazygos veins. The abdominal part drains into the left gastric vein. There is a venous plexus at the distal end that links the upward and downward venous drainage, i.e. the general and portal circulations.

Functions of the mouth, pharynx and oesophagus

Formation of a bolus. When food is taken into the mouth it is masticated, or chewed, by the teeth and moved round the mouth by the tongue and muscles of the cheeks (Fig. 12.17). It is mixed with saliva and formed into a soft mass or bolus ready for swallowing. The length of time that food remains in the mouth depends, to a large extent, on the consistency of the food. Some foods

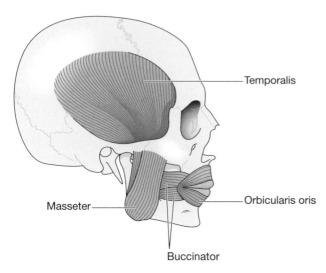

Figure 12.17 The muscles used in chewing.

need to be chewed longer than others before the individual feels that the bolus is ready for swallowing.

Swallowing (deglutition) (Fig. 12.18). This occurs in three stages after mastication is complete and the bolus has been formed. It is initiated voluntarily but completed by a reflex (involuntary) action.

1. The mouth is closed and the voluntary muscles of the tongue and cheeks push the bolus backwards into the pharynx.
2. The muscles of the pharynx are stimulated by a reflex action initiated in the walls of the oropharynx and

coordinated in the medulla and lower pons in the brain stem. Involuntary contraction of these muscles propels the bolus down into the oesophagus. All other routes that the bolus could take are closed. The soft palate rises up and closes off the nasopharynx; the tongue and the pharyngeal folds block the way back into the mouth; and the larynx is lifted up and forward so that its opening is occluded by the overhanging epiglottis preventing entry into the airway (trachea).

3. The presence of the bolus in the pharynx stimulates a wave of peristalsis that propels the bolus through the oesophagus to the stomach.

Peristaltic waves pass along the oesophagus only after swallowing begins (see Fig. 12.4). Otherwise the walls are relaxed. Ahead of a peristaltic wave, the cardiac sphincter guarding the entrance to the stomach relaxes to allow the descending bolus to pass into the stomach. Usually, constriction of the cardiac sphincter prevents reflux of gastric acid into the oesophagus. Other factors preventing gastric reflux include:

- the attachment of the stomach to the diaphragm by the peritoneum
- the maintenance of an acute angle between the oesophagus and the fundus of the stomach, i.e. an acute cardio-oesophageal angle
- increased tone of the cardiac sphincter when intra-abdominal pressure is increased and the pinching effect of diaphragm muscle fibres.

The walls of the oesophagus are lubricated by mucus which assists the passage of the bolus during the peristaltic contraction of the muscular wall.

293

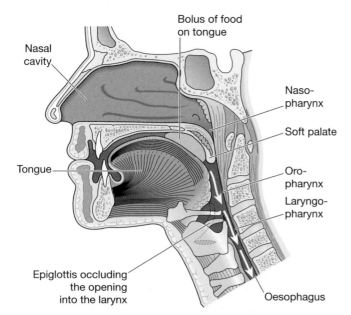

Figure 12.18 Section of the face and neck showing the positions of structures during swallowing.

Stomach

Learning outcomes

After studying this section, you should be able to:

- describe the location of the stomach with reference to surrounding structures

- explain the physiological significance of the layers of the stomach wall

- discuss the digestive functions of the stomach.

The stomach is a J-shaped dilated portion of the alimentary tract situated in the epigastric, umbilical and left hypochondriac regions of the abdominal cavity.

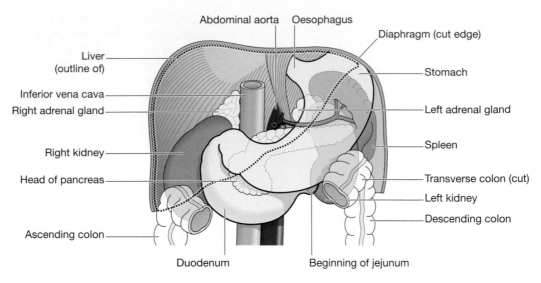

Figure 12.19 **The stomach and its associated structures.**

Organs associated with the stomach

(Fig. 12.19)

Anteriorly – left lobe of liver and anterior abdominal wall

Posteriorly – abdominal aorta, pancreas, spleen, left kidney and adrenal gland

Superiorly – diaphragm, oesophagus and left lobe of liver

Inferiorly – transverse colon and small intestine

To the left – diaphragm and spleen

To the right – liver and duodenum.

Structure of the stomach (Fig. 12.20)

The stomach is continuous with the oesophagus at the cardiac sphincter and with the duodenum at the pyloric sphincter. It has two curvatures. The *lesser curvature* is short, lies on the posterior surface of the stomach and is the downward continuation of the posterior wall of the oesophagus. Just before the pyloric sphincter it curves upwards to complete the J shape. Where the oesophagus joins the stomach the anterior region angles acutely upwards, curves downwards forming the *greater curvature* and then slightly upwards towards the pyloric sphincter.

The stomach is divided into three regions: the fundus, the body and the antrum. At the distal end of the pyloric antrum is the pyloric sphincter, guarding the opening between the stomach and the duodenum. When the stomach is inactive the pyloric sphincter is relaxed and open, and when the stomach contains food the sphincter is closed.

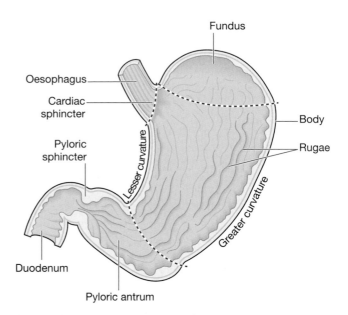

Figure 12.20 **Longitudinal section of the stomach.**

Walls of the stomach

The four layers of tissue that comprise the basic structure of the alimentary canal (Fig. 12.2) are found in the stomach but with some modifications.

Muscle layer (Fig. 12.21). This consists of three layers of smooth muscle fibres:

- an outer layer of longitudinal fibres
- a middle layer of circular fibres
- an inner layer of oblique fibres.

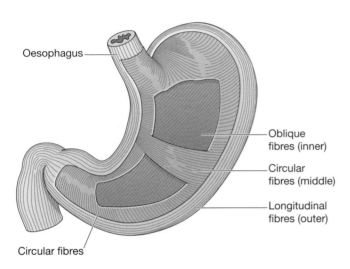

Figure 12.21 The muscle fibres of the stomach wall. Sections have been removed to show the three layers.

In this respect, the stomach is different from other regions of the alimentary tract as it has three layers of muscle instead of two.

This arrangement allows for the churning motion characteristic of gastric activity, as well as peristaltic movement. Circular muscle is strongest in the pyloric antrum and sphincter.

Mucosa. When the stomach is empty the mucous membrane lining is thrown into longitudinal folds or *rugae*, and when full the rugae are 'ironed out' and the surface has a smooth, velvety appearance. Numerous *gastric glands* are situated below the surface in the mucous membrane. They consist of specialised cells that secrete *gastric juice* into the stomach.

Blood supply

Arterial supply to the stomach is by the left gastric artery, a branch of the coeliac artery, the right gastric artery and the gastroepiploic arteries. Venous drainage is through veins of corresponding names into the portal vein. Figures 5.44 and 5.46 show these vessels.

Gastric juice and functions of the stomach

Stomach size varies with the volume of food it contains, which may be 1.5 litres or more in an adult. When a meal has been eaten the food accumulates in the stomach in layers, the last part of the meal remaining in the fundus for some time. Mixing with the gastric juice takes place gradually and it may be some time before the food is sufficiently acidified to stop the action of salivary amylase.

Gastric muscle contraction consists of a churning movement that breaks down the bolus and mixes it with gastric juice, and peristaltic waves that propel the stomach contents towards the pylorus. When the stomach is active the pyloric sphincter closes. Strong peristaltic contraction of the pyloric antrum forces *chyme*, gastric contents after they are sufficiently liquefied, through the pylorus into the duodenum in small spurts. Parasympathetic stimulation increases the motility of the stomach and secretion of gastric juice; sympathetic stimulation has the opposite effect.

Gastric juice

About 2 litres of gastric juice are secreted daily by specialised secretory glands in the mucosa (Fig. 12.22). It consists of:

- water
- mineral salts } secreted by gastric glands
- mucus secreted by goblet cells in the glands and on the stomach surface
- hydrochloric acid
- intrinsic factor } secreted by *parietal cells* in the gastric glands
- inactive enzyme precursors: pepsinogens secreted by *chief cells* in the glands.

Functions of gastric juice

- *Water* further liquefies the food swallowed.
- *Hydrochloric acid*:
  - acidifies the food and stops the action of salivary amylase

295

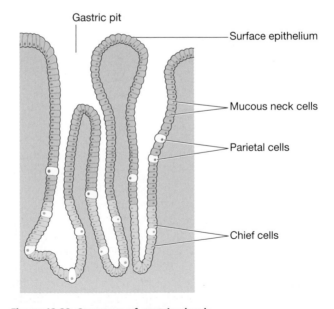

Figure 12.22 Structure of gastric glands.

- kills ingested microbes
- provides the acid environment needed for effective digestion by pepsins.
- *Pepsinogens* are activated to *pepsins* by hydrochloric acid and by pepsins already present in the stomach. They begin the digestion of proteins, breaking them into smaller molecules. Pepsins act most effectively at pH 1.5 to 3.5.
- *Intrinsic factor* (a protein) is necessary for the absorption of vitamin B$_{12}$ from the ileum.
- *Mucus* prevents mechanical injury to the stomach wall by lubricating the contents. It prevents chemical injury by acting as a barrier between the stomach wall and the corrosive gastric juice. Hydrochloric acid is present in potentially damaging concentrations and pepsins digest protein.

Secretion of gastric juice

There is always a small quantity of gastric juice present in the stomach, even when it contains no food. This is known as *fasting juice*. Secretion reaches its maximum level about 1 hour after a meal then declines to the fasting level after about 4 hours.

There are three phases of secretion of gastric juice (Fig. 12.23).

1. *Cephalic phase.* This flow of juice occurs before food reaches the stomach and is due to reflex stimulation of the vagus (parasympathetic) nerves initiated by the sight, smell or taste of food. When the vagus nerves have been cut (vagotomy) this phase of gastric secretion stops. Sympathetic stimulation, e.g. during emotional states, also inhibits gastric activity.
2. *Gastric phase.* When stimulated by the presence of food the *enteroendocrine cells* in the pyloric antrum and duodenum secrete *gastrin*, a hormone which passes directly into the circulating blood. Gastrin, circulating in the blood which supplies the stomach, stimulates the gastric glands to produce more gastric juice. In this way secretion of digestive juice is continued after completion of a meal and the end of the cephalic phase. Gastrin secretion is suppressed when the pH in the pyloric antrum falls to about 1.5.
3. *Intestinal phase.* When the partially digested contents of the stomach reach the small intestine, two hormones, *secretin* and *cholecystokinin*, are produced by endocrine cells in the intestinal mucosa. They slow down the secretion of gastric juice and reduce gastric motility. By slowing the emptying rate of the stomach, the chyme in the duodenum becomes more thoroughly mixed with bile and pancreatic juice. This phase of gastric secretion is most marked following a meal with a high fat content.

The rate at which the stomach empties depends largely on the type of food eaten. A carbohydrate meal leaves the stomach in 2 to 3 hours, a protein meal remains longer and a fatty meal remains in the stomach longest.

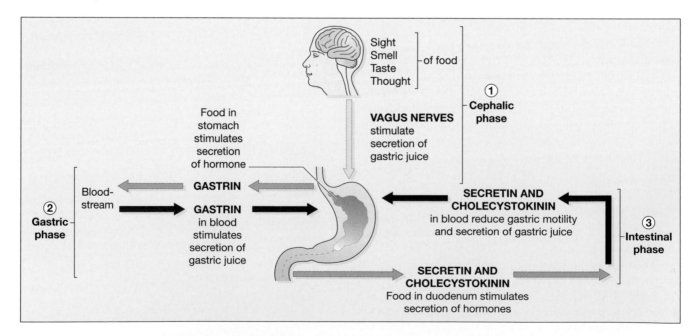

Figure 12.23 The three phases of secretion of gastric juice.

Functions of the stomach

These include:

- temporary storage allowing time for the digestive enzymes, pepsins, to act
- chemical digestion – pepsins convert proteins to polypeptides
- mechanical breakdown – the three smooth muscle layers enable the stomach to act as a churn, gastric juice is added and the contents are liquefied to chyme. Motility and secretion are increased by parasympathetic nerve stimulation
- limited absorption of water, alcohol and some lipid-soluble drugs
- non-specific defence against microbes – provided by hydrochloric acid in gastric juice. Vomiting may occur in response to ingestion of gastric irritants, e.g. microbes or chemicals
- preparation of iron for absorption further along the tract – the acid environment of the stomach solubilises iron salts, which is required before iron can be absorbed
- production and secretion of intrinsic factor needed for absorption of vitamin B_{12} in the terminal ileum
- regulation of the passage of gastric contents into the duodenum. When the chyme is sufficiently acidified and liquefied, the pyloric antrum forces small jets of gastric contents through the pyloric sphincter into the duodenum. The sphincter is normally closed, preventing backflow of chyme into the stomach
- secretion of the hormone gastrin (p. 296).

Small intestine (Figs 12.24 and 12.25)

Learning outcomes

After studying this section, you should be able to:

- describe the location of the small intestine, with reference to surrounding structures
- sketch a villus, labelling its component parts
- discuss the digestive functions of the small intestine and its secretions
- explain how nutrients are absorbed in the small intestine.

The small intestine is continuous with the stomach at the pyloric sphincter and leads into the large intestine at the *ileocaecal valve*. It is a little over 5 metres long and lies in the abdominal cavity surrounded by the large intestine. In the small intestine the chemical digestion of food is completed and most of the absorption of nutrients takes place.

The small intestine comprises three main sections continuous with each other.

The *duodenum* is about 25 cm long and curves around the head of the pancreas. Secretions from the gall bladder and pancreas are released into the duodenum through a common structure, the hepatopancreatic ampulla, and the opening into the duodenum is guarded by the hepatopancreatic sphincter (of Oddi) (see Fig. 12.39).

297

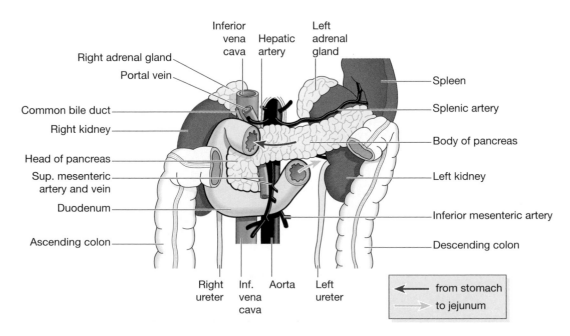

Figure 12.24 The duodenum and its associated structures.

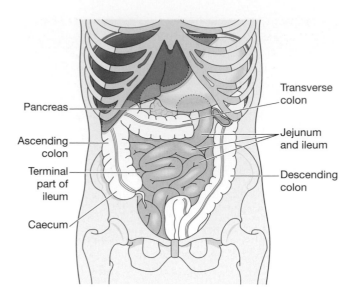

Figure 12.25 The jejunum and ileum and their related structures.

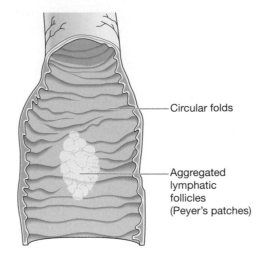

Figure 12.26 Section of a small piece of small intestine (opened out), showing the permanent circular folds.

The *jejunum* is the middle section of the small intestine and is about 2 metres long.

The *ileum*, or terminal section, is about 3 metres long and ends at the ileocaecal valve, which controls the flow of material from the ileum to the *caecum*, the first part of the large intestine, and prevents regurgitation.

Structure of the small intestine

The walls of the small intestine are composed of the four layers of tissue shown in Figure 12.2. Some modifications of the peritoneum and mucosa (mucous membrane lining) are described below.

Peritoneum. A double layer of peritoneum called the *mesentery* attaches the jejunum and ileum to the posterior abdominal wall (see Fig. 12.3A). The attachment is quite short in comparison with the length of the small intestine, therefore it is fan shaped. The large blood vessels and nerves lie on the posterior abdominal wall and the branches to the small intestine pass between the two layers of the mesentery.

Mucosa. The surface area of the small intestine mucosa is greatly increased by permanent circular folds, villi and microvilli.

The *permanent circular folds*, unlike the rugae of the stomach, are not smoothed out when the small intestine is distended (Fig. 12.26). They promote mixing of chyme as it passes along.

The *villi* are tiny finger-like projections of the mucosal layer into the intestinal lumen, about 0.5 to 1 mm long

(Fig. 12.27). Their walls consist of columnar epithelial cells, or *enterocytes*, with tiny *microvilli* (1 μm long) on their free border. *Goblet cells* that secrete mucus are interspersed between the enterocytes. These epithelial cells enclose a network of blood and lymph capillaries.

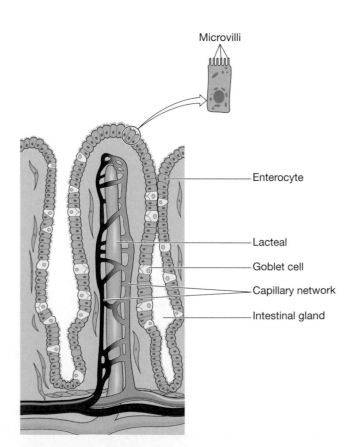

Figure 12.27 A highly magnified view of one complete villus in the small intestine.

298

The lymph capillaries are called *lacteals* because absorbed fat gives the lymph a milky appearance. Absorption and some final stages of digestion of nutrients take place in the enterocytes before entering the blood and lymph capillaries.

The *intestinal glands* are simple tubular glands situated below the surface between the villi. The cells of the glands migrate upwards to form the walls of the villi replacing those at the tips as they are rubbed off by the intestinal contents. The entire epithelium is replaced every 3 to 5 days. During migration, the cells form digestive enzymes that lodge in the microvilli and, together with intestinal juice, complete the chemical digestion of carbohydrates, protein and fats.

Numerous *lymph nodes* are found in the mucosa at irregular intervals throughout the length of the small intestine. The smaller ones are known as *solitary lymphatic follicles*, and about 20 or 30 larger nodes situated towards the distal end of the ileum are called *aggregated lymphatic follicles* (Peyer's patches, Fig. 12.26). These lymphatic tissues, packed with defensive cells, are strategically placed to neutralise ingested antigens (Ch. 15).

Blood supply

The *superior mesenteric artery* supplies the whole of the small intestine, and venous drainage is by the *superior mesenteric vein* that joins other veins to form the portal vein (see Figs 5.45 and 5.46). The portal vein contains a high concentration of absorbed nutrients and this blood passes through the liver before entering the hepatic veins, and, ultimately, into the inferior vena cava (see Fig. 12.37).

Intestinal juice

About 1500 ml of intestinal juice are secreted daily by the glands of the small intestine. It consists of:

- water
- mucus
- mineral salts.

The pH of intestinal juice is usually between 7.8 and 8.0.

Functions of the small intestine

The functions are:

- onward movement of its contents by peristalsis, which is increased by parasympathetic stimulation
- secretion of intestinal juice, also increased by parasympathetic stimulation
- completion of chemical digestion of carbohydrates, protein and fats in the enterocytes of the villi
- protection against infection by microbes that have survived the antimicrobial action of the hydrochloric

acid in the stomach, by the solitary lymph follicles and aggregated lymph follicles
- secretion of the hormones cholecystokinin (CCK) and secretin
- absorption of nutrients.

Chemical digestion in the small intestine

When acid chyme passes into the small intestine it is mixed with *pancreatic juice, bile* and *intestinal juice*, and is in contact with the enterocytes of the villi. In the small intestine digestion of all the nutrients is completed:

- carbohydrates are broken down to monosaccharides
- proteins are broken down to amino acids
- fats are broken down to fatty acids and glycerol.

Pancreatic juice

Pancreatic juice enters the duodenum at the hepato-pancreatic sphincter and consists of:

- water
- mineral salts
- enzymes:
  - amylase
  - lipase
- inactive enzyme precursors:
  - trypsinogen
  - chymotrypsinogen
  - procarboxypeptidase.

Pancreatic juice is alkaline (pH 8) because it contains significant quantities of bicarbonate ions, which are alkaline in solution. When acid stomach contents enter the duodenum they are mixed with pancreatic juice and bile and the pH is raised to between 6 and 8. This is the pH at which the pancreatic enzymes, amylase and lipase, act most effectively.

Functions
Digestion of proteins. Trypsinogen and chymotrypsinogen are inactive enzyme precursors activated by *enterokinase*, an enzyme in the microvilli, which converts them into the active proteolytic enzymes *trypsin* and *chymotrypsin*. These enzymes convert polypeptides to tripeptides, dipeptides and amino acids. It is important that they are produced as inactive precursors and are activated only upon arrival in the duodenum, otherwise they would digest the pancreas.

Digestion of carbohydrates. *Pancreatic amylase* converts all digestible polysaccharides (starches) not acted upon by salivary amylase to disaccharides.

299

Digestion of fats. *Lipase* converts fats to fatty acids and glycerol. To aid the action of lipase, *bile salts* emulsify fats, i.e. reduce the size of the globules, increasing their surface area.

Control of secretion

The secretion of pancreatic juice is stimulated by secretin and CCK, produced by endocrine cells in the walls of the duodenum. The presence in the duodenum of acid chyme from the stomach stimulates the production of these hormones.

Bile

Bile, secreted by the liver, is unable to enter the duodenum when the hepatopancreatic sphincter is closed; therefore it passes from the *hepatic duct* along the *cystic duct* to the gall bladder where it is stored (see Fig. 12.39).

Bile has a pH of around 8 and between 500 and 1000 ml are secreted daily. It consists of:

- water
- mineral salts
- mucus
- bile salts
- bile pigments, mainly bilirubin
- cholesterol.

Functions

- The bile salts emulsify fats in the small intestine.
- Fatty acids are insoluble in water, which makes them very difficult to absorb through the intestinal wall. Bile salts make cholesterol and fatty acids soluble, enabling both these and fat-soluble vitamins (i.e. vitamins A, D, E and K) to be readily absorbed.
- The bile pigment, *bilirubin*, is a waste product of the breakdown of erythrocytes and is excreted in the bile rather than in the urine because of its low solubility in water. Bilirubin is altered by microbes in the large intestine. Some of the resultant *urobilinogen*, which is highly water soluble, is reabsorbed and then excreted in the urine, but most is converted to *stercobilin* and excreted in the faeces.
- Stercobilin colours and deodorises the faeces.

Release from the gall bladder

When a meal has been eaten the duodenum secretes the hormones secretin and CCK during the intestinal phase of gastric secretion (p. 296). They stimulate contraction of the gall bladder and relaxation of the hepatopancreatic sphincter, enabling the bile and pancreatic juice to pass into the duodenum together. Secretion is markedly increased when chyme entering the duodenum contains a high proportion of fat.

Intestinal secretions

The principal constituents of intestinal secretions are water, mucus and mineral salts.

Most of the digestive enzymes in the small intestine are contained in the enterocytes of the walls of the villi. Digestion of carbohydrate, protein and fat is completed by direct contact between these nutrients and the microvilli and within the enterocytes. The enzymes that complete chemical digestion of food in the enterocytes are:

- peptidases
- lipase
- sucrase, maltase and lactase.

Chemical digestion associated with enterocytes

Alkaline intestinal juice (pH 7.8 to 8.0) assists in raising the pH of the intestinal contents to between 6.5 and 7.5.

Enterokinase activates pancreatic peptidases such as trypsin which convert some polypeptides to amino acids and some to smaller peptides. The final stage of breakdown, to amino acids, of all peptides occurs inside the enterocytes.

Lipase completes the digestion of emulsified fats to *fatty acids* and *glycerol* partly in the intestine and partly in the enterocytes.

Sucrase, maltase and *lactase* complete the digestion of carbohydrates by converting disaccharides such as sucrose, maltose and lactose to monosaccharides inside the enterocytes.

Control of secretion

Mechanical stimulation of the intestinal glands by chyme is believed to be the main stimulus for the secretion of intestinal juice, although the hormone secretin may also be involved.

Absorption of nutrients (Fig. 12.28)

Absorption of nutrients occurs by two main processes:

- *Diffusion.* Monosaccharides, amino acids, fatty acids and glycerol diffuse slowly down their concentration gradients into the enterocytes from the intestinal lumen.
- *Active transport.* Monosaccharides, amino acids, fatty acids and glycerol may be actively transported into the villi; this is faster than diffusion. Disaccharides, dipeptides and tripeptides are also actively transported into the enterocytes where their digestion is completed before transfer into the capillaries of the villi.

Monosaccharides and amino acids pass into the capillaries in the villi and fatty acids and glycerol into the lacteals.

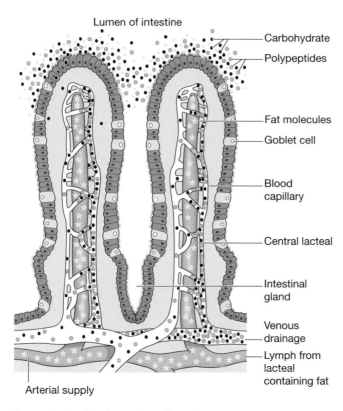

Figure 12.28 **The absorption of nutrients.**

Some proteins are absorbed unchanged, e.g. antibodies present in breast milk and oral vaccines, such as poliomyelitis vaccine. The extent of protein absorption is believed to be limited.

Other nutrients such as vitamins, mineral salts and water are also absorbed from the small intestine into the blood capillaries. Fat-soluble vitamins are absorbed into the lacteals along with fatty acids and glycerol. Vitamin B_{12} combines with intrinsic factor in the stomach and is actively absorbed in the terminal ileum.

The surface area through which absorption takes place in the small intestine is greatly increased by the circular folds of mucous membrane and by the very large number of villi and microvilli present. It has been calculated that the surface area of the small intestine is about five times that of the whole body.

Large amounts of fluid enter the alimentary tract each day (Fig. 12.29). Of this, only about 1500 ml is not absorbed by the small intestine, and passes into the large intestine.

Large intestine (colon), rectum and anal canal

Learning outcomes

After studying this section, you should be able to:

- identify the different sections of the large intestine

- describe the structure and functions of the large intestine, the rectum and the anal canal.

301

The large intestine. This is about 1.5 metres long, beginning at the *caecum* in the right iliac fossa and terminating at the *rectum* and *anal canal* deep in the pelvis.

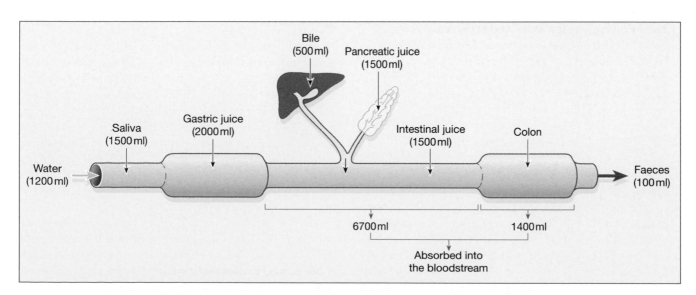

Figure 12.29 **Average volumes of fluid ingested, secreted, absorbed and eliminated from the gastrointestinal tract daily.**

Its lumen is about 6.5 cm in diameter, larger than that of the small intestine. It forms an arch round the coiled-up small intestine (Fig. 12.30).

For descriptive purposes the colon is divided into the caecum, ascending colon, transverse colon, descending colon, sigmoid colon, rectum and anal canal.

The caecum. This is the first part of the colon (Fig. 12.31). It is a dilated region which has a blind end inferiorly and is continuous with the ascending colon superiorly. Just below the junction of the two the *ileocaecal valve* opens from the ileum. The *vermiform appendix* is a fine tube, closed at one end, which leads from the caecum. It is usually about 8 to 9 cm long and has the same structure as the walls of the colon but contains more lymphoid tissue.

The ascending colon. This passes upwards from the caecum to the level of the liver where it curves acutely to the left at the *hepatic flexure* to become the transverse colon.

The transverse colon. This is a loop of colon that extends across the abdominal cavity in front of the duodenum and the stomach to the area of the spleen where it forms the *splenic flexure* and curves acutely downwards to become the descending colon.

The descending colon. This passes down the left side of the abdominal cavity then curves towards the midline. After it enters the true pelvis it is known as the sigmoid colon.

The sigmoid colon. This part describes an S-shaped curve in the pelvis that continues downwards to become the rectum.

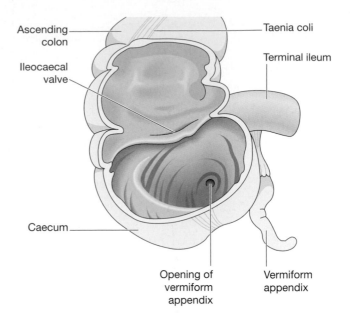

Figure 12.31 Interior of the caecum.

The rectum. This is a slightly dilated section of the colon about 13 cm long. It leads from the sigmoid colon and terminates in the anal canal.

The anal canal. This is a short passage about 3.8 cm long in the adult and leads from the rectum to the exterior. Two sphincter muscles control the anus; the *internal sphincter*, consisting of smooth muscle, is under the control of the autonomic nervous system and the *external sphincter*, formed by skeletal muscle, is under voluntary control (Fig. 12.32).

Structure

The four layers of tissue described in the basic structure of the gastrointestinal tract (Fig. 12.2) are present in the colon, the rectum and the anal canal. The arrangement of the longitudinal muscle fibres is modified in the colon. They do not form a smooth continuous layer of tissue but are instead collected into three bands, called *taeniae coli*, situated at regular intervals round the colon. They stop at the junction of the sigmoid colon and the rectum. As these bands of muscle tissue are slightly shorter than the total length of the colon they give it a sacculated or puckered appearance (Fig. 12.32).

The longitudinal muscle fibres spread out as in the basic structure and completely surround the rectum and the anal canal. The anal sphincters are formed by thickening of the circular muscle layer.

In the submucosal layer there is more lymphoid tissue than in any other part of the alimentary tract, providing

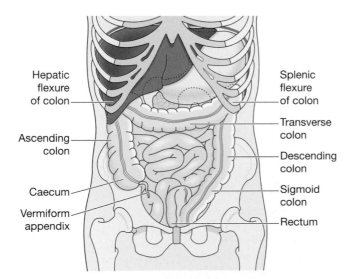

Figure 12.30 The parts of the large intestine (colon) and their positions.

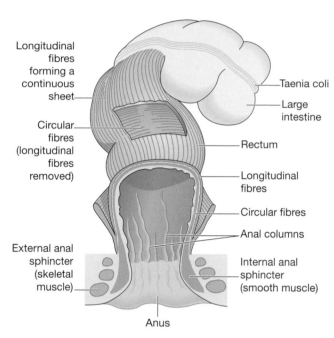

Figure 12.32 Arrangement of muscle fibres in the colon, rectum and anus. Sections have been removed to show the layers.

Labels (left): Longitudinal fibres forming a continuous sheet; Circular fibres (longitudinal fibres removed); External anal sphincter (skeletal muscle)

Labels (right): Taenia coli; Large intestine; Rectum; Longitudinal fibres; Circular fibres; Anal columns; Internal anal sphincter (smooth muscle)

Bottom label: Anus

non-specific defence against invasion by resident and other microbes.

In the mucosal lining of the colon and the upper region of the rectum are large numbers of goblet cells forming simple tubular glands, which secrete mucus. They are not present beyond the junction between the rectum and the anal canal.

The lining membrane of the anal canal consists of stratified squamous epithelium continuous with the mucous membrane lining of the rectum above and which merges with the skin beyond the external anal sphincter. In the upper section of the anal canal the mucous membrane is arranged in 6 to 10 vertical folds, the *anal columns*. Each column contains a terminal branch of the superior rectal artery and vein.

Blood supply

Arterial supply is mainly by the superior and inferior mesenteric arteries (see Fig. 5.45, p. 104). The *superior mesenteric artery* supplies the caecum, ascending and most of the transverse colon. The *inferior mesenteric artery* supplies the remainder of the colon and the proximal part of the rectum. The *middle* and *inferior rectal arteries*, branches of the internal iliac arteries supply the distal section of the rectum and the anus.

Venous drainage is mainly by the *superior* and *inferior mesenteric veins* which drain blood from the parts supplied by arteries of the same names. These veins join the splenic and gastric veins to form the portal vein (see Fig. 5.47, p. 105). Veins draining the distal part of the rectum and the anus join the *internal iliac veins*, meaning that blood from this region returns directly to the inferior cava, bypassing the portal circulation.

Functions of the large intestine, rectum and anal canal

Absorption

The contents of the ileum which pass through the ileocaecal valve into the caecum are fluid, even though some water has been absorbed in the small intestine. In the large intestine absorption of water, by osmosis, continues until the familiar semisolid consistency of faeces is achieved. Mineral salts, vitamins and some drugs are also absorbed into the blood capillaries from the large intestine.

Microbial activity

The large intestine is heavily colonised by certain types of bacteria, which synthesise vitamin K and folic acid. They include *Escherichia coli*, *Enterobacter aerogenes*, *Streptococcus faecalis* and *Clostridium perfringens*. These microbes are *commensals*, i.e. normally harmless, in humans. However, they may become pathogenic if transferred to another part of the body, e.g. *E. coli* may cause cystitis if it gains access to the urinary bladder.

Gases in the bowel consist of some of the constituents of air, mainly nitrogen, swallowed with food and drink and as a feature of some anxiety states. Hydrogen, carbon dioxide and methane are produced by bacterial fermentation of unabsorbed nutrients, especially carbohydrate. Gases pass out of the bowel as *flatus*.

Large numbers of microbes are present in the faeces.

Mass movement

The large intestine does not exhibit peristaltic movement as in other parts of the digestive tract. Only at fairly long intervals (about twice an hour) does a wave of strong peristalsis sweep along the transverse colon forcing its contents into the descending and sigmoid colons. This is known as *mass movement* and it is often precipitated by the entry of food into the stomach. This combination of stimulus and response is called the *gastrocolic reflex*.

Defaecation

Usually the rectum is empty, but when a mass movement forces the contents of the sigmoid colon into the rectum the nerve endings in its walls are stimulated by stretch. In the infant, defaecation occurs by reflex (involuntary) action. However, during the second or third year of life the ability to override the defaecation reflex is developed. In practical terms this acquired voluntary control means that the brain can inhibit the reflex until such time as it is convenient to defaecate. The external anal sphincter is

303

under conscious control through the *pudendal nerve*. Thus defaecation involves involuntary contraction of the muscle of the rectum and relaxation of the internal anal sphincter. Contraction of the abdominal muscles and lowering of the diaphragm increase the intra-abdominal pressure (Valsalva's manoeuvre) and so assist the process of defaecation. When defaecation is voluntarily postponed the need to defaecate tends to fade until the next mass movement occurs and the reflex is initiated again. Repeated suppression of the reflex may lead to constipation.

Constituents of faeces. The faeces consist of a semisolid brown mass. The brown colour is due to the presence of stercobilin (p. 300 and Fig. 12.38).

Even though absorption of water takes place in the large intestine, water still makes up about 60 to 70% of the weight of the faeces. The remainder consists of:

- fibre (indigestible cellular plant and animal material)
- dead and live microbes
- epithelial cells shed from the walls of the tract
- fatty acids
- mucus secreted by the epithelial lining of the large intestine.

Mucus helps to lubricate the faeces and an adequate amount of dietary fibre (roughage) ensures that the contents of the colon are sufficiently bulky to stimulate defaecation.

Pancreas (Fig. 12.33)

Learning outcome

After studying this section, you should be able to:

- differentiate between the structures and functions of the exocrine and endocrine pancreas.

The pancreas is a pale grey gland weighing about 60 grams. It is about 12 to 15 cm long and is situated in the epigastric and left hypochondriac regions of the abdominal cavity (see Figs 3.34 and 3.35, pp. 48 and 49). It consists of a broad head, a body and a narrow tail. The head lies in the curve of the duodenum, the body behind the stomach and the tail lies in front of the left kidney and just reaches the spleen. The abdominal aorta and the inferior vena cava lie behind the gland.

The pancreas is both an exocrine and endocrine gland.

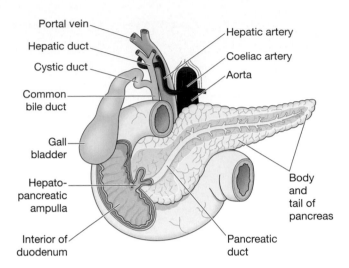

Figure 12.33 The pancreas in relation to the duodenum and biliary tract; part of the anterior wall of the duodenum has been removed.

The exocrine pancreas

This consists of a large number of *lobules* made up of small alveoli, the walls of which consist of secretory cells. Each lobule is drained by a tiny duct and these unite eventually to form the *pancreatic duct*, which extends the whole length of the gland and opens into the duodenum. Just before entering the duodenum the pancreatic duct joins the *common bile duct* to form the hepatopancreatic ampulla. The duodenal opening of the ampulla is controlled by the hepatopancreatic sphincter (of Oddi).

The function of the exocrine pancreas is to produce *pancreatic juice* containing enzymes that digest carbohydrates, proteins and fats (p. 299). As in the alimentary tract, parasympathetic stimulation increases the secretion of pancreatic juice and sympathetic stimulation depresses it.

The endocrine pancreas

Distributed throughout the gland are groups of specialised cells called the pancreatic islets (of Langerhans). The islets have no ducts so the hormones diffuse directly into the blood. The endocrine pancreas secretes the hormones insulin and glucagon, which are principally concerned with control of blood glucose levels (see Ch. 9).

Blood supply

The splenic and mesenteric arteries supply the pancreas, and venous drainage is by veins of the same names that join other veins to form the portal vein.

Liver

Learning outcomes

After studying this section, you should be able to:

- describe the location of the liver in the abdominal cavity
- describe the structure of a liver lobule
- list the functions of the liver.

The liver is the largest gland in the body, weighing between 1 and 2.3 kg. It is situated in the upper part of the abdominal cavity occupying the greater part of the right hypochondriac region, part of the epigastric region and extending into the left hypochondriac region. Its upper and anterior surfaces are smooth and curved to fit the under surface of the diaphragm (Fig. 12.34); its posterior surface is irregular in outline (Fig. 12.35).

Organs associated with the liver

Superiorly and anteriorly	– diaphragm and anterior abdominal wall
Inferiorly	– stomach, bile ducts, duodenum, hepatic flexure of the colon, right kidney and adrenal gland
Posteriorly	– oesophagus, inferior vena cava, aorta, gall bladder, vertebral column and diaphragm
Laterally	– lower ribs and diaphragm.

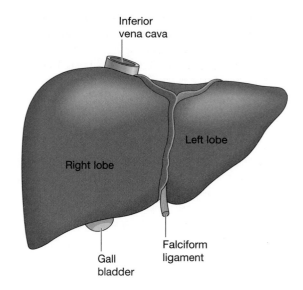

Figure 12.34 The liver: anterior view.

The liver is enclosed in a thin inelastic capsule and incompletely covered by a layer of peritoneum. Folds of peritoneum form supporting ligaments attaching the liver to the inferior surface of the diaphragm. It is held in position partly by these ligaments and partly by the pressure of the organs in the abdominal cavity.

The liver has four lobes. The two most obvious are the large *right lobe* and the smaller, wedge-shaped, *left lobe*. The other two, the *caudate* and *quadrate* lobes, are areas on the posterior surface (Fig. 12.35).

The portal fissure

This is the name given to the region on the posterior surface of the liver where various structures enter and leave the gland.

305

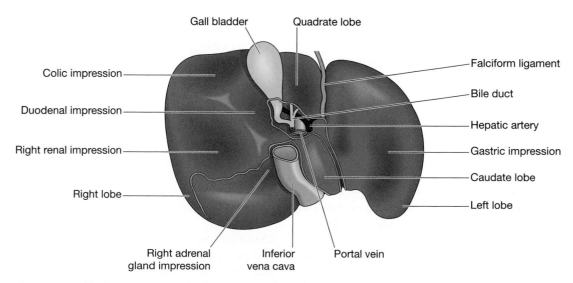

Figure 12.35 The liver, turned up to show the posterior surface.

The *portal vein* enters, carrying blood from the stomach, spleen, pancreas and the small and large intestines.

The *hepatic artery* enters, carrying arterial blood. It is a branch from the coeliac artery, which is a branch from the abdominal aorta.

Nerve fibres, sympathetic and parasympathetic, enter here.

The *right* and *left hepatic ducts* leave, carrying bile from the liver to the gall bladder.

Lymph vessels leave the liver, draining some lymph to abdominal and some to thoracic nodes.

Blood supply (see Figs. 5.44 and 5.46)

The hepatic artery and the portal vein take blood to the liver (see Fig. 12.37). Venous return is by a variable number of hepatic veins that leave the posterior surface and immediately enter the inferior vena cava just below the diaphragm.

Structure

The lobes of the liver are made up of tiny functional units, called *lobules*, which are just visible to the naked eye (Fig. 12.36A). Liver lobules are hexagonal in outline and are formed by cubical-shaped cells, the *hepatocytes*, arranged in pairs of columns radiating from a central vein. Between two pairs of columns of cells are *sinusoids* (blood vessels with incomplete walls) containing a mixture of blood from the tiny branches of the portal vein and hepatic artery (Fig. 12.36B). This arrangement allows the arterial blood and portal venous blood (with a high concentration of nutrients) to mix and come into close contact with the liver cells. Amongst the cells lining the sinusoids are hepatic macrophages (Kupffer cells) whose function is to ingest and destroy worn out blood cells and any foreign particles present in the blood flowing through the liver.

Blood drains from the sinusoids into *central* or *centrilobular veins*. These then join with veins from other lobules, forming larger veins, until eventually they become the hepatic veins, which leave the liver and empty into the inferior vena cava. Figure 12.37 shows the system of blood flow through the liver. One of the functions of the liver is to secrete *bile*. In Figure 12.36B it is seen that *bile canaliculi* run between the columns of liver cells. This means that each column of hepatocytes has a blood sinusoid on one side and a bile canaliculus on the other. The canaliculi join up to form larger bile canals until eventually they form the *right and left hepatic ducts*, which drain bile from the liver.

Lymphoid tissue and a system of lymph vessels are also present in each lobule.

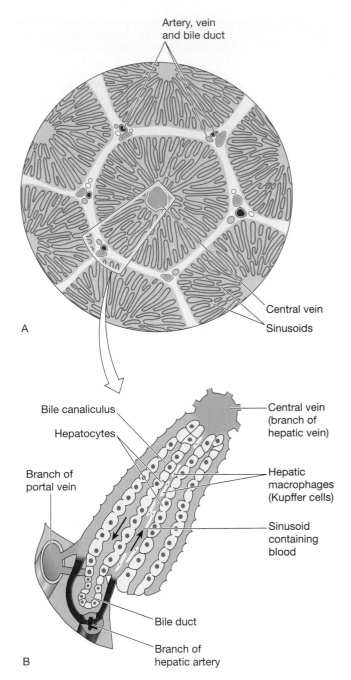

Figure 12.36 A. **A magnified transverse section of a liver lobule.** B. **Direction of the flow of blood and bile in a liver lobule.**

Functions of the liver

The liver is an extremely active organ. Those functions already described are only mentioned here.

Carbohydrate metabolism. The liver has an important role in maintaining plasma glucose levels. After a meal when levels rise, glucose is converted to glycogen for storage under the influence of the hormone insulin. Later,

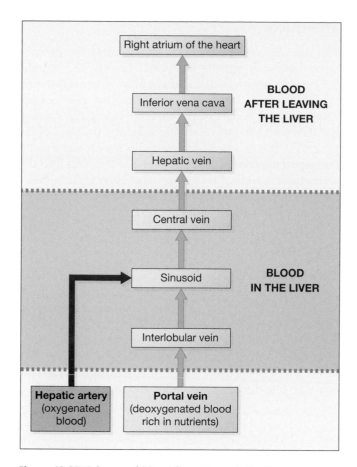

Figure 12.37 Scheme of blood flow through the liver.

Breakdown of erythrocytes and defence against microbes. This is carried out by phagocytic hepatic macrophages (Kupffer cells) in the sinusoids.

Detoxification of drugs and noxious substances. These include ethanol (alcohol) and toxins produced by e.g. microbes.

Inactivation of hormones. These include insulin, glucagon, cortisol, aldosterone, thyroid and sex hormones.

Production of heat. The liver uses a considerable amount of energy, has a high metabolic rate and produces a great deal of heat. It is the main heat-producing organ of the body.

Secretion of bile. The hepatocytes synthesise the constituents of bile from the mixed arterial and venous blood in the sinusoids. These include bile salts, bile pigments and cholesterol.

Storage. The substances include:

- glycogen (see p. 312)
- fat-soluble vitamins: A, D, E, K
- iron, copper
- some water-soluble vitamins, e.g. vitamin B_{12}.

Composition of bile

About 500 ml of bile are secreted by the liver daily. Bile consists of:

- water
- mineral salts
- mucus
- bile pigments, mainly bilirubin
- bile salts, which are derived from the primary bile acids, cholic acid and chenodeoxycholic acid
- cholesterol.

The bile acids, *cholic* and *chenodeoxycholic acid*, are synthesised by hepatocytes from cholesterol, conjugated (combined) with either glycine or taurine, then secreted into bile as sodium or potassium salts. In the small intestine they emulsify fats, aiding their digestion. In the terminal ileum most of the bile salts are reabsorbed and return to the liver in the portal vein. This *enterohepatic circulation*, or recycling of bile salts, ensures that large amounts of bile salts enter the small intestine daily from a relatively small bile acid pool (Fig. 12.38).

Bilirubin is one of the products of haemolysis of erythrocytes by hepatic macrophages (Kupffer cells) in the liver and by other macrophages in the spleen and

307

when glucose levels fall, the hormone glucagon stimulates conversion of glycogen into glucose again, keeping levels within the normal range (see Fig 12.40).

Fat metabolism. Stored fat can be converted to a form in which it can be used by the tissues to provide energy (see Fig. 12.45).

Protein metabolism
Deamination of amino acids. This process:

- removes the nitrogenous portion from the amino acids not required for the formation of new protein; *urea* is formed from this nitrogenous portion which is excreted in urine
- breaks down nucleic acids (genetic material, see p. 433) to form *uric acid*, which is excreted in the urine.

Transamination. Removes the nitrogenous portion of amino acids and attaches it to other carbohydrate molecules forming new non-essential amino acids (see Fig. 12.43).

Synthesis of plasma proteins and most *blood clotting factors* from amino acids.

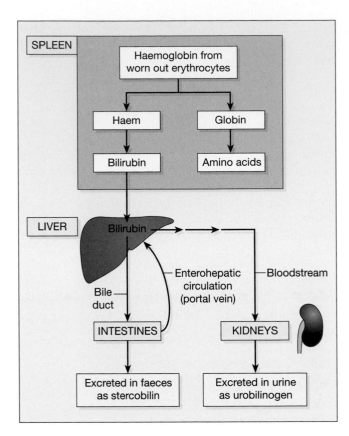

Figure 12.38 Fate of bilirubin from breakdown of worn-out erythrocytes.

bone marrow. In its original form bilirubin is insoluble in water and is carried in the blood bound to albumin. In hepatocytes it is conjugated with glucuronic acid and becomes water soluble before being excreted in bile. Bacteria in the intestine change the form of bilirubin and most is excreted as *stercobilin* in the faeces. A small amount is reabsorbed and excreted in urine as *urobilinogen* (Fig. 12.38). Jaundice is yellow pigmentation of the tissues, seen in the skin and conjunctiva, caused by excess blood bilirubin (p. 333).

Biliary tract

Learning outcomes

After studying this section, you should be able to:

- describe the route taken by bile from the liver, to the gall bladder, and then to the duodenum

- outline the structure and functions of the gall bladder.

Bile ducts (Fig. 12.39)

The *right and left hepatic ducts* join to form the *common hepatic duct* just outside the portal fissure. The hepatic duct passes downwards for about 3 cm where it is joined at an acute angle by the *cystic duct* from the gall bladder. The cystic and hepatic ducts merge forming the *common bile duct*, which passes downwards behind the head of the pancreas. This is joined by the main pancreatic duct at the hepatopancreatic ampulla and the opening into the duodenum is controlled by the hepatopancreatic sphincter (of Oddi). The common bile duct is about 7.5 cm long and has a diameter of about 6 mm.

Structure

The walls of the bile ducts have the same layers of tissue as those described in the basic structure of the alimentary canal (Fig. 12.2). In the cystic duct the mucous membrane lining is arranged in irregular circular folds, which have the effect of a *spiral valve*. Bile passes through the cystic duct twice – once on its way into the gall bladder and again when it is expelled from the gall bladder into the common bile duct and then on to the duodenum.

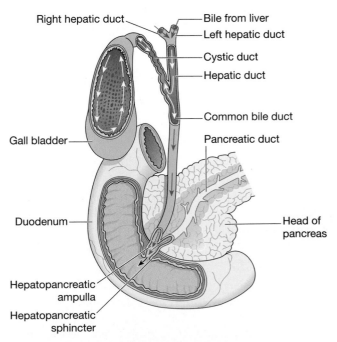

Figure 12.39 Direction of the flow of bile from the liver to the duodenum.

Gall bladder

The gall bladder is a pear-shaped sac attached to the posterior surface of the liver by connective tissue. It has a *fundus* or expanded end, a *body* or main part and a *neck*, which is continuous with the cystic duct.

Structure

The gall bladder has the same layers of tissue as those described in the basic structure of the alimentary canal, with some modifications.

Peritoneum covers only the inferior surface. The gall bladder is in contact with the posterior surface of the right lobe of the liver and is held in place by the visceral peritoneum of the liver.

Muscle layer. There is an additional layer of oblique muscle fibres.

Mucous membrane displays small rugae when the gall bladder is empty that disappear when it is distended with bile.

Blood supply

The *cystic artery*, a branch of the hepatic artery, supplies blood to the gall bladder. Blood is drained away by the *cystic vein* that joins the portal vein.

Functions of the gall bladder

These include:

* reservoir for bile
* concentration of the bile by up to 10- or 15-fold, by absorption of water through the walls of the gall bladder
* release of stored bile.

When the muscle wall of the gall bladder contracts, bile passes through the bile ducts to the duodenum. Contraction is stimulated by:

* the hormone *cholecystokinin* (CCK), secreted by the duodenum
* the presence of fat and acid chyme in the duodenum.

Relaxation of the hepatopancreatic sphincter (of Oddi) is caused by CCK and is a reflex response to contraction of the gall bladder.

Summary of digestion and absorption of nutrients

Learning outcomes

After studying this section, you should be able to:

■ list the principal digestive enzymes, their sites of action, their substrates and their products

■ describe the sites of absorption of the main nutrient groups.

Table 12.2 summarises the main digestive processes of the principal nutrient groups, the locations where these processes occur and the enzymes involved.

Metabolism

Learning outcomes

After studying this section, you should be able to:

■ discuss general principles of metabolism, including anabolism, catabolism, units of energy and metabolic rate

■ compare and contrast the metabolic rates of the body's main energy sources (carbohydrate, protein and fat)

■ describe in simple terms the central metabolic pathways; glycolysis, citric acid cycle and oxidative phosphorylation.

Metabolism constitutes all the chemical reactions that occur in the body, using nutrients to:

* provide energy by chemical oxidation of nutrients
* make new or replacement body substances.

Table 12.2 Summary showing the sites of digestion and absorption of nutrients

	Mouth	Stomach	Small intestine		Large intestine
			Digestion	Absorption	
Carbohydrate	*Salivary amylase*: digestible starches to disaccharides	*Acid* denatures and stops action of salivary amylase	*Pancreatic amylase*: digestible starches to disaccharides *sucrase, maltase, lactase* (in enterocytes): disaccharides to monosaccharides (mainly glucose)	Into blood capillaries of villi	–
Proteins	–	*Acid*: pepsinogen to pepsin *Pepsin*: proteins to polypeptides	*Enterokinase* (in enterocytes): chymotrypsinogen and trypsinogen (from pancreas) to chymotrypsin and trypsin *Chymotrypsin and trypsin*: polypeptides to di- and tripeptides *Peptidases* (in enterocytes): di- and tripeptides to amino acids	Into blood capillaries of villi	–
Fats	–	–	*Bile* (from liver): bile salts emulsify fats *Pancreatic lipase*: fats to fatty acids and glycerol *Lipases* (in enterocytes): fats to fatty acids and glycerol	Into the lacteals of the villi	–
Water	–	Small amount absorbed here	–	Most absorbed here	Remainder absorbed here
Vitamins	–	Intrinsic factor secreted for vitamin B_{12} absorption	–	Water-soluble vitamins absorbed into capillaries; fat-soluble ones into lacteals of villi	Bacteria synthesise vitamin K in colon; absorbed here

Two types of processes are involved.

$$\text{large molecules} \underset{\text{anabolism}}{\overset{\text{catabolism}}{\rightleftharpoons}} \text{small molecules}$$

Catabolism. This process breaks down large molecules into smaller ones releasing *chemical energy*, which is stored as adenosine triphosphate (ATP), and *heat*. Heat is used to maintain core body temperature at the optimum level for chemical activity (36.8 °C). Excess heat is dissipated, mainly through the skin (p. 361).

Anabolism. This is building up, or synthesis, of large molecules from smaller ones and requires a source of energy, usually ATP.

Anabolism and catabolism usually involve a series of chemical reactions, known as *metabolic pathways*. These consist of 'small steps' that permit controlled, efficient and gradual transfer of energy from ATP rather than large intracellular 'explosions'. Metabolic pathways are switched on and off by hormones, providing control of metabolism and meeting individual requirements.

Both processes occur continually in all cells maintaining an energy balance. Very active tissues, such as muscle or liver, need a large energy supply to support their requirements.

Energy

The energy produced in the body may be measured and expressed in units of work (*joules*) or units of heat (kilocalories).

A kilocalorie (kcal) is the amount of heat required to raise the temperature of 1 litre of water by 1 degree Celsius (1 °C). On a daily basis, the body's collective metabolic processes generate a total of about 3 million kilocalories.

1 kcal = 4 184 joules (J) = 4.184 kilojoules (kJ)

The nutritional value of carbohydrates, protein and fats eaten in the diet may be expressed in *kilojoules per gram* or kcal per gram.

1 gram of carbohydrate provides 17 kilojoules (4 kcal)
1 gram of protein provides 17 kilojoules (4 kcal)
1 gram of fat provides 38 kilojoules (9 kcal)

Chapter 11 provides examples of foods providing these nutrients.

Energy balance

Body weight remains constant when energy intake in the form of nutrients is equal to energy use. When intake exceeds requirement, body weight increases. Conversely, body weight decreases when nutrient intake does not meet energy requirements.

Metabolic rate

The metabolic rate is the rate at which energy is released from the fuel molecules inside cells. As most of the processes involved require oxygen and produce carbon dioxide as waste, the metabolic rate can be estimated by measuring oxygen uptake or carbon dioxide excretion.

The *basal metabolic rate* (BMR) is the rate of metabolism when the individual is at rest in a warm environment and is in the *postabsorptive state*, i.e. has not had a meal for at least 12 hours. In this state the release of energy is sufficient to meet only the essential needs of vital organs, such as the heart, lungs, nervous system and kidneys. The postabsorptive state is important because the intake of food, especially protein, increases metabolic rate. Some of the many different factors that affect metabolic rate are shown in Table 12.3.

Most foods contain a mixture of different amounts of carbohydrate, protein, fat, minerals, vitamins, fibre (non-starch polysaccharide) and water (see Ch. 11). Carbohydrates, proteins and fats are the sources of energy

Table 12.3 Factors affecting metabolic rate

Factor	Effect on metabolic rate
Age	Gradually reduced with age
Gender	Higher in men than women
Height, weight	Relatively higher in small people
Pregnancy, menstruation, lactation	Increased
Ingestion of food	Increased
Muscular activity, physical exertion	Increased
Elevated body temperature	Increased
Excess thyroid hormones	Increased
Starvation	Decreased

and they are obtained from the variety of food, usually in the following proportions:

protein   10–15%
fat   15–30%
carbohydrate   55–75%.

Central metabolic pathways

Much of the metabolic effort of cells is concerned with energy production to fuel cellular activities. Certain common pathways are central to this function. Fuel molecules enter these central energy-producing pathways and in a series of steps, during which a series of intermediate molecules are formed and energy is released, these fuel molecules are chemically broken down. The end results of these processes are energy production and carbon dioxide and water (called *metabolic water*) formation. Much of the energy is stored as ATP, although some is lost as heat. The carbon dioxide is excreted through the lungs.

The preferred fuel molecule is glucose, but alternatives should glucose be unavailable include amino acids, fatty acids, glycerol and occasionally nucleic acids. Each of these may enter the central energy-producing pathways and be converted to energy, carbon dioxide and water. There are three central metabolic pathways (see Fig. 12.45):

- glycolysis
- the citric acid (Krebs) cycle
- oxidative phosphorylation.

Products from glycolysis enter the citric acid cycle, and products from the citric acid cycle proceed to oxidative

311

phosphorylation. The fates of the different fuel molecules entering the central metabolic pathways are discussed in the following sections.

Metabolism of carbohydrate

Erythrocytes and neurones can use only glucose for fuel and therefore maintenance of blood glucose levels is needed to provide a constant energy source to these cells. Most other cells can also use other sources of fuel.

Digested carbohydrate, mainly glucose, is absorbed into the blood capillaries of the villi of the small intestine. It is transported by the portal circulation to the liver, where it is dealt with in several ways (Fig. 12.40):

- Glucose may be oxidised to provide the chemical energy, in the form of ATP, necessary for the considerable metabolic activity which takes place in the liver (p. 306).
- Some glucose may remain in the circulating blood to maintain the normal blood glucose of about 3.5 to 8 millimoles per litre (mmol/l) (63 to 144 mg/100ml).
- Some glucose, if in excess of the above requirements, may be converted to the insoluble polysaccharide, *glycogen*, in the liver and in skeletal muscles. *Insulin* is the hormone necessary for this change to take place. The formation of glycogen inside cells is a means of storing carbohydrate without upsetting the osmotic

equilibrium. Before it can be used to maintain blood levels or to provide ATP it must be broken down again into its constituent glucose units. Liver glycogen constitutes a store of glucose used for liver activity and to maintain the blood glucose level. Muscle glycogen stores provide the glucose requirement of muscle activity. *Glucagon, adrenaline (epinephrine)* and *thyroxine* are the main hormones associated with the breakdown of glycogen to glucose. These processes are summarised:

$$\text{glucose} \underset{\text{glucagon}}{\overset{\text{insulin}}{\rightleftharpoons}} \text{glycogen}$$

- Carbohydrate in excess of that required to maintain the blood glucose level and glycogen stores in the tissues is converted to fat and stored in the fat depots.

All body cells require energy to carry out their metabolic processes including multiplication for replacement of worn out cells, contraction of muscle fibres and synthesis of secretions produced by glandular tissues. The oxidation of carbohydrate and fat provides most of the energy required by the body. When glycogen stores are low and more glucose is needed, the body can make glucose from non-carbohydrate sources, e.g. amino acids, glycerol. This is called *gluconeogenesis* (formation of new glucose).

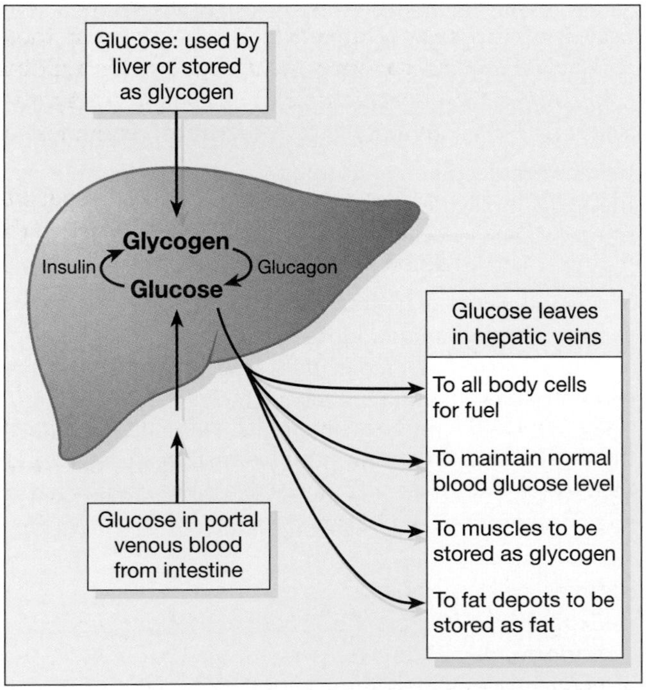

Carbohydrate and energy release (Fig. 12.41)

Glucose is broken down in the body giving energy, carbon dioxide and metabolic water. Catabolism of glucose occurs in a series of steps with a little energy being released at each stage. The total number of ATP molecules which may be generated from the complete breakdown of one molecule of glucose is 38, but for this to be achieved the process must occur in the presence of oxygen (aerobically). In the absence of oxygen (anaerobically) this number is greatly reduced; the process is therefore much less efficient.

Aerobic respiration (catabolism). Aerobic catabolism of glucose can occur only if the oxygen supply is adequate, and is the process by which energy is released during prolonged, manageable exercise. When exercise levels become very intense, the energy requirements of muscles outstrip the oxygen supply, and anaerobic breakdown then occurs. Such high levels of activity can be sustained for only short periods, because there is accumulation of wastes (mainly lactic acid) and reduced efficiency of the energy production process.

The first stage of glucose catabolism is *glycolysis*. This is an anaerobic process that takes place in the cytoplasm of the cell. Through a number of intermediate steps

312

Figure 12.40 Summary of the source, distribution and use of glucose.

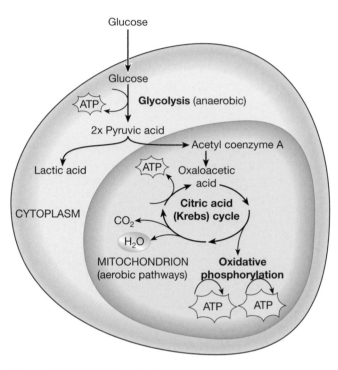

Figure 12.41 Oxidation of glucose.

one glucose molecule is converted to two molecules of pyruvic acid, with the net production of two molecules of ATP. The remainder of the considerable energy stores locked up in the original molecule of glucose is released only if there is enough oxygen to allow the pyruvic acid molecules to enter the biochemical roundabout called the *citric acid cycle* (Fig. 12.41). This takes place in the mitochondria of the cell and is oxygen dependent. For every two molecules of pyruvic acid entering the citric acid cycle, a further two molecules of ATP are formed but this is still far short of the maximum possible 38 ATP molecules. The remaining 34 molecules of ATP come from the third energy-generating process, *oxidative phosphorylation*, a process dependent on hydrogen atoms released during earlier stages of glucose breakdown. Oxidative phosphorylation, like the citric acid cycle, can occur only in the presence of oxygen and takes place in the mitochondria.

Anaerobic catabolism. When oxygen levels in the cell are low, the molecule of glucose still undergoes glycolysis and is split into two molecules of pyruvic acid, because glycolysis is an anaerobic process. However, the pyruvic acid does not enter the citric acid cycle or progress to oxidative phosphorylation; instead it is converted anaerobically to lactic acid. Build-up of lactic acid causes the pain and cramps of overexercised muscles. When oxygen levels are restored, lactic acid is reconverted to pyruvic acid, which may then enter the citric acid cycle.

Fate of the end products of carbohydrate metabolism

Lactic acid. Some of the lactic acid produced by anaerobic catabolism of glucose may be oxidised in the cells to carbon dioxide and water but first it must be changed back to pyruvic acid. If complete oxidation does not take place, lactic acid passes to the liver in the circulating blood where it is converted to glucose and may then take any of the pathways open to glucose (Fig. 12.40).

Carbon dioxide. This is excreted from the body as a gas by the lungs.

Metabolic water. This is added to the considerable amount of water already present in the body; excess is excreted as urine by the kidneys.

Metabolism of protein

Dietary protein consists of a number of amino acids (p. 272). About 20 amino acids have been named and nine of these are described as *essential* because they cannot be synthesised in the body. The others are *non-essential* amino acids because they can be synthesised by many tissues. The enzymes involved in this process are called *transaminases*. Digestion breaks down dietary protein into its constituent amino acids in preparation for absorption into the blood capillaries of the villi in the wall of the small intestine. Amino acids are transported in the portal circulation to the liver and then into the general circulation, thus making them available to all the cells and tissues of the body. Different cells choose from those available the particular amino acids required for building or repairing their specific type of tissue and for synthesising their secretions, e.g. antibodies, enzymes or hormones.

Amino acids not required for building and repairing body tissues cannot be stored and are broken down in the liver (see deamination below).

Amino acid pool (Fig. 12.42)

A small pool of amino acids is maintained within the body. This is the source from which the different cells of the body draw the amino acids they need to synthesise their own materials, e.g. new cells, secretions such as enzymes, hormones and plasma proteins.

Sources of amino acids

Exogenous. These are derived from dietary protein.

Endogenous. These are obtained from the breakdown of body proteins. In adults, about 80 to 100 g of protein are broken down and replaced each day. Intestinal mucosa has the most rapid turnover of cells.

313

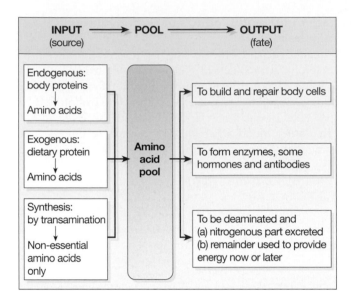

Figure 12.42 Sources and use of amino acids in the body.

Loss of amino acids

Deamination. Amino acids not needed by the body are broken down, or deaminated, mainly in the liver. The *nitrogenous part*, the amino group (NH_2), is converted to ammonia (NH_3) and then combined with carbon dioxide forming *urea*, which is excreted in the urine. The remaining part is used to provide energy, as glucose by gluconeogenesis, or stored as fat, if in excess of immediate requirements.

Excretion. The faeces contain a considerable amount of protein consisting of cells shed from the lining of the alimentary tract.

Endogenous and exogenous amino acids are mixed in the 'pool' and the body is said to be in *nitrogen balance* when the rate of removal from the pool is equal to the additions to it. Unlike carbohydrates, the body has no capacity for the storage of amino acids except for this relatively small pool. Figure 12.43 depicts what happens to amino acids in the body.

Amino acids and energy release

(see Fig. 12.45)

Proteins, in the form of amino acids, are potential fuel molecules that are used by the body only when other energy sources are low, e.g. in starvation. To supply the amino acids for use as fuel, in extreme situations, the body breaks down muscle, its main protein source. Some amino acids can be converted directly to glucose, which enters glycolysis. Other amino acids are changed to intermediate compounds of the central metabolic pathways, e.g. acetyl coenzyme A or oxaloacetic acid, and therefore enter the system at a later stage.

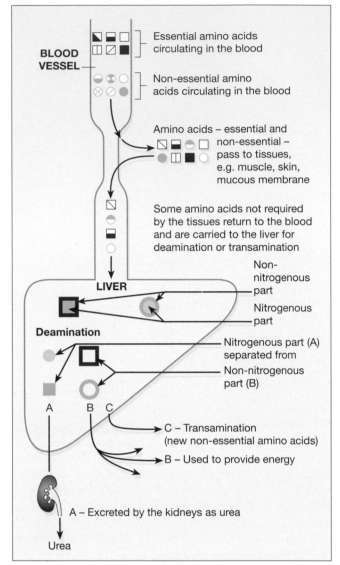

Figure 12.43 The fate of amino acids in the body.

Metabolism of fat (Fig. 12.44)

Fat is synthesised from excess dietary carbohydrates and proteins, and stored in the fat depots, i.e. under the skin, in the omentum or around the kidneys.

Fats that have been digested and absorbed as fatty acids and glycerol into the lacteals are transported via the cisterna chyli and the thoracic duct to the bloodstream and so, by a circuitous route, to the liver. Fatty acids and glycerol circulating in the blood are used by the cells of organs and glands to provide energy and in the synthesis of some of their secretions. In the liver some fatty acids and glycerol are used to provide energy and heat, and some are recombined forming *triglycerides*, the form in which fat is stored. A triglyceride consists of three fatty acids chemically combined with a glycerol molecule

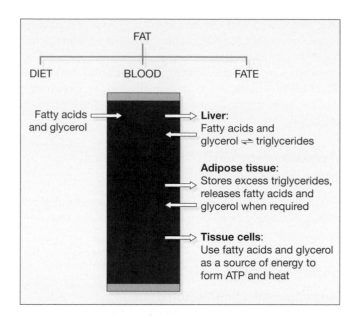

Figure 12.44 Sources, distribution and use of fats in the body.

(see Fig. 2.9, p. 24). When required, triglycerides are converted back to fatty acids and glycerol and used to provide energy. The end products of fat metabolism are energy, heat, carbon dioxide and water.

Fatty acids and energy release

When body tissues are deprived of glucose, as occurs in prolonged fasting, starvation, energy-restricted diets or during strenuous exercise, the body uses alternative energy sources, mainly fat stores. Fatty acids may be converted to acetyl coenzyme A, and enter the energy production pathway in that form. One consequence of this is accumulation of *ketone bodies*, which are produced in the liver from acetyl coenzyme A when levels are too high for processing through the citric acid cycle (see Fig. 12.45). Ketone bodies then enter the blood and can be used by other body tissues, including the brain (which is usually glucose dependent) as a source of fuel. However, at high concentrations, ketone bodies are toxic, particularly to the brain. Ketone bodies consist of a ketone (acetone) and weak organic acids, and are therefore acidic. Normally levels are low because they are used as soon as they are produced. When production exceeds use, in the situations mentioned above, levels rise causing *ketosis*. Excretion is via:

- the urine (ketonuria)
- the lungs, giving the breath a characteristic sweet smell of acetone or 'pear drops'.

In ketosis, compensation is required to maintain acid/base balance. This is achieved by buffer systems that excrete excess acid (hydrogen ions) by the lungs, through hyperventilation, or kidneys. In health, ketosis is self-limiting and ketone body production stops when fasting or exercise ceases. In Type 1 diabetes mellitus, serious metabolic complications occur if there is excessive production of ketone bodies (see p. 233).

Glycerol and energy release (Fig. 12.45)

The body converts glycerol from the degradation of fats into one of the intermediary compounds produced during glycolysis, and in this form it enters the central metabolic pathways.

315

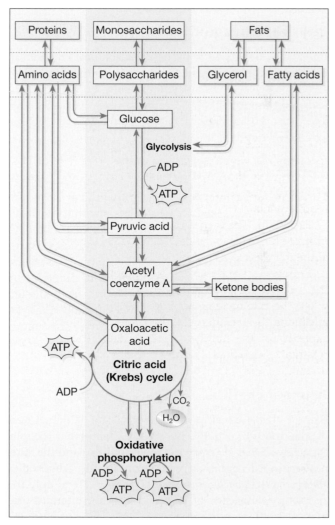

Figure 12.45 Summary of the fates of the three main energy sources in the central metabolic pathways.

Diseases of the mouth

Learning outcomes

After studying this section, you should be able to:

- discuss the main inflammatory and infectious conditions of the mouth

- describe briefly the site and effects of oral squamous cell carcinoma

- distinguish between cleft lip and cleft palate, including describing the anatomical abnormalities involved.

Inflammatory and infectious conditions

Physical damage

Injury may be caused to tissues in and around the mouth by food and other ingested substances, if they are corrosive, abrasive or excessively hot or cold. Corrosive chemicals are the most likely to cause serious tissue damage and acute inflammation. The outcome depends on the extent and depth of the injury.

Thrush (oral candidiasis)

This acute fungal infection of the epithelium of the mouth is caused by the yeast *Candida albicans*. In adults it causes opportunistic infection mainly in debilitated people and in those whose immunity is suppressed by, e.g. steroids, antibiotics or cytotoxic drugs. In babies it may be a severe infection, sometimes causing epidemics in nurseries by cross-infection. It occurs most commonly in bottle-fed babies. *Chronic thrush* may develop, affecting the roof of the mouth in people who wear dentures. The fungus survives in fine grooves on the upper surface of the denture and repeatedly reinfects the epithelium.

Angular cheilitis

Painful cracks develop in folds of tissue at the corners of the mouth, usually in elderly debilitated people, especially if they do not wear their dentures and the folds remain moist. Common causal organisms are *Candida albicans* and *Staphylococcus aureus*.

Dietary deficiency of iron and B group vitamins predispose to this condition.

Acute gingivitis

This is a rare, acute condition previously known as Vincent's infection. There is severe ulceration of the gums that may also affect the lips, mouth, throat and palatine tonsil. It is caused by two commensal organisms acting together, *Borrelia vincenti* and a fusiform bacillus. Both organisms may be present in the mouth and only cause the condition in the presence of malnutrition, debilitating disease, poor dental hygiene or injury caused by previous infection.

Aphthous stomatitis (recurrent oral ulceration)

This common condition features extremely painful ulcers that occur singly or in crops inside the mouth. The cause is unknown.

Viral infections

Acute herpetic gingivostomatitis

This is caused by *Herpes simplex* virus and is the commonest oral virus infection. It is characterised by extensive and very painful ulceration.

Secondary or recurrent herpes lesions (cold sores)

Lesions, caused by *Herpes simplex* virus, occur round the nose and on the lips. After an outbreak the viruses remain dormant within the cells. Later outbreaks, usually at the same site, are precipitated by a variety of stimuli including exposure to UV rays (strong sunlight) and failing immune response in, e.g., old age.

Tumours of the mouth

Squamous cell carcinoma

This is the most common type of malignant tumour in the mouth and carries a poor prognosis. The usual sites are the lower lip and the edge of the tongue. Ulceration occurs frequently and there is early spread to surrounding tissues and cervical lymph nodes.

Developmental defects

Cleft palate and cleft lip (harelip)

During embryonic development, the roof of the mouth (hard palate) develops as two separate (right and left) halves; this occurs from the lips anteriorly to the uvula posteriorly. Before birth, these two halves fuse along the midline. If fusion is incomplete, a cleft (division) occurs, which may be very minor, or it may be substantial. *Cleft lip* (Fig. 12.46B) may be merely a minor notch in the upper lip, or substantial when the lip is completely split in one or two places and the nose is involved. In *cleft palate*, there is a gap between the two halves of the palate, which creates a channel of communication between the mouth

316

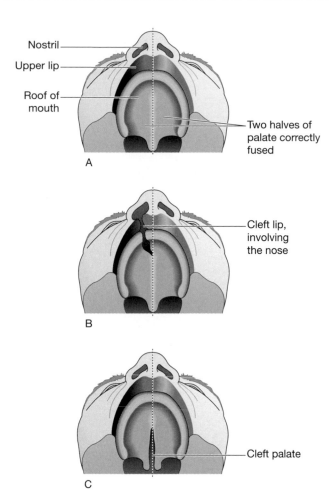

Nostril

Upper lip

Roof of mouth

Two halves of palate correctly fused

A

Cleft lip, involving the nose

B

Cleft palate

C

Figure 12.46 Cleft lip and cleft palate: A. Normal hard palate. **B.** Cleft lip. **C.** Cleft palate.

and the nasal cavity (Fig. 12.46C). Factors believed to play a causative part in these conditions include genetic abnormalities, and fetal exposure to factors such as hypoxia, certain drugs or poor nutrition, between weeks 7 and 10 of pregnancy.

Speech development, and eating and drinking, cannot take place normally until the defect has been surgically repaired.

Diseases of the pharynx

See tonsillitis and diphtheria (p. 257).

Diseases of salivary glands

Learning outcomes

After studying this section, you should be able to:

■ outline the pathophysiology of mumps

■ explain the nature of salivary calculi

■ describe the most common tumours of the salivary glands.

Mumps

This is an acute inflammatory condition of the salivary glands, especially the parotids. It is caused by the mumps virus, one of the parainfluenza group. The virus is inhaled in infected droplets and, during the 18- to 21-day incubation period, viruses multiply elsewhere in the body before spreading to the salivary glands. The virus is present in saliva for about 7 days before and after symptoms appear so the infection may spread to others during this 2-week period. Viruses also occasionally spread to:

- the pancreas, causing pancreatitis
- the testes, causing orchitis after puberty and sometimes atrophy of the glands and sterility
- the brain, causing meningitis or meningoencephalitis.

In developed countries, children are usually vaccinated against mumps in their preschool years.

Calculus formation

Calculi (stones) are formed in the salivary glands by the crystallisation of mineral salts in saliva. They may partially or completely block the ducts, leading to swelling of the gland, a predisposition to infection and, in time, atrophy. The causes are not known.

Tumours of the salivary glands

Mixed tumours (pleomorphic salivary adenoma)

This benign tumour consists of epithelial and connective tissue cells and occurs mainly in the parotid gland. A second tumour may develop in the same gland several years after the first has been removed. It rarely undergoes malignant change.

317

Carcinoma

Malignant tumours usually affect the parotids but may occur in any salivary gland or duct. Some forms have a tendency to infiltrate nerves in the surrounding tissues, causing severe pain. Lymph spread is to the cervical nodes.

Diseases of the oesophagus

Learning outcomes

After studying this section, you should be able to:

- explain how oesophageal varices develop

- discuss the main inflammatory conditions of the oesophagus

- describe the main oesophageal tumours

- define oesophageal atresia and tracheo-oesophageal fistula.

Oesophageal varices (Fig. 12.47)

In conditions such as cirrhosis (p. 331) or venous thrombosis, blood flow into the liver via the portal vein is obstructed and blood pressure within the portal system rises (portal hypertension). This forces blood from the portal vein into anastomotic veins, which redirect (shunt) blood into the systemic venous circulation, bypassing the liver. Fifty per cent or more of the portal blood may be shunted into anastomotic veins, leading to rising pressure in these veins too. One route taken by the shunted blood is into veins of the distal oesophagus, which become distended and weakened by the abnormally high volume of blood. *Varices* develop when the weakest regions of the vessel wall bulge outwards into the lumen of the oesophagus, and, being thin walled and fragile, they are easily eroded or traumatised by swallowed food. Bleeding may be slight, but chronic, leading to iron deficiency anaemia; however, sudden rupture can cause life-threatening haemorrhage.

Inflammatory and infectious conditions

Acute oesophagitis

This arises after caustic materials are swallowed and also if immunocompromised people acquire severe fungal

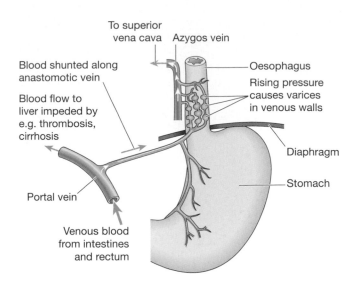

Figure 12.47 Oesophageal varices.

infections, typically candidiasis (p. 316), or viral infections, e.g. *Herpes simplex*. Following severe injury, healing causes fibrosis, and there is a risk of oesophageal stricture developing later, as the fibrous tissue shrinks.

Reflux oesophagitis

This condition, the commonest cause of indigestion (or 'heartburn'), is caused by persistent regurgitation of acidic gastric juice into the oesophagus, causing irritation, inflammation and painful ulceration. Haemorrhage occurs when blood vessels are eroded. Persistent reflux leads to chronic inflammation and if damage is extensive, secondary healing with fibrosis occurs. Shrinkage of mature fibrous tissue may cause stricture of the oesophagus. Reflux of gastric contents is associated with:

- increase in the intra-abdominal pressure, e.g. in pregnancy, constipation and obesity
- high acid content of gastric juice
- low levels of secretion of the hormone gastrin, leading to reduced sphincter action at the lower end of the oesophagus
- the presence of hiatus hernia (p. 327).

Barrett's oesophagus

This condition develops after longstanding reflux oesophagitis. Columnar cells resembling those found in the intestines replace the squamous epithelium of the lower oesophagus and this is a premalignant state carrying an increased risk of subsequent malignancy.

Achalasia

This problem tends to occur in young adults. Peristalsis of the lower oesophagus is impaired and the lower oesophageal sphincter fails to relax during swallowing, causing *dysphagia* (difficulty in swallowing), regurgitation of gastric contents and aspiration pneumonia. The oesophagus becomes dilated and the muscle layer hypertrophies. Autonomic nerve supply to the oesophageal muscle is abnormal, but the cause is not known.

Tumours of the oesophagus

Benign tumours occur rarely.

Malignant tumours

These occur more often in males than females. They are most common in the lower oesophagus but can arise at any level.

Squamous carcinoma usually affects the middle third and is associated with some dietary deficiencies, regular consumption of very hot food and possibly viruses. In developed countries, long-term alcohol consumption and cigarette smoking are also implicated.

Adenocarcinoma develops from Barrett's oesophagus (see above).

Tumours usually begin as an ulcer that spreads round the circumference causing a stricture. Local spread follows and may involve adjacent mediastinal structures, such as lymph nodes. Death is usually due to oesophageal obstruction before metastasis occurs.

Congenital abnormalities

The most common congenital abnormalities of the oesophagus are:

- *oesophageal atresia,* in which the lumen is narrow or blocked
- *tracheo-oesophageal fistula,* in which there is an opening (fistula) between the oesophagus and the trachea through which milk or regurgitated gastric contents are aspirated.

One or both abnormalities may be present. The causes are unknown.

Diseases of the stomach

Learning outcomes

After studying this section, you should be able to:

- compare the main features of chronic and acute gastritis
- discuss the pathophysiology of peptic ulcer disease
- describe the main tumours of the stomach and their consequences
- define the term congenital pyloric stenosis.

Gastritis

This is a common condition that occurs when there is either an excess of acid in the stomach or insufficient mucus to protect the surface epithelium. It may be acute or chronic.

Acute gastritis

Gastritis occurs with varying degrees of severity. The most severe form is *acute haemorrhagic gastritis*. When the surface epithelium of the stomach is exposed to acid gastric juice the cells absorb hydrogen ions which increase their internal acidity, disrupt their metabolic processes and trigger the inflammatory reaction. The causes of acute gastritis include:

- regular prolonged use of aspirin and other anti-inflammatory drugs, especially the non-steroids
- excessive alcohol consumption
- food poisoning caused by, e.g., *Staphylococcus aureus, Salmonella paratyphi* or viruses
- ingestion of corrosive poisons, acids and alkalis
- regurgitation of bile into the stomach.

The outcome depends on the extent of the damage. In many cases recovery is uneventful after the cause is removed. In severe forms there is erosion of the mucosa that may be followed by haemorrhage, accompanied by *haematemesis* (vomiting of blood) and/or *melaena* (passing of black stools containing blood) that sometimes progresses to acute peptic ulceration. Where there has been extensive tissue damage, healing is by fibrosis causing reduced elasticity and peristalsis.

319

Chronic gastritis

Chronic gastritis is a milder longer-lasting form. It is usually associated with *Helicobacter pylori* but is sometimes due to autoimmune disease or chemical injury. It is more common in later life.

Helicobacter-associated gastritis

The microbe *Helicobacter pylori* can survive in the gastric mucosa and is commonly associated with gastric conditions, especially chronic gastritis and peptic ulcer disease.

Autoimmune chronic gastritis

This is a progressive disease. Destructive inflammatory changes that begin on the surface of the mucous membrane may extend to affect its whole thickness, including the gastric glands. When this stage is reached, secretion of hydrochloric acid and intrinsic factor are markedly reduced. The antigens are the gastric parietal cells and the intrinsic factor they secrete. When these cells are destroyed as a result of this abnormal autoimmune condition, the inflammation subsides. The initial causes of the autoimmunity are not known but there is a familial predisposition and an association with chronic thyroiditis, thyrotoxicosis and atrophy of the adrenal glands. Secondary effects include:

- pernicious anaemia due to lack of intrinsic factor (p. 69)
- increased risk of cancer of the stomach.

Peptic ulceration

Ulceration involves the full thickness of the gastrointestinal mucosa. It is caused by disruption of the normal balance between the corrosive effect of gastric juice and the protective effect of mucus on the gastric epithelial cells. It may be viewed as an extension of the gastric erosions found in acute gastritis. The most common sites for ulcers are the stomach and the first few centimetres of the duodenum. More rarely they occur in the oesophagus and round the anastomosis of the stomach and small intestine, following gastrectomy. The underlying causes are not known but, if factors associated with the maintenance of healthy mucosa are impaired, acid gastric juice gains access to the epithelium, causing the initial cell damage that leads to ulceration. The main factors are: normal blood supply, mucus secretion and epithelial cell replacement.

Blood supply

Reduced blood flow and ischaemia may be caused by excessive cigarette smoking and stress, either physical or mental. In stressful situations the accompanying sympa-

thetic activity causes constriction of the blood vessels supplying the alimentary tract.

Secretion of mucus

The composition and the amount of mucus may be altered, e.g.:

- by regular and prolonged use of aspirin and other anti-inflammatory drugs
- by the reflux of bile acids and salts
- in chronic gastritis.

Epithelial cell replacement

There is normally a rapid turnover of gastric and intestinal epithelial cells. This may be reduced:

- by raised levels of steroid hormones, e.g. in response to stress or when they are used as drugs
- in chronic gastritis
- by irradiation and the use of cytotoxic drugs.

In peptic ulcer disease, the alimentary tract is commonly colonised by the bacterium *Helicobacter pylori*, a causative agent in this disorder.

Acute peptic ulcers

These lesions involve tissue to the depth of the submucosa and the lesions may be single or multiple. They are found in many sites in the stomach and in the first few centimetres of the duodenum. The underlying causes are unknown but their development is often associated with severe stress, e.g. severe illness, shock, burns, severe emotional disturbance and following surgery.

Healing without the formation of fibrous tissue usually occurs when the stressor is removed.

Chronic peptic ulcers

These ulcers penetrate through the epithelial and muscle layers of the stomach wall and may include the adjacent pancreas or liver. In the majority of cases they occur singly in the pyloric antrum of the stomach and in the duodenum. Occasionally there are two ulcers facing each other in the duodenum, called kissing ulcers. *Helicobacter pylori* is found in 90% of people with duodenal ulcers and 70% of those with gastric ulcers. The remaining gastric ulcers are almost entirely due to non-steroidal anti-inflammatory drugs (NSAIDs). Smoking predisposes to peptic ulceration and delays healing. Healing occurs with the formation of fibrous tissue and subsequent shrinkage may cause:

- stricture of the lumen of the stomach
- gastric outflow obstruction or stenosis of the pyloric sphincter

- adhesions to adjacent structures, e.g. pancreas, liver, transverse colon.

Complications of peptic ulcers

Haemorrhage. Acid gastric juice may cause the development of many tiny ulcers, or *gastric erosions*, leading to multiple capillary bleeding points and possibly iron deficiency anaemia (p. 68).

When a major artery is eroded a serious and possibly life-threatening haemorrhage may occur, causing shock (p. 322), haematemesis and/or melaena.

Perforation. When an ulcer erodes through the full thickness of the wall of the stomach or duodenum their contents enter the peritoneal cavity, causing acute peritonitis (p. 113).

Infected inflammatory material may collect under the diaphragm, forming a *subphrenic abscess* and the infection may spread through the diaphragm to the pleural cavity.

Gastric outflow obstruction. Also known as pyloric stenosis, fibrous tissue formed as an ulcer in the pyloric region heals, causes narrowing of the pylorus that obstructs outflow from the stomach and results in persistent vomiting.

Development of a malignant tumour. This may complicate gastric ulceration.

Tumours of the stomach

Benign tumours of the stomach occur rarely.

Malignant tumours

This is a common malignancy that occurs more frequently in men than women. The local growth of the tumour gradually destroys the normal tissue so that achlorhydria (reduced hydrochloric acid secretion) and pernicious anaemia are frequently secondary features. As the tumour grows, the surface may ulcerate and become infected, especially when achlorhydria develops. The causes have not been established but there appears to be:

- a link with *Helicobacter pylori* infection
- a familial predisposition
- an association with diet – high-salt diets and regular consumption of smoked or pickled foods increase the risk
- the presence of other diseases, e.g. chronic gastritis, chronic ulceration and pernicious anaemia.

Spread of gastric carcinoma

Local spread. These tumours spread locally to the remainder of the stomach, to the oesophagus, duodenum, omentum, liver and pancreas. The spleen is seldom affected.

Peritoneal spread arises when a tumour includes the full thickness of the stomach wall. Small groups of cells may break off and spread throughout the peritoneal cavity. Metastases may develop in any tissue in the abdominal or pelvic cavity where the fragments settle.

Lymphatic spread. This occurs early in the disease. At first the spread is within the lymph channels in the stomach wall, and then to lymph nodes round the stomach, in the mesentery, omentum and walls of the small intestine and colon.

Blood spread. The common sites for blood-spread metastases are the liver, lungs, brain and bones.

Congenital pyloric stenosis

In this condition there is spasmodic constriction of the pyloric sphincter, characteristic projectile vomiting and failure to put on weight. In an attempt to overcome the spasms, hypertrophy of the muscle of the pyloric antrum develops, causing obstruction of the pylorus 2 to 3 weeks after birth. The reason for the excess stimulation or neuromuscular abnormality of the pylorus is not known but there is a familial tendency and it is more common in boys.

321

Diseases of the intestines

Learning outcomes

After studying this section, you should be able to:

- describe appendicitis and its consequences
- discuss the principal infectious disease of the intestines
- compare and contrast the features of Crohn's disease and ulcerative colitis
- distinguish between diverticulitis and diverticulosis
- describe the main tumours of the intestines
- describe the abnormalities present in hernia, volvulus and intussusception
- list the main causes of intestinal obstruction
- compare the causes and outcomes of primary and secondary malabsorption.

Diseases of the small and large intestines are described together because they have certain characteristics in common and some conditions affect both.

Appendicitis

The lumen of the appendix is very small and there is little room for swelling when it becomes inflamed. The initial cause of inflammation is not always clear. Microbial infection is commonly superimposed on obstruction by, e.g., hard faecal matter (faecoliths), kinking or a foreign body. Inflammatory exudate, with fibrin and phagocytes, causes swelling and ulceration of the mucous membrane lining. In the initial stages, the pain of appendicitis is usually located in the central area of the abdomen. After a few hours, the pain shifts and is localised to the region above the appendix (the right iliac fossa) (see also p. 174). In mild cases the inflammation subsides and healing takes place. In more severe cases microbial growth progresses, leading to suppuration, abscess formation and further congestion. The rising pressure inside the appendix occludes first the veins, then the arteries and ischaemia develops, followed by gangrene and rupture.

Complications of appendicitis

Peritonitis. The peritoneum becomes acutely inflamed, the blood vessels dilate and excess serous fluid is secreted. It occurs as a complication of appendicitis when:

- microbes spread through the wall of the appendix and infect the peritoneum
- an appendix abscess ruptures and pus enters the peritoneal cavity
- the appendix becomes gangrenous and ruptures, discharging its contents into the peritoneal cavity.

Abscess formation. The most common are:

- subphrenic abscess, between the liver and diaphragm, from which infection may spread upwards to the pleura, pericardium and mediastinal structures
- pelvic abscess from which infection may spread to adjacent structures (Fig. 12.48).

Fibrous adhesions. When healing takes place fibrous tissue forms and later shrinkage may cause:

- stricture or obstruction of the bowel
- limitation of the movement of a loop of bowel, which may twist around the adhesion causing a type of bowel obstruction called a *volvulus* (p. 327).

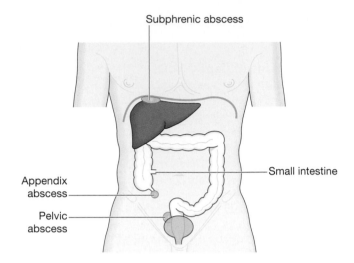

Figure 12.48 Abscess formation; complication of appendicitis.

Microbial diseases (Fig. 12.49)

These conditions represent a major cause of morbidity and mortality worldwide. Contamination of drinking water results in diarrhoeal diseases that are a major cause of infant death in developing countries.

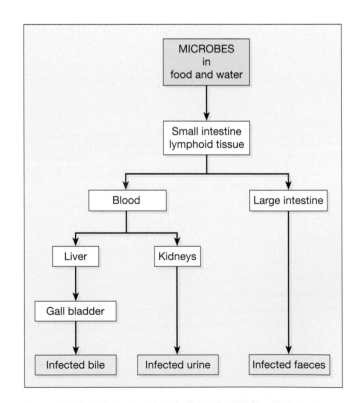

Figure 12.49 The routes of excretion of microbes in enteric fever.

Typhoid fever

This type of enteritis is caused by the bacterium *Salmonella typhi*, ingested in food and water. Humans are its only host so the source of contamination is an individual who is either suffering from the disease or is a carrier.

After infection, there is an incubation period of about 14 days before signs of the disease appear. During this period the microbes invade lymphoid tissue in the walls of the small and large intestines, especially the aggregated lymph follicles (Peyer's patches) and solitary lymph nodes. The microbes then enter the blood vessels and spread to the liver, spleen and gall bladder. In the bacteraemic period acute inflammation develops with necrosis of intestinal lymphoid tissue and ulceration of overlying mucosa. Other effects of *Salmonella typhi* or their endotoxins include:

- typhoid cholecystitis in which the microbes multiply in the gall bladder and are excreted in bile, reinfecting the intestine
- red spots on the skin, especially of the chest and abdomen
- enlargement of the spleen
- myocardial damage and endocarditis
- liver and kidney damage
- reduced resistance to other infections, especially of the respiratory tract, e.g. laryngitis, bronchitis, pneumonia.

Uncomplicated recovery takes place in about 5 weeks with healing of intestinal ulcers and very little fibrosis.

Complications

- The ulcers may perforate a blood vessel, causing haemorrhage, or erode the intestinal wall, leading to acute peritonitis.
- The individual may become a carrier. When this happens the typhoid fever becomes a chronic, asymptomatic infection of the biliary and urinary tracts. Microbes continue to be excreted indefinitely in urine and faeces. Contamination of food and water by carriers is the usual source of infection.

Paratyphoid fever

This disease is caused by *Salmonella paratyphi* A or B spread in the same way as typhoid fever, i.e. in food and drink contaminated by infected urine or faeces. The infection, causing inflammation of the intestinal mucosa, is usually confined to the ileum although the duration is shorter and the symptoms less severe than typhoid fever. Other parts of the body are not usually affected but occasionally chronic infection of the urinary and biliary tracts occurs and the individual becomes an asymptomatic carrier, excreting the microbes in urine and faeces.

Other Salmonella infections

Salmonella typhimurium and *S. enteritidis* are the most common microbes in this group. Generally the effects are confined to the gastrointestinal tract, unlike the infections above. In addition to humans their hosts are domestic animals and birds. The microbes may be present in meat, poultry, eggs and milk, causing infection if cooking does not achieve sterilisation. Mice and rats also carry the organisms and may contaminate food before or after cooking.

The infection is usually of short duration and is usually accompanied by acute abdominal pain and diarrhoea, causing dehydration and electrolyte imbalance. Sometimes vomiting is present. In children and debilitated elderly people the infection may be severe or even fatal. Chronic infection of the biliary and urinary tracts may develop and the individual becomes a carrier, excreting the organisms in urine and faeces (Fig. 12.49).

Escherichia coli (*E. coli*) food poisoning

Common sources of these bacteria include undercooked meat and unpasteurised milk; adequate cooking kills *E. coli*. The severity of the disease depends on the type of *E. coli* responsible; some types are more virulent than others. Outbreaks of *E. coli* food poisoning can cause fatalities, particularly in the young and elderly people.

Staphylococcal food poisoning

This is not an infection in the true sense. *Staphylococcus aureus* in contaminated food produces toxins that cause acute gastroenteritis. Although cooking kills the bacteria, the toxin is heat stable.

There is usually short-term acute inflammation with violent vomiting and diarrhoea, causing dehydration and electrolyte imbalance. In most cases complete recovery occurs within 24 hours.

Clostridium perfringens food poisoning

These microbes, although normally present in the intestines of humans and animals, cause food poisoning when ingested in large numbers. Meat may be contaminated at any stage between slaughter and the consumer. Outbreaks of food poisoning are associated with large-scale cooking, e.g. in institutions. Slow cooling after cooking and/or slow reheating allow microbial multiplication. When they reach the intestines, the bacteria release a toxin that causes diarrhoea and abdominal pain.

323

Campylobacter food poisoning

These Gram-negative bacilli are a common cause of gastroenteritis accompanied by fever, acute pain and sometimes bleeding. They affect mainly young adults and children under 5 years. The microbes are present in the intestines of birds and animals, and are spread in undercooked poultry and meat. They may also be spread in water and milk. Pets, such as cats and dogs, may be a source of infection.

Cholera

Cholera is caused by *Vibrio cholerae* and is spread by contaminated water, faeces, vomit, food, hands and fomites. The only known hosts are humans. A very powerful toxin is produced by the bacteria, which stimulates the intestinal glands to secrete large quantities of water, bicarbonate and chloride. This leads to persistent diarrhoea, severe dehydration and electrolyte imbalance, and may cause death due to hypovolaemic shock. The microbes occasionally spread to the gall bladder where they multiply. They are then excreted in bile and faeces. This carrier state usually lasts for a maximum of about 4 years, providing a reservoir for spread of infection.

Dysentery

Bacillary dysentery

This infection of the colon is caused by bacteria of the *Shigella* group. The severity of the condition depends on the organisms involved. In the UK it is usually a relatively mild condition caused by *Shigella sonnei*. Outbreaks may reach epidemic proportions, especially in institutions. Children and elderly debilitated adults are particularly susceptible. The only host is humans and the organisms are spread by faecal contamination of food, drink, hands and fomites.

The intestinal mucosa becomes inflamed, ulcerated and oedematous with excess mucus secretion. In severe infections, the acute diarrhoea, containing blood and excess mucus, causes dehydration, electrolyte imbalance and anaemia. When healing occurs the mucous membrane is fully restored. Occasionally a chronic infection develops and the individual becomes a carrier, excreting the microbes in faeces. *Shigella dysenteriae* causes the most severe type of infection. It occurs mainly in tropical countries.

Amoebic dysentery

This disease is caused by *Entamoeba histolytica*. The only known hosts are humans and it is spread by faecal contamination of food, water, hands and fomites. Within the colon, the amoebae grow, divide and invade the mucosal cells, causing inflammation and ulceration. In the later stages, destruction of much of the mucosa and sometimes perforation occurs. Diarrhoea containing mucus and blood is persistent and debilitating.

The disease may progress in a number of ways.

- Healing may produce fibrous adhesions, causing partial or complete intestinal obstruction.
- The amoebae may spread to the liver, causing amoebic hepatitis and abscesses.
- Chronic dysentery may develop with intermittent diarrhoea and amoebae in the faeces.

Although most infected people do not develop symptoms they may become carriers.

Inflammatory bowel disease (Table 12.4)

This term includes Crohn's disease and ulcerative colitis. Their aetiology is unknown but both are thought to be triggered by environmental factors in genetically susceptible individuals.

Crohn's disease (regional ileitis)

This chronic inflammatory condition of the alimentary tract usually occurs in young adults. The terminal ileum and the rectum are most commonly affected but the disease may be more widespread. There is chronic patchy inflammation with oedema of the full thickness of the intestinal wall, causing partial obstruction of the lumen, sometimes described as *skip lesions*. There are periods of remission of varying duration. The cause of Crohn's disease is not entirely clear but it may be that immunological abnormality renders the individual susceptible to infection, especially by viruses. Complications include:

- secondary infections, occurring when inflamed areas ulcerate
- fibrous adhesions and subsequent intestinal obstruction caused by the healing process
- fistulae between intestinal lesions and adjacent structures, e.g. loops of bowel, surface of the skin (p. 373)
- perianal fistulae, fissures and skin tags
- megaloblastic anaemia due to malabsorption of vitamin B_{12} and folic acid
- cancer of the small or large intestine.

Ulcerative colitis

This is a chronic inflammatory disease of the mucosa of the colon and rectum, which may ulcerate and become infected. It usually occurs in young adults and begins in the rectum and sigmoid colon. From there it may spread

Table 12.4 Comparison of the main features of Crohn's disease and ulcerative colitis

	Crohn's disease	Ulcerative colitis
Incidence	Usually between 20 and 40 years of age; both sexes affected equally; smokers at higher risk	Usually between 20 and 40 years of age; more women affected than men; smoking not a risk factor
Main sites of lesions	Anywhere in digestive tract from mouth to anus; common in terminal ileum	Rectum always involved, with variable spread along colon
Tissue involved	Entire thickness of the wall inflamed and thickened tissue; ulcers and fistulae common	Only mucosa involved
Nature of lesions	'Skip' lesions, i.e. diseased areas interspersed with regions of normal tissue; ulcers and fistulae common	Continuous lesion; mucosa is red and inflamed
Prognosis	In severe cases, surgery may improve condition, but relapse rate very high	Surgical removal of entire colon cures the condition

to involve a variable proportion of the colon and, sometimes, the entire colon. There are periods of remission lasting weeks, months or years. Individuals may develop other systemic problems affecting e.g. the joints (ankylosing spondylitis, p. 428), skin and liver. In long-standing cases, cancer sometimes develops.

Fulminating ulcerative colitis

This is also called *toxic megacolon*. The colon loses its muscle tone and dilates, the wall becomes thinner and perforation, which can be fatal, may follow. There is sudden onset of acute diarrhoea, with severe blood loss, leading to dehydration, electrolyte imbalance, perforation, hypovolaemic shock and possibly death.

Diverticular disease

Diverticula are small pouches of mucosa that protrude (herniate) into the peritoneal cavity through the circular muscle fibres of the colon between the taeniae coli (Fig. 12.50). The walls consist of mucous membrane with a covering of visceral peritoneum. They occur at the weakest points of the intestinal wall, i.e. where the blood vessels enter, most commonly in the sigmoid colon.

The causes of *diverticulosis* (presence of diverticuli) are not known but it is associated with deficiency of dietary fibre and abnormally active peristalsis. In Western countries, diverticulosis is fairly common after the age of 60 but diverticulitis affects only a small proportion.

Diverticulitis arises when faeces impact in the diverticula and the walls become inflamed and oedematous as secondary infection develops. This reduces the blood

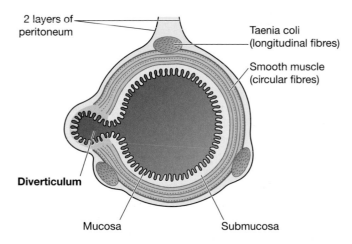

Figure 12.50 Diverticular disease; cross-section of bowel showing one diverticulum.

supply causing ischaemic pain. Occasionally, rupture occurs resulting in peritonitis (p. 322).

Tumours of the small and large intestines

Benign and malignant tumours of the small intestine are rare, compared with their occurrence in the stomach and colon.

Benign tumours

Benign neoplasms may form a broad-based mass or polyp, i.e. develop a pedicle. Occasionally polyps twist

325

upon themselves, causing ischaemia, necrosis and possibly gangrene. Malignant changes may occur in adenomas, which are very common in developed countries.

Malignant tumours

Small intestine. Malignant tumours tend not to obstruct the lumen and may remain unnoticed until symptoms caused by metastases appear. The most common sites of metastases are local lymph nodes, the liver, lungs and brain.

The colon and rectum. This is the most common site of malignancy in the alimentary tract in Western countries. The tumour may be:

- a soft polypoid mass, projecting into the lumen of the colon with a tendency to ulceration, infection and haemorrhage
- a hard fibrous mass encircling the colon, causing reduced elasticity and peristalsis, narrowing of the lumen and obstruction.

The most important predisposing factor for colorectal cancer is thought to be diet. In cultures eating a high-fibre, low-fat diet, the disease is virtually unknown, whereas in Western countries, where large quantities of red meat, saturated animal fat and insufficient fibre are eaten, the disease is much more common. Slow movement of bowel contents may result in conversion of unknown substances present into carcinogenic agents. Predisposing diseases include ulcerative colitis and some benign tumours (usually adenomas).

Local spread of intestinal tumours occurs early but may not be evident until there is severe ulceration and haemorrhage or obstruction. Spread can be outwards through the wall into the peritoneal cavity and adjacent structures.

Lymph-spread metastases occur in mesenteric lymph nodes, the peritoneum and other abdominal and pelvic organs. Pressure caused by enlarged lymph nodes may cause obstruction or damage other structures.

Blood-spread metastases are most common in the liver, brain and bones.

Carcinoid tumours (argentaffinomas)

These tumours are considered, on clinical evidence, to be benign but they spread into the tissues around their original site. They grow very slowly and rarely metastasise. The parent cells are hormone-secreting cells widely dispersed throughout the body, not situated in endocrine glands. Some of these tumours secrete hormones while others do not. They are called APUD cells, an acronym for some of their chemical characteristics. The cells react with silver compounds, hence the name argentaffinomas. Common sites in the intestines for these *apudomas* are the

appendix and ileum although the stomach, colon and rectum can also be affected. The tumours are frequently multiple and larger ones may spread locally, causing obstruction.

Carcinoid syndrome. This is the name given to the effects of the substances secreted by apudomas in the intestine and elsewhere. The secretions include serotonin (5-hydroxytryptamine), histamine and bradykinin, and the effects include flushing attacks, tachycardia, sweating, anxiety and diarrhoea.

Hernias

A hernia is a protrusion of an organ or part of an organ through a weak point or aperture in the surrounding structures. In those affecting the digestive system, a piece of bowel protrudes through a weak point in either the musculature of the anterior abdominal wall or an existing opening (Fig. 12.51A). It occurs when there are intermittent increases in intra-abdominal pressure, most commonly in men who lift heavy loads at work. The underlying causes of the abdominal wall weakness are unknown. Possible outcomes include:

- spontaneous reduction, i.e. the loop of bowel slips back to its correct place when the intra-abdominal pressure returns to normal
- manual reduction, i.e. by applying slight pressure over the abdominal swelling
- strangulation (Fig. 12.51B), when reduction is not possible and the venous drainage from the herniated loop of bowel is obstructed, causing congestion, ischaemia and gangrene. In addition there is intestinal obstruction.

Sites of hernias (Fig. 12.51A)

Inguinal hernia. The weak point is the inguinal canal, which contains the spermatic cord in the male and the round ligament in the female. It occurs more commonly in males than in females.

Femoral hernia. The weak point is the femoral canal through which the femoral artery, vein and lymph vessels pass from the pelvis to the thigh.

Umbilical hernia. The weak point is the umbilicus where the umbilical blood vessels from the placenta enter the fetus.

Incisional hernia. This is caused by repeated stretching of the fibrous tissue formed after previous abdominal surgery.

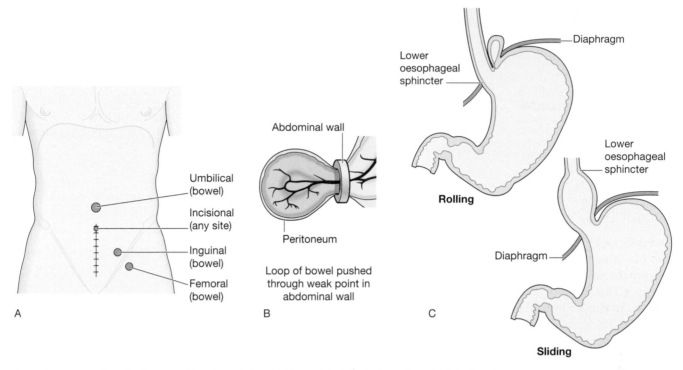

Figure 12.51 Hernias: A. Common sites of herniation. **B.** Strangulated hernia formation. **C.** Hiatus hernia.

327

Diaphragmatic or hiatus hernia (Fig. 12.51C). This is the protrusion of a part of the fundus of the stomach through the oesophageal opening in the diaphragm. The main complication is irritation caused by reflux of acid gastric juice, especially when the individual lies flat or bends down. The long-term effects may be oesophagitis, fibrosis and narrowing of the oesophagus, causing dysphagia. Strangulation does not occur.

Rolling hiatus hernia. An abnormally large opening in the diaphragm allows a pouch of stomach to 'roll' upwards into the thorax beside the oesophagus. This is associated with obesity and increased intra-abdominal pressure.

Sliding hiatus hernia. An unusually short oesophagus that ends above the diaphragm pulls a part of the stomach upwards into the thorax. The abnormality may be congenital or be caused by shrinkage of fibrous tissue formed during healing of a previous oesophageal injury. The sliding movement of the stomach in the oesophageal opening is due to normal shortening of the oesophagus by muscular contraction during swallowing.

Peritoneal hernia. A loop of bowel may herniate through the foramen of Winslow, the opening in the lesser omentum that separates the greater and lesser peritoneal sacs.

Volvulus

This occurs when a loop of bowel twists through 180°, cutting off its blood supply, causing gangrene and obstruction. It occurs in parts of the intestine that are attached to the posterior abdominal wall by a long double fold of visceral peritoneum, the mesentery. The most common site in adults is the sigmoid colon and in children the small intestine. Predisposing factors include:

- an unusually long mesentery
- heavy loading of the pelvic colon with faeces
- a slight twist of a loop of bowel, causing gas and fluid to accumulate and promote further twisting
- adhesions formed following surgery or peritonitis.

Intussusception

In this condition a length of intestine is invaginated into itself (Fig. 12.52). It occurs most commonly in children when a piece of terminal ileum is pushed through the ileocaecal valve. In a child, infection, usually by viruses, causes swelling of the lymphoid tissue in the intestinal wall. The overlying mucosa bulges into the lumen, creating a partial obstruction and a rise in pressure inside

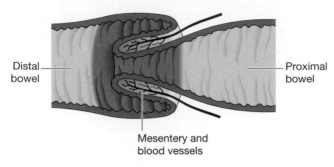

Distal bowel — Proximal bowel

Mesentery and blood vessels

Figure 12.52 Intussusception

the intestine proximal to the swelling. Strong peristaltic waves develop in an attempt to overcome the partial obstruction. These push the swollen piece of bowel into the lumen of the section immediately distal to it, creating the intussusception. The pressure on the veins in the invaginated portion is increased, causing congestion, further swelling, ischaemia and possibly gangrene. Complete intestinal obstruction may occur. In adults tumours that bulge into the lumen, e.g. polyps, together with the strong peristalsis, may be the cause.

Intestinal obstruction

This is not a disease in itself. The following is a summary of the main causes of obstruction with some examples.

Mechanical causes of obstruction
These include:

- constriction of the intestine by, e.g., strangulated hernia, intussusception, volvulus, peritoneal adhesions; partial obstruction may suddenly become complete
- stenosis and thickening of the intestinal wall, e.g. in diverticulosis, Crohn's disease and malignant tumours; there is usually a gradual progression from partial to complete obstruction
- obstruction by, e.g., a large gallstone or a tumour growing into the lumen
- pressure on the intestine from outside, e.g. a large tumour in any pelvic or abdominal organ, such as a uterine fibroid; this is most likely to occur inside the confined space of the bony pelvis.

Neurological causes of obstruction
Partial or complete loss of peristaltic activity produces the effects of obstruction. *Paralytic ileus* is the most common form. The mechanisms are not clear but there are well-recognised predisposing conditions including:

- peritonitis, especially when large amounts of exotoxin are released from dead microbes

- following surgery when there has been considerable handling of the intestines
- severe intestinal infection, especially if there is acute toxaemia, e.g. following ruptured appendix.

Secretion of water and electrolytes continues although intestinal mobility is lost and absorption impaired. This causes distension and electrolyte imbalance, leading to hypovolaemic shock. Growth and multiplication of microbes may also occur.

Vascular causes of obstruction
When the blood supply to a segment of bowel is cut off, ischaemia is followed by infarction, gangrene and obstruction. The causes may be:

- atheromatous changes in the blood vessel walls, with thrombosis (p. 115)
- embolism (p. 115)
- mechanical obstruction of the bowel, e.g. strangulated hernia (p. 326).

Malabsorption

Impaired absorption of nutrients and water from the intestines is not a disease in itself, but the result of diseases causing one or more of the following changes:

- atrophy of the villi of the mucosa of the small intestine
- incomplete digestion of food
- interference with the transport of absorbed nutrients from the small intestine to the blood.

Primary malabsorption

Disease of the intestinal mucous membrane
Atrophy of the villi is the main cause, varying in severity from minor abnormality to almost complete loss of function. The most common underlying diseases are coeliac disease and tropical sprue.

Coeliac disease. This disease is due to an abnormal, genetically determined immunological reaction to the protein *gluten*, present in wheat. When it is removed from the diet, recovery is complete. There is marked villous atrophy and malabsorption characterised by the passage of loose, pale-coloured, fatty stools (steatorrhoea).

There may be abnormal immune reaction to other antigens. Atrophy of the spleen is common and malignant lymphoma of the small intestine may develop. It often presents in infants after weaning but can affect any age.

Tropical sprue. This disease is endemic in subtropical and tropical countries except Africa south of the Sahara.

After leaving the endemic area most people suffering from sprue recover, but others may not develop symptoms until months or even years later.

There is partial villous atrophy with malabsorption, chronic diarrhoea, severe wasting and pernicious anaemia due to deficient absorption of vitamin B_{12} and folic acid. The cause is unknown but it may be that bacterial growth in the small intestine is a factor.

Secondary malabsorption

This is associated with incomplete digestion of food, impaired transport of absorbed nutrients and following extensive small bowel resection.

Incomplete digestion

This occurs in a variety of conditions:

- disease of the liver and pancreas
- following extensive resection of small intestine in, e.g. Crohn's disease
- following surgery if microbes grow in a blind end of intestine.

Impaired transport of nutrients

This occurs when there is:

- lymphatic obstruction by, e.g., lymph node tumours, removal of nodes at surgery, tubercular disease of lymph nodes
- impairment of mesenteric blood flow by, e.g., arterial or venous thrombosis, pressure caused by a tumour
- obstruction of blood flow through the liver, e.g. in cirrhosis.

Diseases of the pancreas

Learning outcomes

After studying this section, you should be able to:

- compare and contrast the causes and effects of acute and chronic pancreatitis
- outline the main pancreatic tumours and their consequences.

Acute pancreatitis

Proteolytic enzymes produced by the pancreas are secreted in inactive forms, which are not activated until they reach the intestine; this protects the pancreas from digestion by its own enzymes. If these precursor enzymes are activated while still in the pancreas, pancreatitis results. The severity of the disease is directly related to the amount of pancreatic tissue destroyed.

Mild forms are more common and damage only those cells near the ducts.

Severe forms cause widespread damage with necrosis and haemorrhage. Common complications include infection, suppuration, and local venous thrombosis. Pancreatic enzymes, especially amylase, enter and circulate in the blood, causing similar damage to other structures. In severe cases there is a high mortality rate.

The causes of acute pancreatitis are not clear but known predisposing factors are gallstones and alcoholism. Other associated conditions include:

- cancer of the ampulla or head of pancreas
- virus infections, notably mumps
- chronic renal failure
- kidney and liver transplantation
- hyperparathyroidism
- severe hypothermia
- drugs, e.g. corticosteroids, cytotoxic agents.

Chronic pancreatitis

This is due to repeated attacks of acute pancreatitis or may arise gradually without evidence of pancreatic disease. It is frequently associated with fibrosis and distortion of the main pancreatic duct. There is intestinal malabsorption when pancreatic secretions are reduced and diabetes mellitus (p. 232) occurs when severe damage affects the β-islet cells.

Protein material secreted by the acinar cells blocks the tiny acinar ducts. This eventually leads to the formation of cysts which may rupture into the peritoneal cavity. Intact cysts may cause obstruction of the:

- common bile duct, causing jaundice
- portal vein, causing venous congestion in the organs drained by its tributaries.

The causes of these changes are associated mainly with excessive alcohol consumption.

Cystic fibrosis (see p. 266)

Tumours of the pancreas

Benign tumours are very rare.

Malignant tumours

These are relatively common and affect more men than women. They occur most frequently in the head of the pancreas, obstructing the flow of bile and pancreatic juice into the duodenum. Jaundice, sometimes accompanied by itching, develops. Weight loss is the result of impaired digestion and absorption of fat, although anorexia and metabolic effects of the tumour may also play a role. Tumours in the body and tail of the gland rarely cause symptoms until the disease is advanced. Metastases are often recognised before the primary tumour and the prognosis is generally poor. There is an association with cigarette smoking and diabetes mellitus.

Diseases of the liver

Learning outcomes

After studying this section, you should be able to:

- compare and contrast the causes, forms and effects of chronic and acute hepatitis

- describe the main non-viral inflammatory conditions of the liver

- discuss the causes and consequences of liver failure

- describe the main liver tumours.

New liver cells develop only when needed to replace damaged cells. Capacity for regeneration is considerable and damage is usually extensive before it is evident. The effects of disease or toxic agents are seen when:

- regeneration of hepatocytes (liver cells) does not keep pace with damage, leading to hepatocellular failure
- there is a gradual replacement of damaged cells by fibrous tissue, leading to portal hypertension.

In most liver disease both conditions are present.

Acute hepatitis

Areas of necrosis develop as groups of hepatocytes die and the eventual outcome depends on the size and number of these areas. Causes of the damage may be a variety of conditions, including:

- viral infections
- toxic substances
- circulatory disturbances.

Viral hepatitis

Viral infections are the commonest cause of acute liver injury and include Type A, Type B and Type C. The types are distinguished serologically, i.e. by the antibodies produced to combat the infection. The severity of the ensuing disease caused by the different virus types varies considerably, but the pattern is similar. The viruses enter the liver cells, causing degenerative changes. An inflammatory reaction ensues, accompanied by production of an exudate containing lymphocytes, plasma cells and granulocytes. There is reactive hyperplasia of the hepatic macrophages (Kupffer cells) in the walls of the sinusoids.

As groups of cells die, necrotic areas of varying sizes develop, phagocytes remove the necrotic material and the lobules collapse. The basic lobule framework (Fig. 12.36) becomes distorted and blood vessels develop kinks. These changes interfere with the circulation of blood to the remaining hepatocytes and the resultant hypoxia causes further damage. Fibrous tissue develops in the damaged area, and adjacent hepatocytes proliferate. The effect of these changes on the overall functioning of the liver depends on the size of the necrotic areas, the amount of fibrous tissue formed and the extent to which the blood and bile channels are distorted.

Type A virus (infectious hepatitis)

This type occurs endemically, affecting mainly children, causing a mild illness. Infection is spread by hands, food, water and fomites contaminated by infected faeces. The incubation period is 15 to 40 days and the viruses are excreted in the faeces for 7 to 14 days before clinical symptoms appear and for about 7 days after. Antibodies develop and immunity persists after recovery. Subclinical disease may occur but not carriers.

Type B virus (serum hepatitis)

Infection occurs at any age, but mostly in adults. The incubation period is 50 to 180 days. The virus enters the blood and is spread by blood and blood products. People at greatest risk of infection are those who come in contact with blood and blood products in their daily work, e.g. people in the health, ambulance and fire services. The virus is also spread by body fluids, i.e. saliva, semen, vaginal secretions and from mother to fetus. Others at risk include intravenous drug users and homosexual men. Antibodies are formed and immunity persists after recovery. Infection usually leads to severe illness lasting 2 to 6 weeks, often followed by a protracted convalescence. Carriers may, or may not, have had clinical disease. Type B virus may cause massive liver necrosis and death. In less severe cases recovery may be complete. In chronic hepatitis (p. 331) that may develop, live viruses continue to circulate in the blood and other body fluids. The condition is thought to predispose to liver cancer.

Hepatitis C

This virus is spread by blood and blood products. It is prevalent in IV drug users and also occurs as a complication of blood transfusion. The infection can be asymptomatic as a carrier state occurs. When hepatitis develops, it is often recurrent and may result in chronic liver disease, especially cirrhosis.

Toxic substances

Many drugs undergo chemical change in the liver before excretion in bile or by other organs. They may damage the liver cells in their original form or while in various intermediate stages. Some substances always cause liver damage (predictably toxic) while others only do so when hypersensitivity develops (unpredictably toxic). In both types the extent of the damage depends on the size of the dose and/or the duration of exposure (Box 12.1).

Circulatory disturbances

The intensely active hepatocytes are particularly vulnerable to damage by hypoxia, which is usually due to impaired blood supply caused by:

- fibrosis in the liver following inflammation
- compression of the portal vein, hepatic artery or vein by a tumour
- acute general circulatory failure and shock
- venous congestion caused by acute or chronic right-sided heart failure.

Chronic hepatitis

This is defined as any form of hepatitis which persists for more than 6 months. It may be caused by viruses or drugs, but in some cases the cause is unknown.

Chronic persistent hepatitis

This is a mild, persistent inflammation following acute viral hepatitis. There is usually little or no fibrosis.

Box 12.1 Some hepatotoxic substances

Predictable group (dose related)	Unpredictable group (individual idiosyncrasy)
Chloroform	Phenothiazine compounds
Tetracyclines	Halothane
Cytotoxic drugs	Methyldopa
Anabolic steroids	Indometacin
Alcohol	Chlorpropamide
Paracetamol	Thiouracil
Some fungi	Sulphonamides

Chronic active hepatitis

This is a continuing progressive inflammation with cell necrosis and the formation of fibrous tissue that may lead to cirrhosis of the liver. There is distortion of the liver blood vessels and hypoxia, leading to further hepatocyte damage. This condition is commonly associated with Types B and C viral hepatitis, with some forms of autoimmunity and unpredictable (idiosyncratic) drug reactions.

Non-viral inflammation of the liver

Pyogenic

Ascending cholangitis. Infection, usually by *E. coli*, may spread from the biliary tract and may result in liver abscesses. The most common predisposing factor is obstruction of the common bile duct by gallstones.

Liver abscess. Septic emboli from infective foci in the abdomen and pelvis may lodge in branches of the portal vein and cause multiple abscesses or infect the vein itself. Common sources of this type of infection are acute appendicitis, diverticulitis and inflamed haemorrhoids.

Cirrhosis of the liver

This is the result of long-term inflammation caused by a wide variety of agents. The most common causes are:

- alcoholism
- hepatitis B and C virus infections
- the effects of bile retained in hepatocytes due to obstruction of bile flow or chronic inflammation
- congenital metabolic abnormalities.

As the inflammation subsides, destroyed liver tissue is replaced by fibrous tissue. There is hyperplasia of hepatocytes adjacent to the damaged area, in an attempt to compensate for the destroyed cells. This leads to the formation of nodules consisting of hepatocytes confined within sheets of fibrous tissue.

As the condition progresses portal hypertension develops, leading to congestion in the organs drained by the tributaries of the portal vein, to ascites and possibly to the development of oesophageal varices (p. 318).

Liver failure may occur when hyperplasia is unable to keep pace with cell destruction, and there is increased risk of liver cancer developing.

Liver failure

This occurs when liver function is reduced to such an extent that other body activities are impaired. It may be acute or chronic and may be the outcome of a wide variety of disorders, e.g.:

- acute viral hepatitis
- extensive necrosis due to poisoning, e.g. some drug overdoses, hepatotoxic chemicals, adverse drug reactions
- cirrhosis of the liver
- following some medical procedures, e.g. abdominal paracentesis, portacaval shunt operations.

Liver failure has serious effects on other parts of the body.

Hepatic encephalopathy

The cells affected are the astrocytes in the brain. The condition is characterised by apathy, disorientation, muscular rigidity, confusion and coma. Several factors may be involved, e.g.:

- nitrogenous bacterial metabolites absorbed from the colon, which are normally detoxified in the liver, reach the brain via the blood
- other metabolites, normally present in trace amounts, e.g. ammonia, may reach toxic concentrations and change the permeability of the cerebral blood vessels and the effectiveness of the blood–brain barrier
- hypoxia and electrolyte imbalance.

Blood coagulation defects

The liver fails to synthesise substances needed for blood clotting, i.e. prothrombin, fibrinogen and factors II, V, VII, IX and X. Purpura, bruising and bleeding may occur.

Oliguria and renal failure

Portal hypertension may cause the development of oesophageal varices. If these rupture, bleeding may lead to a fall in blood pressure sufficient to reduce the renal blood flow, causing progressive oliguria and renal failure.

Oedema and ascites

These may be caused by the combination of two factors:

- portal hypertension raises the capillary hydrostatic pressure in the organs drained by the tributaries of the portal vein (see Fig. 5.46, p. 105)
- diminished production of serum albumin and clotting factors reduces the plasma osmotic pressure.

Together these changes cause the movement of excess fluid into the interstitial spaces where it causes *oedema*. Eventually free fluid accumulates in the peritoneal cavity and the resultant *ascites* may be severe.

Anaemia

This is usually due to the combined effect of a number of factors:

- disturbed metabolism of folic acid and vitamin B_{12}
- chronic blood loss from oesophageal varices, causing iron deficiency anaemia
- increased breakdown of red blood cells in the congested spleen, causing haemolytic anaemia (p. 70).

Jaundice

The following factors may cause jaundice as liver failure develops:

- inability of the hepatocytes to conjugate and excrete bilirubin
- obstruction to the movement of bile through the bile channels by fibrous tissue that has distorted the structural framework of liver lobules.

Tumours of the liver

Benign tumours are very rare.

Malignant tumours

In many cases cancer of the liver is associated with cirrhosis but the relationship between them is not clear. It may be that both cirrhosis and cancer are caused by the same agents or that the carcinogenic action of other agents is promoted by cirrhotic changes. Malignancy sometimes develops in acute hepatitis caused by Types B and C virus. The most common sites of metastases are the abdominal lymph nodes, the peritoneum and the lungs.

Secondary malignant tumours in the liver are very common, especially from primary tumours in the gastrointestinal tract, the lungs and the breast. They tend to grow rapidly and are often the cause of death.

Diseases of the gall bladder and bile ducts

Learning outcomes

After studying this section, you should be able to:

- describe the causes and consequences of gallstones
- compare and contrast acute and chronic cholecystitis
- briefly outline the common sites and consequences of biliary tract tumours
- discuss the main causes and effects of jaundice.

Gallstones (cholelithiasis)

Gallstones consist of deposits of the constituents of bile, most commonly cholesterol. Many small stones or one large stone may form but they do not necessarily produce symptoms. Predisposing factors include:

- changes in the composition of bile that affect the solubility of its constituents
- high levels of blood and dietary cholesterol
- diabetes mellitus when associated with high blood cholesterol levels
- female gender
- obesity
- long-term use of oral contraceptives
- several pregnancies in young women especially when accompanied by obesity.

Complications

Biliary colic. If a gallstone becomes impacted (stuck) in the cystic or common bile duct there is strong peristaltic contraction of the smooth muscle in the wall of the duct (spasm) in an effort to move the stone onwards. The severe pain associated with biliary colic is due to ischaemia of the duct wall over the stone during the smooth muscle spasm.

Inflammation. Gallstones can cause irritation and inflammation of the walls of the gall bladder and also the cystic and common bile ducts. There may be superimposed microbial infection.

Impaction. Blockage of the cystic duct by a gallstone leads to distension of the gall bladder and *cholecystitis*. This does not cause jaundice because bile from the liver can still pass directly into the duodenum. Obstruction of the common bile duct leads to retention of bile, jaundice and *cholangitis* (inflammation of the bile ducts) that predisposes to secondary infection.

Acute cholecystitis

This is usually a complication of gallstones or an exacerbation of chronic cholecystitis, especially if there has been partial or intermittent obstruction of the cystic duct. Inflammation develops, followed by secondary microbial infections spread from a focus of infection elsewhere in the body, e.g. they may be blood-borne or pass directly from the adjacent colon. Those most commonly involved are *E. coli* and *Streptococcus faecalis*. In severe cases there may be fibrinous exudate into the gall bladder, suppuration, gangrene, perforation, peritonitis, local abscess formation, disruption of gall bladder

activity, gallstone formation and the infection may spread to the bile ducts and the liver.

Chronic cholecystitis

The onset is usually insidious, sometimes following repeated acute attacks. Gallstones are invariably present and there may be accompanying biliary colic. Pain is due to the spasmodic contraction of muscle, causing ischaemia when the gall bladder is packed with gallstones. There is usually secondary infection with suppuration. Ulceration of the tissues between the gall bladder and the duodenum or colon may occur with fistula formation and, later, fibrous adhesions.

Tumours of the biliary tract

Benign tumours are rare.

Malignant tumours
These are relatively rare but when they do occur the most common sites are the neck of the gall bladder, the junction of the cystic and bile ducts, and the ampulla of the bile duct.

Local spread to the liver, the pancreas and other adjacent organs is common. Lymph and blood spread lead to widespread metastases. Early sites include the liver, lungs, abdominal lymph nodes and the peritoneum.

Jaundice

This is not a disease in itself, but is a sign of abnormal bilirubin metabolism and excretion. Bilirubin, produced from the breakdown of haemoglobin, is usually conjugated in the liver and excreted in the bile. Conjugation, the process of adding certain groups to the bilirubin molecule, makes it water soluble and greatly enhances its removal from the blood, an essential step in excretion.

Unconjugated bilirubin, which is fat soluble, has a toxic effect on brain cells. However, it is unable to cross the blood–brain barrier until the plasma level rises above 340 µmol/l, but when it does it may cause neurological damage, seizures (fits) and mental impairment. Serum bilirubin may rise to 40 to 50 µmol/l before the yellow coloration of jaundice is evident in the skin and conjunctiva (normal 3 to 13 µmol/l).

Jaundice develops when there is an abnormality at some stage in the metabolic sequence caused by one or more factors, e.g.:

- excess haemolysis of red blood cells with the production of more bilirubin than the liver can deal with

333

- abnormal liver function that may cause:
  - incomplete uptake of unconjugated bilirubin by hepatocytes
  - ineffective conjugation of bilirubin
  - interference with bilirubin secretion into the bile
- obstruction to the flow of bile from the liver to the duodenum.

Types of jaundice

Whatever stage in bilirubin processing is affected, the end result is rising blood bilirubin levels.

Haemolytic jaundice

This is due to increased haemolysis of red blood cells (see Fig. 12.38 and p. 62) in the spleen. Circulating bilirubin is increased and if hypoxia develops the efficiency of hepatocyte activity is reduced.

Neonatal haemolytic jaundice occurs in many babies, especially in those born prematurely where the normal high haemolysis is coupled with shortage of conjugating enzymes in the hepatocytes.

Obstructive jaundice

Obstruction to the flow of bile in the biliary tract is caused by, e.g.:

- gallstones in the common bile duct
- tumour of the head of the pancreas
- fibrosis of the bile ducts, following inflammation or injury by cholangitis or the passage of gallstones.

Effects of raised serum bilirubin include:

- pruritus (itching) caused by the irritating effects of bile salts on the skin
- pale faeces due to absence of stercobilin (p. 304)
- dark urine due to the presence of increased amounts of bilirubin.

Hepatocellular jaundice

This is the result of damage to the liver itself by, e.g.:

- viral hepatitis
- toxic substances, such as drugs
- amoebiasis (amoebic dysentery)
- cirrhosis.

The damaged hepatocytes may be unable to remove unconjugated bilirubin from the blood, or conjugate bilirubin, or secrete conjugated bilirubin into bile canaliculi.

The urinary system

13

The urinary system is the main excretory system and consists of the following structures:

- 2 *kidneys*, which secrete urine
- 2 *ureters*, which convey the urine from the kidneys to the urinary bladder
- the *urinary bladder* where urine collects and is temporarily stored
- the *urethra* through which the urine is discharged from the urinary bladder to the exterior.

Figure 13.1 shows an overview of the urinary system.

The urinary system plays a vital part in maintaining homeostasis of water and electrolyte concentrations within the body. The kidneys produce urine that contains metabolic waste products, including the nitrogenous compounds urea and uric acid, excess ions and some drugs.

The main functions of the kidneys are:

- formation and secretion of urine
- production and secretion of erythropoietin, the hormone that controls formation of red blood cells (p. 62)
- production and secretion of renin, an important enzyme in the control of blood pressure (p. 221).

Urine is stored in the bladder and excreted by the process of *micturition*.

Kidneys

Learning outcomes

After studying this section you should be able to:

- identify the organs associated with the kidneys
- outline the gross structure of the kidneys
- describe the structure of a nephron
- explain the processes involved in the formation of urine
- explain how body water and electrolyte balance is maintained.

The kidneys (Fig. 13.2) lie on the posterior abdominal wall, one on each side of the vertebral column, behind the peritoneum and below the diaphragm. They extend from the level of the 12th thoracic vertebra to the 3rd lumbar vertebra, receiving some protection from the lower rib cage. The right kidney is usually slightly lower than the left, probably because of the considerable space occupied by the liver.

Kidneys are bean-shaped organs, about 11 cm long, 6 cm wide, 3 cm thick and weigh 150 g. They are embedded in, and held in position by, a mass of fat. A sheath of fibroelastic *renal fascia* encloses the kidney and the renal fat.

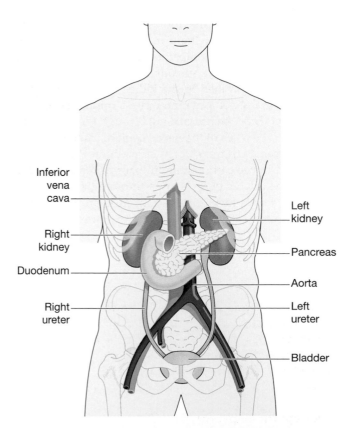

Figure 13.1 The parts of the urinary system (excluding the urethra) and some associated structures.

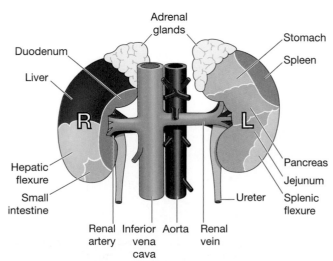

Figure 13.2 Anterior view of the kidneys showing the areas of contact with associated structures.

Organs associated with the kidneys

(Figs 13.1, 13.2 and 13.3)

As the kidneys lie on either side of the vertebral column, each is associated with a different group of structures.

Right kidney

Superiorly – the right adrenal gland

Anteriorly – the right lobe of the liver, the duodenum and the hepatic flexure of the colon

Posteriorly – the diaphragm, and muscles of the posterior abdominal wall

Left kidney

Superiorly – the left adrenal gland

Anteriorly – the spleen, stomach, pancreas, jejunum and splenic flexure of the colon

Posteriorly – the diaphragm and muscles of the posterior abdominal wall

Gross structure of the kidney

There are three areas of tissue that can be distinguished when a longitudinal section of the kidney is viewed with the naked eye (Fig. 13.4):

- a *fibrous capsule*, surrounding the kidney
- the *cortex*, a reddish-brown layer of tissue immediately below the capsule and outside the pyramids

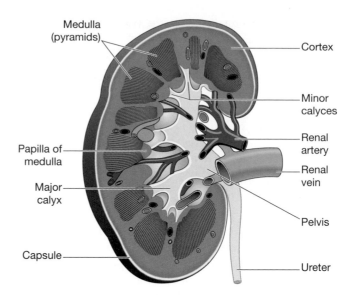

Figure 13.4 A longitudinal section of the right kidney.

- the *medulla*, the innermost layer, consisting of pale conical-shaped striations, the *renal pyramids*.

The hilum is the concave medial border of the kidney where the renal blood and lymph vessels, the ureter and nerves enter.

The renal pelvis is the funnel-shaped structure that acts as a receptacle for the urine formed by the kidney (Fig. 13.4). It has a number of distal branches called *calyces*, each of which surrounds the apex of a renal pyramid. Urine formed in the kidney passes through a *papilla* at the apex of a pyramid into a minor calyx, then into a major calyx before passing through the pelvis into the ureter. The walls of the pelvis contain smooth muscle and are lined with transitional epithelium. Peristalsis of the smooth muscle originating in pacemaker cells in the walls of the calyces propels urine through the pelvis and ureters to the bladder. This is an intrinsic property of the smooth muscle, and is not under nerve control.

Microscopic structure of the kidney

The kidney is composed of about 1 million functional units, the *nephrons*, and a smaller number of *collecting ducts*. The collecting ducts transport urine through the pyramids to the renal pelvis, giving them their striped appearance. The tubules are supported by a small amount of connective tissue, containing blood vessels, nerves and lymph vessels.

The nephron (Fig. 13.5)

The nephron consists of a tubule closed at one end, the other end opening into a collecting tubule. The closed or

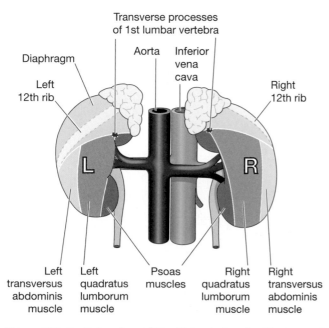

Figure 13.3 Posterior view of the kidneys showing the areas of contact with associated structures.

337

blind end is indented to form the cup-shaped *glomerular capsule* (Bowman's capsule), which almost completely encloses a network of arterial capillaries, the *glomerulus*. Continuing from the glomerular capsule, the remainder of the nephron is about 3 cm long and is described in three parts:

- the proximal convoluted tubule
- the medullary loop (loop of Henle)
- the distal convoluted tubule, leading into a collecting duct.

The collecting ducts unite, forming larger ducts that empty into the minor calyces.

After entering the kidney at the hilum the renal artery divides into smaller arteries and arterioles. In the cortex an arteriole, the *afferent arteriole*, enters each glomerular capsule and then subdivides into a cluster of capillaries, forming the glomerulus. Between the capillary loops are

connective tissue phagocytic *mesangial cells*, which are part of the monocyte–macrophage system (p. 65). The blood vessel leading away from the glomerulus is the *efferent arteriole*. It breaks up into a second capillary network, and exchange across capillary walls regulates the composition of the blood and supplies local tissues with oxygen and nutrients (Fig. 13.6). Venous blood drained from this capillary bed eventually leaves the kidney in the renal vein, which empties into the inferior vena cava. The blood pressure in the glomerulus is higher than in other capillaries because the diameter of the afferent arteriole is greater than that of the efferent arteriole.

The walls of the glomerulus and the glomerular capsule consist of a single layer of flattened epithelial cells (Fig. 13.7). The glomerular walls are more permeable than those of other capillaries. The remainder of the nephron and the collecting tubule are formed by a single layer of highly specialised cells.

The blood vessels of the kidney are supplied by both sympathetic and parasympathetic nerves. The presence of both branches of the autonomic nervous system controls renal blood vessel diameter and renal blood flow independently of autoregulation.

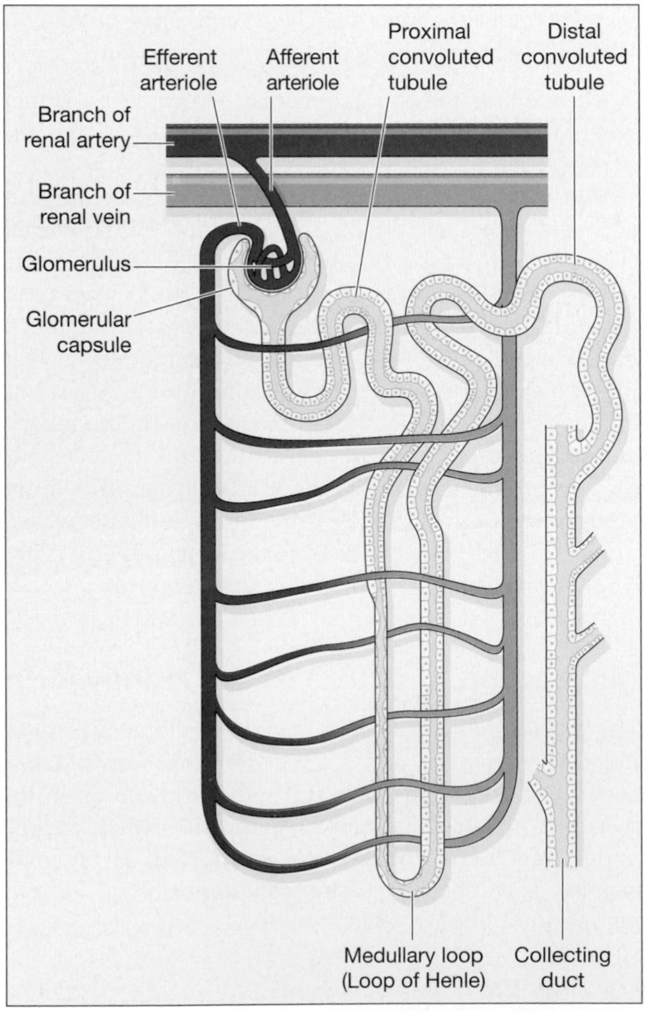

338

Figure 13.5 A nephron and associated blood vessels.

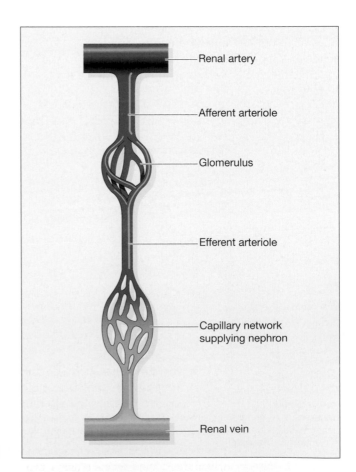

Figure 13.6 The series of blood vessels in the kidney.

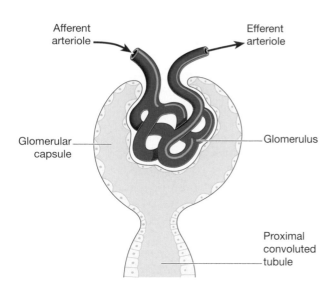

Figure 13.7 The glomerulus and glomerular capsule.

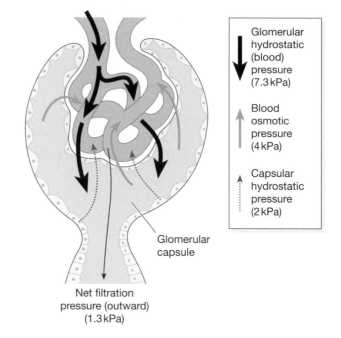

Figure 13.8 Filtration in the nephron.

Functions of the kidney

Formation of urine

The kidneys form urine, which passes through the ureters to the bladder for storage prior to excretion. The composition of urine reflects exchange of substances between the nephron and the blood in the renal capillaries. Waste products of protein metabolism are excreted, electrolyte levels are controlled and pH (acid–base balance) is maintained by excretion of hydrogen ions. There are three processes involved in the formation of urine:

- filtration
- selective reabsorption
- secretion.

Filtration (Fig. 13.8)

This takes place through the semipermeable walls of the glomerulus and glomerular capsule. Water and other small molecules pass through, although some are reabsorbed later. Blood cells, plasma proteins and other large molecules are too large to filter through and therefore remain in the capillaries (see Box 13.1). The filtrate in the glomerulus is very similar in composition to plasma with the important exception of plasma proteins.

Filtration is assisted by the difference between the blood pressure in the glomerulus and the pressure of the filtrate in the glomerular capsule. Because the efferent arteriole is narrower than the afferent arteriole, a *capillary hydrostatic pressure* of about 7.3 kPa (55 mmHg) builds up in the glomerulus. This pressure is opposed by the *osmotic pressure* of the blood, provided mainly by plasma proteins, about 4 kPa (30 mmHg), and by *filtrate hydrostatic*

Box 13.1 Constituents of glomerular filtrate and glomerular capillaries

Blood constituents in glomerular filtrate	Blood constituents remaining in glomerular capillaries
Water	Leukocytes
Mineral salts	Erythrocytes
Amino acids	Platelets
Ketoacids	Plasma proteins
Glucose	Some drugs
Some hormones	
Creatinine	
Urea	
Uric acid	
Some toxins	
Some drugs	

339

pressure of about 2 kPa (15 mmHg) in the glomerular capsule. The net *filtration pressure* is, therefore:

$$7.3 - (4 + 2) = 1.3 \text{ kPa, or}$$
$$55 - (30 + 15) = 10 \text{ mmHg.}$$

The volume of filtrate formed by both kidneys each minute is called the *glomerular filtration rate* (GFR). In a healthy adult the GFR is about 125 ml/min; i.e. 180 litres of filtrate are formed each day by the two kidneys. Nearly all of the filtrate is later reabsorbed with less than 1%, i.e. 1 to 1.5 litres, excreted as urine. The differences in volume and concentration are due to selective reabsorption of some filtrate constituents and tubular secretion of others.

Autoregulation of filtration. Renal blood flow is protected by a mechanism called *autoregulation*, whereby renal blood flow is maintained at a constant pressure across a wide range of systolic blood pressures (from 80 to 200 mmHg). Autoregulation operates independently of nervous control; i.e. if the nerve supply to the renal blood vessels is interrupted, autoregulation continues to operate. It is therefore a property inherent in renal blood vessels; it may be stimulated by changes in blood pressure in the renal arteries or by fluctuating levels of certain metabolites, e.g. prostaglandins.

In severe shock, when the systolic blood pressure falls below 80 mmHg, autoregulation fails and renal blood flow and the hydrostatic pressure decrease, impairing filtration within the nephrons.

Selective reabsorption (Fig. 13.9)

Selective reabsorption is one process by which the composition and volume of the glomerular filtrate are altered during its passage through the convoluted tubules, the medullary loop and the collecting tubule. This process enables reabsorption, into the blood, of those filtrate constituents needed to maintain fluid and electrolyte balance and the pH of the blood. Active transport takes place at carrier sites in the epithelial membrane, using chemical energy to transport substances against their concentration gradients (p. 33).

Some constituents of glomerular filtrate (e.g. glucose, amino acids) do not normally appear in urine because they are completely reabsorbed unless blood levels are excessive. The kidneys' maximum capacity for reabsorption of a substance is the *transport maximum*, or renal threshold. For example, the normal blood glucose level is 3.5 to 8 mmol/l (63 to 144 mg/100 ml) and if this rises above the transport maximum of about 9 mmol/l (160 mg/100 ml), glucose appears in the urine. This occurs because all the carrier sites are occupied and the mechanism for active transport out of the tubules is overloaded. Other substances reabsorbed by active transport include sodium, calcium, potassium, phosphate and chloride.

Some ions, e.g. sodium and chloride, can be absorbed by both active and passive mechanisms depending on the site in the nephron.

The transport maximum, or renal threshold, of some substances varies according to body need at a particular time, and in some cases reabsorption is regulated by hormones.

Parathyroid hormone from the parathyroid glands and *calcitonin* from the thyroid gland together regulate reabsorption of calcium and phosphate.

Antidiuretic hormone (ADH) from the posterior lobe of the pituitary gland increases the permeability of the distal convoluted tubules and collecting ducts, increasing water reabsorption (Fig. 13.10).

Aldosterone, secreted by the adrenal cortex, increases the reabsorption of sodium and excretion of potassium (Fig. 13.11).

Atrial natriuretic peptide (ANP), secreted by the atria of the heart in response to stretching of the atrial wall, decreases reabsorption of sodium and water in the proximal convoluted tubules and collecting ducts (Fig. 13.12). It also inhibits secretion of ADH and aldosterone.

Reabsorption of nitrogenous waste products, such as urea and uric acid is very limited.

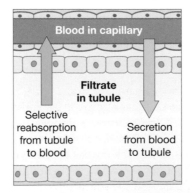

Figure 13.9 Directions of selective reabsorption and secretion in the nephron.

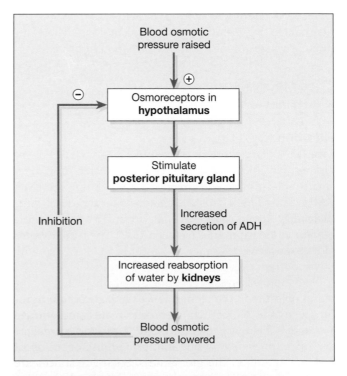

Figure 13.10 Negative feedback regulation of secretion of antidiuretic hormone (ADH).

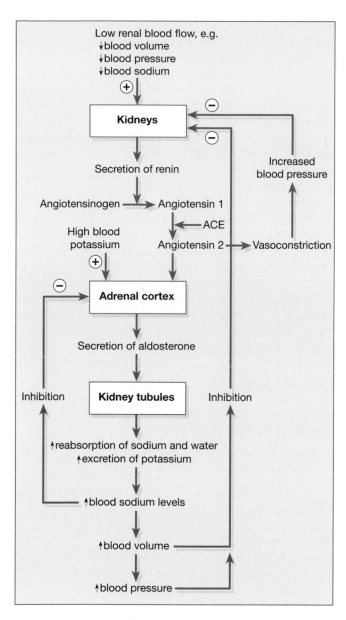

Figure 13.11 Negative feedback regulation of aldosterone secretion. ACE = angiotensin converting enzyme.

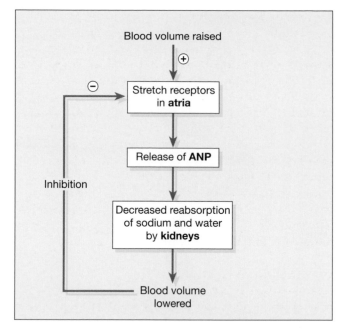

Figure 13.12 Negative feedback regulation of secretion of atrial natriuretic peptide (ANP).

341

hydrogen ions (H⁺) is important in maintaining normal blood pH.

Summary of urine formation
The three processes involved – filtration, selective reabsorption and tubular secretion – are described above and summarised in Figure 13.13.

Composition of urine

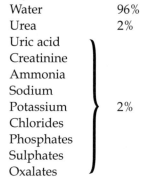

Water	96%	
Urea	2%	
Uric acid		
Creatinine		
Ammonia		
Sodium		
Potassium	2%	
Chlorides		
Phosphates		
Sulphates		
Oxalates		

Urine is clear and amber in colour due to the presence of urobilin, a bile pigment altered in the intestine, reabsorbed then excreted by the kidneys (see Fig. 12.38, p. 308). The specific gravity is between 1020 and 1030, and the pH is around 6 (normal range of 4.5 to 8). A healthy adult passes 1000 to 1500 ml per day. The amount of urine produced and the specific gravity vary according to fluid intake and the amount of solute excreted. Urine production is decreased during sleep and exercise.

Substances not normally found in blood are not reabsorbed. If blood passes through the glomerulus too quickly for filtration to clear such substances, the tubules secrete them into the filtrate.

Tubular secretion (Fig. 13.9)
Filtration occurs as the blood flows through the glomerulus. Substances not required and foreign materials, e.g. drugs including penicillin and aspirin, may not be cleared from the blood by filtration because of the short time it remains in the glomerulus. Such substances are cleared by secretion into the convoluted tubules and excreted from the body in the urine. Tubular secretion of

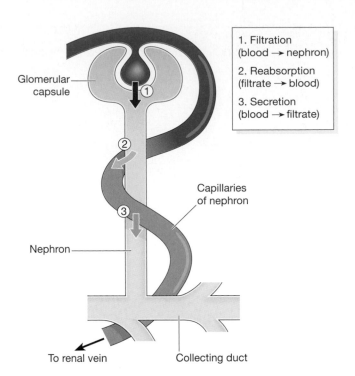

1. Filtration
(blood → nephron)

2. Reabsorption
(filtrate → blood)

3. Secretion
(blood → filtrate)

Glomerular capsule

Capillaries of nephron

Nephron

To renal vein

Collecting duct

Figure 13.13 Summary of the three processes that form urine.

Water balance and urine output

The source of most body water is dietary food and fluid, and a small amount (called 'metabolic water') is formed by metabolic processes. Water is excreted as the main constituent of urine, in expired air, faeces and through the skin as sweat. The amount lost in expired air and faeces is fairly constant, and the amount of sweat produced is associated with environmental and body temperatures (p. 362).

The balance between fluid intake and output is controlled by the kidneys. The minimum urinary output, i.e., the smallest volume required to excrete body waste products, is about 500 ml per day. Urinary volume in excess of this is controlled mainly by antidiuretic hormone (ADH) released into the blood by the posterior lobe of the pituitary gland. The posterior pituitary is closely related to the hypothalamus in the brain (see Fig. 9.3A and B, p. 214).

Sensory nerve cells in the hypothalamus (*osmoreceptors*) detect changes in the osmotic pressure of the blood. Nerve impulses from the osmoreceptors stimulate the posterior pituitary to release ADH. When the osmotic pressure is raised, ADH output is increased and as a result, water reabsorption by the cells in distal convoluted tubules and collecting ducts is increased, reducing the blood osmotic pressure and ADH output. This nega-

tive feedback mechanism maintains the blood osmotic pressure (and therefore sodium and water concentrations) within normal limits (see Fig. 13.10).

The feedback mechanism may be suppressed when there is an excessive amount of a dissolved substance in the blood. For example, in diabetes mellitus when the blood glucose level is above the transport maximum of the renal tubules, excess water is excreted with the excess glucose. This *polyuria* may lead to dehydration despite increased production of ADH but is usually accompanied by acute thirst and increased water intake.

When blood volume is increased, stretch receptors in the atria of the heart release atrial natriuretic hormone (ANP). This reduces reabsorption of sodium and water by the proximal convoluted tubules and collecting ducts, meaning that more sodium and water are excreted. In turn, this lowers blood volume and reduces atrial stretching, and through the negative feedback mechanism ANP secretion is switched off (see Fig. 13.12). Raised ANP levels also inhibit secretion of ADH and aldosterone, further promoting loss of sodium and water.

Electrolyte balance

Changes in the concentration of electrolytes in the body fluids may be due to changes in:

- the body water content, or
- electrolyte levels.

There are several mechanisms that maintain the balance between water and electrolyte concentration.

Sodium and potassium balance

Sodium is the most common cation (positively charged ion) in extracellular fluid and potassium is the most common intracellular cation.

Sodium is a constituent of almost all foods and salt is often added to food during cooking. This means that intake is usually in excess of the body's needs. It is excreted mainly in urine and sweat.

The amount of sodium excreted in sweat is insignificant except when sweating is excessive. This may occur when there is pyrexia, a high environmental temperature or during sustained physical exercise. Normally the renal mechanism described below maintains the concentration of sodium and potassium within physiological limits. When excessive sweating is sustained, e.g. living in a hot climate or working in a hot environment, acclimatisation occurs in about 7 to 10 days and the amount of electrolytes lost in sweat is reduced.

Sodium and potassium occur in high concentrations in digestive juices – sodium in gastric juice and potassium in pancreatic and intestinal juice. Normally these ions are reabsorbed by the colon, but following acute and prolonged diarrhoea they may be excreted in large quantities with resultant electrolyte imbalance.

Renin–angiotensin–aldosterone system (Fig. 13.11). Sodium is a normal constituent of urine and the amount excreted is regulated by the hormone *aldosterone*, secreted by the adrenal cortex. Cells in the afferent arteriole of the nephron are stimulated to produce the enzyme *renin* by sympathetic stimulation, low blood volume or by low arterial blood pressure. Renin converts the plasma protein *angiotensinogen*, produced by the liver, to *angiotensin 1*. *Angiotensin converting enzyme* (ACE), formed in small quantities in the lungs, proximal convoluted tubules and other tissues, converts angiotensin 1 into angiotensin 2, which is a very potent vasoconstrictor and increases blood pressure. Renin and raised blood potassium levels also stimulate the adrenal gland to secrete aldosterone. Water is reabsorbed with sodium and together they increase the blood volume, leading to reduced renin secretion through the negative feedback mechanism. When sodium reabsorption is increased potassium excretion is increased, indirectly reducing intracellular potassium.

As described above, ANP is also involved in the regulation of sodium levels.

Calcium balance

Regulation of calcium levels is achieved by coordinated secretion of parathyroid hormone (p. 220) and calcitonin (p. 219). The distal collecting tubules reabsorb more calcium in response to PTH secretion, and reabsorb less calcium in response to secretion of calcitonin.

pH balance

In order to maintain the normal blood pH (acid–base balance), the cells of the proximal convoluted tubules secrete hydrogen ions. In the filtrate they combine with buffers (p. 22):

- bicarbonate, forming carbonic acid
  ($H^+ + HCO_3^- \rightarrow H_2CO_3$)
- ammonia, forming ammonium ions
  ($H^+ + NH_3 \rightarrow NH_4^+$)
- hydrogen phosphate, forming dihydrogen phosphate
  ($H^+ + HPO_3^{2-} \rightarrow H_2PO_3^-$).

Carbonic acid is converted to carbon dioxide (CO_2) and water (H_2O), and the CO_2 is reabsorbed, maintaining the buffering capacity of the blood. Hydrogen ions are excreted in the urine as ammonium salts and hydrogen phosphate. The normal pH of urine varies from 4.5 to 8 depending on diet, time of day and a number of other factors. Individuals whose diet contains a large amount of animal proteins tend to produce more acidic urine (lower pH) than vegetarians.

Ureters

Learning outcome

After studying this section you should be able to:

- outline the structure and function of the ureters.

The ureters are the tubes that convey urine from the kidneys to the urinary bladder (Fig. 13.14). They are about 25 to 30 cm long with a diameter of about 3 mm.

The ureter is continuous with the funnel-shaped renal pelvis. It passes downwards through the abdominal cavity, behind the peritoneum in front of the psoas muscle into the pelvic cavity, and passes obliquely through the posterior wall of the bladder (Fig. 13.15). Because of this arrangement, when urine accumulates and the pressure in the bladder rises, the ureters are compressed and the openings occluded. This prevents reflux of urine into the ureters (towards the kidneys) as the bladder fills and during micturition, when pressure increases as the muscular bladder wall contracts.

343

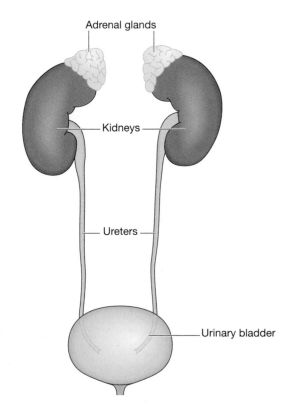

Figure 13.14 **The ureters and their relationship to the kidneys and bladder.**

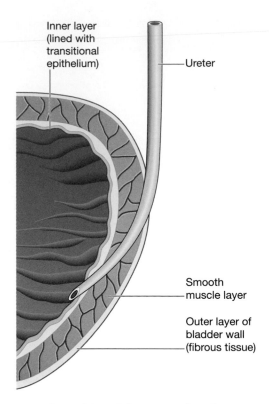

Inner layer
(lined with
transitional
epithelium)

Ureter

Smooth
muscle layer

Outer layer of
bladder wall
(fibrous tissue)

Figure 13.15 The position of the ureter where it passes through the bladder wall.

344

Structure

The ureters consist of three layers of tissue:

- an outer covering of *fibrous tissue*, continuous with the fibrous capsule of the kidney
- a middle *muscular layer* consisting of interlacing smooth muscle fibres that form a functional unit spiralling round the ureter, some in clockwise and some in anticlockwise directions and an additional outer longitudinal layer in the lower third
- an inner layer, the *mucosa*, composed of transitional epithelium (see p. 35).

Function

The ureters propel urine from the kidneys into the bladder by peristaltic contraction of the smooth muscle layer. This is an intrinsic property of the smooth muscle and is not under autonomic nerve control. Peristalsis originates in a pacemaker in the minor calyces. Peristaltic waves occur several times per minute, increasing in frequency with the volume of urine produced, and send little spurts of urine into the bladder.

Urinary bladder

Learning outcome

After studying this section you should be able to:

- describe the structure of the bladder.

The urinary bladder is a reservoir for urine. It lies in the pelvic cavity and its size and position vary, depending on the volume of urine it contains. When distended, the bladder rises into the abdominal cavity.

Organs associated with the bladder
(Fig. 13.16)

Structure (Fig. 13.17)

The bladder is roughly pear shaped, but becomes more oval as it fills with urine. The posterior surface is the *base*. The bladder opens into the urethra at its lowest point, the *neck*.

The peritoneum covers only the superior surface before it turns upwards as the parietal peritoneum, lining the anterior abdominal wall. Posteriorly it surrounds the uterus in the female and the rectum in the male.

The bladder wall is composed of three layers:

- the outer layer of loose connective tissue, containing blood and lymphatic vessels and nerves, covered on the upper surface by the peritoneum
- the middle layer, consisting of a mass of interlacing smooth muscle fibres and elastic tissue loosely arranged in three layers. This is called the *detrusor muscle* and when it contracts, it empties the bladder
- the mucosa, composed of transitional epithelium (p. 35).

When the bladder is empty the inner lining is arranged in folds, or rugae, which gradually disappear as it fills. The bladder is distensible but when it contains 300 to 400 ml, awareness of the need to pass urine is felt. The total capacity is rarely more than about 600 ml.

The three orifices in the bladder wall form a triangle or *trigone* (Fig. 13.17). The upper two orifices on the posterior wall are the openings of the ureters. The lower orifice is the opening into the urethra. The *internal urethral sphincter*, a thickening of the urethral smooth muscle layer in the upper part of the urethra, controls outflow of urine from the bladder. This sphincter is not under voluntary control.

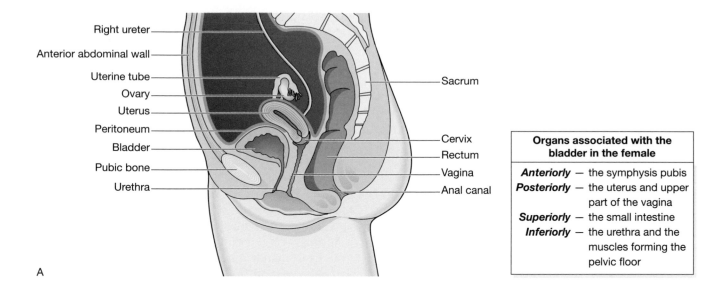

Right ureter
Anterior abdominal wall
Uterine tube
Ovary
Uterus
Peritoneum
Bladder
Pubic bone
Urethra

Sacrum
Cervix
Rectum
Vagina
Anal canal

Organs associated with the bladder in the female	
Anteriorly —	the symphysis pubis
Posteriorly —	the uterus and upper part of the vagina
Superiorly —	the small intestine
Inferiorly —	the urethra and the muscles forming the pelvic floor

A

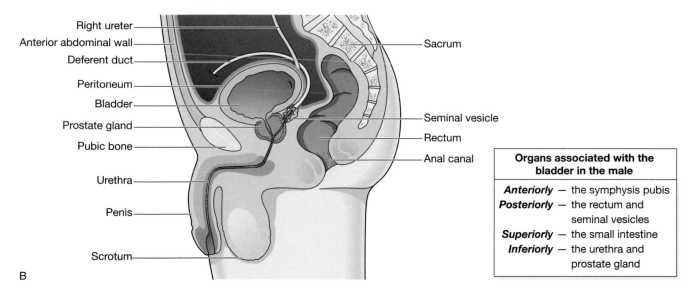

Right ureter
Anterior abdominal wall
Deferent duct
Peritoneum
Bladder
Prostate gland
Pubic bone
Urethra
Penis
Scrotum

Sacrum
Seminal vesicle
Rectum
Anal canal

Organs associated with the bladder in the male	
Anteriorly —	the symphysis pubis
Posteriorly —	the rectum and seminal vesicles
Superiorly —	the small intestine
Inferiorly —	the urethra and prostate gland

B

Figure 13.16 The pelvic organs associated with the bladder and the urethra in: A. The female. B. The male.

345

Urethra

Learning outcome

After studying this section you should be able to:

■ outline the structure and function of the urethra in males and females.

The urethra is a canal extending from the neck of the bladder to the exterior, at the external urethral orifice. It is longer in the male than in the female. The male urethra is associated with the urinary and the reproductive systems, and is described in Chapter 18.

The female urethra is approximately 4 cm long. It runs downwards and forwards behind the symphysis pubis and opens at the *external urethral orifice* just in front of the vagina. The external urethral orifice is guarded by the *external urethral sphincter*, which is under voluntary control.

The male urethra is described in detail in Chapter 18, but in both sexes the basic structure is the same. Its walls consist of three layers of tissue.

• The *muscle layer* is continuous with that of the bladder. At its origin is the internal urethral sphincter,

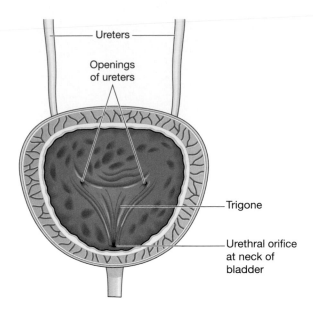

Figure 13.17 Section of the bladder showing the trigone.

346

consisting mainly of elastic tissue and smooth muscle fibres, under autonomic nerve control. Slow and continuous contraction of this sphincter keeps the urethra closed. In the middle third is skeletal muscle surrounding the urethra, under voluntary nerve control, that forms the external urethral sphincter.

- The *submucosa* is a spongy layer containing blood vessels and nerves.
- The *mucosa* is continuous with that of the bladder in the upper part of the urethra. In the lower part the lining consists of stratified squamous epithelium, continuous externally with the skin of the vulva.

Micturition

Learning outcome

After studying this section you should be able to:

- compare and contrast the process of micturition in babies and adults.

The urinary bladder acts as a reservoir for urine. When 300 to 400 ml of urine have accumulated, afferent autonomic nerve fibres in the bladder wall sensitive to stretch are stimulated. In the infant this initiates a *spinal reflex* (see p. 160) and micturition occurs (Fig. 13.18). Micturition occurs when autonomic efferent fibres convey impulses

to the bladder, causing contraction of the detrusor muscle and relaxation of the internal urethral sphincter.

When the nervous system is fully developed, the micturition reflex is stimulated but sensory impulses also pass upwards to the brain and there is awareness of the need to pass urine. By learned and conscious effort, contraction of the external urethral sphincter and muscles of the pelvic floor will inhibit micturition for a limited period (Fig. 13.19).

In adults, micturition occurs when the detrusor muscle contracts, and there is reflex relaxation of the internal sphincter and voluntary relaxation of the external sphincter. It can be assisted by increasing the pressure within the pelvic cavity, achieved by lowering the diaphragm and contracting the abdominal muscles (Valsalva's manoeuvre). Overdistension of the bladder is extremely painful, and when this stage is reached there is a tendency for involuntary relaxation of the external sphincter to occur allowing a small amount of urine to escape, provided there is no mechanical obstruction.

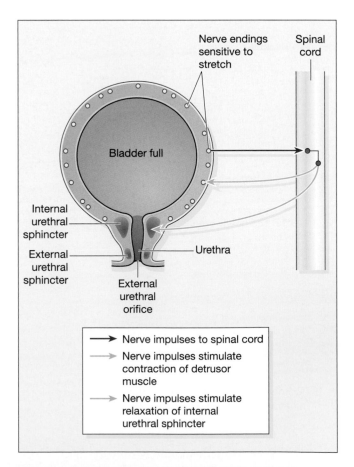

Figure 13.18 Reflex control of micturition when conscious effort cannot override the reflex action.

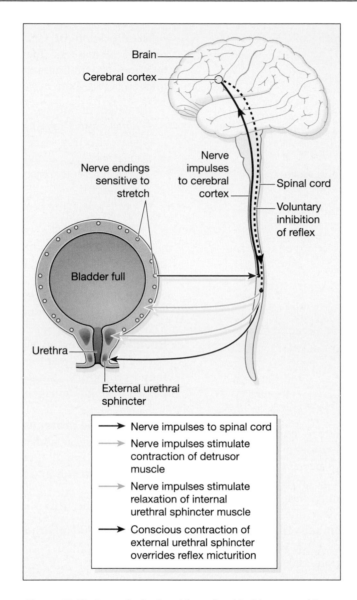

Figure 13.19 Control of micturition after bladder control is established.

347

Diseases of the kidneys

Learning outcomes

After studying this section you should be able to:

■ outline the principal effects of glomerulonephritis

■ describe the effects of diabetes mellitus and hypertension on kidney function

■ discuss the sources and consequences of kidney infections

■ explain the causes and implications of acute and chronic renal failure

■ describe the pathogenesis of kidney stones

■ list common congenital abnormalities of the kidneys

■ outline the development and spread of common kidney tumours.

Glomerulonephritis (GN)

This term suggests inflammatory conditions of the glomerulus, but there are several types of GN and inflammatory changes are not always present. In many cases immune complexes damage the glomeruli. These are formed when antigens and antibodies combine either within the kidney or elsewhere in the body, and they circulate in the blood. When immune complexes lodge in the walls of the glomeruli they often cause an inflammatory response that impairs glomerular function. Other immune mechanisms are also implicated in GN.

Classification of GN is complex and based on a number of features: the cause, immunological characteristics and findings on microscopy. Microscopic distinction is based on:

- the extent of damage:
  - *diffuse:* affecting all glomeruli
  - *focal:* affecting some glomeruli
- appearance:
  - *proliferative:* increased number of cells in the glomeruli
  - *membranous:* thickening of the glomerular basement membrane.

Examples of different types of GN, their features and prognoses are shown in Table 13.1.

Effects of glomerulonephritis

These depend on the type and are listed below.

Haematuria. This is usually painless and not accompanied by other symptoms. When microscopic, it may be found on routine urinalysis when red blood cells have passed through damaged glomeruli into the filtrate.

Asymptomatic proteinuria. This may also be found on routine urinalysis and, at low levels, does not cause nephrotic syndrome. It occurs as protein passes through damaged glomeruli into the filtrate.

Acute nephritis. This is characterised by the presence of:

- oliguria (<400 ml urine/day in adults)
- hypertension
- haematuria
- uraemia (p. 351).

Table 13.1 Glomerulonephritis: features and prognosis of different types

Type	Presenting features	Prognosis
Diffuse proliferative GN	Acute nephritis Haematuria Proteinuria	Good in children; less good in adults, up to 40% develop hypertension or chronic renal failure
Focal proliferative GN	Acute nephritis Haematuria Proteinuria	Variable
Membranous GN	Nephrotic syndrome Haematuria Proteinuria	Variable, but most cases progress to chronic renal failure as sclerosis of glomeruli progresses
Minimal change GN	Nephrotic syndrome Haematuria Proteinuria	Good in children, but recurrences are common in adults

Loin pain, headache and malaise are also common.

Nephrotic syndrome. (See below.)

Chronic renal failure. This occurs when nephrons are progressively and irreversibly damaged after the renal reserve is lost.

Nephrotic syndrome

This is not a disease in itself but is an important feature of several kidney diseases. The main characteristics are:

- marked proteinuria
- hypoalbuminaemia
- generalised oedema
- hyperlipidaemia.

When glomeruli are damaged, the permeability of the glomerular membrane is increased and plasma proteins pass through into the filtrate. Albumin is the main protein lost because it is the most common and is the smallest of the plasma proteins. When the daily loss exceeds the rate of production by the liver there is a significant fall in the total plasma protein level. The consequent low plasma osmotic pressure leads to widespread oedema and reduced plasma volume (see Fig. 5.61, p. 121). This reduces the renal blood flow and stimulates the renin–angiotensin–aldosterone system, causing increased reabsorption of water and sodium from the renal tubules. The reabsorbed water further reduces the osmotic pressure, increasing the oedema. The key factor is the loss of albumin across the glomerular membrane and as long as this continues, the vicious circle is perpetuated (Fig. 13.20). Levels of nitrogenous waste products, i.e. uric acid, urea and creatinine, usually remain normal. Hyperlipidaemia, especially hypercholesterolaemia, also occurs but the cause is unknown.

The nephrotic syndrome occurs in a number of diseases. In children the most common cause is minimal-change glomerulonephritis. In adults it may complicate:

- most forms of glomerulonephritis
- diabetic nephropathy
- systemic lupus erythematosus
- infections, e.g. malaria, syphilis, hepatitis B
- drug treatment, e.g. penicillamine, gold, captopril, phenytoin.

Diabetic nephropathy

Renal failure is the commonest cause of death in young people with diabetes mellitus (p. 232) and is more common if hypertension and severe, long-standing hypergly-

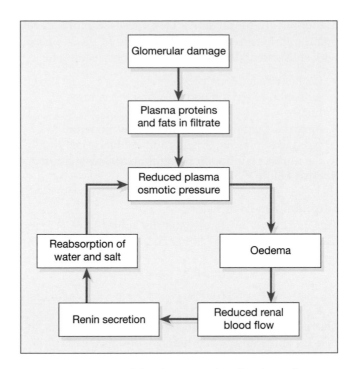

Figure 13.20 Stages of development of nephrotic syndrome.

caemia are present. Diabetes causes widespread blood vessel damage and the effects vary between individuals. In the kidney, these are known collectively as *diabetic nephropathy* or *diabetic kidney* and include:

- progressive glomerulosclerosis, proteinuria and nephrotic syndrome
- ascending infection leading to acute pyelonephritis, sometimes complicated by renal papillary necrosis
- atheroma (see Ch. 5) of the renal arteries and their branches leading to renal ischaemia and hypertension
- chronic renal failure.

Hypertension and the kidneys

Hypertension can be the cause or the result of renal disease. Essential and secondary hypertension (p. 128) both affect the kidneys when there is renal blood vessel damage, causing ischaemia. The reduced blood flow stimulates the renin–angiotensin–aldosterone system (see Fig. 13.11), raising the blood pressure still further.

Essential hypertension
Benign hypertension. This causes gradual and progressive sclerosis and fibrosis of the glomeruli, leading to renal failure or, more commonly, to malignant hypertension.

349

Malignant hypertension. This causes rapidly developing arteriolosclerosis which spreads to the glomeruli with subsequent destruction of nephrons, leading to:

- further rise in blood pressure
- reduction in renal blood flow and the volume of filtrate
- increased permeability of the glomeruli, with the passage of plasma proteins and red blood cells into the filtrate resulting in proteinuria and haematuria
- renal failure.

Secondary hypertension

This is caused by long-standing kidney diseases and leads to chronic renal ischaemia, further hypertension and renal failure.

Acute pyelonephritis

This is acute bacterial infection of the renal pelvis and calyces, spreading to the kidney substance causing formation of small abscesses. The infection may travel up the urinary tract from the perineum or be blood-borne. It is accompanied by fever, malaise and loin pain.

Ascending infection

Upward spread of microbes from the bladder (see cystitis, p. 353) is the most common cause of this condition. Reflux of infected urine into the ureters when the bladder contracts during micturition predisposes to upward spread of infection to the renal pelves and kidney substance.

Blood-borne infection

The source of microbes may be from septicaemia or elsewhere in the body, e.g. respiratory tract infections, infected wounds or abscesses.

When the infection spreads into the kidney tissue it causes suppuration and destruction of nephrons. The prognosis depends on the amount of healthy kidney remaining after the infection subsides. Necrotic tissue is eventually replaced by fibrous tissue but there may be some hypertrophy of healthy nephrons. There are a number of outcomes: healing, recurrence, especially if there is a structural abnormality of the urinary tract, and reflux nephropathy. Perinephric abscess and papillary necrosis are complications, usually if the condition is untreated.

Reflux nephropathy

Previously known as chronic pyelonephritis, this is almost always associated with reflux of urine from the bladder to the ureter enabling microbes to gain access to the kidneys. A congenital abnormality of the angle of insertion of the ureter into the bladder predisposes to reflux of urine, but it is sometimes caused by an obstruction that develops later in life. Progressive loss of functioning nephrons leads to chronic renal failure and concurrent hypertension is common. Occasionally it follows repeated episodes of acute pyelonephritis.

Renal failure

Acute renal failure

There is a sudden and severe reduction in the glomerular filtration rate and kidney function that is usually reversible over days or weeks when treated. This occurs as a complication of a variety of conditions not necessarily associated with the kidneys. The causes of acute renal failure are classified as:

- *prerenal*: the result of reduced renal blood flow, especially severe and prolonged shock
- *renal*: damage to the kidney itself due to, e.g., acute tubular necrosis, glomerulonephritis
- *postrenal*: obstruction to the outflow of urine, e.g. tumour of the bladder, uterus or cervix, large calculus in the renal pelvis.

Acute tubular necrosis (ATN)

This is the most common cause of acute renal failure. There is severe damage to the tubular epithelial cells caused by ischaemia or, less often, by nephrotoxic substances (Box 13.2).

Oliguria (less than 400 ml of urine per day in adults), *severe oliguria* (less than 100 ml of urine per day in adults) or *anuria* (absence of urine) may last for a few weeks, followed by diuresis. There is reduced glomerular filtration and, selective reabsorption and secretion by the tubules, leading to:

Box 13.2 Some causes of ATN

Ischaemia – severe shock, dehydration, haemorrhage, trauma; extensive burns; myocardial infarction; prolonged and complex surgery, especially in older people

Drugs – aminoglycoside antibiotics, non-steroidal anti-inflammatory drugs, ACE inhibitors, lithium compounds, paracetamol overdose

Haemoglobinaemia – accumulation of haemoglobin, released by haemolysis of red blood cells e.g. incompatible blood transfusion, malaria

Myoglobinaemia – myoglobin released from damaged muscle raises blood levels e.g. following crush injury (p. 430).

- generalised and pulmonary oedema
- accumulation of urea and other metabolic waste products
- electrolyte imbalance which may be exacerbated by the retention of potassium (hyperkalaemia) released from damaged cells anywhere in the body
- acidosis due to hydrogen ion retention.

Profound diuresis (the diuretic phase) occurs during the healing process when the epithelial cells of the tubules have regenerated but are still incapable of selective reabsorption and secretion. Diuresis may lead to acute dehydration, complicating the existing high plasma urea, acidosis and electrolyte imbalance. If the patient survives the initial acute phase, a considerable degree of renal function is usually restored over several weeks.

Chronic renal failure

This occurs when there is irreversible damage to about 75% of nephrons. Onset is usually slow and asymptomatic, progressing over several years. The main causes are glomerulonephritis, diabetes mellitus, reflux nephropathy and hypertension.

The effects on glomerular filtration rate (GFR), selective reabsorption and secretion are significant. GFR and filtrate volumes are greatly reduced, and reabsorption of water is also seriously impaired. This results in production of up to 10 litres of urine per day (Table 13.2). Reduced glomerular filtration leads to accumulation of waste substances in the blood, notably urea and creatinine. When the signs and symptoms of renal failure become evident, they are referred to as *uraemia*. Some of these are outlined below.

Polyuria. Large volumes of dilute urine (with a low specific gravity) are passed, because water reabsorption is impaired. Nocturia is a common presenting symptom.

Acidosis. As the kidney buffer system that normally controls the pH of body fluids fails, hydrogen ions accumulate.

Electrolyte imbalance. This is also the result of impaired tubular reabsorption and secretion.

Anaemia. Deficiency of erythropoietin (p. 62) occurs after a few months, causing anaemia that is usually exacerbated by dialysis. If untreated, anaemia results in fatigue, and may also lead to dyspnoea and cardiac failure. Tiredness and breathlessness are sometimes the initial symptoms of chronic renal failure.

Hypertension. This is often a consequence, if not a cause, of renal failure.

When death is likely without renal replacement therapy, such as haemodialysis, peritoneal dialysis or a kidney transplant, the condition is referred to as *end-stage renal failure*. Anorexia, nausea and very deep (Kussmaul's) respirations occur as uraemia progresses. In the final stages there may be hiccoughs, itching, vomiting, muscle twitching, seizures, drowsiness and coma.

Renal calculi

Calculi (stones) form in the kidneys and bladder when urinary constituents normally in solution are precipitated. The solutes involved are usually oxalates and phosphates. They are more common in males and after 30 years of age. Most originate in the collecting tubules or renal papillae. They then pass into the renal pelvis where they may increase in size. Some become too large to pass through the ureter and may obstruct the outflow of urine, causing renal failure. Others pass to the bladder and are either excreted or increase in size and obstruct the urethra. Sometimes stones originate in the bladder, usually in developing countries and often in children. Predisposing factors include:

- *Dehydration*. This leads to increased reabsorption of water from the tubules but does not change solute reabsorption, resulting in a reduced volume of highly concentrated filtrate in the collecting tubules.

351

Table 13.2 Polyuria in chronic renal failure		
	Normal kidney	**End-stage kidney**
GFR	125 ml/min or 180 l/day	10 ml/min or 14 l/day
Reabsorption of water	> 99%	Approx. 30%
Urine output	< 1ml/min or 1.5 l/day	Approx. 7 ml/min or 10 l/day

- *pH of urine*. When the normally acid filtrate becomes alkaline, some substances may be precipitated, e.g. phosphates. This occurs when the kidney buffering system is impaired and in some infections.
- *Infection*. Necrotic material and pus provide foci upon which solutes in the filtrate may be deposited and the products of infection may alter the pH of the urine. Infection sometimes leads to alkaline urine (see above).
- *Metabolic conditions*. These include hyperparathyroidism and gout.

Small calculi

These may pass through or become impacted in a ureter and damage the epithelium, leading to haematuria and after healing, fibrosis and stricture. In ureteric obstruction, usually unilateral, there is spasmodic contraction of the ureter, causing acute intermittent ischaemic pain (*renal colic*) as the ureter contracts over the stone. Stones reaching the bladder may be passed in urine or increase in size and eventually obstruct the urethra. Consequences include retention of urine and bilateral *hydronephrosis* (p. 353), infection proximal to the blockage, pyelonephritis and severe kidney damage.

Large calculi (staghorn calculus)

One large stone may form, usually over many years, filling the renal pelvis and the calyces (see Fig. 13.21). It causes stagnation of urine, predisposing to infection, hydronephrosis and occasionally kidney tumours. It may cause chronic renal failure.

Congenital abnormalities of the kidneys

Misplaced (ectopic) kidney

One or both kidneys may develop in abnormally low positions. Misplaced kidneys function normally if the blood vessels are long enough to provide an adequate blood supply but a kidney in the pelvic cavity may cause problems during pregnancy as the expanding uterus compresses renal blood vessels or the ureters. If the ureters become kinked there is increased risk of infection as there is a tendency for reflux and backflow to the kidney. There may also be difficulties during childbirth.

Polycystic disease

The *infantile form* is very rare and is usually fatal in early childhood.

Adult polycystic kidney disease. This is inherited as an autosomal dominant condition (p. 437) that becomes apparent in adulthood. Both kidneys are affected. Dilatations (cysts) form at the junction of the distal convoluted tubules and collecting ducts. The cysts slowly enlarge and pressure causes ischaemia and destruction of nephrons. The disease is progressive and secondary hypertension is common; chronic renal failure affects about 50% of patients. Death may be due to chronic renal failure, cardiac failure or subarachnoid haemorrhage due to increased incidence of berry aneurysms of the circulus arteriosus. Cysts may also develop in the liver, spleen and pancreas.

Tumours of the kidney

Benign tumours are relatively uncommon.

Malignant tumours

Renal cell carcinoma

Previously known as hypernephroma or Grawitz's tumour, this tumour of tubular epithelium is more common after 50 years of age, especially in males. Local spread involves the renal vein and leads to early bloodspread of tumour fragments, most commonly to the lungs and bones. The causes are unknown although there is an increased incidence in cigarette smokers.

Nephroblastoma (Wilms' tumour)

This is one of the most common malignant tumours in children, usually occurring in the first 3 years. It is usually unilateral but rapidly becomes very large and invades the renal blood vessels, causing early bloodspread to the lungs.

Diseases of the renal pelvis, ureters, bladder and urethra

Learning outcomes

After studying this section you should be able to:

- describe the causes and implications of urinary obstruction
- explain the pathological features of urinary tract infections
- outline the characteristics of the main bladder tumours
- discuss the principal causes of urinary incontinence.

These structures are considered together because their combined functions are to collect and store urine prior to

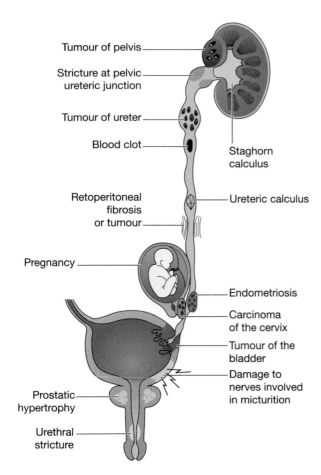

Tumour of pelvis

Stricture at pelvic ureteric junction

Tumour of ureter

Blood clot

Staghorn calculus

Retoperitoneal fibrosis or tumour

Ureteric calculus

Pregnancy

Endometriosis

Carcinoma of the cervix

Tumour of the bladder

Damage to nerves involved in micturition

Prostatic hypertrophy

Urethral stricture

Figure 13.21 Summary of obstructions of the urinary tract.

excretion from the body. Obstruction and infection are the main problems (Fig. 13.21).

Obstruction to the outflow of urine

Hydronephrosis

This is dilatation of the renal pelvis and calyces caused by accumulation of urine above an obstruction of the urinary tract (Fig. 13.21). It leads to destruction of the nephrons, fibrosis and atrophy of the kidney. One or both kidneys may be involved, depending on the cause and site. When there is an abnormality of the bladder or urethra, both kidneys are affected whereas an obstruction above the bladder is more common and affects only one kidney. The effects depend on the site and extent of the obstruction. Stasis of urine within the urinary tract predisposes to infection.

Complete sustained obstruction

In this condition hydronephrosis develops quickly, pressure in the nephrons rises and urine production stops. The most common causes are a large calculus or tumour.

The outcome depends on whether one or both kidneys are involved (homeostasis can be maintained by one kidney).

Partial or intermittent obstruction

This may progress undetected for many years. It leads to progressive hydronephrosis and is caused by, e.g.:

- a succession of renal calculi in a ureter, eventually moved onwards by peristalsis
- constriction of a ureter or the urethra by fibrous tissue, following epithelial inflammation caused by the passage of a stone or by infection
- a tumour in the urinary tract or in the abdominal or pelvic cavity
- enlarged prostate gland in the male.

Spinal lesions

The immediate effect of transverse spinal cord lesions that damage the nerve supply to the bladder is that micturition does not occur. When the bladder fills, the rise in pressure causes overflow incontinence, back pressure into the ureters and hydronephrosis. Reflex micturition is usually re-established after a time, but loss of voluntary control may be irreversible. Pressure on the spinal cord and other abnormalities, e.g. spina bifida, can also impair micturition.

Infections of the urinary tract

Infection of any part of the tract may spread upwards causing pyelonephritis (p. 350) and kidney damage.

Ureteritis

Inflammation of a ureter is usually due to the upward spread of infection in cystitis.

Cystitis

This is inflammation of the bladder and may be due to:

- spread of microbes that are commensals of the bowel (*Escherichia coli* and *Streptococcus faecalis*) from the perineum, especially in women because of the short urethra, its proximity to the anus and the moist perineal conditions
- trauma, with or without infection, following healthcare interventions, e.g. radiotherapy, insertion of a urinary catheter or instrument.

The effects are inflammation, with oedema and small haemorrhages of the mucosa, which may be accompanied by *haematuria*. The sensory nerve endings in the bladder wall become hypersensitive and are stimulated before the bladder has filled, leading to *frequency of micturition* and *dysuria* (a burning sensation on micturition). The urine may appear cloudy and have an unpleasant smell.

353

Lower abdominal pain often accompanies cystitis. If untreated, upward spread may cause acute pyelonephritis (see p. 350) or septicaemia.

Cystitis is *uncomplicated* when it occurs in otherwise healthy individuals with a normal urinary tract. When it affects people with structural or functional abnormalities of the urinary tract or those with pre-existing conditions, e.g. diabetes mellitus or urinary outflow obstruction, it is described as *complicated*. Complicated UTIs sometimes cause permanent renal damage, whereas this is very rare in uncomplicated infections. Recurrence is fairly common, especially in women, either when the original infection is not eradicated or reinfection occurs.

Predisposing factors. The most important are coliform microbes in the perineal region, and stasis of urine in the bladder. Sexual intercourse may cause trauma to the urethra and transfer of microbes from the perineum, especially in the female. Hormones associated with pregnancy relax perineal muscle, and cause relaxation and kinking of the ureters. Towards the end of pregnancy, pressure caused by the fetus may obstruct the outflow of urine. In the male, prostatitis provides a focus of local infection or an enlarged prostate gland may cause progressive urethral obstruction.

Urethritis

This is inflammation of the urethra. A common cause is *Neisseria gonorrhoeae* (gonococcus) spread by sexual intercourse directly to the urethra in the male and indirectly from the perineum in the female. It may also be caused by a calculus or urinary catheter but many cases have no known cause and are described as *non-specific urethritis* (Ch. 18).

Tumours of the bladder

It is not always clear whether bladder tumours are benign or malignant. Tumours are often multiple and recurrence is common. Predisposing factors include cigarette smoking, taking high doses of analgesics over a long period and occupational exposure to some chemicals, e.g. aniline dyes used in the textile and printing industries.

Papillomas

These tumours arise from transitional epithelium and are often benign. They consist of a stalk with fine-branching fronds, which tend to break off causing painless bleeding and haematuria. Papillomas commonly recur, even when benign. Sometimes the tumour cells are well differentiated and non-invasive but in other cases they behave as carcinomas and invade surrounding blood and lymph vessels.

Solid tumours

These are all malignant to some degree. At an early stage the more malignant and solid tumours rapidly invade the bladder wall and spread in lymph and blood to other parts of the body. If the surface ulcerates there may be haemorrhage and necrosis.

Urinary incontinence

In this condition there is involuntary loss of urine and several types are recognised.

Stress incontinence

This is leakage of urine when intra-abdominal pressure is raised, e.g. on coughing, laughing, sneezing or lifting. It usually affects women when there is weakness of the pelvic floor muscles or pelvic ligaments, e.g. after childbirth or as part of the ageing process.

Urge incontinence

Leakage of urine follows a sudden and intense urge to void and may be due to a urinary tract infection, calculus, tumour or overactivity of the detrusor muscle.

Overflow incontinence

This occurs when there is overfilling of the bladder and may be due to:

- retention of urine due to obstruction of urinary outflow, e.g. enlarged prostate gland or urethral stricture, or
- a neurological abnormality affecting the nerves involved in micturition, e.g. stroke, spinal cord injury or multiple sclerosis.

The bladder becomes distended and when the pressure inside overcomes the resistance of the external urethral sphincter, urine dribbles from the urethra. The individual may be unable to initiate and/or maintain micturition.

Protection and survival

The skin

The skin

Learning outcomes

After studying this section you should be able to:

- describe the structure of the skin

- explain the principal functions of the skin

- compare and contrast the processes of primary and secondary wound healing.

The skin completely covers the body and is continuous with the membranes lining the body orifices. It:

- protects the underlying structures from injury and from invasion by microbes
- contains sensory (*somatic*) nerve endings of pain, temperature and touch
- is involved in the regulation of body temperature.

Structure of the skin

The skin is the largest organ in the body and has a surface area of about 1.5 to 2 m^2 in adults and it contains glands, hair and nails. There are two main layers:

- epidermis
- dermis.

Between the skin and underlying structures is a layer of subcutaneous fat.

Epidermis (Fig. 14.1)

The epidermis is the most superficial layer of the skin and is composed of *stratified keratinised squamous epithelium* (see Fig. 3.10, p. 35), which varies in thickness in different parts of the body. It is thickest on the palms of the hands and soles of the feet. There are no blood vessels or nerve endings in the epidermis, but its deeper layers are bathed in interstitial fluid from the dermis, which provides oxygen and nutrients, and is drained away as lymph.

There are several layers (strata) of cells in the epidermis which extend from the deepest *germinative layer* to the surface *stratum corneum* (a thick horny layer). The cells on the surface are flat, thin, non-nucleated, dead cells, or *squames*, in which the cytoplasm has been replaced by the fibrous protein *keratin*. These cells are constantly being rubbed off and replaced by cells that originated in the germinative layer and have undergone gradual change as they progressed towards the surface.

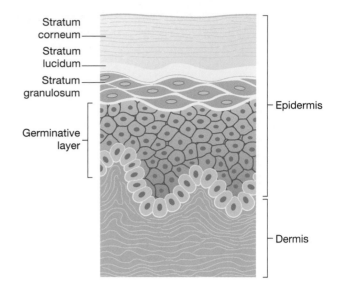

Figure 14.1 The skin showing the main layers of the epidermis.

Complete replacement of the epidermis takes about a month.

The maintenance of healthy epidermis depends upon three processes being synchronised:

- desquamation (shedding) of the keratinised cells from the surface
- effective keratinisation of the cells approaching the surface
- continual cell division in the deeper layers with newly formed cells being pushed to the surface.

Hairs, secretions from sebaceous glands and ducts of sweat glands pass through the epidermis to reach the surface.

The surface of the epidermis is ridged by projections of cells in the dermis called *papillae*. The pattern of ridges is different in every individual and the impression made by them is the 'fingerprint'. The downward projections of the germinative layer between the papillae are believed to aid nutrition of epidermal cells and stabilise the two layers, preventing damage due to shearing forces. *Blisters* develop when trauma causes separation of the dermis and epidermis and serous fluid collects between the two layers.

Skin colour is affected by various factors.

- Melanin, a dark pigment derived from the amino acid tyrosine and secreted by *melanocytes* in the deep germinative layer, is absorbed by surrounding epithelial cells. The amount is genetically determined and varies between different parts of the body, between people of the same ethnic origin and between ethnic groups. The number of melanocytes is fairly constant so the differences in colour depend on the amount of melanin secreted. It protects the skin from the harmful effects of sunlight. Exposure to sunlight promotes synthesis of melanin.

- The percentage saturation of haemoglobin (p. 60) and the amount of blood circulating in the dermis give white skin its pink colour.
- Excessive levels of bile pigments in blood and carotenes in subcutaneous fat give the skin a yellowish colour.

Dermis (Fig. 14.2)

The dermis is tough and elastic. It is formed from connective tissue and the matrix contains *collagen fibres* interlaced with *elastic fibres*. Rupture of elastic fibres occurs when the skin is overstretched, resulting in permanent *striae*, or stretch marks, that may be found in pregnancy and obesity. Collagen fibres bind water and give the skin its tensile strength, but as this ability declines with age, wrinkles develop. Fibroblasts, macrophages and mast cells are the main cells found in the dermis. Underlying its deepest layer there is areolar tissue and varying amounts of adipose (fat) tissue. The structures in the dermis are:

- blood vessels
- lymph vessels
- sensory (somatic) nerve endings
- sweat glands and their ducts
- hairs, arrector pili muscles and sebaceous glands.

Blood vessels. Arterioles form a fine network with capillary branches supplying sweat glands, sebaceous glands, hair follicles and the dermis. The epidermis has no blood supply. It obtains nutrients and oxygen from interstitial fluid derived from blood vessels in the papillae of the dermis.

Lymph vessels. These form a network throughout the dermis.

Sensory nerve endings. Sensory receptors (specialised nerve endings) sensitive to *touch*, *temperature*, *pressure* and *pain* are widely distributed in the dermis. Incoming stimuli activate different types of sensory receptors (Fig. 14.2, Box 14.1). The skin is an important sensory organ through which individuals receive information about their environment. Nerve impulses, generated in the sensory receptors in the dermis, are conveyed to the spinal cord by sensory (somatic cutaneous) nerves, then to the sensory area of the cerebrum where the sensations are perceived (see Fig. 7.18B).

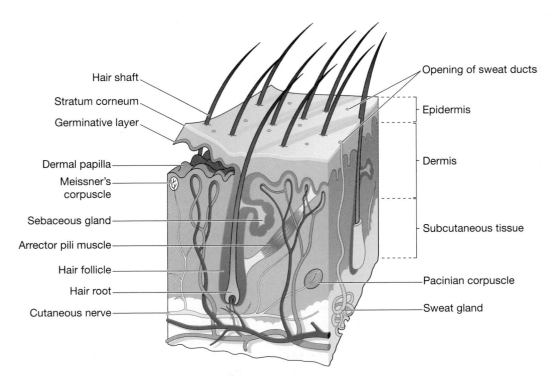

Figure 14.2 The skin showing the main structures in the dermis.

Sweat glands

Sweat glands are widely distributed throughout the skin and are most numerous in the palms of the hands, soles of the feet, axillae and groins. They are composed of epithelial cells. The bodies of the glands lie coiled in the subcutaneous tissue. Some ducts open onto the skin surface at tiny depressions, or pores, and others open into hair follicles. Glands opening into hair follicles do not become active until puberty. In the axilla they secrete an odourless milky fluid which, if decomposed by surface microbes, causes an unpleasant odour. The functions of this secretion are not known. Sweat glands are stimulated by sympathetic nerves in response to raised body temperature and fear.

The most important function of sweat secreted by glands opening on to the skin surface is in the regulation of body temperature. Evaporation of sweat from body surfaces takes heat from the body core and the amount of sweat produced is governed by the temperature-regulating centre in the hypothalamus. Excessive sweating may lead to dehydration and serious depletion of sodium chloride unless intake of water and salt is appropriately increased. After 7 to 10 days' exposure to high environmental temperatures the amount of salt lost is substantially reduced but water loss remains high.

Hairs

These are formed by a down-growth of epidermal cells into the dermis or subcutaneous tissue, called *hair follicles*. At the base of the follicle is a cluster of cells called the *bulb*. The hair is formed by multiplication of cells of the bulb and as they are pushed upwards, away from their source of nutrition, the cells die and become keratinised. The part of the hair above the skin is the *shaft* and the remainder, the *root* (Fig. 14.2).

The colour of the hair is genetically determined and depends on the amount of melanin present. White hair is the result of the replacement of melanin by tiny air bubbles.

The arrector pili (Fig. 14.2). These are little bundles of smooth muscle fibres attached to the hair follicles. Contraction makes the hair stand erect and raises the skin around the hair, causing 'goose flesh'. The muscles are stimulated by sympathetic nerve fibres in response to fear and cold. Erect hairs trap air, which acts as an insulating layer. This is an efficient warming mechanism especially when accompanied by shivering, i.e. involuntary contraction of skeletal muscles.

The sebaceous glands (Fig. 14.2). These consist of secretory epithelial cells derived from the same tissue as the hair follicles. They secrete an oily substance, *sebum*, into the hair follicles and are present in the skin of all parts of the body except the palms of the hands and the soles of the feet. They are most numerous in the skin of the scalp, face, axillae and groins. In regions of transition from one type of superficial epithelium to another, such as lips, eyelids, nipple, labia minora and glans penis, there are sebaceous glands that are independent of hair follicles, secreting sebum directly onto the surface.

Sebum keeps the hair soft and pliable and gives it a shiny appearance. On the skin it provides some waterproofing and acts as a bactericidal and fungicidal agent, preventing infection. It also prevents drying and cracking of skin, especially on exposure to heat and sunshine. The activity of these glands increases at puberty and is less at the extremes of age, rendering infants and older adults prone to the effects of excessive moisture (maceration).

Nails (Fig. 14.3)

Human nails are equivalent to the claws, horns and hoofs of animals. They are derived from the same cells as epidermis and hair and consist of hard, horny keratin plates. They protect the tips of the fingers and toes.

The *root* of the nail is embedded in the skin, is covered by the *cuticle* and forms the hemispherical pale area called the *lunula*.

The *nail plate* is the exposed part that has grown out from the germinative zone of the epidermis called the *nail bed*.

Finger nails grow more quickly than toe nails and growth is quicker when the environmental temperature is high.

Functions of the skin

Protection

The skin forms a relatively waterproof layer, provided mainly by its keratinised epithelium, which protects the deeper and more delicate structures. As an important non-specific defence mechanism it acts as a barrier against:

- invasion by microbes
- chemicals
- physical agents, e.g. mild trauma, ultraviolet light
- dehydration.

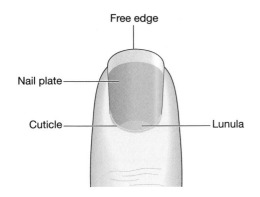

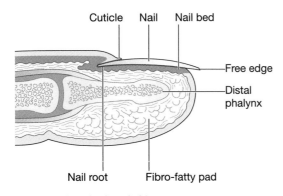

Figure 14.3 The nail and related skin.

The epidermis contains specialised immune cells called Langerhans cells. They phagocytose intruding antigens and travel to lymphoid tissue, where they present antigen to T-lymphocytes, thus stimulating an immune response (p. 375).

Due to the presence of the sensory nerve endings in the skin the body reacts by reflex action to unpleasant or painful stimuli, protecting it from further injury (p. 160).

The pigment melanin affords some protection against harmful ultraviolet rays in sunlight.

Regulation of body temperature

The temperature of the body remains fairly constant at about 36.8 °C across a wide range of environmental temperatures. In health, variations are usually limited to between 0.5 and 0.75 °C, although it is raised slightly in the evening, during exercise and in women just after ovulation. When metabolic rate increases, body temperature rises, and when it decreases body temperature falls. To ensure this constant temperature, a balance is maintained between heat produced in the body and heat lost to the environment.

Heat production

Some of the energy released in the cells during metabolic activity is in the form of heat and the most active organs produce the most heat. The principal organs involved are as follows.

- *The muscles* – contraction of skeletal muscles produces a large amount of heat and the more strenuous the muscular exercise, the greater the heat produced. Shivering also involves skeletal muscle contraction and produces heat when there is the risk of the body temperature falling below normal.
- *The liver* is very metabolically active, and heat is produced as a by-product. Metabolic rate and heat production are increased after eating.
- *The digestive organs* produce heat during peristalsis and during the chemical reactions involved in digestion.

Heat loss

Most heat loss from the body occurs through the skin. Small amounts are lost in expired air, urine and faeces. Only heat loss through the skin can be regulated; there is no control over heat lost by the other routes.

Heat loss through the skin is affected by the difference between body and environmental temperatures, the amount of the body surface exposed to the air and the type of clothes worn. Air is a poor conductor of heat and when layers of air are trapped in clothing and between the skin and clothing they act as effective insulators against excessive heat loss. For this reason several layers of lightweight clothes provide more effective insulation against a low environmental temperature than one heavy garment. A balance is maintained between heat production and heat loss.

Mechanisms of heat loss. In *evaporation*, the body is cooled when heat is used to convert the water in sweat to water vapour.

In *radiation*, exposed parts of the body radiate heat away from the body.

In *conduction*, clothes and other objects in contact with the skin take up heat.

In *convection*, air passing over the exposed parts of the body is heated and rises, cool air replaces it and convection currents are set up. Heat is also lost from the clothes by convection.

Control of body temperature

Nervous control. The *temperature regulating centre* in the hypothalamus is responsive to the temperature of circulating blood. This centre controls body temperature through autonomic nerve stimulation of the sweat glands when body temperature rises.

The *vasomotor centre* in the medulla oblongata controls the diameter of the small arteries and arterioles, and therefore the amount of blood which circulates in the capillaries in the dermis. The vasomotor centre is influenced by the temperature of its blood supply and by nerve impulses from the hypothalamus. When body temperature rises, the skin capillaries dilate and the extra blood near the surface increases heat loss by radiation, conduction and convection. The skin is warm and pink in colour. When body temperature falls arteriolar constriction conserves heat and the skin is whiter and feels cool.

Activity of the sweat glands. When the temperature of the body is increased by 0.25 to 0.5 °C the sweat glands are stimulated to secrete sweat, brought to the surface by ducts. When sweat droplets can be seen on the skin, the rate of production is exceeding the rate of evaporation. This is most likely to happen when air is humid and the temperature high.

Loss of heat from the body by unnoticeable evaporation of water through the skin and expired air occurs even when the environmental temperature is low. This is called *insensible water loss* (around 500 ml per day) and is accompanied by insensible heat loss.

Effects of vasodilatation and vasoconstriction. The amount of heat lost from the skin depends to a great extent on the amount of blood in the vessels in the dermis. As heat production increases, the arterioles become dilated and more blood enters the capillary network in the skin. In addition to increasing the amount of sweat produced, the temperature of the skin is raised and there is an increase in the amount of heat lost by radiation, conduction and convection.

If the environmental temperature is low or if heat production is decreased, vasoconstriction is stimulated by sympathetic nerves. This decreases the blood flow near the body surface, conserving heat.

Fever. This is often the result of infection and is caused by release of chemicals (*pyrogens*) from damaged tissue and the cells involved in inflammation. Pyrogens act on the hypothalamus, which releases prostaglandins that reset the hypothalamic thermostat to a higher temperature. The body responds by activating heat-promoting mechanisms, e.g. shivering and vasoconstriction until the new higher temperature is reached. When the thermostat is reset to the normal level, heat-loss mechanisms are activated. There is profuse sweating and vasodilatation accompanied by warm, pink (flushed) skin until body temperature falls to the normal range again.

Hypothermia. This is present when core temperature, e.g. the rectal temperature, is below 35 °C. At a core temperature below 32 °C, compensatory mechanisms to restore body temperature usually fail, e.g. shivering is replaced by muscle rigidity and cramps, vasoconstriction fails and blood pressure, pulse and respiration rates fall. Mental confusion and disorientation occur. Death usually occurs when the temperature falls below 25 °C.

Individuals at the extremes of age are prone to hypothermia.

Formation of vitamin D

7-dehydrocholesterol is a lipid-based substance in the skin, and ultraviolet light from the sun converts it to vitamin D. This circulates in the blood and is used, with calcium and phosphate, in the formation and maintenance of bone.

Cutaneous sensation

Sensory receptors consist of nerve endings in the dermis that are sensitive to touch, pressure, temperature or pain. Stimulation generates nerve impulses in sensory nerves that are transmitted to the cerebral cortex (see Fig. 7.18B, p. 153). Some areas have more sensory receptors than others causing them to be especially sensitive, e.g. the lips and fingertips.

Absorption

This property is limited but substances that can be absorbed include:

- some drugs, in transdermal patches, e.g. hormone replacement therapy during the menopause, nicotine as an aid to stopping smoking
- some toxic chemicals, e.g. mercury.

Excretion

The skin is a minor excretory organ for some substances including:

- sodium chloride in sweat; excess sweating may lead to low blood sodium levels (hyponatraemia)
- urea, especially when kidney function is impaired
- aromatic substances, e.g. garlic and other spices.

Wound healing

Conditions required for wound healing

Systemic factors. These include good nutritional status and general health. Infection, impaired immunity, poor blood supply and systemic conditions, e.g. diabetes mellitus and cancer, reduce the rate of wound healing.

Local factors. Local factors that facilitate wound healing include a good blood supply to provide oxygen and nutrients and remove waste products, and freedom from contamination by, e.g., microbes, foreign bodies or toxic chemicals.

Primary healing (healing by first intention)

This method of healing follows minimal destruction of tissue when the damaged edges of a wound are in close apposition (Fig. 14.4). There are several overlapping stages in the repair process.

Inflammation. The cut surfaces become inflamed and blood clot and cell debris fill the gap between them in the first few hours. Phagocytes and fibroblasts migrate into the blood clot:

- phagocytes begin to remove the clot and cell debris stimulating fibroblast activity
- fibroblasts secrete collagen fibres which begin to bind the surfaces together.

Proliferation. Epithelial cells proliferate across the wound, through the clot. The epidermis meets and grows upwards until full thickness is restored. The clot above the new tissue becomes the scab and separates after 3 to 10 days. *Granulation tissue*, consisting of new capillary buds, phagocytes and fibroblasts, develops, invading

the clot and restoring the blood supply to the wound. Fibroblasts continue to secrete collagen fibres as the clot and any bacteria are removed by phagocytosis.

Maturation. The granulation tissue is replaced by fibrous scar tissue. Rearrangement of collagen fibres occurs and the strength of the wound increases. In time the scar becomes less vascular, appearing after a few months as a fine line.

The channels left when stitches are removed heal by the same process.

Secondary healing (healing by second intention)

This method of healing follows destruction of a large amount of tissue or when the edges of a wound cannot be brought into apposition, e.g. varicose ulcers and pressure (decubitus) ulcers (Fig. 14.5). The stages of secondary healing are the same as in primary healing (see below) and the time taken for healing depends on the effective removal of the cause and on the size of the wound.

Inflammation. This develops on the surface of the healthy tissue and separation of necrotic tissue (*slough*) begins, due mainly to the action of phagocytes in the inflammatory exudate. The inflammatory process is described on page 371.

363

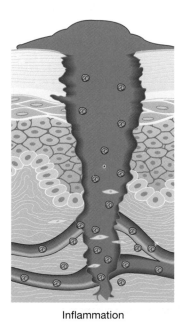 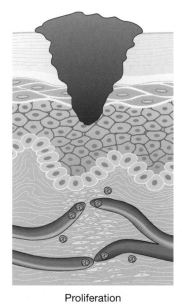 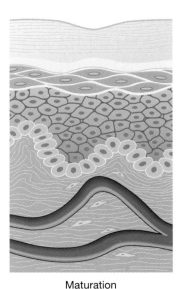

Inflammation Proliferation Maturation

Fibroblast
Phagocyte

Figure 14.4 Stages in primary wound healing.

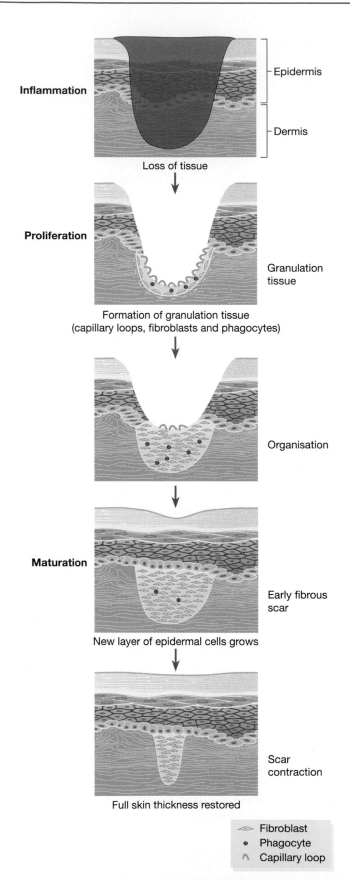

Proliferation. This begins as granulation tissue, consisting of capillary buds, phagocytes and fibroblasts, and develops at the base of the cavity. It grows towards the surface, probably stimulated by macrophages. Phagocytes in the plentiful blood supply tend to prevent infection of the wound by ingesting bacteria after separation of the slough. Some fibroblasts in the wound develop a limited ability to contract, reducing the size of the wound and healing time. When granulation tissue reaches the level of the dermis, epithelial cells at the edges proliferate and grow towards the centre.

Maturation. This occurs by *fibrosis*, in which scar tissue replaces granulation tissue, usually over several months until the full thickness of the skin is restored. Scar tissue is shiny and does not contain sweat glands, hair follicles or sebaceous glands.

Figure 14.5 **Stages in secondary wound healing.**

Disorders of the skin

> **Learning outcomes**
>
> After studying this section you should be able to:
>
> ■ list the causes of diseases in this section
>
> ■ explain the pathological features and effects of common skin conditions.

Infections

Viral infections

Human papilloma virus (HPV)

This causes *warts* or *veruccas* that are spread by direct contact, e.g. from another lesion, or another infected individual. There is proliferation of the epidermis and development of a small firm growth. Common sites are the hands, the face and soles of the feet.

Herpes viruses

Chicken pox and shingles (p. 183) are caused by the herpes zoster virus. Other herpes viruses cause *cold sores* (HSV1) and *genital herpes* (HSV2). The latter cause genital warts affecting the genitalia and/or anus and are spread by direct contact during sexual intercourse.

Bacterial infections

Impetigo

This is a highly infectious condition commonly caused by *Staphylococcus aureus*. Superficial pustules develop, usually round the nose and mouth. It is spread by direct contact and affects mainly children and immuno-suppressed individuals. When caused by *Streptococcus pyogenes* (group A β-haemolytic streptococcus) the infection may be complicated, a few weeks later, by an immune reaction causing glomerulonephritis (p. 348).

Cellulitis

This is a spreading infection caused by some anaerobic microbes or by *Streptococcus pyogenes* or *Clostridium perfringens*. The spread of infection is facilitated by the formation of enzymes that break down the connective tissue that normally isolates an area of inflammation. The microbes enter the body through a break in the skin. If untreated, the microbes may enter the blood causing septicaemia. In severe cases *necrotising fasciitis* may occur. There is oedema and necrosis of subcutaneous tissue that usually includes the fascia in the affected area.

Fungal infections

Ringworm and tinea pedis

These are superficial infections of the skin. In ringworm there is an outward spreading ring of inflammation. It most commonly affects the scalp and is found in cattle from which infection is spread.

Tinea pedis (athlete's foot) affects the area between the toes. Both infections are spread by direct contact.

Non-infective inflammatory conditions

Eczema and dermatitis

These two terms are synonymous and describe inflammatory conditions which can be acute or chronic. In acute dermatitis there is redness, swelling and exudation of serous fluid usually accompanied by *pruritis* (itching). This is often followed by crusting and scaling. If the condition becomes chronic, the skin thickens and may become leathery due to long-term scratching. Scratching may cause infection.

Atopic dermatitis is caused by allergens and commonly affects atopic individuals, i.e. those prone to hypersensitivity disorders (p. 379). Children, who may also suffer from hay fever or asthma (pp. 258 and 259), are often affected.

Contact dermatitis may be caused by:

- direct contact with irritants, e.g. cosmetics, soap, detergent, strong acids or alkalis, industrial chemicals
- a hypersensitivity reaction (see Fig. 15.9, p. 380) to, e.g., latex rubber, nickel, dyes and other chemicals.

Psoriasis

This condition is genetically determined and characterised by exacerbations and periods of remission of varying duration. It is common, especially between the ages of 15 and 40 years. Cells of the basal layers of the epidermis proliferate and the more rapid upward progress of these cells through the epidermis results in incomplete maturation of the upper layer. The skin is shiny, silver coloured and scaly. Bleeding may occur when scales are scratched or rubbed off. The elbows, knees and scalp are common sites but other parts can also be affected. Triggering factors that lead to exacerbation of the condition include trauma, infection and sunburn. Sometimes psoriasis is associated with arthritis (p. 428).

Acne vulgaris

This is common in adolescents and is thought to be caused by increased levels of male sex hormones after puberty. Sebaceous glands in hair follicles become

365

blocked and then infected, leading to inflammation and pustule formation. In severe cases permanent scarring may result. The most common sites are the face, chest and upper back.

Pressure ulcers

Also known as *decubitus ulcers* or *bedsores*, these occur over 'pressure points', areas where the skin may be compressed for long periods between a bony prominence and a hard surface, e.g. a bed or chair. When this occurs, blood flow to the affected area is impaired and ischaemia develops. Initially the skin reddens, and later as ischaemia and necrosis occur the skin sloughs and an ulcer forms that may then enlarge into a cavity. If infection occurs, this can result in septicaemia. Healing takes place by second intention (p. 363).

Predisposing factors
These may be:

- extrinsic, e.g. pressure, shearing forces, trauma, immobility, moisture, infection
- intrinsic, e.g. poor nutritional status, emaciation, incontinence, infection, concurrent illness, sensory impairment, poor circulation, old age.

Burns

These may be caused by many types of trauma including: heat, cold, electricity, ionising radiation and corrosive chemicals, including strong acids or alkalis.

Local damage occurs disrupting the structure and functions of the skin. Infection is a common complication of any burn as the outer barrier formed by the epidermis is lost.

Burns are classified according to their depth:

- *partial thickness* (superficial) when only the epidermis is involved. There are signs of inflammation (p. 371) and sometimes blistering
- *full thickness* (deep) when the epidermis and dermis are destroyed. These burns are usually relatively painless as the sensory nerve endings in the dermis are destroyed. After a few days the destroyed tissue coagulates and forms an *eschar*, or thick scab, which sloughs off after 2 to 3 weeks. In *circumferential burns*, which encircle any area of the body, complications may arise from constriction of the part by eschar, e.g. respiratory impairment may follow circumferential burns of the chest, or the circulation to the distal part of an affected limb may be seriously impaired. Skin grafting is required except for small injuries. Otherwise, healing, which is prolonged, occurs by second intention (p. 363) and there is no regeneration

of sweat glands, hair follicles or sebaceous glands. Resultant scar tissue often limits movement of affected joints.

The extent of burns in adults is roughly estimated using the 'rule of nines' (Fig. 14.6). In adults, hypovolaemic shock usually develops when 15% of the surface area is affected. Fatality is likely, in adults with full thickness burns if the surface area affected is added to the patient's age and the total is greater than 80.

Complications of burns
Although burns affect the skin, when extensive, their systemic consequences can also be life threatening or fatal.

Dehydration and hypovolaemia. These may occur in extensive burns due to excessive leakage of water and plasma proteins from the surface of the damaged skin.

Shock. This may accompany severe hypovolaemia.

Hypothermia. This develops when excessive heat is lost.

Infection. This may result in septicaemia.

Renal failure. This occurs when the kidney tubules cannot deal with the amount of waste from haemolysed erythrocytes and damaged tissue.

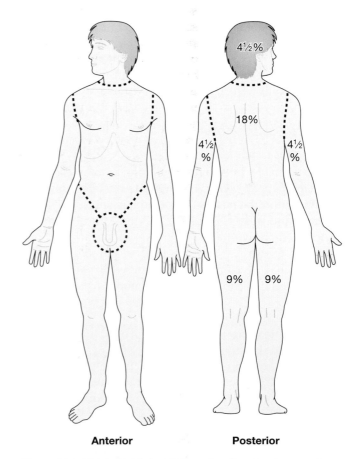

Figure 14.6 The 'rule of nines' for estimating the extent of burns in adults.

Contractures. These may develop later as fibrous scar tissue contracts distorting the limbs, e.g. the hands, and impairing function.

Malignant tumours

Basal cell carcinoma

This is the least malignant and most common type of skin cancer. It is associated with long-term exposure to sunlight and is therefore most likely to occur on sun-exposed sites, usually the head or neck. It appears as a shiny nodule and later this breaks down, becoming an ulcer with irregular edges, commonly called a *rodent ulcer*. This is locally invasive but seldom metastasises.

Malignant melanoma

This is malignant proliferation of melanocytes, usually originating in a mole that may have an irregular outline.

It may ulcerate and bleed and most commonly affects young and middle-aged adults. Predisposing factors are a fair skin and recurrent episodes of intensive exposure to sunlight including repeated episodes of sunburn, especially in childhood. Sites for this tumour show a gender bias, with the lower leg being the commonest site in females and the torso being a common site in males. Metastases usually develop early and are frequently found in lymph nodes. The most common sites of blood-spread metastases are the liver, brain, lungs, bowel and bone marrow.

Kaposi's sarcoma

In this rare condition, a malignant tumour arises in the walls of lymphatic vessels. A small red-blue patch or nodule develops usually on the lower limbs.

It is also an AIDS-related disease and has thus become more common. In such cases, multiple lesions may occur and affect many sites of the body.

Resistance and immunity

Every individual is under constant attack from an enormous range of potentially harmful invaders, from the months spent in the womb to the end of his life. These threats include such diverse entities as bacteria, viruses, cancer cells, parasites and foreign (non-self) cells, e.g. in tissue transplant. The body therefore has developed a wide selection of protective measures, which can be divided into two categories.

Non-specific defence mechanisms. These protect against any of an enormous range of possible dangers.

Specific defence mechanisms. These are grouped together under the term *immunity*. Resistance is directed against only one specific invader. In addition, *immunological memory* develops, which confers long-term immunity to specific infections. An *antigen* is anything that stimulates an immune response.

Non-specific defence mechanisms

Learning outcomes

After studying this section, you should be able to:

- identify the body's main non-specific defence cells
- describe the functions and features of the inflammatory response
- discuss the process of phagocytosis
- list the main antimicrobial substances of the body.

These are the first lines of general defence; they prevent entry and minimise further passage of microbes and other foreign material into the body.

There are five main non-specific defence mechanisms:

- defence at body surfaces
- phagocytosis
- natural antimicrobial substances
- the inflammatory response
- immunological surveillance.

Defence at body surfaces

When skin and mucous membrane are intact and healthy, they provide an efficient physical barrier to invading microbes. The outer layer of skin can be penetrated by only a few types of microbe, and the mucus secreted by mucous membranes traps microbes and other foreign material on its sticky surface. Sebum and sweat secreted

onto the skin surface contain antibacterial and antifungal substances.

Hairs in the nose act as a coarse filter, and the sweeping action of cilia in the respiratory tract moves mucus and inhaled foreign materials towards the throat. Then it is coughed up or swallowed.

The one-way flow of urine from the bladder minimises the risk of microbes ascending through the urethra into the bladder.

Phagocytosis

The process of phagocytosis (cell eating) is shown in Figure 4.10, page 64. Phagocytic defence cells such as macrophages and neutrophils migrate to sites of inflammation and infection (chemotaxis), because neutrophils themselves and invading microbes release chemicals that attract them (chemoattractants). Phagocytes trap particles either by engulfing them with their body mass or by extending long pseudopodia towards them, which grasp them and reel them in (Fig. 15.1). These cells are non-selective in their targets; they will bind, engulf and digest foreign cells or particles.

Macrophages have an important role as a link between the non-specific and specific defence mechanisms. After ingestion and digestion of an antigen, they act as *antigen-presenting cells*, displaying their antigen on their own cell surface to stimulate T-lymphocytes and activate the immune response (p. 375).

Natural antimicrobial substances

Hydrochloric acid
This is present in high concentrations in gastric juice, and kills the majority of ingested microbes.

Lysozyme
This is a small protein with antibacterial properties present in granulocytes, tears, and other body secretions, but not in sweat, urine or cerebrospinal fluid.

Antibodies
These are present in nasal secretions and saliva, and inactivate microbes (p. 375).

Saliva
This is secreted into the mouth and washes away food debris that may otherwise encourage bacterial growth. Its slightly acid medium is antibacterial.

Interferons
These are substances produced by T-lymphocytes and by cells that have been invaded by viruses. They prevent

viral replication within infected cells, and the spread of viruses to healthy cells.

Complement

Complement is a system of about 20 proteins found in the blood and tissues. It is activated by the presence of *immune complexes* (an antigen and antibody bound together) and by foreign sugars on bacterial cell walls. Complement:

- binds to, and damages, bacterial cell walls, thus destroying the microbe
- binds to bacterial cell walls, stimulating phagocytosis by neutrophils and macrophages
- attracts phagocytic cells such as neutrophils into an area of infection, i.e. stimulates chemotaxis.

The inflammatory response

This is the physiological response to tissue damage and is accompanied by a characteristic series of local changes (Fig. 15.1). It most commonly takes place when microbes have overcome other non-specific defence mechanisms. Its purpose is protective: to isolate, inactivate and remove both the causative agent and damaged tissue so that healing can take place.

Inflammatory conditions are recognised by their Latin suffix '-itis'; for example, appendicitis is inflammation of the appendix and laryngitis is inflammation of the larynx.

Causes of inflammation

The numerous causes of inflammation may be classified as follows:

- microbes, e.g. bacteria, viruses, protozoa, fungi
- physical agents, e.g. heat, cold, mechanical injury, ultraviolet and ionising radiation
- chemical agents
  - organic, e.g. microbial toxins and organic poisons, such as weedkillers
  - inorganic, e.g. acids, alkalis.

Acute inflammation

Episodes of acute inflammation are usually of short duration, e.g. days to a few weeks, and may range from mild to very severe. The cardinal signs of inflammation are:

- redness
- heat
- pain
- swelling
- loss of function.

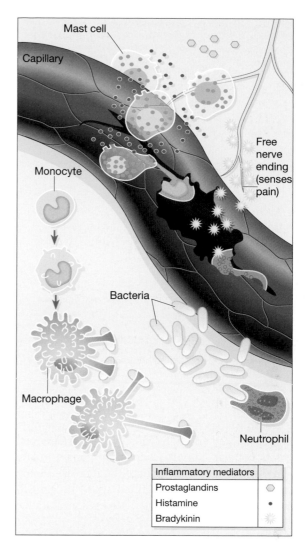

Figure 15.1 **The inflammatory response.**

371

Most aspects of the inflammatory response are hugely beneficial, promoting removal of the harmful agent and setting the scene for healing to follow.

The acute inflammatory response is described here as a collection of overlapping events: increased blood flow, accumulation of tissue fluid, migration of leukocytes, increased core temperature, pain and suppuration.

Some of the most important substances released in inflammation are summarised in Table 15.1.

Increased blood flow

Following injury, both the arterioles supplying the damaged area and the local capillaries dilate, increasing blood flow to the site.

This is caused mainly by the local release of a number of chemical mediators from damaged cells, e.g. histamine

Table 15.1 Summary of the principal substances released in inflammation

Substance	Made by	Trigger for release	Main pro-inflammatory actions
Histamine	Mast cells (in most tissues), basophils (blood); stored in cytoplasmic granules	Binding of antibody to mast cells and basophils	Vasodilatation, itching, ↑vascular permeability, degranulation, smooth muscle contraction (e.g. bronchoconstriction)
Serotonin (5-HT)	Platelets Mast cells and basophils (stored in granules) Also in CNS (acts as neurotransmitter)	When platelets are activated, and when mast cells/basophils degranulate	Vasoconstriction, ↑vascular permeability
Prostaglandins (PGs)	Nearly all cells; not stored, but made from cell membranes as required	Many different stimuli, e.g. drugs, toxins, other inflammatory mediators, hormones, trauma	Diverse, sometimes opposing, e.g. fever, pain, vasodilatation or vasoconstriction, ↑vascular permeability
Heparin	Liver, mast cells, basophils (stored in cytoplasmic granules)	Released when cells degranulate	Anticoagulant (prevents blood clotting), which maintains blood supply (nutrients, O_2) to injured tissue and washes away microbes and wastes
Bradykinin	Tissues and blood	When blood clots, in trauma and inflammation	Pain Vasodilatation

and serotonin. Increased blood flow to the area of tissue damage provides more oxygen and nutrients for the increased cellular activity that accompanies inflammation. Increased blood flow causes the increased temperature and reddening of an inflamed area, and contributes to the swelling and oedema associated with inflammation.

Increased tissue fluid formation

One of the cardinal signs of inflammation is swelling (oedema) of the tissues involved, which is caused by fluid leaving local blood vessels and entering the interstitial spaces.

This is partly due to increased capillary permeability caused by inflammatory mediators such as histamine, serotonin and prostaglandins, and partly due to elevated pressure inside the vessels because of increased flow. Most of the excess tissue fluid drains away in the lymphatic vessels, and takes damaged tissue, dead and dying cells, and toxins with it.

Plasma proteins, normally retained within the bloodstream, also escape into the tissues through the leaky capillary walls; this increases the osmotic pressure of the tissue fluid and draws more fluid out of the blood. These proteins include antibodies, which combat infection, and fibrinogen, a clotting protein. Fibrinogen in the tissues is converted by *thromboplastin* to fibrin, which forms an insoluble mesh within the interstitial space, walling off the inflamed area and helping to limit the spread of any infection. Some pathogens e.g. *Streptococcus pyogenes*, which causes throat and skin infections, release toxins that break down this fibrin network and promote spread of infection into adjacent, healthy tissue.

Sometimes tissue oedema can be harmful. For instance, swelling around respiratory passages can obstruct breathing, and significant swelling often causes pain. On the other hand, the swelling around a joint cushions it and limits movement, which encourages healing.

Migration of leukocytes

Loss of fluid from the blood thickens it, slowing flow and allowing the normally fast-flowing white blood cells to make contact with, and adhere to, the vessel wall. In the acute stages, the most important leukocyte is the neutrophil, which adheres to the blood vessel lining, squeezes between the endothelial cells and enters the tissues (see Fig. 4.10, p. 64), where its main function is in phagocytosis of antigens.

Phagocyte activity is promoted by the raised temperatures (local and systemic) associated with inflammation.

After about 24 hours, macrophages become the predominant cell type at the inflamed site, and they persist in the tissues if the situation is not resolved, leading to chronic inflammation. Macrophages are larger and longer lived than the neutrophils. They phagocytose dead/dying tissue, microbes and other antigenic material, and dead/dying neutrophils. Some microbes resist digestion and provide a possible source of future infection, e.g. *Mycobacterium tuberculosis*.

Chemotaxis. This is the chemical attraction of leukocytes, including neutrophils and macrophages, to an area of inflammation.

It may be that chemoattractants act to retain passing leukocytes in the inflamed area, rather than actively attracting them from distant areas of the body. Known chemoattractants include microbial toxins, chemicals released from leukocytes, prostaglandins from damaged cells and complement proteins.

Increased core temperature

The inflammatory response may be accompanied by a rise in body temperature (pyrexia), especially if there is significant infection. Body temperature rises when an endogenous pyrogen (interleukin 1) is released from macrophages and granulocytes in response to microbial toxins or immune complexes. Interleukin 1 is a chemical mediator that resets the temperature thermostat in the hypothalamus at a higher level, causing pyrexia and other symptoms that may also accompany inflammation, e.g. fatigue and loss of appetite. Pyrexia increases the metabolic rate of cells in the inflamed area and, consequently, there is an increased need for oxygen and nutrients. The increased temperature of inflamed tissues has the twin benefits of inhibiting the growth and division of microbes, whilst promoting the activity of phagocytes.

Pain

This occurs when local swelling compresses sensory nerve endings. It is exacerbated by chemical mediators of the inflammatory process, e.g. bradykinin, prostaglandins that potentiate the sensitivity of the sensory nerve endings to painful stimuli. Although pain is an unpleasant experience, it may indirectly promote healing, because it encourages protection of the damaged site.

Suppuration (pus formation)

Pus consists of dead phagocytes, dead cells, cell debris, fibrin, inflammatory exudate and living and dead microbes. It is contained within a membrane of new blood capillaries, phagocytes and fibroblasts. The most common causative pyogenic (pus-forming) microbes are *Staphylococcus aureus* and *Streptococcus pyogenes*. Small amounts of pus form *boils* and larger amounts form abscesses. *S. aureus* produces the enzyme coagulase, which converts fibrinogen to fibrin, localising the pus. *S. pyogenes* produces toxins that break down tissue, causing spreading infection. Healing, following pus formation, is by second intention (see Ch. 14).

Superficial abscesses tend to rupture and discharge pus through the skin. Healing is usually complete unless tissue damage is extensive.

Deep-seated abscesses may have a variety of outcomes. There may be:

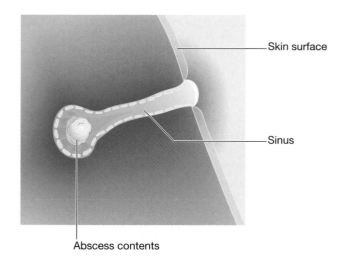

Figure 15.2 **Sinus between an abscess and the surface of the body.**

- early rupture with complete discharge of pus on to the surface, followed by healing
- rupture and limited discharge of pus on to the surface, followed by the development of a chronic abscess with an infected open channel or *sinus* (Fig. 15.2)
- rupture and discharge of pus into an adjacent organ or cavity, forming an infected channel open at both ends or *fistula* (Fig. 15.3)
- eventual removal of pus by phagocytes, followed by healing
- enclosure of pus by fibrous tissue that may become calcified, harbouring live organisms which may become a source of future infection
- formation of fibrous adhesions between adjacent membranes, e.g. pleura, peritoneum

373

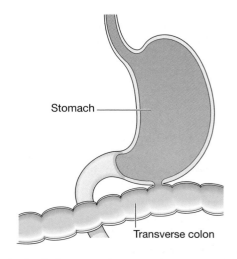

Figure 15.3 **Fistula between the stomach and the colon.**

- shrinkage of fibrous tissue as it ages, which may reduce the lumen or obstruct a tube, e.g. oesophagus, bowel, blood vessel.

Outcomes of acute inflammation

Resolution. This occurs when the cause has been successfully overcome. Damaged cells and residual fibrin are removed, being replaced with new healthy tissue, and repair is complete, with or without scar formation.

Development of chronic inflammation. Acute inflammation may become chronic if resolution is not complete, e.g. if live microbes remain at the site, as in some deep-seated abscesses, wound infections and bone infections.

Chronic inflammation

The processes involved are very similar to those of acute inflammation but, because the process is of longer duration, considerably more tissue is likely to be destroyed. The inflammatory cells are mainly lymphocytes instead of neutrophils, and fibroblasts are activated, leading to the laying down of collagen, and *fibrosis*. If the body defences are unable to clear the infection, they may try to wall it off instead, forming nodules called *granulomas*, within which are collections of defensive cells. Tuberculosis is an example of an infection that frequently becomes chronic, leading to granuloma formation. The causative bacterium, *Mycobacterium tuberculosis*, is resistant to body defences and so pockets of organisms are sealed up in granulomas within the lungs.

Chronic inflammation may either be a complication of acute inflammation (see above) or follow chronic exposure to an irritant.

Fibrosis (scar formation)

Fibrous tissue is formed during healing when there is loss of tissue or the cells destroyed do not regenerate, e.g. following chronic inflammation, persistent ischaemia, suppuration or large-scale trauma. The process begins with formation of granulation tissue, then, over time, the new capillaries and inflammatory material are removed leaving only the collagen fibres secreted by the fibroblasts. Fibrous tissue may have long-lasting damaging effects.

Adhesions. These consist of fibrous tissue and may limit movement, e.g. between the layers of pleura, preventing inflation of the lungs; between loops of bowel, interfering with peristalsis.

Fibrosis of infarcts. Blockage of a vessel by a thrombus or an embolus causes an infarction (p. 115). Fibrosis of

one large infarct or of numerous small infarcts may follow, leading to varying degrees of organ dysfunction, e.g. in heart, brain, kidneys, liver.

Tissue shrinkage. This occurs as fibrous tissue ages. The effects depend on the site and extent of the fibrosis, e.g.:

- Small tubes, such as blood vessels, air passages, ureters, the urethra and ducts of glands may become narrow or obstructed and lose their elasticity
- Contractures (bands of shrunken fibrous tissue) may extend across joints, e.g. in a limb or digit there may be limitation of movement or, following burns of the neck, the head may be pulled to one side.

Immunological surveillance

A population of lymphocytes, called natural killer (NK) cells, constantly patrol the body searching for abnormal cells. Cells that have been infected with a virus, or mutated cells that might become malignant, frequently display unusual markers on their cell membranes, which are recognised by NK cells. Having detected an abnormal cell, the NK cell immediately kills it. Although NK cells are lymphocytes, they are much less selective about their targets than the other two types discussed in this chapter (T- and B-cells).

Immunity

Learning outcomes

After studying this section, you should be able to:

- discuss the roles of the different types of T-lymphocyte in providing cell-mediated immunity
- describe the process of antibody-mediated immunity
- distinguish between artificially and naturally acquired immunity, giving examples of each
- distinguish between active and passive immunity, giving examples of each.

The cell type involved in immunity is the lymphocyte (p. 65). This white blood cell is manufactured in the bone marrow, and has a characteristically large, single nucleus. Once released into the bloodstream from the bone marrow, lymphocytes are further processed to make two functionally distinct types: the T-lymphocyte and the B-lymphocyte.

T-lymphocytes

These are processed by the thymus gland (p. 136), which lies between the heart and the sternum. The hormone thymosin, produced by the thymus, is responsible for promoting the processing, which leads to the formation of fully specialised (differentiated), mature, functional T-lymphocytes. It is important to recognise that a mature T-lymphocyte has been programmed to recognise only one type of antigen, and during its subsequent travels through the body will react to no other antigen, however dangerous it might be. Thus, a T-lymphocyte manufactured to recognise the chickenpox virus will not react to a measles virus, a cancer cell, or a tuberculosis bacterium.

T-lymphocytes provide *cell-mediated immunity*, discussed below.

B-lymphocytes

These are both produced and processed in the bone marrow. Their role is in production of antibodies (immunoglobulins), which are proteins designed to bind to, and destroy, an antigen. As with T-lymphocytes, each B-lymphocyte targets one specific antigen; the antibody released reacts with one type of antigen and no other. B-lymphocytes provide *antibody-mediated immunity*, discussed below.

From this description of T- and B-lymphocytes, it is clear that for every one of the millions of possible antigens that might be encountered in life there is one corresponding T- and B-lymphocyte. There is therefore a vast number of different T- and B-lymphocytes in the body, each capable of responding to only one antigen.

Cell-mediated immunity

T-lymphocytes that have been activated in the thymus gland are released into the circulation. When they encounter their antigen for the first time, they become sensitised to it. If the antigen has come from outside the body, it needs to be 'presented' to the T-lymphocyte on the surface of an antigen-presenting cell. There are different types of antigen-presenting cell, including macrophages. Macrophages are part of the non-specific defences, because they engulf and digest antigens indiscriminately, but they also participate in immune responses. To do this, after digesting the antigen they transport the most antigenic fragment to their own cell membrane and display it on their surface (Fig. 15.4). On their journey around the body, still displaying the antigen fragment, they eventually come into contact with the T-lymphocyte that has been processed to target that particular antigen.

If the antigen is an abnormal body cell, such as a cancer cell, it too will be displaying foreign (non-self) material on its cell membrane that will stimulate the T-lymphocyte. Whichever way the antigen is presented to the T-lymphocyte, it stimulates the division and proliferation (*clonal expansion*) of the T-lymphocyte (Fig. 15.4). Four main types of specialised T-lymphocyte are produced, each of which is still directed against the original antigen, but which will tackle it in different ways.

Memory T-cells

These long-lived cells survive after the threat has been neutralised, and provide *cell-mediated immunity* by responding rapidly to another encounter with the same antigen.

Cytotoxic T-cells

These directly inactivate any cells carrying antigens. They attach themselves to the target cell and release powerful toxins, which are very effective because the two cells are so close together. The main role of cytotoxic T-lymphocytes is in destruction of abnormal body cells, e.g. infected cells and cancer cells.

Helper T-cells

These are essential for correct functioning of not only cell-mediated immunity, but also antibody-mediated immunity. Their central role in immunity is emphasised in situations where they are destroyed, as by the human immunodeficiency virus (HIV). When helper T-lymphocyte numbers fall significantly, the whole immune system is compromised. T-helpers are the commonest of the T-lymphocytes; their main functions include:

- production of special chemicals called *cytokines*, e.g. interleukins and interferons, which support and promote cytotoxic T-lymphocytes and macrophages
- cooperating with B-lymphocytes to produce antibodies; although B-lymphocytes are responsible for antibody manufacture, they require to be stimulated by a helper T-lymphocyte first.

Suppressor T-cells

These cells act as 'brakes', turning off activated T- and B-lymphocytes. This limits the powerful and potentially damaging effects of the immune response.

Antibody-mediated (humoral) immunity

B-lymphocytes, unlike T-lymphocytes, which are free to circulate around the body, are fixed in lymphoid tissue (e.g. the spleen and lymph nodes). B-lymphocytes, unlike T-lymphocytes, recognise and bind antigen particles without having to be presented with them by an antigen-presenting cell. Once its antigen has been detected and bound, and with the help of a helper T-lymphocyte, the

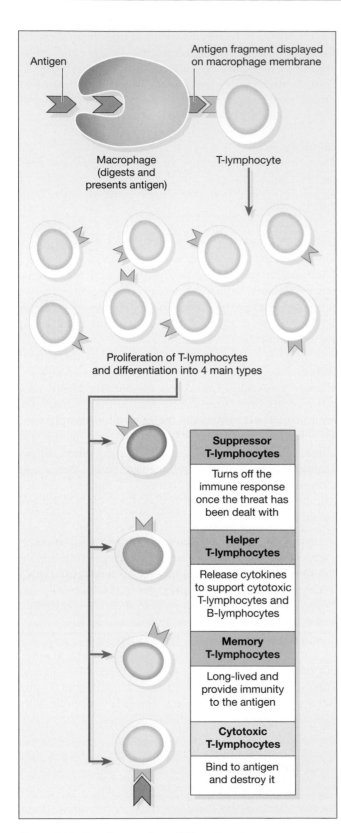

Figure 15.4 Clonal expansion of T-lymphocytes.

B-lymphocyte enlarges and begins to divide (clonal expansion, Fig. 15.5). It produces two functionally distinct types of cell, plasma cells and memory B-cells.

Plasma cells

These secrete antibodies (immunoglobulins) into the blood. Antibodies are carried throughout the tissues, while the B-lymphocytes themselves remain fixed in lymphoid tissue. Plasma cells live no longer than a day, and produce only one type of antibody, which targets the specific antigen that originally bound to the B-lymphocyte. Antibodies:

- bind to antigens, labelling them as targets for other defence cells such as cytotoxic T-lymphocytes and macrophages

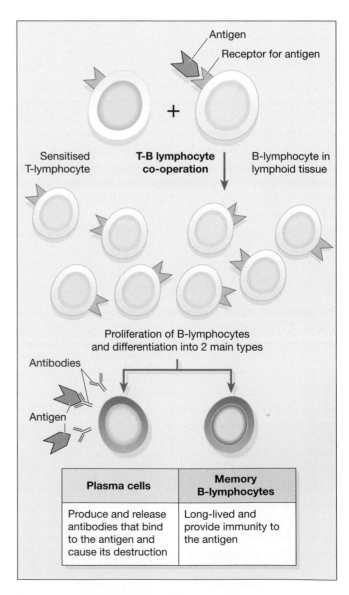

Figure 15.5 Clonal expansion of B-lymphocytes.

- bind to bacterial toxins, neutralising them
- activate complement (p. 371).

There are five main types of antibody, summarised in Table 15.2.

Memory B-cells

Like memory T-cells, these cells remain in the body long after the initial episode has been dealt with, and rapidly respond to another encounter with the same antigen by stimulating the production of antibody-secreting plasma cells.

The interdependence of the two parts of the immune system is summarised in Figure 15.6.

The fact that the body does not normally develop immunity to its own cells is due to the fine balance that exists between the immune reaction and its suppression. *Autoimmune diseases* are due to the disturbance of this balance.

Acquired immunity

When antigens, e.g. microbes, are encountered for the first time, a *primary response* follows, in which a low level of antibodies can be detected in the blood after about 2 weeks. Although the response may be sufficient to deal with the antigen, the antibody levels then fall unless there is another encounter with the same antigen within a short period of time (2 to 4 weeks). The second encounter produces a *secondary response* characterised by a rapid memory B-cell response, resulting in a marked increase in

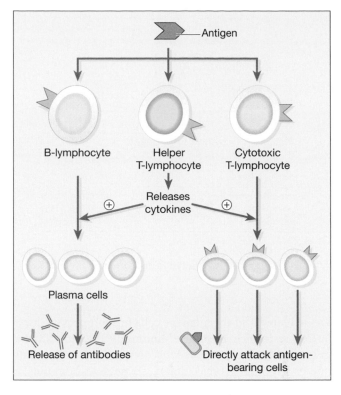

Figure 15.6 Interdependence of the T- and B-lymphocyte systems in the immune response.

antibody production (Fig. 15.7). Further increases can be achieved by later encounters but eventually a maximum is reached. This principle is used in active immunisation against infectious diseases.

Immunity may be acquired *naturally* or *artificially* and both forms may be *active* or *passive* (Fig. 15.8). Active immunity means that the individual has responded to an antigen and produced his own antibodies, lymphocytes

Table 15.2 The five types of antibody

Type of antibody	Function
IgA	Found in body secretions like breast milk and saliva, and prevent antigens crossing epithelial membranes and invading deeper tissues.
IgD	This is made by B-cells and displayed on their surfaces. Antigens bind here to activate B-cells.
IgE	Found on cell membranes of e.g. basophils and mast cells, and if it binds its antigen, activates the inflammatory response. This antibody is often found in excess in allergy.
IgG	This is the largest and most common antibody type. It attacks many different pathogens, and crosses the placenta to protect the fetus.
IgM	Produced in large quantities in the primary response and is a potent activator of complement.

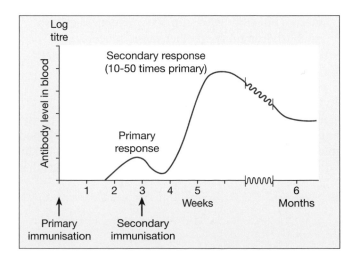

Figure 15.7 The antibody responses to immunisation.

377

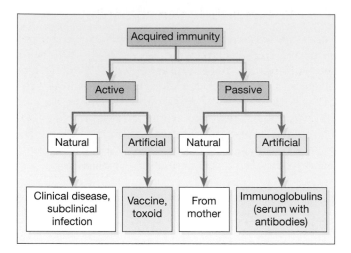

Figure 15.8 Summary of the types of acquired immunity.

are activated and the memory cells formed provide long-lasting resistance. In passive immunity the individual is given antibodies produced by someone else. The antibodies eventually break down, so passive immunity is relatively brief.

Active naturally acquired immunity

The body may be stimulated to produce its own antibodies by:

- *Having the disease.* During the course of the illness, B-lymphocytes develop into plasma cells that produce antibodies in sufficient quantities to overcome the infection. After recovery, the memory B-cells retain the ability to produce more plasma cells that produce the specific antibodies, conferring immunity to future infection by the same microbe or strain of microbe.
- *Having a subclinical infection.* Sometimes the microbial infection is not sufficiently severe to cause clinical disease but stimulates sufficient memory B-cells to establish immunity. In other cases, subclinical infection may be too mild to stimulate an adequate response for immunity to develop.

Active artificially acquired immunity

This type of immunity develops in response to the administration of dead or live artificially weakened microbes (*vaccines*) or deactivated toxins (*toxoids*). The vaccines and toxoids retain the antigenic properties that

Box 15.1 Diseases preventable by vaccination

- Anthrax
- Cholera
- Diphtheria
- Hepatitis B
- Measles
- Mumps
- Poliomyelitis
- Rubella
- Smallpox
- Tetanus
- Tuberculosis
- Typhoid
- Whooping cough

stimulate the development of immunity but they cannot cause the disease. Many infectious diseases can be prevented by artificial immunisation. Examples are shown in Box 15.1.

Active immunisation against some infectious disorders gives lifelong immunity, e.g. diphtheria, whooping cough or mumps. In other infections the immunity may last for a number of years or for only a few weeks before revaccination is necessary. Apparent loss of immunity may be due to infection with a different strain of the same microbe, which has different antigenic properties but causes the same clinical illness, e.g. viruses that cause the common cold and influenza. In older or poorly nourished individuals, lymphocyte production, especially B-lymphocytes, is reduced and the primary and secondary response may be inadequate.

Passive naturally acquired immunity

This type of immunity is acquired before birth by the passage of maternal antibodies across the placenta to the fetus, and to the baby in breast milk. The variety of different antibodies provided depends on the mother's active immunity. The baby's lymphocytes are not stimulated and the immunity is short lived.

Passive artificially acquired immunity

In this type, ready-made antibodies, in human or animal serum, are injected into the recipient. The source of the antibodies may be an individual who has recovered from the infection, or animals, commonly horses, that have been artificially actively immunised. Specific immunoglobulins (antiserum) may be administered *prophylactically* to prevent the development of disease in people who have been exposed to the infection, or *therapeutically* after the disease has developed.

Abnormal immune function

Learning outcomes

After studying this section, you should be able to:

- describe, with examples, the four types of allergic response
- describe the basis of autoimmune disease
- discuss the specific examples of autoimmune disease
- discuss the cause and effects of acquired immune deficiency syndrome (AIDS).

Hypersensitivity (allergy)

Allergy is powerful immune response to an antigen (allergen). The allergen itself is usually harmless (e.g. house dust, animal dander, grass pollen). It is therefore usually the immune response that causes the damage to the body, not the allergen itself. Upon initial exposure to the allergen the individual becomes sensitised to it, and on second and subsequent exposures the immune system mounts a response entirely out of proportion to the perceived threat. It should be noted that these responses are exaggerated versions of normal immune function. Sometimes symptoms are mild, if annoying, e.g. the running nose and streaming eyes of hay fever. Occasionally the reaction can be extreme, overwhelming body systems and causing death, e.g. anaphylactic shock, see below.

There are four mechanisms of hypersensitivity, which are classified according to what parts of the immune system are involved. They are summarised in Figure 15.9.

Type I, anaphylactic hypersensitivity

This occurs in individuals who have inherited very high levels of immunoglobulin E (IgE). When exposed to an allergen, e.g. house dust, these high levels of antibody activate mast cells and basophils (p. 65), which release their granular contents. The most important substance released is histamine, which constricts some smooth muscle, e.g. airway smooth muscle, causes vasodilatation and increases vascular permeability (leading to exudation of fluid and proteins into the tissues). Examples of type I reactions include the serious situation of anaphylaxis. There is profound bronchoconstriction and shock (p. 113) due to extensive vasodilatation. The condition can lead to death.

Type II, cytotoxic hypersensitivity

When an antibody reacts with an antigen on a cell surface, that cell is marked for destruction by a number of mechanisms, e.g. phagocytosis, or destruction by lytic enzymes. This is the usual procedure in the elimination of, for example, bacteria, but if the antibodies are directed against self-antigens the result is destruction of the body's own tissues (autoimmune disease). Type II mechanisms cause other conditions, e.g. haemolytic disease of the newborn (p. 70) and transfusion reactions (p. 62).

Type III, immune-complex-mediated hypersensitivity

Antibody–antigen complexes (immune complexes) are usually cleared efficiently from the blood by phagocytosis. If they are not, for example when there is phagocyte failure or an excessive production of immune complexes (e.g. in chronic infections), they can be deposited in tissues, e.g. kidneys, skin, joints and the eye, where they set up an inflammatory reaction. The kidney is a common site of deposition because it receives a large proportion of the cardiac output and filters the blood. Immune complexes collecting here lodge in and block the glomeruli (p. 337), impairing kidney function (glomerulonephritis). Sensitivity to penicillin is also a type III reaction; antibodies bind to penicillin (the antigen), and the symptoms are the result of deposition of immune complexes in tissues – rashes, joint pains and sometimes haematuria.

Type IV, delayed type hypersensitivity

Unlike types I–III, type IV hypersensitivity does not involve antibodies, but is an overreaction of T-lymphocytes to an antigen. When an antigen is detected by memory T-lymphocytes, it provokes clonal expansion of the T-lymphocyte (Fig. 15.4), and large numbers of cytotoxic T-lymphocytes are released to eliminate the antigen. Usually this system is controlled and the T-lymphocyte response is appropriate. If not, the actively aggressive cytotoxic T-lymphocytes damage normal tissues.

An example of this is contact dermatitis (p. 365). Graft rejection is also caused by T-lymphocytes; an incompatible skin graft, for instance, will become necrotic and slough off in the days following application of the graft.

Autoimmune diseases

Normally, an immune response is mounted only against foreign (non-self) antigens, but occasionally the body fails to recognise its own tissues and attacks itself. The resulting autoimmune disorders, examples of type II

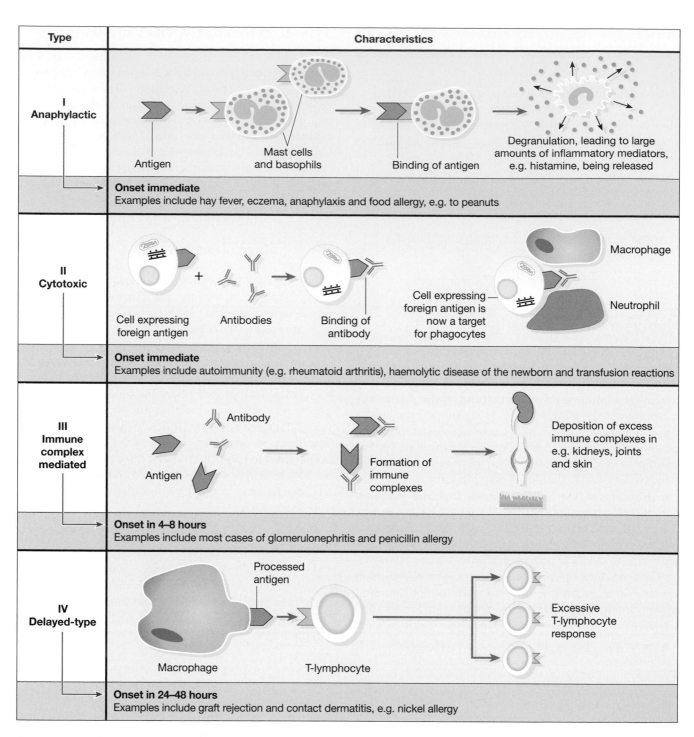

Figure 15.9 The four types of hypersensitivity.

hypersensitivity, include a number of relatively common conditions.

Rheumatoid arthritis (p. 427)
The body produces antibodies to the synovial membranes (p. 407). In most sufferers, the antibody can be detected in the blood. Called *rheumatoid factor*, it binds to the synovial membrane, leading to chronically inflamed joints that are stiff, painful and swollen.

Hashimoto's disease (p. 228)
The body makes antibodies to thyroglobulin, leading to destruction of thyroid hormone, and hyposecretion of the thyroid.

Graves' disease
The body makes antibodies to thyroid cells. Unlike Hashimoto's disease, however, the effect of the antibodies is to stimulate the gland, with a resultant hyperthyroidism (p. 227).

Autoimmune haemolytic anaemia (p. 71)
In this, individuals make antibodies to their own red blood cells, leading to haemolytic anaemia.

Myasthenia gravis
This autoimmune condition of unknown origin affects more women than men, and usually those between 20 and 40 years. Antibodies are produced that bind to and block the acetylcholine receptors of neuromuscular junctions. The transmission of nerve impulses to muscle fibres is therefore blocked. This causes progressive and extensive muscle weakness, although the muscles themselves are normal. Extrinsic and eyelid muscles are affected first, causing *ptosis* (drooping of the eyelid) or *diplopia* (double vision), followed by those of the neck (possibly affecting chewing, swallowing and speech) and limbs. There are periods of remission, relapses being precipitated by, for example, strenuous exercise, infections or pregnancy.

Immunodeficiency

When the immune system is compromised, there is a tendency to recurrent infections, often by microbes not normally pathogenic in humans (*opportunistic infections*). Immunodeficiency is classified as *primary* (usually occurring in infancy and genetically mediated) or *secondary*, that is, acquired in later life as the result of another disease, e.g. protein deficiency, acute infection, chronic renal failure, bone marrow diseases, following splenectomy or acquired immune deficiency syndrome (AIDS).

Acquired immune deficiency syndrome (AIDS)

This condition is caused by the human immunodeficiency virus (HIV), an RNA retrovirus which produces the enzyme *reverse transcriptase* inside the cells of the infected person (host cells). This enzyme transforms viral RNA to DNA and this new DNA, called the provirus, is incorporated into the host cell DNA. The host cell then produces new copies of the virus that pass out into tissue fluid and blood and infect other host cells. When infected host cells divide, copies of the provirus are integrated into the DNA of daughter cells, spreading the disease within the body.

HIV has an affinity for cells that have a protein receptor called CD_4 in their membrane, including T-lymphocytes, monocytes, macrophages, some B-lymphocytes and, possibly, cells in the gastrointestinal tract and neuroglial cells in the brain. Helper T-cells (Fig. 15.4) are the main cells involved. When infected their number is reduced, causing suppression of both antibody-mediated and cell-mediated immunity with the consequent development of widespread opportunistic infections, often by microbes of relatively low pathogenicity.

HIV has been isolated from semen, cervical secretions, lymphocytes, plasma, cerebrospinal fluid, tears, saliva, urine and breast milk. The secretions known to be especially infectious are semen, cervical secretions, blood and blood products.

Infection is spread by:

- sexual intercourse, vaginal and anal
- contaminated needles used:
  - during treatment of patients
  - when drug abusers share needles.
- an infected mother to her child:
  - across the placenta before birth
  - during childbirth
  - possibly by breast milk.

The presence of antibodies to HIV indicates that the individual has been exposed to the virus but *not* that a naturally acquired immunity has developed. Not all those who have antibodies in their blood develop AIDS although they may act as carriers and spread the infection to others.

A few weeks after initial infection there may be an acute influenza-like illness with no specific features, followed by a period of two or more years without symptoms.

Chronic HIV infection may cause persistent generalised lymphadenopathy (PGL). Some patients may then develop AIDS-related complex (ARC) and experience chronic low-grade fever, diarrhoea, weight loss, anaemia and leukopenia.

When AIDS develops, the main complications are widespread recurrent opportunistic infections and tumours. Outstanding features include the following.

- Pneumonia, commonly caused by *Pneumocystis carinii*, but many other microbes may be involved.
- Persistent nausea, diarrhoea and weight loss due to recurrent infections of the alimentary tract by a wide variety of microbes.
- Meningitis, encephalitis and brain abscesses may be recurrent, either caused by opportunistic microbes or possibly by HIV.
- Neurological function may deteriorate, characterised by forgetfulness, loss of concentration, confusion, apathy, dementia, limb weakness, ataxia and incontinence.
- Skin eruptions, often widespread, may occur, e.g. eczema, psoriasis, cellulitis, impetigo, warts, shingles and cold sores.
- Generalised lymphadenopathy may occur, i.e. non-infective enlargement of lymph nodes.
- Development of malignant tumours is not uncommon, because of the progressive failure of immunological surveillance as the virus destroys the T-cell population. Typical cancers include:
  - lymphomas, i.e. tumours of lymph nodes
  - Kaposi's sarcoma, consisting of tumours under the skin and in internal organs (p. 367).

The musculoskeletal system

16

The musculoskeletal system consists of the bones of the skeleton, their joints and the skeletal (voluntary) muscles that move the body. The characteristics and properties of joints, and of bone and muscle tissue, are discussed in this chapter.

Bone

Learning outcomes

After studying this section you should be able to:

■ state the functions of bones

■ list five types of bones and give an example of each

■ outline the general structure of a long bone

■ describe the structure of compact and spongy bone tissue

■ describe the development of bone

■ explain the process of bone healing

■ identify the factors that delay bone healing

■ describe two complications of fractures

■ outline the factors that determine bone growth.

Although bones are often thought to be static or permanent, they are highly vascular living structures that are continuously being remodelled.

Functions of bones

The functions of bones include:

- provision of the framework of the body
- giving attachment to muscles and tendons
- allowing movement of the body as a whole and of parts of the body, by forming joints that are moved by muscles
- forming the boundaries of the cranial, thoracic and pelvic cavities, protecting the organs they contain
- haemopoiesis, the production of blood cells in red bone marrow (p. 60)
- mineral storage, especially calcium phosphate – the mineral reservoir within bone is essential for maintenance of blood calcium levels, which must be tightly controlled.

Types of bones

Bones are classified as long, short, irregular, flat and sesamoid.

Long bones. These consist of a shaft and two extremities. As the name suggests, these bones are longer than they are wide. Examples include the femur, tibia and fibula.

Short, irregular, flat and sesamoid bones. These have no shafts or extremities and are diverse in shape and size. Examples include:

- short bones – carpals (wrist)
- irregular bones – vertebrae and some skull bones
- flat bones – sternum, ribs and most skull bones
- sesamoid bones – patella (knee cap).

Bone structure

General structure of a long bone

These have a *diaphysis* or shaft and two *epiphyses* or extremities (Fig. 16.1). The diaphysis is composed of *compact bone* with a central medullary canal, containing fatty *yellow bone marrow*. The epiphyses consist of an

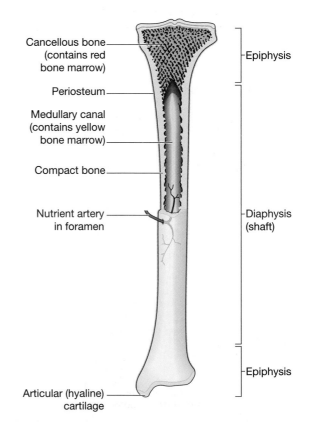

Cancellous bone (contains red bone marrow)

Periosteum

Medullary canal (contains yellow bone marrow)

Compact bone

Nutrient artery in foramen

Articular (hyaline) cartilage

Epiphysis

Diaphysis (shaft)

Epiphysis

Figure 16.1 A mature long bone – partially sectioned.

outer covering of compact bone with *spongy (cancellous) bone* inside. The diaphysis and epiphyses are separated by *epiphyseal cartilages*, which ossify when growth is complete. Thickening of a bone occurs by the deposition of new bone tissue under the periosteum.

Long bones are almost completely covered by a vascular membrane, the *periosteum*, which has two layers. The outer layer is tough and fibrous, and protects the bone underneath. The inner layer contains osteoblasts and osteoclasts, the cells responsible for bone production and breakdown (see below), and is important in repair and remodelling of the bone. The periosteum covers the whole bone except within joint cavities, allows attachments of tendons and is continuous with the joint capsule. *Hyaline cartilage* replaces periosteum on bone surfaces that form joints. Blood supply to the shaft of the bone derives from one or more nutrient arteries; the epiphyses have their own blood supply, although in the mature bone the capillary networks arising from the two are heavily interconnected.

Structure of short, irregular, flat and sesamoid bones

These have a relatively thin outer layer of compact bone with cancellous bone inside containing *red bone marrow* (Fig. 16.2). They are enclosed by periosteum except the inner layer of the cranial bones where it is replaced by dura mater.

Microscopic structure of bone

Bone is a strong and durable type of connective tissue. Its major constituent (65%) is a mixture of calcium salts,

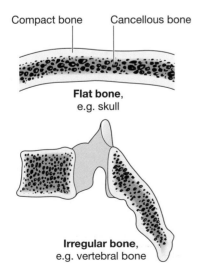

Figure 16.2 Sections of flat and irregular bones.

mainly calcium phosphate. This inorganic matrix gives bone great hardness, but on its own would be brittle and prone to shattering. The remaining third is organic material, called *osteoid*, which is composed mainly of collagen. Collagen is very strong and gives bone slight flexibility. The cellular component of bone contributes less than 2% of bone mass.

Bone cells

The cells responsible for bone formation are *osteoblasts* (these later mature into *osteocytes*). Osteoblasts and *chondrocytes* (cartilage-forming cells) develop from the same parent fibrous tissue cells. Differentiation into *osteogenic cells*, rather than *chondroblasts*, is believed to depend upon an adequate oxygen supply. This may be a factor affecting healing of fractures, i.e. if the oxygen supply is deficient there may be a preponderance of chondroblasts, resulting in a cartilaginous union of the fracture.

Osteoblasts
These are the bone-forming cells that secrete collagen and other constituents of bone tissue. They are present:

- in the deeper layers of periosteum
- in the centres of ossification of immature bone
- at the ends of the diaphysis adjacent to the epiphyseal cartilages of long bones
- at the site of a fracture.

Osteocytes
As bone develops, osteoblasts become trapped within the newly formed bone. They stop forming new bone at this stage and are called *osteocytes*. These are the mature bone cells that monitor and maintain bone tissue, and are nourished by tissue fluid in the canaliculi that radiate from the central canals.

Osteoclasts
Their function is resorption of bone to maintain the optimum shape. This takes place at bone surfaces:

- under the periosteum, to maintain the shape of bones during growth and to remove excess callus formed during healing of fractures (p. 389)
- round the walls of the medullary canal during growth and to canalise callus during healing.

A fine balance of osteoblast and osteoclast activity maintains normal bone structure and functions.

Compact (cortical) bone

Compact bone makes up about 80% of the body bone mass. It is made up of a large number of tube-shaped

385

units called *osteons* (Haversian systems), each of which is made up of a central canal surrounded by a series of expanding rings, similar to the growth rings of a tree (Fig. 16.3). Osteons tend to be aligned the same way that force is applied to the bone, so for example in the femur (thigh bone), they run from one epiphysis to the other. This gives the bone great strength.

The central canal contains nerves, lymphatics and blood vessels, and each central canal is linked with neighbouring canals by tunnels running at right angles between them, called *perforating canals*. The series of cylindrical plates of bone arranged around each central canal are called *lamellae*. Between the adjacent lamellae of the osteon are strings of little cavities called *lacunae*, in each of which sits an osteocyte. Lacunae communicate with each other through a series of tiny channels called *canaliculi*, which allows the circulation of interstitial fluid through the bone, and direct contact between the osteocytes, which extend fine processes into them.

Between the osteons are *interstitial lamellae*, the remnants of older systems partially broken down during remodelling or growth of bone.

Spongy (cancellous, trabecular) bone

To the naked eye, spongy bone looks like a honeycomb. Microscopic examination reveals a framework formed from *trabeculae* (meaning 'little beams'), which consist of a few lamellae and osteocytes interconnected by canaliculi (Fig. 16.4). The spaces between the trabeculae contain red bone marrow.

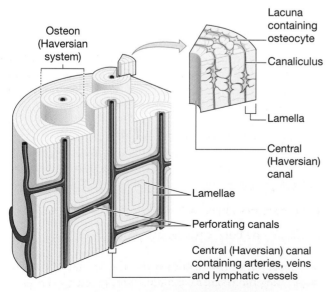

Figure 16.3 Microscopic structure of compact bone.

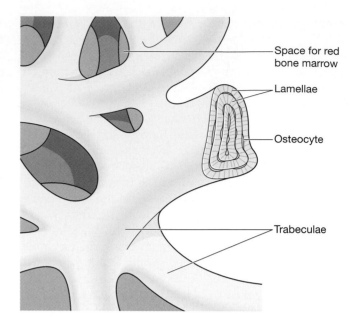

Figure 16.4 Microscopic structure of spongy bone.

Development of bone tissue

Also called *osteogenesis* or *ossification*, this begins before birth and is not complete until about the 21st year of life (Fig. 16.5). Long, short and irregular bones develop from rods of cartilage, *cartilage models*. Flat bones develop from *membrane models* and sesamoid bones from *tendon models*.

During the process of bone development, osteoblasts secrete osteoid, which gradually replaces the initial model; then this osteoid is progressively calcified, also by osteoblast action. As the bone grows, the osteoblasts become trapped in the matrix of their own making and become osteocytes.

Development of long bones

In long bones the focal points from which ossification begins are small areas of osteogenic cells, or *centres of ossification* in the cartilage model. This is accompanied by development of a bone collar at about 8 weeks of gestation. Later the blood supply develops and bone tissue replaces cartilage as osteoblasts secrete osteoid components in the shaft. The bone lengthens as ossification continues and spreads to the epiphyses. Around birth, secondary centres of ossification develop in the epiphyses, and the medullary canal forms when osteoclasts break down the central bone tissue in the middle of the shaft. After birth, the bone grows in length by ossification of the diaphyseal surface of the epiphyseal cartilages and lengthways growth is complete when the cartilages become completely ossified (Fig. 16.5).

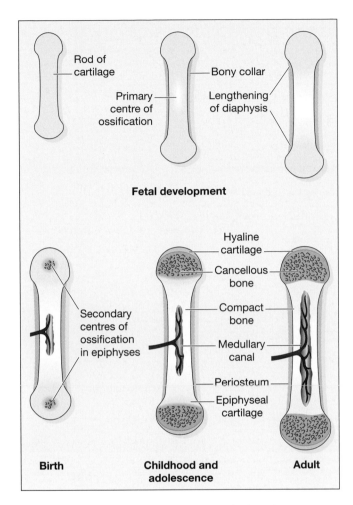

Figure 16.5 The stages of development of a long bone.

Hormonal regulation of bone growth

Hormones that regulate the growth, size and shape of bones include the following:

- *Growth hormone* and the thyroid hormones, *thyroxine* and *tri-iodothyronine*, are especially important during infancy and childhood; deficient or excessive secretion of these results in abnormal development of the skeleton.

- *Testosterone* and *oestrogens* influence the physical changes that occur at puberty and help maintain bone structure throughout life. Rising levels of these hormones are responsible for the growth spurt of puberty, but later stimulate closure of the epiphyseal plates, so that bone growth lengthways stops (although bones can grow in thickness throughout life). Oestrogens are responsible for the wider female pelvis that develops during puberty, and for maintaining bone mass in the adult female. Falling oestrogen levels at menopause can put postmenopausal women at higher risk of bone fracture.

- *Calcitonin* and *parathyroid hormone* (p. 219) control blood levels of calcium by regulating its uptake into and release from bone. Calcitonin increases calcium uptake into bone, and parathormone decreases it.

Although the length and shape of bones does not normally change after ossification is complete, bone tissue is continually being remodelled and replaced when damaged. Osteoblasts continue to lay down osteoid and osteoclasts reabsorb it. The rate in different bones varies, e.g. the distal part of the femur is replaced gradually over a period of 5 to 6 months.

Exercise and bone

Although bone growth lengthways permanently ceases once the epiphyseal plates have ossified, thickening of bone is possible throughout life. This involves the laying down of new osteons at the periphery of the bone through the action of osteoblasts in the inner layer of the periosteum. Weight-bearing exercise stimulates thickening of bone, strengthening it and making it less liable to fracture. Lack of exercise reverses these changes, leading to lighter, weaker bones.

Diet and bone

Healthy bone tissue requires adequate dietary calcium and vitamins A, C and D. Calcium, and smaller amounts of other minerals such as phosphate, iron and manganese, is essential for adequate mineralisation of bone. Vitamin A is needed for osteoblast activity. Vitamin C is used in collagen synthesis, and vitamin D is required for calcium and phosphate absorption from the intestinal tract.

Bone markings

Most bones have rough surfaces, raised protuberances and ridges that give attachment to muscle tendons and ligaments. These are not included in the following descriptions of individual bones unless they are of particular note, but many are marked on illustrations. Related terminology is defined in Table 16.1.

Healing of bone

Bone fractures are classified as:

- *simple*: the bone ends do not protrude through the skin
- *compound*: the bone ends protrude through the skin
- *pathological*: fracture of a bone weakened by disease.

387

Table 16.1 Terminology related to the skeleton

Term	Meaning
Articulating surface	The part of the bone that enters into the formation of a joint
Articulation	A joint between two or more bones
Bony sinus	A hollow cavity within a bone
Border	A ridge of bone separating two surfaces
Condyle	A smooth rounded projection of bone that forms part of a joint
Facet	A small, generally rather flat, articulating surface
Fissure or cleft	A narrow slit
Foramen (plural: foramina)	A hole in a structure
Fossa (plural: fossae)	A hollow or depression
Meatus	A tube-shaped cavity within a bone
Septum	A partition separating two cavities
Spine, spinous process or crest	A sharp ridge of bone
Styloid process	A sharp downward projection of bone that gives attachment to muscles and ligaments
Suture	An immovable joint, e.g. between the bones of the skull
Trochanter, tuberosity or tubercle	Roughened bony projections, usually for attachment of muscles or ligaments. The different names are used according to the size of the projection. Trochanters are the largest and tubercles the smallest

Following a fracture, the broken ends of bone are joined by the deposition of new bone. This occurs in several stages (Fig. 16.6).

1. A haematoma forms between the ends of bone and in surrounding soft tissues.
2. There follows development of acute inflammation and accumulation of inflammatory exudate, containing macrophages that phagocytose the haematoma and small fragments of bone without blood supply (this takes about 5 days). Fibroblasts migrate to the site; granulation tissue and new capillaries develop.
3. New bone forms as large numbers of osteoblasts secrete spongy bone, which unites the broken ends, and is protected by an outer layer of bone and cartilage; these new deposits of bone and cartilage are called *callus*.
4. Over the next few weeks, the callus matures, and the cartilage is gradually replaced with new bone.
5. Reshaping of the bone continues and gradually the medullary canal is reopened through the callus (in weeks or months). In time the bone heals completely with the callus tissue completely replaced with mature compact bone. Often the bone is thicker and stronger at the repair site than originally, and a second fracture is more likely to occur at a different site.

Factors that delay healing of fractures

Tissue fragments between bone ends. Splinters of dead bone (*sequestrae*) and soft tissue fragments not removed by phagocytosis delay healing.

Deficient blood supply. This delays growth of granulation tissue and new blood vessels. Hypoxia also reduces the number of osteoblasts and increases the number of chondrocytes that develop from their common parent cells. This may lead to cartilaginous union of the fracture, which results in a weaker repair. The most vulnerable sites, because of their normally poor blood supply, are the neck of femur, the scaphoid and the shaft of tibia.

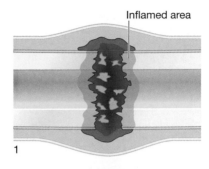

Inflamed area

Haematoma and bone fragments

1

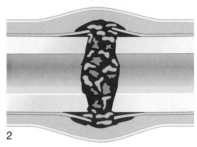

Phagocytosis of clot and debris. Growth of granulation tissue begins

2

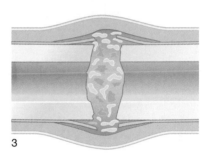

Osteoblasts begin to form new bone (callus)

3

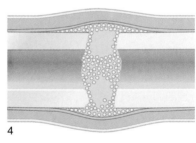

Gradual spread and mineralisation of callus to bridge the gap

4

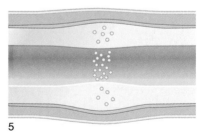

Bone almost healed. Osteoclasts reshape and canalise new bone

5

Figure 16.6 Stages in bone healing.

Poor alignment of bone ends. This may result in the formation of a large and irregular callus that heals slowly and often results in permanent disability.

Continued mobility of bone ends. Continuous movement results in fibrosis of the granulation tissue followed by fibrous union of the fracture.

Miscellaneous. These include:

• infection (see below)
• systemic illness
• malnutrition
• drugs, e.g. corticosteroids
• ageing.

Complications of fractures

Infection (osteomyelitis). Pathogens enter through broken skin, although they may occasionally be blood-borne (p. 428). Healing will not occur until the infection resolves.

Fat embolism. Emboli consisting of fat from the marrow in the medullary canal may enter the circulation through torn veins. They are most likely to lodge in the lungs.

389

Axial skeleton

Learning outcomes

After studying this section you should be able to:

■ identify the bones of the skull (face and cranium)

■ list the functions of the sinuses and fontanelles of the skull

■ outline the characteristics of a typical vertebra

■ describe the structure of the vertebral column

■ explain the movements and functions of the vertebral column

■ identify the bones forming the thoracic cage.

The bones of the skeleton are divided into two groups: the *axial skeleton* and the *appendicular skeleton* (Fig. 16.7).

The axial skeleton consists of the *skull, vertebral column, ribs* and *sternum*. Together the bones forming these structures constitute the central bony core of the body, the axis.

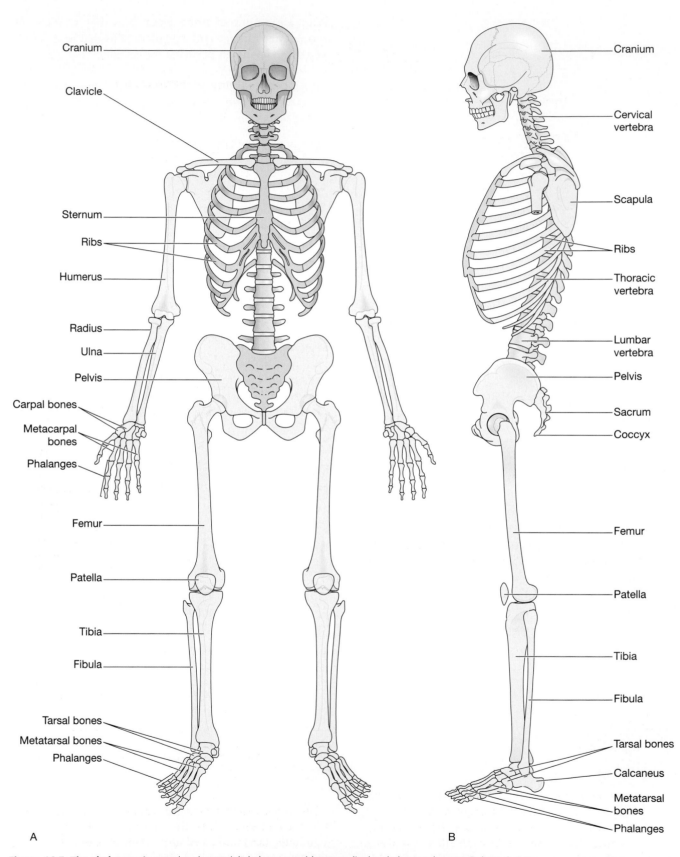

Cranium

Clavicle

Sternum

Ribs

Humerus

Radius

Ulna

Pelvis

Carpal bones

Metacarpal bones

Phalanges

Femur

Patella

Tibia

Fibula

Tarsal bones

Metatarsal bones

Phalanges

Cranium

Cervical vertebra

Scapula

Ribs

Thoracic vertebra

Lumbar vertebra

Pelvis

Sacrum

Coccyx

Femur

Patella

Tibia

Fibula

Tarsal bones

Calcaneus

Metatarsal bones

Phalanges

A

B

Figure 16.7 The skeleton. A: anterior view; axial skeleton – gold, appendicular skeleton – brown. B: lateral view.

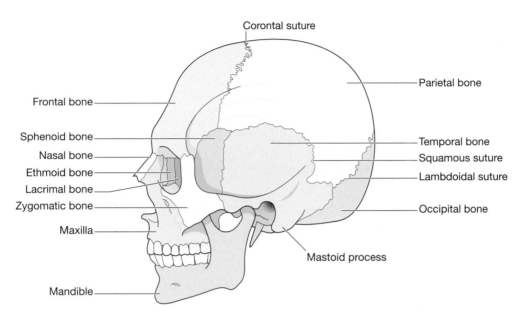

Figure 16.8 The bones of the skull and their sutures (joints).

Skull (Figs 16.8 and 16.9)

The skull rests on the upper end of the vertebral column and its bony structure is divided into two parts: the cranium and the face.

Cranium

The cranium is formed by a number of flat and irregular bones that provide a bony protection for the brain. It has a *base* upon which the brain rests and a *vault* that surrounds and covers it. The periosteum lining the inner surface of the skull bones forms the outer layer of dura mater. In the mature skull the joints (*sutures*) between the bones are immovable (fibrous). The bones have numerous perforations (e.g. foramina, fissures) through which nerves, blood and lymph vessels pass. The bones of the cranium are:

- 1 frontal bone
- 2 parietal bones
- 2 temporal bones
- 1 occipital bone
- 1 sphenoid bone
- 1 ethmoid bone.

Frontal bone

This is the bone of the forehead. It forms part of the *orbital cavities* (eye sockets) and the prominent ridges above the eyes, the *supraorbital margins*. Just above the supraorbital margins, within the bone, are two air-filled cavities or *sinuses* lined with ciliated mucous membrane, which open into the nasal cavity.

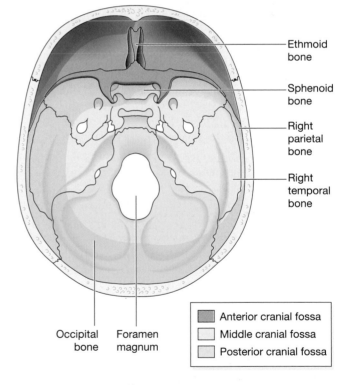

Figure 16.9 The bones forming the base of the skull and the cranial fossae – viewed from above.

The *coronal suture* joins the frontal and parietal bones and other fibrous joints are formed with the sphenoid, zygomatic, lacrimal, nasal and ethmoid bones. The bone originates in two parts joined in the midline by the *frontal suture* (see Fig. 16.16).

391

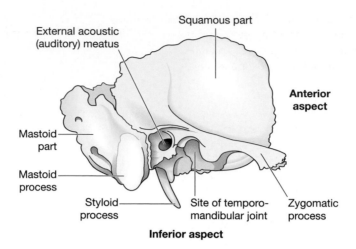

External acoustic
(auditory) meatus

Squamous part

**Anterior
aspect**

Mastoid
part

Mastoid
process

Styloid
process

Site of temporo-
mandibular joint

Zygomatic
process

Inferior aspect

Figure 16.10 **The right temporal bone.** Lateral view.

392

Parietal bones

These bones form the sides and roof of the skull. They articulate with each other at the *sagittal suture*, with the frontal bone at the coronal suture, with the occipital bone at the *lambdoidal suture* and with the temporal bones at the *squamous sutures*. The inner surface is concave and is grooved by the brain and blood vessels.

Temporal bones (Fig. 16.10)

These bones lie one on each side of the head and form fibrous immovable joints with the parietal, occipital, sphenoid and zygomatic bones. Each temporal bone has several important features.

The *squamous part* is the thin fan-shaped area that articulates with the parietal bone. *The zygomatic process* articulates with the zygomatic bone to form the zygomatic arch (cheekbone).

The *mastoid part* contains the *mastoid process*, a thickened region behind the ear. It contains a large number of very small air sinuses that communicate with the middle ear and are lined with squamous epithelium.

The *petrous portion* forms part of the base of the skull and contains the organs of hearing (the spiral organ) and balance.

The temporal bone articulates with the mandible at the *temporomandibular joint*, the only movable joint of the skull. Immediately behind this articulating surface is the *external acoustic meatus* (auditory canal), which passes inwards towards the petrous portion of the bone.

The styloid process projects from the lower process of the temporal bone, and supports the hyoid bone and muscles associated with the tongue and pharynx.

Occipital bone (Fig. 16.11)

This bone forms the back of the head and part of the base of the skull. It has immovable fibrous joints with the parietal, temporal and sphenoid bones. Its inner surface is deeply concave and the concavity is occupied by the occipital lobes of the cerebrum and by the cerebellum. The occiput has two articular condyles that form condy-

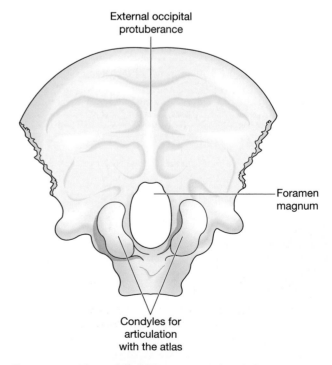

External occipital
protuberance

Foramen
magnum

Condyles for
articulation
with the atlas

Figure 16.11 **The occipital bone** – viewed from below.

loid joints (p. 408) with the first bone of the vertebral column, the atlas. This joint permits nodding movements of the head. Between the condyles is the *foramen magnum* (meaning 'large hole') through which the spinal cord passes into the cranial cavity.

Sphenoid bone (Fig. 16.12)

This bone occupies the middle portion of the base of the skull and it articulates with the occipital, temporal, parietal and frontal bones (Fig. 16.9). It links the cranial and facial bones, and cross-braces the skull. On the superior surface in the middle of the bone is a little saddle-shaped depression, the *hypophyseal fossa* (*sella turcica*) in which the *pituitary gland* rests. The body of the bone contains some fairly large air sinuses lined with ciliated mucous membrane with openings into the nasal cavity.

Ethmoid bone (Fig. 16.13)

The ethmoid bone occupies the anterior part of the base of the skull and helps to form the orbital cavity, the nasal septum and the lateral walls of the nasal cavity. On each side are two projections into the nasal cavity, the *upper* and *middle conchae* or *turbinated processes*. It is a very delicate bone containing many air sinuses lined with ciliated epithelium and with openings into the nasal cavity. The horizontal flattened part, the *cribriform plate*, forms the roof of the nasal cavity and has numerous small foramina through which nerve fibres of the *olfactory nerve* (sense of smell) pass upwards from the nasal cavity to the brain. There is also a very fine *perpendicular plate* of bone that forms the upper part of the *nasal septum*.

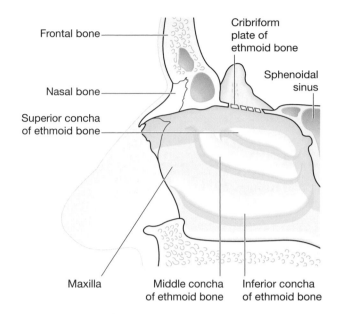

Figure 16.13 The right ethmoid bone and its related structures.

Face

The skeleton of the face is formed by 13 bones, in addition to the frontal bone, already described. Figure 16.14 shows the relationships between the bones:

- 2 zygomatic (cheek) bones
- 1 maxilla (originated as 2)
- 2 nasal bones
- 2 lacrimal bones

393

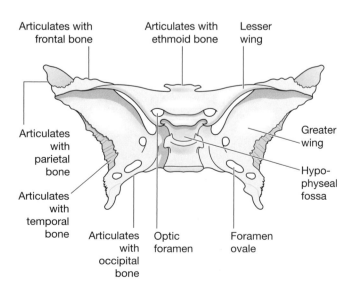

Figure 16.12 The sphenoid bone – viewed from above.

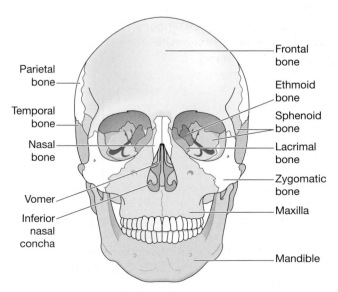

Figure 16.14 The bones of the face. Anterior view.

- 1 vomer
- 2 palatine bones
- 2 inferior conchae
- 1 mandible (originated as 2).

Zygomatic (cheek) bones

The zygomatic bones form the prominences of the cheeks and part of the floor and lateral walls of the orbital cavities.

Maxilla (upper jaw bone)

This originates as two bones, but fusion takes place before birth. The maxilla forms the upper jaw, the anterior part of the roof of the mouth, the lateral walls of the nasal cavity and part of the floor of the orbital cavities. The *alveolar ridge*, or *process*, projects downwards and carries the upper teeth. On each side is a large air sinus, the *maxillary sinus*, lined with ciliated mucous membrane and with openings into the nasal cavity.

Nasal bones

These are two small flat bones that form the greater part of the lateral and superior surfaces of the bridge of the nose.

Lacrimal bones

These two small bones are posterior and lateral to the nasal bones and form part of the medial walls of the orbital cavities. Each is pierced by a foramen for the passage of the *nasolacrimal duct* that carries the tears from the medial canthus of the eye to the nasal cavity.

Vomer

The vomer is a thin flat bone that extends upwards from the middle of the hard palate to form most of the inferior part of the nasal septum. Superiorly it articulates with the perpendicular plate of the ethmoid bone.

Palatine bones

These are two small L-shaped bones. The horizontal parts unite to form the posterior part of the hard palate and the perpendicular parts project upwards to form part of the lateral walls of the nasal cavity. At their upper extremities they form part of the orbital cavities.

Inferior conchae

Each concha is a scroll-shaped bone, which forms part of the lateral wall of the nasal cavity and projects into it below the middle concha. The superior and middle conchae are parts of the ethmoid bone. The conchae collectively increase the surface area in the nasal cavity, allowing inspired air to be warmed and humidified more effectively.

Mandible (Fig. 16.15)

This is the lower jaw, the only movable bone of the skull. It originates as two parts that unite at the midline. Each half consists of two main parts: a *curved body* with the *alveolar ridge* containing the lower teeth and a *ramus*, which projects upwards almost at right angles to the posterior end of the body.

At the upper end the ramus divides into the *condylar process* which articulates with the temporal bone to form the *temporomandibular* joint (see Fig. 16.10) and the *coronoid process*, which gives attachment to muscles and ligaments that close the jaw. The point where the ramus joins the body is the *angle* of the jaw.

Hyoid bone

This is an isolated horseshoe-shaped bone lying in the soft tissues of the neck just above the *larynx* and below the *mandible* (see Fig. 10.4, p. 240). It does not articulate with any other bone, but is attached to the styloid process of the temporal bone by ligaments. It supports the larynx and gives attachment to the base of the tongue.

Sinuses

Sinuses containing air are present in the sphenoid, ethmoid, maxillary and frontal bones. They all communicate with the nasal cavity and are lined with ciliated mucous membrane. Their functions are to give resonance to the voice and to reduce the weight of the skull, making it easier to carry.

Fontanelles of the skull (Fig. 16.16)

At birth, ossification of the cranial sutures is incomplete. Where three or more bones meet there are distinct membranous areas, or *fontanelles*. The two largest are the

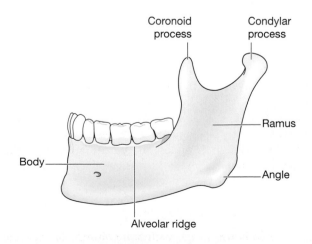

Figure 16.15 The left mandible. Lateral view.

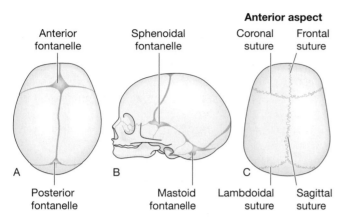

Figure 16.16 The skull showing the fontanelles and sutures.
A: Fontanelles viewed from above. B: Fontanelles viewed from the side. C: Main sutures viewed from above when ossification is complete.

anterior fontanelle, not fully ossified until the child is 12 to 18 months old, and the *posterior fontanelle*, usually ossified 2 to 3 months after birth. The skull bones do not fuse earlier to allow for moulding of the baby's head during childbirth.

Functions of the skull

The various parts of the skull have specific and different functions:

- The *cranium* protects the delicate tissues of the brain.
- The *bony eye sockets* provide the eyes with some protection against injury and give attachment to the muscles that move the eyes.
- The *temporal bone* protects the delicate structures of the ear.
- Some bones of the face and the base of the skull give resonance to the voice because they have cavities called sinuses, containing air. The sinuses have tiny openings into the nasal cavity.
- The bones of the face form the walls of the posterior part of the nasal cavities. They keep the air passages open, facilitating breathing.
- The *maxilla* and the *mandible* provide alveolar ridges in which the teeth are embedded.
- The mandible (jawbone) is the only movable bone of the skull, and chewing food is the result of coordinated activity of certain muscles of the face, the muscles of mastication, which move the mandible.

Vertebral column (Fig. 16.17)

There are 26 bones in the vertebral column. 24 separate vertebrae extend downwards from the occipital bone of

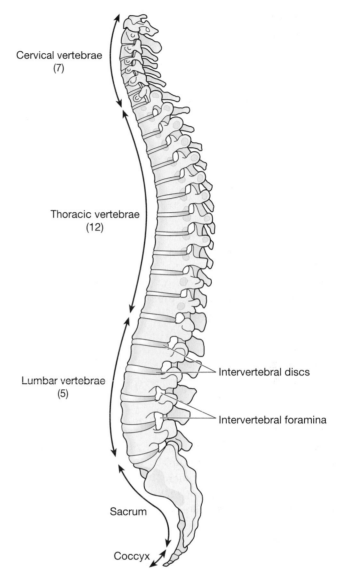

Figure 16.17 The vertebral column. Lateral view.

the skull; then there is the *sacrum*, formed from five fused vertebrae, and lastly the *coccyx*, or tail, which is formed from between three to five small fused vertebrae. The vertebral column is divided into different regions. The first seven vertebrae, in the neck, form the cervical spine; the next twelve vertebrae are the thoracic spine, and the next five the lumbar spine, the lowest vertebra of which articulates with the sacrum. Each vertebra is identified by the first letter of its region in the spine, followed by a number indicating its position. For example, the topmost vertebra is called C1, and the third lumbar vertebra is called L3.

The movable vertebrae have many characteristics in common, but some groups have distinguishing features.

395

Characteristics of a typical vertebra

(Fig. 16.18)

The body. The body of each vertebra is situated anteriorly. The size varies with the site. They are smallest in the cervical region and become larger towards the lumbar region.

The vertebral (neural) arch. This encloses a large *vertebral foramen*. It is the area behind the body, and forms the posterior and lateral walls of the vertebral foramen. The lateral walls are formed from plates of bone called *pedicles*, and the posterior walls are formed from *laminae*. Projecting from the regions where the pedicle meets the lamina is a lateral prominence called a *transverse process*, and where the two laminae meet at the back is a process called the *spinous process*. These are the bony prominences that can be felt through the skin along the length of the spine. The neural arch has four articular surfaces: two articulate with the vertebra above and two with the one below. The vertebral foramina form the vertebral (neural) canal that contains the spinal cord.

Region-specific vertebral characteristics

Cervical vertebrae (Fig. 16.19)

These are the smallest vertebrae. The transverse processes have a foramen through which a vertebral artery passes upwards to the brain. The first two cervical vertebrae, the *atlas* and the *axis*, are atypical.

The first cervical vertebra, the *atlas*, is the bone on which the skull rests. Below the atlas is the *axis*, the second cervical vertebra (C2).

The atlas (Fig. 16.20A) is essentially a ring of bone, with no distinct body or spinous process, although it has

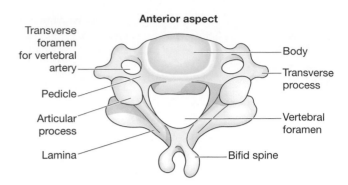

Figure 16.19 A cervical vertebra, showing typical features – viewed from above.

two short transverse processes. It possesses two flattened facets that articulate with the occipital bone; these are condyloid joints (p. 408) and they permit nodding of the head.

The axis (Fig. 16.20B) sits below the atlas, and has a small body with a small superior projection called the *odontoid process* (also called the dens, meaning tooth). This occupies part of the posterior foramen of the atlas above, and is held securely within it by the transverse ligament (Fig. 16.20C). The head pivots (i.e. turns from side to side) on this joint.

The seventh cervical vertebra, C7, is also known as the *vertebra prominens*. It possesses a long spinous prominence terminating in a swollen tubercle, which is easily felt at the base of the neck.

Thoracic vertebrae (Fig. 16.21)

The thoracic vertebrae are larger than the cervical vertebrae because this section of the vertebral column has to support more body weight. The bodies and transverse processes have facets for articulation with the ribs.

Lumbar vertebrae (Fig. 16.18)

These are the largest of the vertebrae because they have to support the weight of the upper body. They have substantial spinous processes for muscle attachment.

Sacrum (Fig. 16.22)

This consists of five rudimentary vertebrae fused to form a triangular or wedge-shaped bone with a concave anterior surface. The upper part, or base, articulates with the 5th lumbar vertebra. On each side it articulates with the ilium to form a *sacroiliac joint*, and at its inferior tip it articulates with the coccyx. The anterior edge of the base, the *promontory*, protrudes into the pelvic cavity. The vertebral foramina are present, and on each side of the bone there is a series of foramina for the passage of nerves.

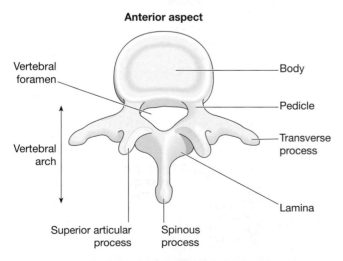

Figure 16.18 A lumbar vertebra showing the features of a typical vertebra – viewed from above.

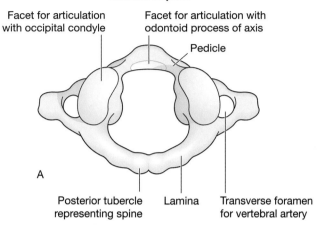

Anterior aspect

Facet for articulation with occipital condyle

Facet for articulation with odontoid process of axis

Pedicle

A

Posterior tubercle representing spine

Lamina

Transverse foramen for vertebral artery

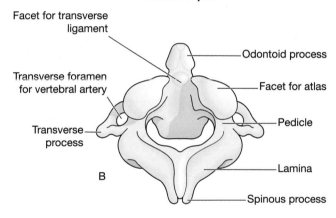

Anterior aspect

Facet for transverse ligament

Transverse foramen for vertebral artery

Transverse process

Odontoid process

Facet for atlas

Pedicle

Lamina

Spinous process

B

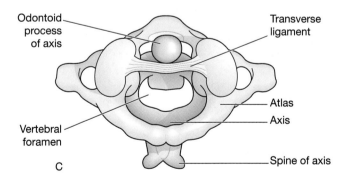

Odontoid process of axis

Transverse ligament

Vertebral foramen

Atlas

Axis

Spine of axis

C

Figure 16.20 The upper cervical vertebrae – viewed from above. **A:** the atlas; **B:** the axis; **C:** the atlas and axis in position showing the transverse ligament.

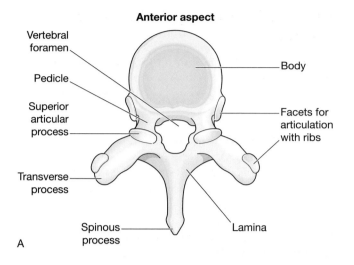

Anterior aspect

Vertebral foramen

Pedicle

Superior articular process

Transverse process

Spinous process

Body

Facets for articulation with ribs

Lamina

A

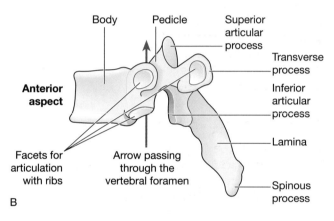

Body   Pedicle   Superior articular process

Anterior aspect

Facets for articulation with ribs

Arrow passing through the vertebral foramen

Transverse process

Inferior articular process

Lamina

Spinous process

B

Figure 16.21 A thoracic vertebra. A: viewed from above. **B:** viewed from the side.

397

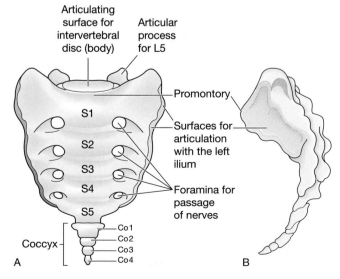

Articulating surface for intervertebral disc (body)

Articular process for L5

Promontory

Surfaces for articulation with the left ilium

Foramina for passage of nerves

S1
S2
S3
S4
S5

Co1
Co2
Co3
Co4

Coccyx

A

B

Figure 16.22 The sacrum and coccyx. A: Anterior view. **B:** Lateral view.

Coccyx (Fig. 16.22)

This consists of the four terminal vertebrae fused to form a very small triangular bone, the broad base of which articulates with the tip of the sacrum.

Features of the vertebral column

Intervertebral discs

The bodies of adjacent vertebrae are separated by *intervertebral discs*, consisting of an outer rim of fibrocartilage (*annulus fibrosus*) and a central core of soft gelatinous material (*nucleus pulposus*) (Fig. 16.23). They are thinnest in the cervical region and become progressively thicker towards the lumbar region, as spinal loading increases. The posterior longitudinal ligament in the vertebral canal helps to keep them in place. They have a shock-absorbing function and the cartilaginous joints they form contribute to the flexibility of the vertebral column as a whole.

Intervertebral foramina

When two adjacent vertebrae are viewed from the side, a foramen formed by a gap between the vertebral pedicles can be seen. Half of the wall is formed by the vertebra above, and half by the one below (Fig. 16.24).

Throughout the length of the column there is an intervertebral foramen on each side between every pair of vertebrae, through which the spinal nerves, blood vessels and lymph vessels pass.

Ligaments of the vertebral column (Fig. 16.23)

These ligaments hold the vertebrae together and keep the intervertebral discs in position.

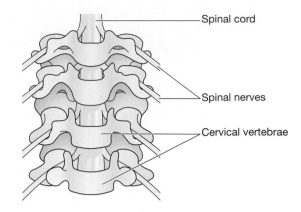

Figure 16.24 Lower cervical vertebrae separated to show the spinal cord and spinal nerves emerging through the intervertebral foramina. Anterior view.

The *transverse ligament* maintains the odontoid process of the axis in the correct position in relation to the atlas (Fig. 16.20C).

The *anterior longitudinal ligament* extends the whole length of the column and lies in front of the vertebral bodies.

The *posterior longitudinal ligament* lies inside the vertebral canal and extends the whole length of the vertebral column in close contact with the posterior surface of the bodies of the bones.

The *ligamenta flava* connect the laminae of adjacent vertebrae.

The *ligamentum nuchae* and the *supraspinous ligament* connect the spinous processes, extending from the occiput to the sacrum.

Curves of the vertebral column (Fig. 16.25)

When viewed from the side, the vertebral column presents four curves: two *primary* and two *secondary*.

The fetus in the uterus lies curled up so that the head and the knees are more or less touching. This position shows the *primary curvature*. The secondary *cervical curve* develops when the child can hold up his head (after about 3 months) and the secondary *lumbar curve* develops when he stands upright (after 12 to 15 months). The thoracic and sacral primary curves are retained.

Movements of the vertebral column

The movements between the individual bones of the vertebral column are very limited. However, the movements of the column as a whole are quite extensive and include *flexion* (bending forward), *extension* (bending backward), *lateral flexion* (bending to the side) and *rotation*. There is more movement in the cervical and lumbar regions than elsewhere.

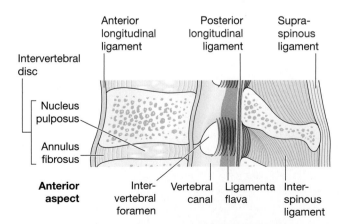

Figure 16.23 Section of the vertebral column showing the ligaments, intervertebral discs and intervertebral foramina.

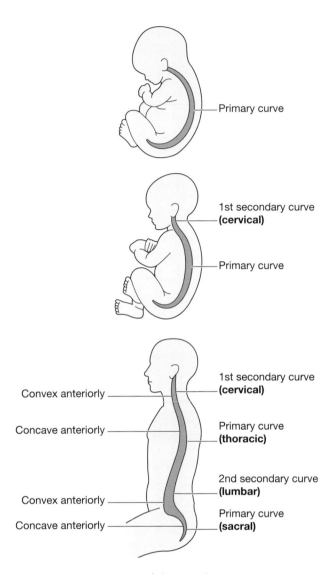

Figure 16.25 **Development of the spinal curves.**

Functions of the vertebral column

These include the following.

- Collectively the vertebral foramina form the vertebral canal, which provides a strong bony protection for the delicate spinal cord lying within it.
- The pedicles of adjacent vertebrae form intervertebral foramina, one on each side, providing access to the spinal cord for spinal nerves, blood vessels and lymph vessels.
- The numerous individual bones enable a certain amount of movement.
- It supports the skull.
- The intervertebral discs act as shock absorbers, protecting the brain.

- It forms the axis of the trunk, giving attachment to the ribs, shoulder girdle and upper limbs, and the pelvic girdle and lower limbs.

Thoracic cage (Fig. 16.26)

The thorax (thoracic cage) is formed by the sternum anteriorly, twelve pairs of ribs forming the lateral bony cages, and the twelve thoracic vertebrae.

Sternum (breast bone) (Fig. 16.27)

This flat bone can be felt just under the skin in the middle of the front of the chest.

The *manubrium* is the uppermost section and articulates with the clavicles at the *sternoclavicular joints* and with the first two pairs of ribs.

The *body* or *middle portion* gives attachment to the ribs.

The *xiphoid process* is the tip of the bone. It gives attachment to the diaphragm, muscles of the anterior abdominal wall and the *linea alba*.

Ribs

The 12 pairs of ribs form the lateral walls of the thoracic cage (Fig. 16.26). They are elongated curved bones (Fig. 16.28) that articulate posteriorly with the vertebral column. Anteriorly, the first 7 pairs of ribs articulate directly with the sternum and are known as the *true ribs*. The next 3 pairs articulate only indirectly. In both cases,

399

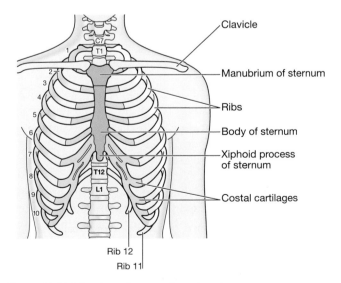

Figure 16.26 **The thoracic cage.** Anterior view.

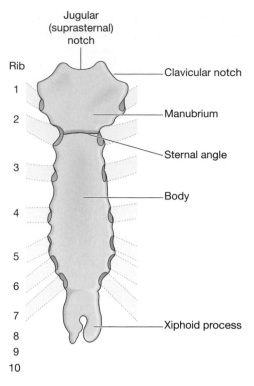

Figure 16.27 **The sternum and its attachments.**

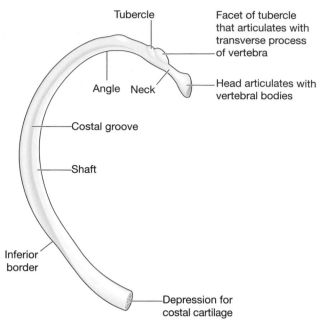

Figure 16.28 **A typical rib** – viewed from below.

costal cartilages attach the ribs to the sternum. The lowest 2 pairs of ribs, referred to as *floating ribs,* do not join the sternum at all, their anterior tips being free.

Each rib forms up to three joints with the vertebral column. Two of these joints are formed between facets on the head of the rib and facets on the bodies of two vertebrae, the one above the rib and the one below. Ten of the ribs also form joints between the tubercle of the rib and the transverse process of (usually) the lower vertebra.

The inferior surface of the rib is deeply grooved, providing a channel along which intercostal nerves and blood vessels run. Between each rib and the one below are the intercostal muscles, essential for breathing.

Because of the arrangement of the ribs, and the quantity of cartilage present in the ribcage, it is a flexible structure that can change its shape and size during breathing. The first rib is firmly fixed to the sternum and to the first thoracic vertebra, and does not move during inspiration. Because it is a fixed point, when the intercostal muscles contract, they pull the entire ribcage upwards towards the first rib. The mechanism of breathing is described on page 251.

Appendicular skeleton

Learning outcomes

After studying this section you should be able to:

- identify the bones forming the appendicular skeleton
- state the characteristics of the bones forming the appendicular skeleton
- outline the differences in structure between the male and female pelves.

The appendicular skeleton consists of the shoulder girdle with the upper limbs and the pelvic girdle with the lower limbs (Fig. 16.6).

Shoulder girdle and upper limb

The upper limb forms a joint with the trunk via the shoulder (pectoral) girdle.

Shoulder girdle

The shoulder girdle consists of two scapulae and two clavicles.

400

Clavicle (collar bone) (Fig. 16.29)

The clavicle is an S-shaped long bone. It articulates with the manubrium of the sternum at the *sternoclavicular joint* and forms the *acromioclavicular joint* with the *acromion process* of the scapula. The clavicle provides the only bony link between the upper limb and the axial skeleton.

Scapula (shoulder blade) (Fig. 16.30)

The scapula is a flat triangular-shaped bone, lying on the posterior chest wall superficial to the ribs and separated from them by muscles.

At the lateral angle is a shallow articular surface, the *glenoid cavity*, which, with the *head of the humerus*, forms the *shoulder joint*.

On the posterior surface runs a rough ridge called the *spine*, which extends beyond the lateral border of the scapula and overhangs the glenoid cavity. The prominent overhang, which can be felt through the skin as the highest point of the shoulder, is called the *acromion process*

and forms a joint with the clavicle, the *acromioclavicular joint*, a slightly movable synovial joint that contributes to the mobility of the shoulder girdle. The *coracoid process*, a projection from the upper border of the bone, gives attachment to muscles that move the shoulder joint.

The upper limb

Humerus (Fig. 16.31)

This is the bone of the upper arm. The head sits within the glenoid cavity of the scapula, forming the shoulder joint. Distal to the head are two roughened projections of bone, the *greater* and *lesser tubercles*, and between them there is a deep groove, the *bicipital groove* or *intertubercular sulcus*, occupied by one of the tendons of the biceps muscle.

The distal end of the bone presents two surfaces that articulate with the radius and ulna to form the elbow joint.

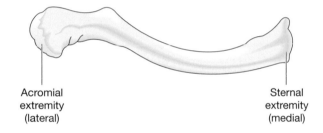

Figure 16.29 **The right clavicle.**

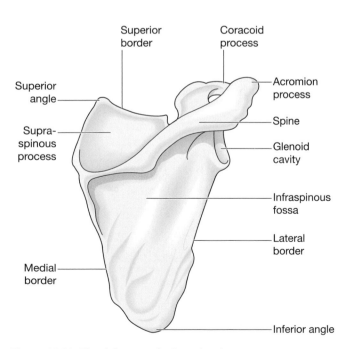

Figure 16.30 **The right scapula.** Posterior view.

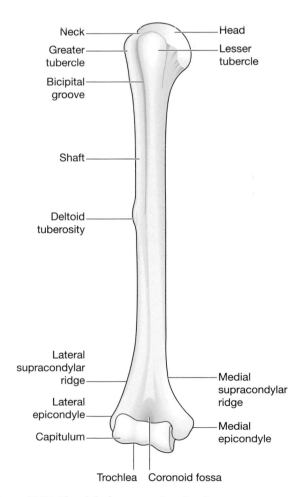

Figure 16.31 **The right humerus.** Anterior view.

401

Ulna and radius (Fig. 16.32)

These are the two bones of the forearm. The ulna is longer than and medial to the radius and when the arm is in the anatomical position, i.e. with the palm of the hand facing forward, the two bones are parallel. They articulate with the humerus at the *elbow joint*, the carpal bones at the *wrist joint* and with each other at the *proximal* and *distal radioulnar* joints. In addition, an interosseous membrane, a fibrous joint, connects the bones along their shafts, stabilising their association and maintaining their relative positions despite forces applied from the elbow or wrist.

Carpal (wrist) bones (Fig. 16.33)

There are eight carpal bones arranged in two rows of four. From outside inwards they are:

- *proximal row*: scaphoid, lunate, triquetral, pisiform
- *distal row*: trapezium, trapezoid, capitate, hamate.

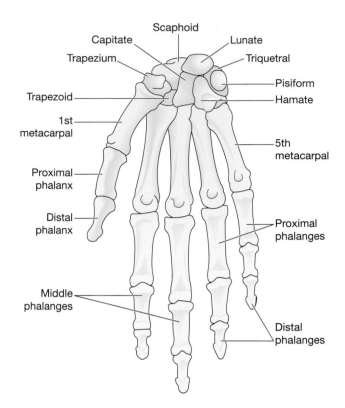

Figure 16.33 The bones of the hand, wrist and fingers. Anterior view.

402

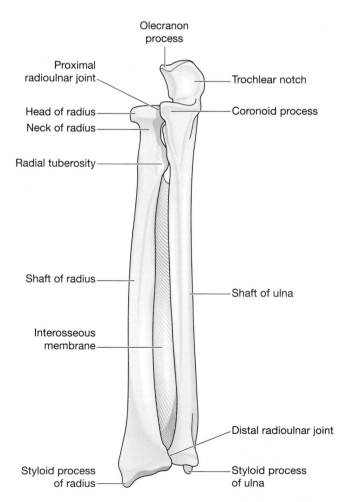

Figure 16.32 The right radius and ulna with the interosseous membrane. Anterior view.

These bones are closely fitted together and held in position by ligaments that allow a limited amount of movement between them. The bones of the proximal row are associated with the wrist joint and those of the distal row form joints with the metacarpal bones. Tendons of muscles lying in the forearm cross the wrist and are held close to the bones by strong fibrous bands, called retinacula (see Fig. 16.48, p. 412).

Metacarpal bones (bones of the hand)

These five bones form the palm of the hand. They are numbered from the thumb side inwards. The proximal ends articulate with the carpal bones and the distal ends with the phalanges.

Phalanges (finger bones)

There are 14 phalanges, three in each finger and two in the thumb. They articulate with the metacarpal bones and with each other, by hinge joints.

Pelvic girdle and lower limb

The lower limb forms a joint with the trunk at the pelvic girdle.

The pelvic girdle

The pelvic girdle is formed from two innominate (hip) bones. The *pelvis* is the term given to the basin-shaped structure formed by the pelvic girdle and its associated sacrum.

Innominate (hip) bones (Fig. 16.34)
Each hip bone consists of three fused bones: the *ilium, ischium* and *pubis*. On its lateral surface is a deep depression, the *acetabulum*, which forms the hip joint with the almost-spherical head of femur.

The *ilium* is the upper flattened part of the bone and it presents the *iliac crest*, the anterior curve of which is called the *anterior superior iliac spine*. The ilium forms a synovial joint with the sacrum, the *sacroiliac joint*, a strong joint capable of absorbing the stresses of weight bearing and which tends to become fibrosed in later life.

The *pubis* is the anterior part of the bone and it articulates with the pubis of the other hip bone at a cartilaginous joint, the *symphysis pubis*.

The *ischium* is the inferior and posterior part. The rough inferior projections of the ischia, the *ischial tuberosities*, bear the weight of the body when seated.

The union of the three parts takes place in the *acetabulum*.

The pelvis (Fig. 16.35)
The pelvis is formed by the hip bones, the sacrum and the coccyx. It is divided into upper and lower parts by the *brim of the pelvis*, consisting of the promontory of the sacrum and the *iliopectineal lines* of the innominate bones. The *greater* or *false pelvis* is above the brim and the *lesser* or *true pelvis* is below.

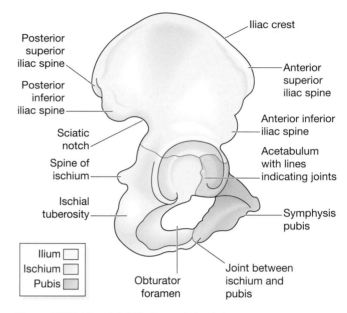

Figure 16.34 The right hip bone. Lateral view.

Differences between male and female pelves (Fig. 16.36). The shape of the female pelvis allows for the passage of the baby during childbirth. In comparison with the male pelvis, the female pelvis has lighter bones, is more shallow and rounded and is generally roomier.

The lower limb

Femur (thigh bone) (Fig. 16.37)
The femur is the longest and heaviest bone of the body. The head is almost spherical and fits into the *acetabulum* of the hip bone to form the *hip joint*. The neck extends

403

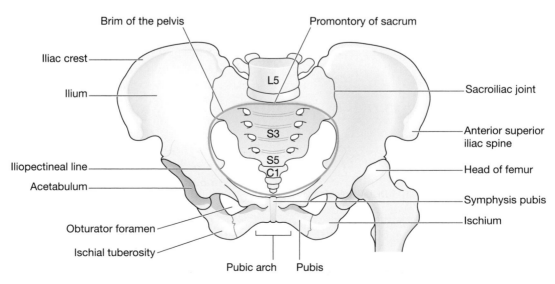

Figure 16.35 The bones of the pelvis and the upper part of the left femur.

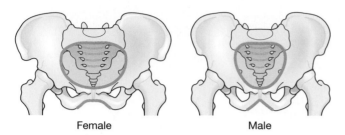

Female   Male

Figure 16.36 The difference in shape of the male and female pelves.

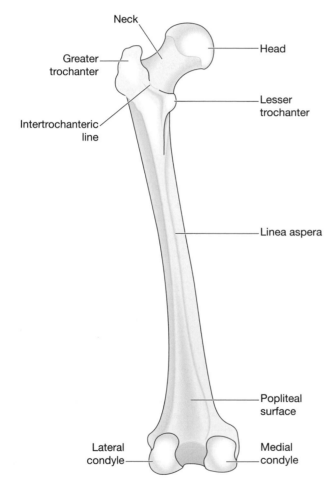

Figure 16.37 The left femur. Posterior view.

404

outwards and slightly downwards from the head to the shaft and most of it is within the capsule of the hip joint.

The posterior surface of the lower third forms a flat triangular area called the *popliteal surface*. The distal extremity has two articular *condyles*, which, with the tibia and patella, form the knee joint. The function of the femur is to transmit the weight of the body through the bones below the knee to the foot.

Tibia (shin bone) (Fig. 16.38)

The tibia is the medial of the two bones of the lower leg. The proximal extremity is broad and flat and presents two *condyles* for articulation with the femur at the *knee joint*. The head of the fibula articulates with the inferior aspect of the lateral condyle, forming the *proximal tibiofibular* joint.

The distal extremity of the tibia forms the *ankle joint* with the *talus* and the fibula. The *medial malleolus* is a downward projection of bone medial to the ankle joint.

Fibula (Fig. 16.38)

The fibula is the long slender lateral bone in the leg. The head or upper extremity articulates with the lateral condyle of the tibia, forming the proximal tibiofibular joint, and the lower extremity articulates with the tibia, and projects beyond it to form the *lateral malleolus*. This helps to stabilise the ankle joint.

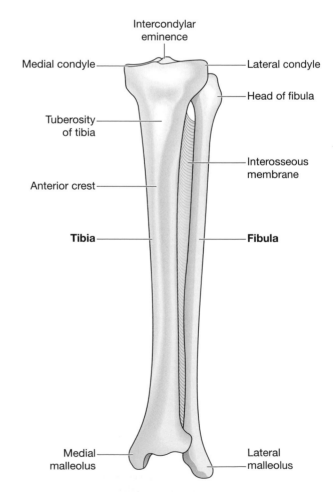

Figure 16.38 The left tibia and fibula with the interosseous membrane. Anterior view.

Patella (knee cap)

This is a roughly triangular-shaped *sesamoid* bone associated with the knee joint. Its posterior surface articulates with the patellar surface of the femur in the knee joint and its anterior surface is in the *patellar tendon*, i.e. the tendon of the quadriceps femoris muscle.

Tarsal (ankle) bones (Fig. 16.39)

The seven tarsal bones forming the posterior part of the foot (ankle) are the *talus, calcaneus, navicular, cuboid* and three *cuneiform* bones. The *talus* articulates with the tibia and fibula at the ankle joint. The *calcaneus* forms the heel of the foot. The other bones articulate with each other and with the metatarsal bones.

Metatarsals (bones of the foot) (Fig. 16.39)

These are five bones, numbered from inside out, which form the greater part of the dorsum of the foot. At their proximal ends they articulate with the tarsal bones and at their distal ends, with the phalanges. The enlarged distal head of the 1st metatarsal bone forms the 'ball' of the foot.

Phalanges (toe bones) (Fig. 16.39)

There are 14 phalanges arranged in a similar manner to those in the fingers, i.e. two in the great toe (the *halux*) and three in each of the other toes.

Arches of the foot. The arrangement of bones in the foot, supported by associated ligaments and action of associated muscles, gives the sole of the foot an arched or curved shape (Figs. 16.39 and 16.40). The curve running from heel to toe is called the *longitudinal* arch, and the curve running across the foot is called the *transverse* arch.

In the normal longitudinal arch, only the calcaneus and the distal ends of the metatarsals should touch the ground, the bones in between lifted clear. This gives a conventional footprint shape. If, however, the concavity

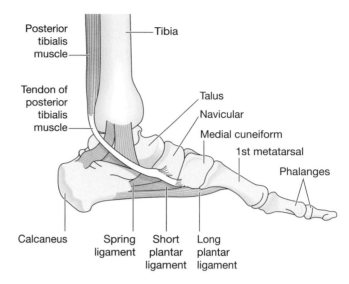

Figure 16.40 **The tendons and ligaments supporting the arches of the left foot.** Medial view.

of the sole is lost because of sagging ligaments or tendons, the arch sinks and much more of the sole of the foot is in contact with the ground: this is called flat foot. Because the arches of the foot are important in distributing the weight of the body evenly whilst upright, whether stationary or moving, the flat foot loses the springiness of normal foot structure and leads to sore feet when standing, walking or running for long periods. As there are movable joints between all the bones of the foot, very strong muscles and ligaments are necessary to maintain the strength, resilience and stability of the foot during walking, running and jumping.

Posterior tibialis muscle. This is the most important muscular support of the longitudinal arch. It lies on the posterior aspect of the lower leg, originates from the middle third of the tibia and fibula and its tendon passes behind the medial malleolus to be inserted into the navicular, cuneiform, cuboid and metatarsal bones. It acts as a sling or 'suspension apparatus' for the arch.

Short muscles of the foot. This group of muscles is mainly concerned with the maintenance of the longitudinal and transverse arches. They make up the fleshy part of the sole of the foot.

Plantar calcaneonavicular ligament ('spring' ligament). This is a very strong thick ligament stretching from the calcaneus to the navicular bone. It plays an important part in supporting the medial longitudinal arch.

Plantar ligaments and interosseous membranes. These structures support the lateral and transverse arches.

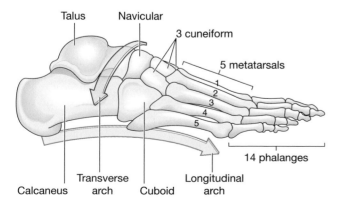

Figure 16.39 **The bones of the foot.** Lateral view.

405

Joints

A joint is the site at which any two or more bones articulate or come together. Joints allow flexibility and movement of the skeleton and allow attachment between bones.

Fibrous joints

The bones forming these joints are linked with tough, fibrous material. Such an arrangement often permits no movement. The joints between the skull bones, the *sutures*, are completely immovable (Fig. 16.41), and the healthy tooth is cemented into the mandible by the periodontal ligament. The tibia and fibula in the leg are held together along their shafts by a sheet of fibrous tissue called the interosseous membrane (Fig. 16.38). This is a fibrous joint that allows a limited amount of movement and stabilises the alignment of the bones.

Cartilaginous joints

These joints are formed by a pad of fibrocartilage, a tough material that acts as a shock absorber. The joint may be

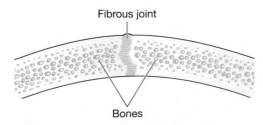

Figure 16.41 Suture (fibrous joint) of the skull.

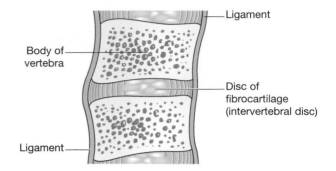

Figure 16.42 The cartilaginous joint between adjacent vertebral bodies.

immovable, as in the cartilaginous epiphyseal plates, which in the growing child link the diaphysis of a long bone to the epiphysis (p. 387). In other joints, a limited degree of movement may take place, as between the vertebrae, which are separated by the intervertebral discs (Fig. 16.42), or at the symphysis pubis (Fig. 16.35), which is softened by circulating hormones during pregnancy to allow for childbirth.

Synovial joints

Synovial joints are characterised by the presence of a space or capsule between the articulating bones (Fig. 16.43). The ends of the bones are held close together by a sleeve of fibrous tissue, and the capsule is lubricated with a small amount of fluid. Most synovial joints permit a range of movement.

Characteristics of a synovial joint

All synovial joints have certain characteristics in common (Fig. 16.43).

Articular or hyaline cartilage

The parts of the bones which are in contact are always covered with hyaline cartilage (see Fig. 3.17, p. 38). This provides a smooth articular surface and is strong enough to absorb compression forces and bear the weight of the body. The cartilage lining, which is up to 7 mm thick in young people, becomes thinner and less compressible with age. This leads to increasing stress on other structures in the joint. Cartilage has no blood supply and receives its nourishment from synovial fluid.

Capsule or capsular ligament

The joint is surrounded and enclosed by a sleeve of fibrous tissue which holds the bones together. It is sufficiently loose to allow freedom of movement but strong enough to protect it from injury.

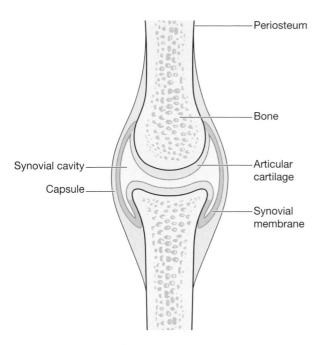

Figure 16.43 The basic structure of a synovial joint.

Synovial membrane

This is composed of epithelial cells and is found:

- lining the capsule
- covering those parts of the bones within the joint not covered by articular cartilage
- covering all intracapsular structures that do not bear weight.

Synovial fluid

This is a thick sticky fluid, of egg-white consistency, secreted by synovial membranes into the *synovial cavity*, and it:

- provides nutrients for the structures within the joint cavity
- contains phagocytes, which remove microbes and cellular debris
- acts as a lubricant
- maintains joint stability
- prevents the ends of the bones from being separated, as does a little water between two glass surfaces.

Little sacs of synovial fluid or *bursae* are present in some joints, e.g. the knee. They act as cushions to prevent friction between a bone and a ligament or tendon, or skin where a bone in a joint is near the surface.

Other intracapsular structures

Some joints have structures within the capsule, but outside the synovial membrane, which assist in maintenance of stability, e.g. fat pads and menisci in the knee joint.

When these structures do not bear weight they are covered by synovial membrane.

Extracapsular structures

- *Ligaments* that blend with the capsule provide additional stability at most joints.
- *Muscles* or their *tendons* also provide stability and stretch across the joints they move. When the muscle contracts it shortens, pulling one bone towards the other.

Nerve and blood supply

Nerves and blood vessels crossing a joint usually supply the capsule and the muscles that move it.

Movements at synovial joints

Movement at any given joint depends on various factors, such as the tightness of the ligaments holding the joint together, how well the bones fit and the presence or absence of intracapsular structures. Generally, the more stable the joint, the less mobile it is. The main movements possible are summarised in Table 16.2 and Figure 16.44.

Types of synovial joint

Synovial joints are classified according to the range of movement possible (Table 16.2) or to the shape of the articulating parts of the bones involved.

Ball and socket joints. The head of one bone is ball-shaped and articulates with a cup-shaped socket of another. The joint allows for a wide range of movement, including flexion, extension, adduction, abduction, rotation and circumduction. Examples are the shoulder and hip.

Hinge joints. The articulating ends of the bones form an arrangement like a hinge on a door, and movement is therefore restricted to flexion and extension. The elbow joint is one example, permitting only flexion and extension of the forearm. Other hinge joints include the knee, ankle and the joints between the phalanges of the fingers and toes (interphalangeal joints).

Gliding joints. The articular surfaces are flat or very slightly curved and glide over one another, but the amount of movement possible is very restricted; this group of joints is the least movable of all the synovial joints. Examples include the joints between the carpal bones in the wrist, the tarsal bones in the foot, and between the processes of the spinal vertebrae (note that the joints between the vertebral bodies are the cartilaginous discs, Fig. 16.42).

Pivot joints. These joints allow a bone or a limb to rotate. One bone fits into a hoop-shaped ligament that holds it close to another bone and allows it to rotate in the

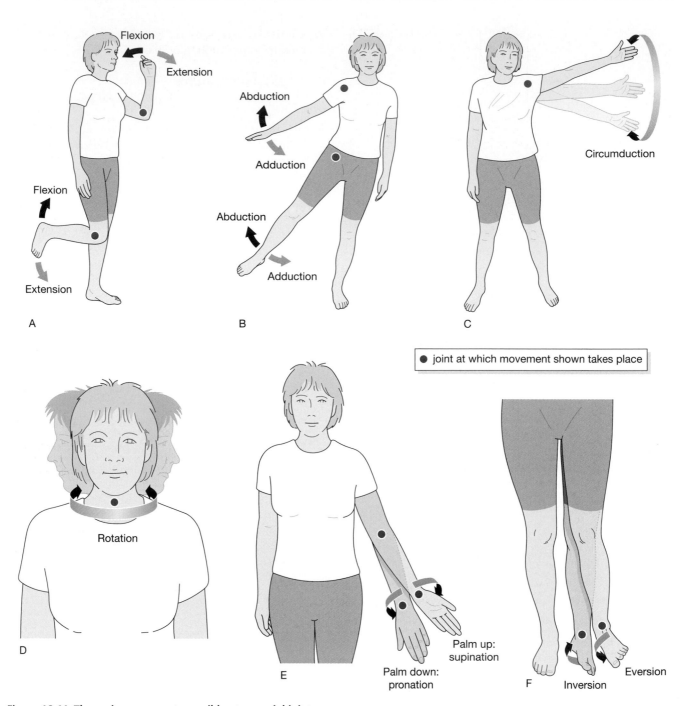

Figure 16.44 **The main movements possible at synovial joints.**

● joint at which movement shown takes place

ring thus formed. For example, the head rotates on the pivot joint formed by the dens of the axis held within the ring formed by the transverse ligament and the odontoid process of the atlas (Fig. 16.20).

Condyloid joints. A condyle is a smooth, rounded projection on a bone and in a condyloid joint it sits within a cup-shaped depression on the other bone. Examples include the joint between the condylar process of the mandible and the temporal bone, and the joints between the metacarpal and phalangeal bones of the hand, and between the metatarsal and phalangeal bones of the foot. These joints permit flexion, extension, abduction, adduction and circumduction.

Saddle joints. The articulating bones fit together like a man sitting on a saddle. The most important saddle joint is at the base of the thumb, between the trapezium of the

408

Table 16.2 Movements possible at synovial joints

Movement	Definition
Flexion	Bending, usually forward but occasionally backward, e.g. knee joint
Extension	Straightening or bending backward
Abduction	Movement away from the midline of the body
Adduction	Movement towards the midline of the body
Circumduction	Movement of a limb or digit so that it describes the shape of a cone
Rotation	Movement round the long axis of a bone
Pronation	Turning the palm of the hand down
Supination	Turning the palm of the hand up
Inversion	Turning the sole of the foot inwards
Eversion	Turning the sole of the foot outwards

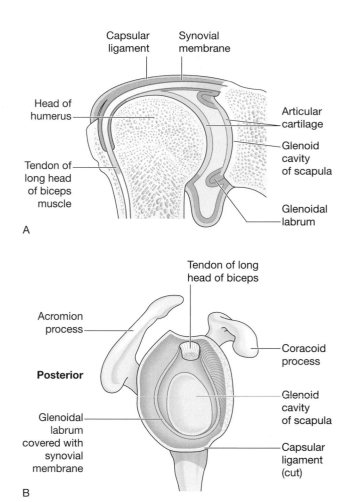

A

B

wrist and the first metacarpal bone (Fig. 16.33). The range of movement is similar to that at a condyloid joint but with additional flexibility; *opposition* of the thumb, the ability to touch each of the fingertips on the same hand, is due to the nature of the thumb joint.

Main synovial joints of the limbs

Individual synovial joints have the characteristics described above, so only their distinctive features are included in this section.

Shoulder joint (Fig. 16.45)

This ball and socket joint is the most mobile in the body, and consequently is the least stable and prone to dislocation, especially in children. It is formed by the glenoid cavity of the scapula and the head of the humerus, and is well padded with protective bursae. The capsular ligament is very loose inferiorly to allow for the free movement normally possible at this joint. The glenoid cavity is deepened by a rim of fibrocartilage, the *glenoidal labrum*, which provides additional stability without limiting movement. The tendon of the long head of the *biceps muscle* is held in the intertubercular (bicipital) groove of the humerus by the transverse humeral ligament. It

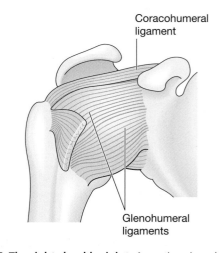

C

Figure 16.45 The right shoulder joint. A: section viewed from the front. **B:** the position of glenoidal labrum with the humerus removed, viewed from the side. **C:** the supporting ligaments viewed from the front.

409

extends through the joint cavity and attaches to the upper rim of the glenoid cavity.

Synovial membrane forms a sleeve round the part of the tendon of the long head of the biceps muscles within the capsular ligament and covers the glenoidal labrum.

The joint is stabilised partly by a number of ligaments (the glenohumeral, coracohumeral and transverse humeral) but mainly by the muscles (and their tendons) present in the shoulder. The stability of the joint may be reduced if these structures, together with the tendon of the biceps muscle, are stretched by repeated dislocations of the joint.

Muscles and movements (see Fig. 16.61)

The muscles that move the arm are described in more detail on page 422, and Table 16.3 summarises the muscles and movements possible at the shoulder joint.

Elbow joint (Fig. 16.46)

This hinge joint is formed by the trochlea and the capitulum of the humerus, and the trochlear notch of the ulna and the head of the radius. It is an extremely stable joint because the humeral and ulnar surfaces interlock, and the capsule is very strong.

Extracapsular structures consist of anterior, posterior, medial and lateral strengthening ligaments, which contribute to joint stability.

Muscles and movements (see Fig. 16.61)

Because of the structure of the elbow joint, the only two movements it allows are flexion and extension. The biceps is the main flexor of the forearm, aided by the brachialis; the triceps extends it (p. 422–3).

Table 16.3 Muscles and movements at the shoulder joint	
Extension	Latissimus dorsi, teres major
Flexion	Coracobrachialis, pectoralis major
Abduction	Deltoid
Adduction	Latissimus dorsi, pectoralis major
Lateral rotation	Teres minor, posterior part of deltoid
Medial rotation	Latissimus dorsi, pectoralis major, teres major and anterior part of deltoid
Circumduction	Combination of actions of above muscles

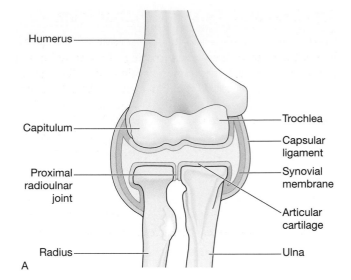

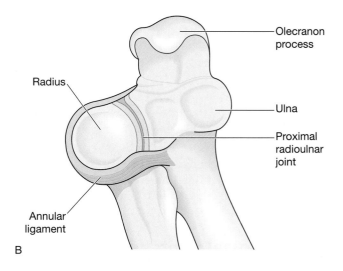

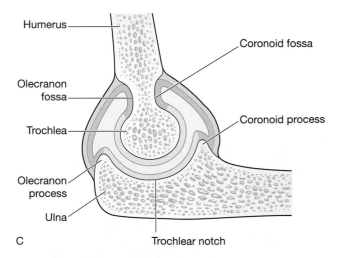

Figure 16.46 The elbow and proximal radioulnar joints. A: section viewed from the front. **B:** the proximal radioulnar joint, viewed from above. **C:** section of the elbow joint, partly flexed, viewed from the side.

410

Proximal and distal radioulnar joints

The *proximal radioulnar joint* is a pivot joint formed by the rim of the head of the radius rotating in the radial notch of the ulna, and is in the same capsule as the elbow joint. The *annular ligament* is a strong extracapsular ligament that encircles the head of the radius and keeps it in contact with the radial notch of the ulna (Fig. 16.46B).

The distal *radioulnar joint* is a pivot joint between the distal end of the radius and the head of the ulna (Fig. 16.47).

Note, in addition, the presence of a fibrous membrane linking the bones along their shafts; this interosseous membrane is an example of a fibrous joint and prevents separation of the bones when force is applied at either end, i.e. at the wrist or elbow.

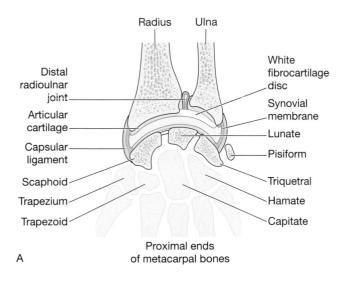

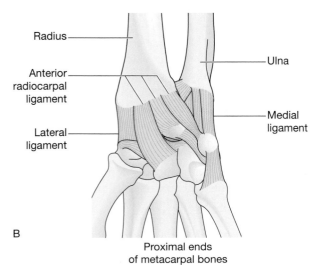

Figure 16.47 The wrist and distal radioulnar joints. Anterior view. **A:** section. **B:** supporting ligaments.

Muscles and movements (Fig. 16.61)

The forearm may be pronated (turned palm down) or supinated (turned palm up). Pronation is caused by the action of the pronator teres (p. 423) and supination by the supinator and biceps muscles (p. 422–3).

Wrist joint (Fig. 16.47)

This is a condyloid joint between the distal end of the radius and the proximal ends of the scaphoid, lunate and triquetral. A disc of white fibrocartilage separates the ulna from the joint cavity and articulates with the carpal bones. It also separates the inferior radioulnar joint from the wrist joint.

Extracapsular structures consist of medial and lateral ligaments and anterior and posterior radiocarpal ligaments.

Muscles and movements (see Fig. 16.61)

The wrist can be flexed, extended, abducted and adducted. The muscles that perform these movements are described in more detail on page 423–4. Table 16.4 summarises the main muscles that move the wrist.

Joints of the hands and fingers

There are synovial joints between the carpal bones, between the carpal and metacarpal bones, between the metacarpal bones and proximal phalanges and between the phalanges. Movement at the hand and finger joints are controlled by muscles in the forearm and smaller muscles within the hand. There are no muscles in the fingers; finger movements are produced by tendons extending from muscles in the forearm and the hand.

The joint at the base of the thumb is a saddle joint, unlike the corresponding joints of the other fingers, which are condyloid. This means that the thumb is more mobile than the fingers and the thumb can be flexed, extended, circumducted, abducted and adducted. In addition, the thumb can be moved across the palm to touch the tips of each of the fingers on the same hand

411

Table 16.4 **Muscles and movements at the wrist joint**	
Flexion	Flexor carpi radialis, flexor carpi ulnaris
Extension	Extensors carpi radialis (longus and brevis), extensor carpi ulnaris
Adduction	Flexor carpi radialis, extensor carpi radialis
Abduction	Flexor carpi ulnaris, extensor carpi ulnaris

(opposition), an ability that confers great manual dexterity and allows, for example, the holding of a pen and the fine manipulation of objects held in the hand.

The joints between the wrist and finger bones allow movement of the fingers. The fingers may be flexed, extended, adducted, abducted and circumducted, with the first finger having the greatest flexibility of movement. The finger joints are hinge joints, and allow only flexion and extension.

The *flexor retinaculum* is a strong fibrous band that stretches across the front of the carpal bones, enclosing their concavity and forming the *carpal tunnel*. The tendons of flexor muscles of the wrist joint and the fingers and the median nerve pass through the carpal tunnel, the retinaculum holding them close to the bones. Synovial membrane forms sleeves around these tendons in the carpal tunnel and extends some way into the palm of the hand. Synovial sheaths also enclose the tendons on the flexor surfaces of the fingers. Their synovial fluid prevents friction that might damage the tendons as they move over the bones (Fig. 16.48).

The *extensor retinaculum* is a strong fibrous band that extends across the back of the wrist. Tendons of muscles that extend the wrist and finger joints are encased in synovial membrane under the retinaculum. The synovial sheaths are less extensive than on the flexor aspect. The synovial fluid secreted prevents friction.

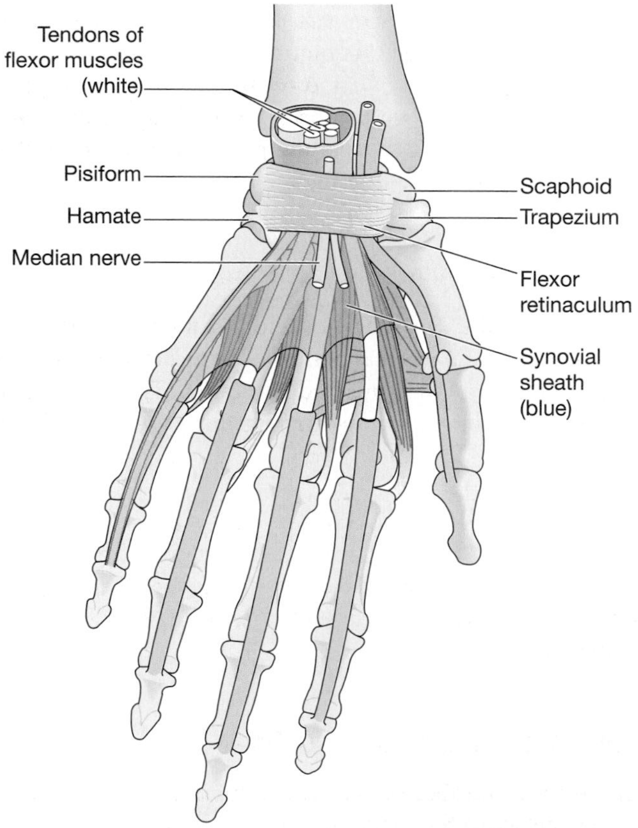

Hip joint (Fig. 16.49)

This ball and socket joint is formed by the cup-shaped acetabulum of the innominate (hip) bone and the almost spherical head of the femur. The capsular ligament encloses the head and most of the neck of the femur. The cavity is deepened by the *acetabular labrum*, a ring of fibrocartilage attached to the rim of the acetabulum, which stabilises the joint without limiting its range of movement. The hip joint is necessarily a sturdy and powerful joint, since it bears all body weight when standing upright. It is stabilised by its surrounding musculature, but its ligaments are also important. The three main external ligaments are the *iliofemoral*, *pubofemoral* and *ischiofemoral* ligaments, which are localised thickenings of the joint capsule (Fig. 16.49B). Within the joint, the *ligament of the head of the femur (ligamentum teres)* attaches the femoral head to the acetabulum (Fig. 16.49A and C).

Muscles and movements (see Fig. 16.62)

The lower limb can be extended, flexed, abducted, adducted, rotated and circumducted at the hip joint (Table 16.5).

Knee joint (Fig. 16.50)

This is the largest and most complex joint. It is a hinge joint formed by the condyles of the femur, the condyles of the tibia and the posterior surface of the patella. The anterior part of the capsule is formed by the tendon of the quadriceps femoris muscle, which also supports the patella. Intracapsular structures include two *cruciate ligaments* that cross each other, extending from the *intercondylar notch* of the femur to the *intercondylar eminence* of the tibia. They help to stabilise the joint.

Semilunar cartilages or *menisci* are incomplete discs of white fibrocartilage lying on top of the articular condyles of the tibia. They are wedge shaped, being thicker at their outer edges, and provide stability. They prevent lateral displacement of the bones, and cushion the moving joint by shifting within the joint space according to the relative positions of the articulating bones.

Bursae and pads of fat are numerous. They prevent friction between a bone and a ligament or tendon and between the skin and the patella. Synovial membrane covers the cruciate ligaments and the pads of fat. The menisci are not covered with synovial membrane because

412

Figure 16.48 The carpal tunnel and synovial sheaths in the wrist and hand in blue; tendons in white. Palmar view, left hand.

Labels:
Tendons of flexor muscles (white)
Pisiform
Hamate
Median nerve
Scaphoid
Trapezium
Flexor retinaculum
Synovial sheath (blue)

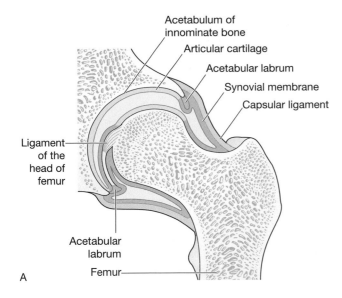

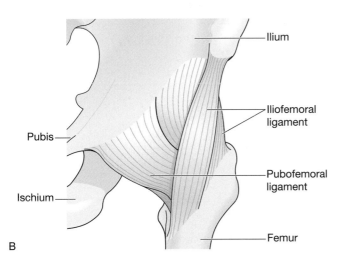

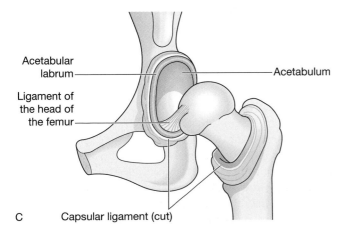

Figure 16.49 The hip joint. A: section. B: supporting ligaments. C: head of femur and acetabulum separated to show acetabular labrum and ligament of head of femur.

Table 16.5 Muscles and movements at the hip joint	
Flexion	Psoas, iliacus, sartorius
Extension	Gluteus maximus, hamstrings
Abduction	Gluteus medius and minimus, sartorius
Adduction	Adductor group (longus, brevis and magnus)
Medial rotation	Gluteus medius and minimus, adductor group
Lateral rotation	Gluteus maximus, quadratus femoris, obturators

they are weight bearing. External ligaments of the joint provide further support, making it a hard joint to dislocate. The main ligaments are the patellar ligament, an extension of the quadriceps tendon, the popliteal ligaments at the back of the knee and the collateral ligaments to each side.

Muscles and movements (see Fig. 16.62)
Possible movements at this joint are flexion, extension and a rotatory movement that 'locks' the joint when it is fully extended. When the joint is locked, it is possible to stand upright for long periods of time without tiring the knee extensors. The main muscles extending the knee are the quadriceps femoris, and the principal flexors are the gastrocnemius and hamstrings.

Ankle joint (Fig. 16.51)

This hinge joint is formed by the distal end of the tibia and its malleolus (medial malleolus), the distal end of the fibula (lateral malleolus) and the talus. There are four important ligaments strengthening this joint: the deltoid and anterior, posterior, medial and lateral ligaments.

Muscles and movements (see Fig. 16.62)
The movements of *inversion* and *eversion* occur between the tarsal bones and not at the ankle joint. Ankle joint movements and the related muscles are shown in Table 16.6.

Joints of the foot and toes

There are a number of synovial joints between the tarsal bones, between the tarsal and metatarsal bones, between the metatarsals and proximal phalanges and between the phalanges. Movements are produced by muscles in

413

414

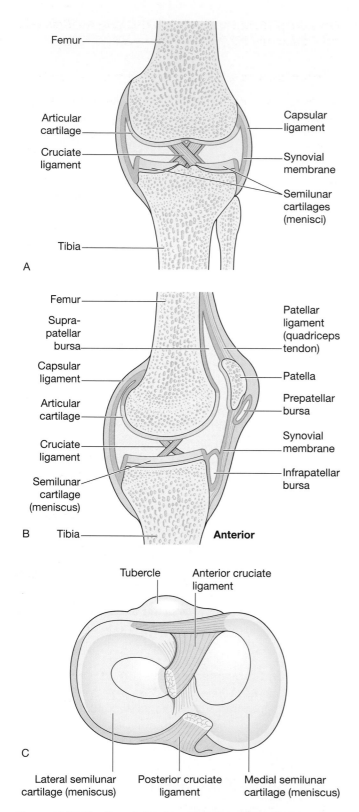

Figure 16.50 The knee joint. A: section viewed from the front. B: section viewed from the side. C: the superior surface of the tibia, showing the semilunar cartilages and the cruciate ligaments.

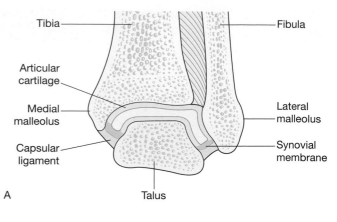

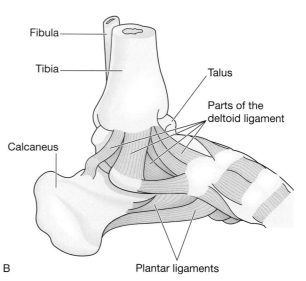

Figure 16.51 The left ankle joint. A: section viewed from the front. B: supporting ligaments, medial view.

the leg with long tendons that cross the ankle joint, and by muscles of the foot. The tendons crossing the ankle joint are encased in synovial sheaths and are held close to the bones by strong transverse ligaments. They move smoothly within their sheaths as the joints move. In addition to moving the joints of the foot, these muscles support the arches of the foot and help to maintain body balance.

Table 16.6 Muscles and movements at the ankle joint	
Dorsiflexion (lifting toes towards calf)	Anterior tibialis and toe extensors
Plantar flexion (rising on tiptoe)	Gastrocnemius, soleus and toe flexors

Muscle tissue

Learning outcomes

After studying this section you should be able to:

- identify the main characteristics of skeletal muscle

- relate the structure of skeletal muscle fibres to their contractile activity

- describe the nature of muscle tone and fatigue

- discuss the factors that affect the performance of skeletal muscle.

Muscle cells are specialised contractile cells, also called *fibres*. Three types of muscle tissue are identified: *smooth, cardiac* and *skeletal*, each differing in structure, location and physiological function.

Smooth muscle

Smooth muscle (involuntary or non-striated) muscle is not under conscious control. The cells are small, have one nucleus and are spindle shaped (see Fig. 3.21, p. 40). Unlike skeletal and cardiac muscle, smooth muscle cells do not have a striped appearance under the microscope. Smooth muscle forms sheets in the walls of hollow organs and tubular structures to regulate diameter and propel substances through tracts (p. 39). Some smooth muscle units have the ability to initiate their own contraction independently of nerve stimulation (automaticity); cardiac muscle has this property too. Both are normally innervated by branches of the autonomic nervous system (p. 170). In addition some hormones and local metabolites may influence contraction; for example, adrenaline (epinephrine) from the adrenal medulla dilates the airways.

Cardiac muscle

Cardiac muscle is found exclusively in the wall of the heart (see also p. 39 and Fig. 5.11, p. 82).

Skeletal muscle

This type of muscle is also called *voluntary muscle* because there is conscious control over it; these muscles are attached to bone via tendons, and are used to move the skeleton. It is also referred to as *striped* or *striated* muscle

because of the characteristic banded pattern of the cells seen under the microscope.

Organisation of skeletal muscle (Fig. 16.52)

A muscle consists of a large number of muscle fibres. The entire muscle is covered in a connective tissue sheath called the *epimysium*. Within the muscle, the cells are collected into separate bundles called *fascicles*, and each fascicle is covered in its own connective tissue sheath called the *perimysium*. Within the fascicles are the individual muscle cells, each wrapped in a fine connective tissue layer called the *endomysium*. Each of these connective tissue layers runs the length of the muscle. They bind the fibres into a highly organised structure, and blend together at each end of the muscle to form the *tendon*, which secures the muscle to the bone. Often the tendon is rope-like, but sometimes it takes the form of a broad

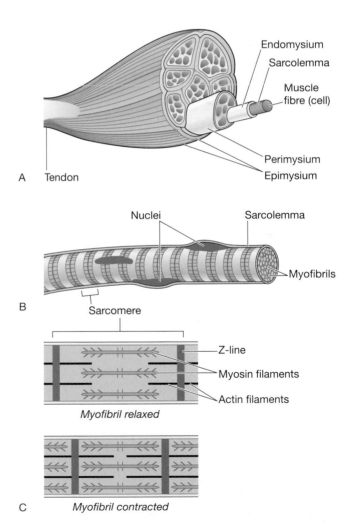

Figure 16.52 Organisation within a skeletal muscle. A: a skeletal muscle and its connective tissue. B: a muscle fibre (cell). C: a myofibril, relaxed and contracted.

415

sheet called an *aponeurosis*. The multiple connective tissue layers throughout the muscle are important for transmitting the force of contraction from each individual muscle cell to its points of attachment to the skeleton.

The fleshy part of the muscle is called the *belly*, and when the muscle contracts it bulges and becomes shorter.

Skeletal muscle fibres

Contraction of a whole skeletal muscle occurs because of coordinated contraction of its individual fibres.

Structure

When skeletal muscle is examined microscopically, the cells are seen to be roughly cylindrical in shape, lying parallel to one another, with a distinctive banded appearance consisting of alternate dark and light stripes (16.52B). Individual fibres may be very long, up to 35 cm in the longest muscles. Each cell has several nuclei (because the cells are so large), which are situated just under the cell membrane (the *sarcolemma*). The cytoplasm of muscle cells, also called *sarcoplasm*, is packed with tiny filaments running longitudinally along the length of the muscle; these are the contractile filaments. There are also many mitochondria, essential for producing ATP from glucose and oxygen to power the contractile mechanism. Also present is a specialised oxygen-binding substance called *myoglobin*, which is similar to the haemoglobin of red blood cells and stores oxygen within the muscle. In addition, there are extensive intracellular stores of calcium, which is released into the sarcoplasm by nervous stimulation of muscle and is essential for the contractile activity of the myofilaments.

Actin, myosin and sarcomeres. There are two types of contractile myofilament within the muscle fibre, called thick and thin, arranged in repeating units called *sarcomeres* (Fig. 16.52C). The thick filaments, which are made of a protein called *myosin*, correspond to the dark bands seen under the microscope. The thin filaments are made of a protein called *actin*. Where only these are present, the bands are lighter in appearance.

Each sarcomere is bounded at each end by a dense stripe called the Z-line, to which the myosin fibres are attached, and lying in the middle of the sarcomere are the actin filaments, overlapping with the myosin.

Contraction

The skeletal muscle cell contracts in response to stimulation from a nerve fibre, which supplies the muscle cell usually about halfway along its length. The region where the nerve and muscle come into closest proximity and the transmission of the action potential takes place is called the *neuromuscular junction*. When the action potential spreads from the nerve along the sarcolemma, it penetrates deep into the muscle cell through a special network of channels that run through the sarcoplasm, and releases calcium from the intracellular stores. Calcium triggers the binding of myosin to the actin filament next to it, forming so-called cross bridges. ATP then provides the energy for the two filaments to slide over each other, pulling the Z-lines at each end of the sarcomere closer to one another, shortening the sarcomere (Fig. 16.52C). If enough fibres are stimulated to do this at the same time, the whole muscle will shorten (contract). This is called the *sliding filament theory*.

The muscle relaxes when nerve stimulation stops. Calcium is pumped back into its intracellular storage areas, which breaks the cross-bridges between the actin and myosin filaments. They then slide back into their starting positions, lengthening the sarcomeres and returning the muscle to its original length.

The neuromuscular junction

The axons of *motor neurones*, carrying impulses to skeletal muscle to produce contraction, divide into fine filaments terminating in minute pads called *motor end-plates* (Fig. 16.53). At the point where the nerve reaches the muscle, the myelin sheath is absent and the fine filament passes to a sensitive area on the surface of the muscle fibre. Each muscle fibre is stimulated through a single motor end-plate, and one motor nerve has many motor end-plates. The motor end-plate and the sensitive area of muscle fibre through which it is stimulated is analogous to the synapse between neurones and is called the neuromuscular junction. The nerve impulse is passed across the gap between the motor end-plate and the muscle fibre by the neurotransmitter, *acetylcholine*. One nerve fibre and the muscle fibres it supplies constitute a

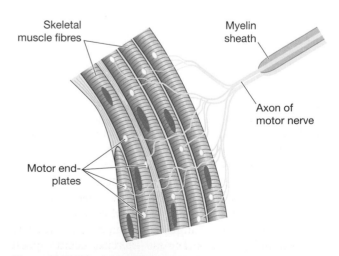

Figure 16.53 The neuromuscular junction.

motor unit. Nerve impulses cause serial contraction of motor units in a muscle, and each unit contracts to its full capacity. The *strength* of the contraction depends on the *number* of motor units in action at a particular time.

Function of skeletal muscle

Muscle function is characterised by alternate phases of contraction and relaxation, but control of their activity depends upon the type of muscle involved. Skeletal muscle contracts in response to motor nerve impulses originating in the brain or spinal cord, and arriving at the neuromuscular junction.

Muscle tone

When each muscle fibre contracts, it obeys the *all-or-none law*; i.e., the whole fibre either contracts completely or not at all. The degree of contraction achieved by a whole muscle depends therefore on the number of fibres within it that are contracting at any one time, as well as how often they are stimulated. Powerful contractions involve a larger proportion of available fibres than weaker ones; to lift a heavy weight, more muscle fibres are required to contract than to lift a lighter one. *Muscle tone* is sustained, partial muscle contraction that allows posture to be maintained without fatiguing the muscles involved. For instance, keeping the head upright requires constant activity of the muscles of the neck and shoulders. Groups of muscle fibres within these muscles take it in turns to contract, so that at any one time, some fibres are contracted and others are resting. This allows the effort required to hold the head upright to be distributed throughout the muscles involved. Good muscle tone protects joints and gives a muscle firmness and shape, even when relaxed.

Muscle fatigue

To work at sustained levels, muscles need an adequate supply of oxygen and fuel molecules such as glucose. Fatigue occurs when a muscle works at a level that exceeds these supplies. The muscle response will become depressed and eventually cease altogether.

The chemical energy (ATP) that muscles require is usually derived from the breakdown of carbohydrate and fat; protein may be used if supplies of fat and carbohydrate are exhausted. An adequate oxygen supply is needed to release fully all the energy stored within these fuel molecules; without it, the body uses anaerobic metabolic pathways (p. 313) that are less efficient and lead to lactic acid production. Fatigue resulting from inadequate oxygen supply, as in strenuous exercise, occurs when lactic acid accumulates in working muscles. Fatigue may

also occur because energy stores are exhausted, or due to physical injury to muscle, which may occur after prolonged episodes of strenuous activity e.g. marathon running.

Muscle recovery

After exercise, muscle needs a period of time to recover, to replenish its ATP and glycogen stores and to repair any damaged fibres. For some time following exercise, depending on the degree of exertion, the *oxygen debt* remains (an extended period of increased oxygen demand), as the body converts excess lactic acid to pyruvic acid and replaces its energy stores.

Factors affecting skeletal muscle performance

Skeletal muscle performs better when it is regularly exercised. Training improves endurance and power. Anaerobic training, such as weightlifting, increases muscle bulk because it increases the size of individual fibres within the muscle (hypertrophy). Ageing reduces the size of muscle fibres as well as their endurance and strength.

Action of skeletal muscles

In order to move a body part, the muscle or its tendon must stretch across at least one joint. When it contracts, the muscle then pulls one bone towards another. For example, when the elbow is bent during flexion of the forearm, the main mover is the biceps brachii, which is anchored on the scapula at one end and on the radius at the other. When it contracts, its shortening pulls on the radius, moving the forearm up toward the upper arm and bending the elbow.

This example also illustrates another feature of muscle arrangement: that of *antagonistic pairs*. Many muscles/muscle groups of the body are arranged so that their actions oppose one another. Using the example of bending the elbow, when the main flexors on the front of the upper arm contract, the muscles at the back of the upper arm must simultaneously relax to prevent injury.

Isometric and isotonic contraction

Contraction of a muscle usually results in its shortening, as happens for instance to the biceps muscle if the forearm is used to pick up a cup. The power generated by the muscle is used to lift the manageable weight, and tension in the muscle remains constant. In this situation, the contraction is said to be *isotonic* (iso = same; tonic = tension). However, imagine trying to lift an 80 kg man with one hand. Most people would be unable to perform this task, but the muscles of the arm and shoulder would still be working hard as they attempted it. In this situation, because the resistance from the man's weight is too great for him to be moved by the efforts of the lifter, the muscles would be unable to shorten, and the power generated increases the muscle tension instead. This is *isometric* contraction (iso = same; metric = length).

Muscle terminology

Muscles are named according to various characteristics (Table 16.7), and becoming familiar with the principal ones makes it much easier to identify unfamiliar muscles.

The *origin* of a muscle is (usually) its proximal attachment; this is generally the bone that remains still when the muscle contracts, giving it an anchor to pull against. The *insertion* is (usually) the distal attachment site, generally on the bone that is moved when the muscle contracts.

Principal skeletal muscles

Learning outcomes

After studying this section you should be able to:

- name the main muscles of the body regions described in this section
- outline the functions of the main muscles described in this section.

This section considers the main muscles that move the limbs, as well as the major muscles of the face and neck, back, chest, pelvic floor and abdominal wall.

Muscles of the face and neck (Fig. 16.54)

Muscles of the face

There are many muscles involved in changing facial expression and with movement of the lower jaw during chewing and speaking. Only the main muscles are described here. Except where indicated the muscles are present in pairs, one on each side.

Occipitofrontalis (unpaired). This consists of a posterior muscular part over the occipital bone (*occipitalis*), an anterior part over the frontal bone (*frontalis*) and an extensive flat tendon or *aponeurosis* that stretches over the dome of the skull and joins the two muscular parts. It raises the eyebrows.

Levator palpebrae superioris. This muscle extends from the posterior part of the orbital cavity to the upper eyelid. It raises the eyelid.

Orbicularis oculi. This muscle surrounds the eye, eyelid and orbital cavity. It closes the eye and when strongly contracted 'screws up' the eyes.

Buccinator. This flat muscle of the cheek draws the cheeks in towards the teeth in chewing and in forcible expulsion of air from the mouth ('the trumpeter's muscle').

Table 16.7 Muscle terminology

Characteristic	Example	Comment
Shape	Trapezius	Trapezium shaped
Fibre direction	Oblique muscles of abdomen	Fibres run obliquely
Muscle position	Tibialis	Found close to tibia in the leg
Movement produced	Extensor carpi ulnaris	Attached to the carpal bones of the wrist and the ulna, and extends the wrist
Number of points of attachment	Biceps brachii	Bi = 2; this muscle has two points of attachment at the shoulder
Bones to which muscle is attached	Carpi radialis muscles	Attached to the carpal bones of the wrist and the radius of the forearm

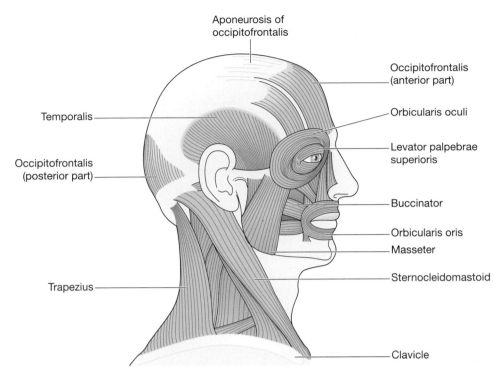

Figure 16.54 **The main muscles on the right side of the face, head and neck.**

Orbicularis oris (unpaired). This muscle surrounds the mouth and blends with the muscles of the cheeks. It closes the lips and, when strongly contracted, shapes the mouth for whistling.

Masseter. This is a broad muscle, extending from the zygomatic arch to the angle of the jaw. In chewing it draws the mandible up to the maxilla, closing the jaw, and exerts considerable pressure on the food.

Temporalis. This muscle covers the squamous part of the temporal bone. It passes behind the zygomatic arch to be inserted into the coronoid process of the mandible. It closes the mouth and assists with chewing.

Pterygoid. This muscle extends from the sphenoid bone to the mandible. It closes the mouth and pulls the lower jaw forward.

Muscles of the neck

There are many muscles in the neck, but only the two largest are considered here.

Sternocleidomastoid. This muscle arises from the manubrium of the sternum and the clavicle and extends upwards to the mastoid process of the temporal bone. It

assists in turning the head from side to side. When the muscle on one side contracts it draws the head towards the shoulder. When both contract at the same time they flex the cervical vertebrae or draw the sternum and clavicles upwards when the head is maintained in a fixed position, e.g. in forced respiration.

Trapezius. This muscle covers the shoulder and the back of the neck. The upper attachment is to the occipital protuberance, the medial attachment is to the transverse processes of the cervical and thoracic vertebrae and the lateral attachment is to the clavicle and to the spinous and acromion processes of the scapula. It pulls the head backwards, squares the shoulders and controls the movements of the scapula when the shoulder joint is in use.

Muscles of the trunk

These muscles stabilise the association between the appendicular and axial skeletons at the pectoral girdle, and stabilise and allow movement of the shoulders and upper arms.

Muscles of the back

There are six pairs of large muscles in the back, in addition to those forming the posterior abdominal wall

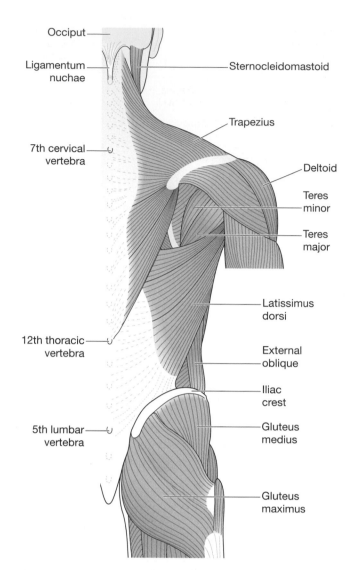

Figure 16.55 The main muscles of the back.

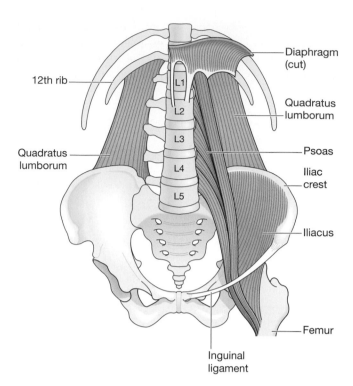

Figure 16.56 The deep muscles of the posterior abdominal wall.

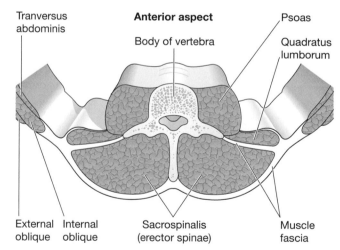

Figure 16.57 Transverse section of the posterior abdominal wall: a lumbar vertebra and its associated muscles.

(Figs 16.55, 16.56 and 16.57). The arrangement of these muscles is the same on each side of the vertebral column. They are:

- trapezius (see above)
- latissimus dorsi
- teres major
- psoas (p. 424)
- quadratus lumborum
- sacrospinalis.

Latissimus dorsi. This arises from the posterior part of the iliac crest and the spinous processes of the lumbar and lower thoracic vertebrae. It passes upwards across the back then under the arm to be inserted into the bicipital groove of the humerus. It adducts, medially rotates and extends the arm.

Teres major. This originates from the inferior angle of the scapula and is inserted into the humerus just below the shoulder joint. It extends, adducts and medially rotates the arm.

Quadratus lumborum. This muscle originates from the iliac crest, then it passes upwards, parallel and close to the vertebral column and it is inserted into the 12th rib

(Fig. 16.56). Together the two muscles fix the lower rib during respiration and cause extension of the vertebral column (bending backwards). If one muscle contracts it causes lateral flexion of the lumbar region of the vertebral column.

Sacrospinalis (erector spinae). This is a group of muscles lying between the spinous and transverse processes of the vertebrae (Fig. 16.57). They originate from the sacrum and are finally inserted into the occipital bone. Their contraction causes extension of the vertebral column.

Muscles of the abdominal wall

Five pairs of muscles form the abdominal wall (Figs 16.58 and 16.59). From the surface inwards they are:

- rectus abdominis
- external oblique
- internal oblique
- transversus abdominis
- quadratus lumborum (see above).

The anterior abdominal wall is divided longitudinally by a very strong midline tendinous cord, the *linea alba* (meaning 'white cord') which extends from the xiphoid process of the sternum to the symphysis pubis. The structure of the abdominal wall on each side of the linea alba is identical.

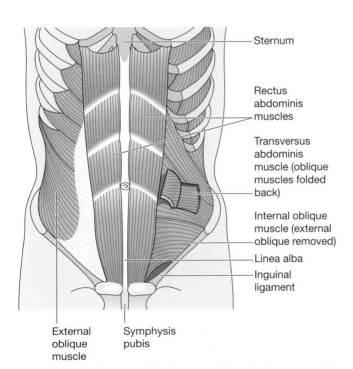

Figure 16.58 The muscles of the anterior abdominal wall.

Sternum

Rectus abdominis muscles

Transversus abdominis muscle (oblique muscles folded back)

Internal oblique muscle (external oblique removed)

Linea alba

Inguinal ligament

External oblique muscle

Symphysis pubis

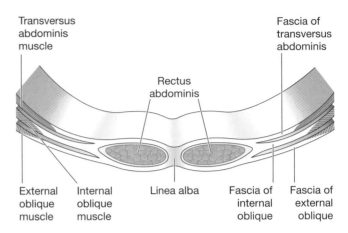

Transversus abdominis muscle

Fascia of transversus abdominis

Rectus abdominis

External oblique muscle

Internal oblique muscle

Linea alba

Fascia of internal oblique

Fascia of external oblique

Figure 16.59 Transverse section of the muscles and fasciae of the anterior abdominal wall.

Rectus abdominis. This is the most superficial muscle. It is broad and flat, originating from the transverse part of the pubic bone then passing upwards to be inserted into the lower ribs and the xiphoid process of the sternum. Medially the two muscles are attached to the linea alba.

External oblique. This muscle extends from the lower ribs downwards and forward to be inserted into the iliac crest and, by an aponeurosis, to the linea alba.

Internal oblique. This muscle lies deep to the external oblique. Its fibres arise from the iliac crest and by a broad band of fascia from the spinous processes of the lumbar vertebrae. The fibres pass upwards towards the midline to be inserted into the lower ribs and, by an aponeurosis, into the linea alba. The fibres are at right angles to those of the external oblique.

Transversus abdominis. This is the deepest muscle of the abdominal wall. The fibres arise from the iliac crest and the lumbar vertebrae and pass across the abdominal wall to be inserted into the linea alba by an aponeurosis. The fibres are at right angles to those of the rectus abdominis.

Functions

The main function of these paired muscles is to form the strong muscular anterior wall of the abdominal cavity. When the muscles contract together they:

- compress the abdominal organs
- flex the vertebral column in the lumbar region (Fig. 16.57).

Contraction of the muscles on one side only bends the trunk towards that side. Contraction of the oblique muscles on one side rotates the trunk.

421

Inguinal canal

This canal is 2.5 to 4 cm long and passes obliquely through the abdominal wall. It runs parallel to and immediately in front of the transversalis fascia and part of the inguinal ligament (Fig. 16.56). In the male it contains the *spermatic cord* and in the female, the *round ligament*. It constitutes a weak point in the otherwise strong abdominal wall through which herniation may occur.

Muscles of the thorax

These muscles are concerned with respiration, and are discussed in Chapter 10 (p. 250).

Muscles of the pelvic floor (Fig. 16.60)

The pelvic floor is divided into two identical halves that unite along the midline. Each half consists of fascia and muscle. The muscles are:

- levator ani
- coccygeus.

Levator ani. This is a pair of broad flat muscles, forming the anterior part of the pelvic floor. They originate from the inner surface of the true pelvis and unite in the midline. Together they form a sling that supports the pelvic organs.

Coccygeus. This is a paired triangular sheet of muscle and tendinous fibres situated behind the levator ani. They originate from the medial surface of the ischium and are inserted into the sacrum and coccyx. They complete the formation of the pelvic floor, which is

perforated in the male by the urethra and anus, and in the female by the urethra, vagina and anus.

Functions

The pelvic floor supports the organs of the pelvis and maintains continence, i.e. it resists raised intrapelvic pressure during micturition and defaecation.

Muscles of the shoulder and upper limb
(Fig. 16.61)

These muscles stabilise the association between the appendicular and axial skeletons at the pectoral girdle, and stabilise and allow movement of the shoulders and upper arms.

Deltoid. These muscle fibres originate from the clavicle, acromion process and spine of scapula and radiate over the shoulder joint to be inserted into the deltoid tuberosity of the humerus. It forms the fleshy and rounded contour of the shoulder and the main function is movement of the arm. The anterior part causes flexion, the middle or main part abduction and the posterior part extends and laterally rotates the shoulder joint.

Pectoralis major. This lies on the anterior thoracic wall. The fibres originate from the middle third of the clavicle and from the sternum and are inserted into the lip of the intertubercular groove of the humerus. It draws the arm forward and towards the body, i.e. flexes and adducts.

Coracobrachialis. This lies on the upper medial aspect of the arm. It arises from the coracoid process of the scapula, stretches across in front of the shoulder joint and is inserted into the middle third of the humerus. It flexes the shoulder joint.

Biceps. This lies on the anterior aspect of the upper arm. At its proximal end it is divided into two parts (heads) each of which has its own tendon. The short head rises from the coracoid process of the scapula and passes in front of the shoulder joint to the arm. The long head originates from the rim of the glenoid cavity and its tendon passes through the joint cavity and the bicipital groove of the humerus to the arm. It is retained in the bicipital groove by a transverse humeral ligament that stretches across the groove. The distal tendon crosses the elbow joint and is inserted into the radial tuberosity. It helps to stabilise and flex the shoulder joint and at the elbow joint it assists with flexion and supination.

Brachialis. This lies on the anterior aspect of the upper arm deep to the biceps. It originates from the shaft of the

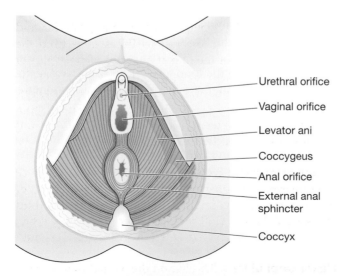

Urethral orifice

Vaginal orifice

Levator ani

Coccygeus

Anal orifice

External anal sphincter

Coccyx

Figure 16.60 The muscles of the female pelvic floor.

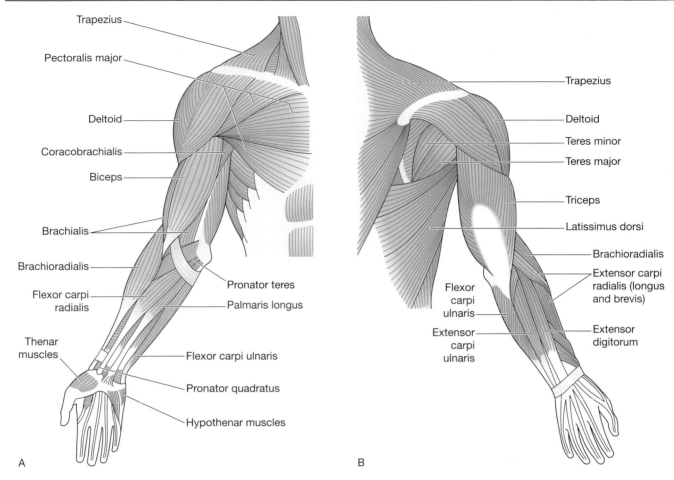

Trapezius

Pectoralis major

Deltoid

Coracobrachialis

Biceps

Brachialis

Brachioradialis

Flexor carpi
radialis

Thenar
muscles

Pronator teres

Palmaris longus

Flexor carpi ulnaris

Pronator quadratus

Hypothenar muscles

A

Trapezius

Deltoid

Teres minor

Teres major

Triceps

Latissimus dorsi

Brachioradialis

Extensor carpi
radialis (longus
and brevis)

Flexor
carpi
ulnaris

Extensor
carpi
ulnaris

Extensor
digitorum

B

Figure 16.61 The main muscles of the shoulder and upper limb. A: anterior view. B: posterior view.

humerus, extends across the elbow joint and is inserted into the ulna just distal to the joint capsule. It is the main flexor of the elbow joint.

Triceps. This lies on the posterior aspect of the humerus. It arises from three heads, one from the scapula and two from the posterior surface of the humerus. The insertion is by a common tendon to the olecranon process of the ulna. It helps to stabilise the shoulder joint, assists in adduction of the arm and extends the elbow joint.

Brachioradialis. The brachioradialis spans the elbow joint, originating on the distal end of the humerus and inserts on the lateral epicondyle of the radius. When it contracts, it flexes the elbow joint.

Pronator quadratus. This square-shaped muscle is the main muscle causing pronation of the hand and has attachments on the lower sections of both the radius and the ulna.

Pronator teres. This lies obliquely across the upper third of the front of the forearm. It arises from the medial

epicondyle of the humerus and the coronoid process of the ulna and passes obliquely across the forearm to be inserted into the lateral surface of the shaft of the radius. It rotates the radioulnar joints, changing the hand from the anatomical to the writing position, i.e. pronation.

Supinator. This lies obliquely across the posterior and lateral aspects of the forearm. Its fibres arise from the lateral epicondyle of the humerus and the upper part of the ulna and are inserted into the lateral surface of the upper third of the radius. It rotates the radioulnar joints, often with help form the biceps, changing the hand from the writing to the anatomical position, i.e. supination. It lies deep to the muscles shown in Figure 16.61.

Flexor carpi radialis. This lies on the anterior surface of the forearm. It originates from the medial epicondyle of the humerus and is inserted into the second and third metacarpal bones. It flexes the wrist joint, and when acting with the extensor carpi radialis, abducts the joint.

Flexor carpi ulnaris. This lies on the medial aspect of the forearm. It originates from the medial epicondyle of the humerus and the upper parts of the ulna and is inserted into the pisiform, the hamate and the fifth metacarpal bones. It flexes the wrist, and when acting with the extensor carpi ulnaris, adducts the joint.

Extensor carpi radialis longus and brevis. These lie on the posterior aspect of the forearm. The fibres originate from the lateral epicondyle of the humerus and are inserted by a long tendon into the second and third metacarpal bones. They extend and abduct the wrist.

Extensor carpi ulnaris. This lies on the posterior surface of the forearm. It originates from the lateral epicondyle of the humerus and is inserted into the fifth metacarpal bone. It extends and adducts the wrist.

Palmarus longus. This muscle resists shearing forces that might pull the skin and fascia of the palm away from the underlying structures, and flexes the wrist. Its origin is on the medial epicondyle of the humerus, and it inserts on tendons on the palm of the hand.

Extensor digitorum. This muscle originates on the lateral epicondyle of the humerus and spans both the elbow and wrist joints; in the wrist, it divides into four tendons, one for each finger. Action of this muscle can extend any of the joints across which it passes, i.e. the elbow, wrist or finger joints.

Muscles that control finger movements. Large muscles in the forearm that extend to the hand give power to the hand and fingers, but not the delicacy of movement needed for fine and dextrous finger control. Smaller muscles, which originate on the carpal and metacarpal bones, control tiny and precise finger movements via tendinous attachments on the phalanges; muscle fibres do not extend into the fingers.

Muscles of the hip and lower limb

(Fig. 16.62)

The biggest muscles of the body are found here, since their function is largely in weight bearing. The lower parts of the body are designed to transmit the force of body weight in walking, running etc evenly throughout weight-bearing structures, and as shock absorbers.

Psoas. This arises from the transverse processes and bodies of the lumbar vertebrae. It passes across the flat part of the ilium and behind the inguinal ligament to be inserted into the femur. Together with the iliacus it flexes the hip joint (see Fig. 16.56).

Iliacus. This lies in the iliac fossa of the innominate bone. It originates from the iliac crest, passes over the iliac fossa and joins the tendon of the psoas muscle to be inserted into the lesser trochanter of the femur. The combined action of the iliacus and psoas flexes the hip joint.

Quadriceps femoris. This is a group of four muscles lying on the front and sides of the thigh. They are the *rectus femoris* and three *vasti*: lateralis, medialis and intermedius (this last muscle is not shown in Fig. 16.62 because it lies deep to the other two). The rectus femoris originates from the ilium and the three vasti from the upper end of the femur. Together they pass over the front of the knee joint to be inserted into the tibia by the patellar tendon. Only the rectus femoris flexes the hip joint. Together, the group acts as a very strong extensor of the knee joint.

Obturators. The obturators, deep muscles of the buttock, have their origins in the rim of the obturator foramen of the pelvis and insert into the proximal femur. Their main function lies in lateral rotation at the hip joint.

Gluteals. These consist of the *gluteus maximus, medius* and *minimus*, which together form the fleshy part of the buttock. They originate from the ilium and sacrum and are inserted into the femur. They cause extension, abduction and medial rotation at the hip joint.

Sartorius. This is the longest muscle in the body and crosses both the hip and knee joints. It originates from the anterior superior iliac spine and passes obliquely across the hip joint, thigh and knee joint to be inserted into the medial surface of the upper part of the tibia. It is associated with flexion and abduction at the hip joint and flexion at the knee.

Adductor group. This lies on the medial aspect of the thigh. They originate from the pubic bone and are inserted into the linea aspera of the femur. They adduct and medially rotate the thigh.

Hamstrings. These lie on the posterior aspect of the thigh. They originate from the ischium and are inserted into the upper end of the tibia. They are the *biceps femoris*, *semimembranosus* and *semitendinosus muscles*. They flex the knee joint.

Gastrocnemius. This forms the bulk of the calf of the leg. It arises by two heads, one from each condyle of the femur, and passes down behind the tibia to be inserted into the calcaneus by the *calcanean tendon* (*Achilles tendon*). It crosses both knee and ankle joints, causing flexion at

424

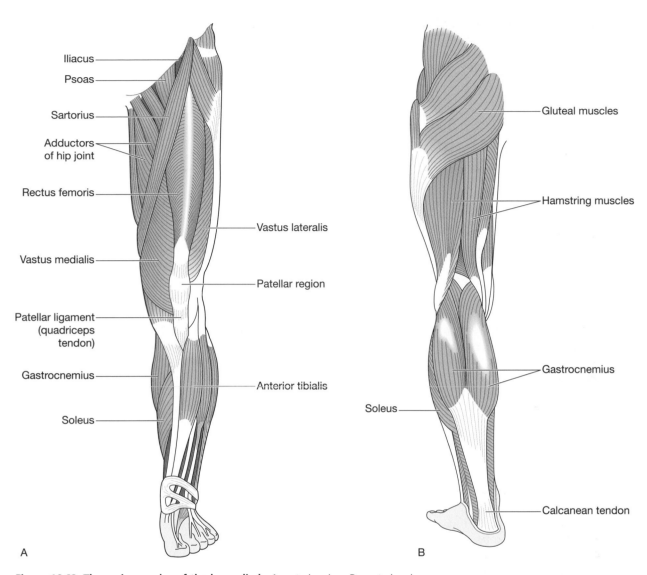

Figure 16.62 The main muscles of the lower limb. A: anterior view. B: posterior view.

425

the knee and plantarflexion (rising onto the ball of the foot) at the ankle.

Anterior tibialis. This originates from the upper end of the tibia, lies on the anterior surface of the leg and is inserted into the middle cuneiform bone by a long tendon. It is associated with dorsiflexion of the foot.

Soleus. This is one of the main muscles of the calf of the leg, lying immediately deep to the gastrocnemius. It originates from the heads and upper parts of the fibula and the tibia. Its tendon joins that of the gastrocnemius so that they have a common insertion into the calcaneus by the calcanean (Achilles) tendon. It causes plantarflexion at the ankle and helps to stabilise the joint when standing.

Labels on Figure A:
- Iliacus
- Psoas
- Sartorius
- Adductors of hip joint
- Rectus femoris
- Vastus medialis
- Patellar ligament (quadriceps tendon)
- Gastrocnemius
- Soleus
- Vastus lateralis
- Patellar region
- Anterior tibialis

Labels on Figure B:
- Gluteal muscles
- Hamstring muscles
- Gastrocnemius
- Soleus
- Calcanean tendon

A

B

Diseases of bone

Learning outcomes

After studying this section you should be able to:

- explain the pathological features of osteoporosis, Paget's disease, rickets and osteomalacia
- outline the causes and effects of osteomyelitis
- describe abnormalities of bone development
- explain the effects of bone tumours.

Osteoporosis

In this condition, bone density (the amount of bone tissue) is reduced because its deposition does not keep pace with resorption. Although the bone is adequately mineralised, it is fragile and microscopically abnormal, with loss of internal structure. Peak bone mass occurs around 35 years and then gradually declines in both sexes. Lowered oestrogen levels after the menopause are associated with a period of accelerated bone loss in women. Thereafter bone density in women is less than in men for any given age. A range of environmental factors and diseases are also associated with decreased bone mass and are implicated in development of osteoporosis (Box 16.1). Some can be influenced by changes in lifestyle. Exercise and calcium intake during childhood and adolescence are thought to be important in determining eventual bone mass of an individual, and therefore the risk of osteoporosis in later life. As bone mass decreases, susceptibility to fractures increases. Immobility causes reversible osteoporosis, the extent of which corresponds to the length and extent of immobility. For instance,

during prolonged periods of unconsciousness, osteoporotic changes are uniform throughout the skeleton, but immobilisation of a particular joint following fracture leads to local osteoporotic changes in involved bones only.

Common features of osteoporosis are:

- skeletal deformity – gradual loss of height with age, caused by compression of vertebrae
- bone pain
- fractures – especially of the hip (neck of femur), wrist (Colles' fracture) and vertebrae.

Paget's disease

Paget's disease is a disorder of bone remodelling, where the normal balance between bone building and bone breakdown becomes disorganised and both osteoblasts and osteoclasts become abnormally active. The bone deposited is soft and structurally abnormal. This predisposes to deformities and fractures, commonly of the pelvis, femur, tibia and skull. Most cases occur after 40 years of age and the incidence increases with age. The cause is unknown and it often goes undetected until complications arise. The disease increases the risk of osteoarthritis and osteosarcoma.

Rickets and osteomalacia

The underlying abnormality in osteomalacia and rickets is inadequate mineralisation of bone, usually because of vitamin D deficiency, or sometimes because of defective vitamin D metabolism. In children, whose bones are still growing, this leads to characteristic bowing and deformity of the lower limbs, and is called rickets. In the adult, who still requires vitamin D for normal turnover of bone, deficiency leads to osteomalacia, which is associated with increased risk of fracture and bone pain.

Deficiency may be caused by poor diet, or by limited exposure to sunlight (needed for normal vitamin D metabolism). Some people are genetically unable to metabolise vitamin D normally, leading to poor bone mineralisation, and occasionally malabsorption may also lead to deficiency.

Osteomyelitis

The general term for bacterial infection of bone is osteomyelitis. This may follow an open fracture or surgical procedures, which allow microbial entry through broken skin. It may also be a consequence of blood-borne infection from a focus elsewhere, such as the ear, throat or skin; this is most commonly seen in children. If promptly and adequately treated, the infection can resolve without

---

Box 16.1 Causes of decreased bone mass

Risk factors	Drugs
Female gender	Corticosteroids
Increasing age	
White ethnic origin	**Diseases**
Family history	Cushing's syndrome
Lack of exercise/	Hyperparathyroidism
immobility	Type I diabetes mellitus
Diet (low calcium)	Rheumatoid arthritis
Smoking	Chronic renal failure
Excess alcohol intake	Chronic liver disease
Early menopause/	Anorexia nervosa
oophorectomy	Certain cancers
Thin build (small bones)	

permanent damage, but if not, it may become chronic, with sinus formation draining pus to the skin, fever and pain.

Developmental abnormalities of bone

Achondroplasia

This is caused by a genetic abnormality that affects the proper ossification of bones that develop from cartilage models, such as the long bones of the limbs, leading to short limbs and characteristic dwarfism.

Osteogenesis imperfecta ('brittle bone syndrome')

This is a group of conditions in which there is a congenital defect of collagen synthesis, resulting in failure of ossification. The bones are brittle and fracture easily, either spontaneously or following very slight trauma.

Tumours of bone

Benign tumours

Single or multiple tumours may develop for unknown reasons in bone and cartilage. They may cause pathological fractures or pressure damage to soft tissues, e.g. a benign vertebral tumour may damage the spinal cord or a spinal nerve. Benign tumours of cartilage have a tendency to undergo malignant change.

Malignant tumours

Metastatic tumours

The most common malignancies of bone are metastases of primary carcinomas of the breast, lungs, thyroid, kidneys and prostate gland. The usual sites are those with the best blood supply, i.e. spongy bone, especially the bodies of the lumbar vertebrae and the epiphyses of the humerus and femur. Tumour fragments are spread in blood, and possibly along the walls of the veins from pelvic tumours to vertebrae. Tumour growth erodes and weakens normal bone tissue, leading to pain, pathological fractures and destruction of normal bone architecture.

Primary tumours

Primary malignant tumours of bone are relatively rare.

Osteosarcoma. This is a rapidly growing and often metastatic tumour believed to develop from the precursors of osteogenic cells. In young people between 10 and 25 years of age the tumour develops most commonly in the medullary canal of long bones, especially the femur. It is usually well advanced before it becomes evident. In older people, usually over 60 years of age, it is often

associated with Paget's disease and the bones most commonly affected are the vertebrae, skull and pelvis.

Chondrosarcoma. These relatively slow-growing tumours are usually the result of malignant change in benign tumours of cartilage cells. They occur mainly between the ages of 40 and 70 years.

Disorders of joints

Learning outcomes

After studying this section you should be able to:

- relate the features of the diseases in this section to abnormal anatomy and physiology
- compare and contrast the features of rheumatoid arthritis and osteoarthritis.

The tissues involved in diseases of the synovial joints are synovial membrane, hyaline cartilage and bone.

Inflammatory joint disease (arthritis)

Rheumatoid arthritis (RA, rheumatoid disease)

This is a chronic progressive inflammatory autoimmune disease mainly affecting peripheral synovial joints. It is a systemic disorder where inflammatory changes affect not only joints but also many other sites including the heart, blood vessels and skin.

It is more common in females than males and can affect all ages, including children (Still's disease), although it usually develops between the ages of 35 and 55 years. The cause is not clearly understood but development of autoimmunity may be initiated by microbial infection, possibly by viruses, in genetically susceptible people. Risk factors include:

- age – risk increases with age
- gender – premenopausal women are affected three times as commonly as men
- genetic risk – there is a strong familial link in some cases, and some markers on the surface membranes of white blood cells have also been associated with higher risk of the disease.

Almost always (up to 90% of cases), affected individuals have rheumatoid factor (RF) in their body fluids. High levels of RF, especially early in the disease, are strongly associated with accelerated and more severe disease. Symptoms include joint pain and stiffness, particularly in the morning and after rest. Joints can be visibly swollen, hot and tender.

Acute exacerbations of rheumatoid arthritis are usually accompanied by fever, and are interspersed with periods of remission. The joints most commonly affected are those of the hands and feet, but in severe cases most synovial joints may be involved. With each exacerbation there is additional and cumulative damage to the joints, leading to increasing deformity, pain and loss of function. The early changes, which may be reversible, include hypertrophy and hyperplasia of synovial cells and fibrinous inflammatory effusion into the joint. Progression of the disease usually leads to permanent tissue damage. Growth of inflammatory granulation tissue, called *pannus*, distorts the joint and destroys articular cartilage, exposing the bone below and causing further damage. Fibrosis of the pannus reduces joint mobility. Pain, stiffness and deformity severely restrict the use of affected joints, and as a result the associated muscles start to waste. About a third of patients, usually those with the most aggressive form of the disease, develop nodules of connective tissue (rheumatoid nodules), usually in the forearm or elbow. Extra-articular symptoms can include anaemia, peripheral neuropathy, cardiac abnormalities, pleurisy and vasculitis.

In the later stages of the disease, the inflammation and fever are less marked. The extent of disability varies from slight to severe. Table 16.8 highlights differences between osteoarthritis and rheumatoid arthritis.

Other types of polyarthritis

This group of autoimmune inflammatory arthritic diseases has many characteristics similar to rheumatoid arthritis but the rheumatoid factor is absent. The causes are not known but genetic features may be involved.

Ankylosing spondylitis. This tends to occur in young adults, and affects the joints of the vertebral column. Calcification of the intervertebral joints and laying down of new bone leads to reduced spinal flexibility and permanent deformity.

Psoriatic arthritis. This occurs in a proportion of people who suffer from psoriasis, especially if the nails are involved. The joints most commonly affected are those of the fingers and toes.

Reiter's syndrome (polyarthritis with urethritis and conjunctivitis). This syndrome, it is believed, may be precipitated by infection with *Chlamydia trachomatis*; the affected joints are usually those of the lower limb.

Rheumatic fever. Rheumatic fever (p. 124) is a diffuse inflammatory condition that affects many connective tissues. Polyarthritis is a common presenting feature, often involving the wrists, elbows, knees and ankles. Unlike cardiac effects, arthritis usually resolves spontaneously without complications.

Infective arthritis

Joint infection (septic arthritis) usually results from a blood-borne systemic infection (septicaemia, mainly staphylococcal), although it may also be caused by a penetrating joint injury. Often the joint has been damaged by pre-existing disease, making it more susceptible to infection. Normally, only one joint is involved, which becomes acutely inflamed, and the patient is likely to be ill from the associated septicaemia. Complete resolution

Table 16.8 Features of the two main types of arthritis

	Osteoarthritis	Rheumatoid arthritis
Type of disease	Degenerative	Inflammatory and autoimmune
Tissue affected	Articular cartilage	Synovial membrane
Age of onset	Late middle age	Any age, mainly 30 to 55 years, occasionally children
Joints affected	Weight bearing, e.g. hip, knee; often only a single joint	Small, e.g. hands, feet; often many joints

is possible if treatment is prompt, but permanent joint damage occurs early in the disease.

Traumatic injury to joints

Sprains, strains and dislocations

These damage the soft tissues, tendons and ligaments round the joint without penetrating the joint capsule. In dislocations there may be additional damage to intracapsular structures by stretching, e.g. to the long head of biceps muscle in the shoulder joint, the cruciate ligaments in the knee joint, or the ligament of head of femur in the hip joint. If repair is incomplete there may be some loss of stability, which increases the risk of repeated injury.

Penetrating injuries

These may be caused by a compound fracture of one of the articulating bones, or trauma caused by, e.g., gunshot. Healing may be uneventful or it may be delayed by the presence of fragments of damaged or torn joint tissue (bone, cartilage or ligaments), which cannot be removed or repaired by normal body mechanisms and prevent full joint recovery. Infection is another risk. Development of chronic inflammation can lead to permanent degenerative changes in the joint.

Osteoarthritis (osteoarthrosis, OA)

This is a degenerative non-inflammatory disease that results in pain and restricted movement of affected joints. Osteoarthrosis is the more appropriate name but is less commonly used. In its early stages, OA is often asymptomatic. It is very common, with the majority of over-65s showing some degree of osteoarthritic changes. Articular cartilage gradually becomes thinner because its renewal does not keep pace with its breakdown. Eventually the bony articular surfaces come in contact and the bones begin to degenerate. Bone repair is abnormal and the articular surfaces become misshapen. This is often the reason for reduced mobility of the joint. Chronic inflammation develops with effusion into the joint, possibly due to irritation caused by tissue debris not removed by phagocytes. Sometimes there is abnormal outgrowth of cartilage at the edges of bones that becomes ossified, forming *osteophytes*.

In most cases, the cause of OA is unknown (primary OA), but risk factors include excessive repetitive use of the affected joints, female gender, increasing age, obesity and heredity. Secondary OA occurs when the joint is already affected by disease or abnormality, e.g. trauma or gout. Osteoarthritis usually develops in late middle age and affects large weight-bearing joints, i.e. the hips, knees and joints of the cervical and lower lumbar spine. In many cases only one joint is involved.

Gout

This condition is more prevalent in males than females and there is a familial tendency. It is caused by the deposition of sodium urate crystals in joints and tendons, provoking an acute inflammatory response. Risk factors include obesity, heredity, hyperuricaemia and high alcohol intake. *Primary* gout, the commonest form, occurs almost always in men and is associated with reduced ability to excrete urate or increased urate production. *Secondary* gout occurs usually as a consequence of diuretic treatment or kidney failure, both of which reduce urate excretion.

In many cases only one joint is involved (monoarthritis) and it is typically red, hot and extremely painful. The sites most commonly affected are the metatarsophalangeal joint of the big toe and the ankle, knee, wrist and elbow joints. Episodes of arthritis lasting days or weeks are interspersed with periods of remission. After repeated acute attacks, permanent damage may occur with chronic deformity and loss of function of the affected joints. Gout is sometimes complicated by the development of renal calculi.

Connective tissue diseases

This group of disorders has common features. They:

- affect many systems of the body, especially the joints, skin and subcutaneous tissues
- tend to occur in early adult life
- usually affect more females than males
- are chronic conditions
- are autoimmune diseases in which abnormal autoantibodies are formed that attack the individual's tissues.

These disorders include the following.

- *Systemic lupus erythematosus* (SLE) – in this the affected joints are usually the hands, knees and ankles. A characteristic red 'butterfly' rash may occur on the face. Kidney involvement is common and can result in glomerulonephritis that may be complicated by chronic renal failure.

- *Systemic sclerosis (scleroderma)* – this is a group of disorders in which there is progressive thickening of connective tissue. There is increased production of collagen that affects many organs. In the skin there is dermal fibrosis and tightness that impairs the functioning of joints, especially of the hands. It also affects the walls of blood vessels, intestinal tract and other organs.
- *Rheumatoid arthritis* (p. 427).
- *Ankylosing spondylitis* (p. 428).
- *Reiter's syndrome* (p. 428).

Carpal tunnel syndrome

This occurs when the median nerve is compressed in the wrist as it passes through the carpal tunnel (see Fig. 16.48). It is a common condition, especially in women, between the ages of 30 and 50 years. There is pain and numbness in the hand and wrist affecting the thumb, index and middle fingers, and half of the ring finger. Many cases are idiopathic or secondary to other conditions, e.g. rheumatoid arthritis, diabetes mellitus, acromegaly and hypothyroidism. Repetitive flexion and extension of the wrist joint also cause the condition, e.g. following prolonged keyboard use.

Diseases of muscle

Learning outcomes

After studying this section you should be able to:

- list the causes of the diseases in this section

- compare and contrast the characteristics of different types of muscular dystrophy.

Myasthenia gravis

See page 381.

Muscular dystrophies

In this group of inherited diseases there is progressive degeneration of groups of muscles. The main differences in the types are:

- age of onset

- rate of progression
- groups of muscles involved.

Duchenne muscular dystrophy

Inheritance of this condition is sex linked, the affected gene being carried on the long X chromosome of female carriers. Their children may be affected by the condition if they are males (50% chance), or be carriers if they are females (50% chance) (see Fig. 17.9, p. 438).

The muscle abnormality is present before birth but may not be evident until the child is about 5 years of age. Wasting and weakness begin in muscles of the lower limbs then spread to the upper limbs, progressing rapidly without remission. Death usually occurs in adolescence, often from respiratory failure, cardiac arrhythmias or cardiomyopathy.

Facioscapulohumeral dystrophy

This disease affects both sexes. It usually begins in adolescence and the younger the age of onset the more rapidly it progresses. Muscles of the face and shoulders are affected first. This is a chronic condition that usually progresses slowly and may not cause complete disability. Life expectancy is normal.

Myotonic dystrophy

This disease usually begins in adult life and affects both genders. Muscles contract and relax slowly, often seen as difficulty in releasing an object held in the hand. Muscles of the tongue and the face are first affected, then muscles of the limbs. Systemic conditions associated with myotonic dystrophy include:

- cataracts
- atrophy of the gonads
- cardiomyopathy
- glucose intolerance.

The disease progresses without remission and with increasing disability. Death usually occurs in middle age from respiratory or cardiac failure.

Crush syndrome

Sustained pressure, on the trunk or a limb, causes ischaemia resulting in massive muscle necrosis. When pressure is relieved and circulation restored, myoglobin and other necrotic products are released from damaged muscle and enter the blood. This material is highly toxic to the kidneys and acute renal failure may develop. A common complication is infection, especially by anaerobic microbes, e.g. *Clostridium perfringens*, causing *gas gangrene*.

Introduction to genetics

All living organisms, including human beings, need to reproduce, so that at the end of their lifespan they have produced at least one, probably many, other individuals to replace themselves. This ensures the continuation of their species. Babies inherit from their parents a copy of all information needed to develop into a functioning member of their species; this information is carried as deoxyribonucleic acid (DNA), mainly within the cell nucleus. DNA is organised into functional units called *genes*, which themselves are part of much bigger structures, the *chromosomes*. The name given to all the genetic material in a cell is the *genome*. *Genetics* is the study of genes, and advancing knowledge in this area has a profound effect on many aspects of daily life, e.g. for genetic counselling in families carrying inherited diseases and the production of human insulin from genetically engineered microbes.

Chromosomes, genes and DNA

Learning outcomes

After studying this section you should be able to:

- explain the structural relationship between chromosomes, genes and DNA

- describe the molecular structure of DNA

- explain the terms autosomes and sex chromosomes

- define the terms genome, haploid, diploid and karyotype.

Chromosomes

Nearly every body cell contains, within its nucleus, an identical copy of the entire complement of the individual's genetic material. Two important exceptions are red blood cells (which have no nucleus) and the gametes or sex cells. In a resting cell, the *chromatin* (genetic material, see Fig. 3.3, p. 32) is diffuse and hard to see under the microscope, but when the cell prepares to divide, it is collected into highly visible, compact, sausage-shaped structures called *chromosomes*. Each chromosome is one of a pair, one inherited from the mother and one from the father, so the human cell has 46 chromosomes that can be arranged as 23 pairs. A cell with 23 pairs of chromosomes is termed *diploid*. Gametes (spermatozoa and ova), with only half of the normal complement, i.e. 23 chromosomes instead of 46, are described as *haploid*. Chromosomes belonging to the same pair are called *homologous* chromo-

somes. The complete set of chromosomes from a cell is its *karyotype* (Fig. 17.1).

Each pair of chromosomes is numbered, the largest pair being no. 1. The first 22 pairs are collectively known as *autosomes*, and the chromosomes of each pair are identical. The chromosomes of pair 23 are called the *sex chromosomes* because they determine the individual's gender. Unlike autosomes, these two chromosomes are not necessarily identical; the Y chromosome is much shorter than the X and is carried only by males. A child inheriting two X chromosomes (XX) from her parents is female, and a child inheriting an X from his mother and a Y from his father (XY) is male.

Genes

Along the length of the chromosomes are the genes. Each gene contains information in code that allows the cell to make (almost always) a specific protein, the so-called *gene product*. Each gene codes for one specific protein, and research puts the number of genes within the human genome at 24 500 – that means 24 500 different proteins.

Genes normally exist in pairs, because each gene site (locus) is present at corresponding sites on both homologous chromosomes (p. 437).

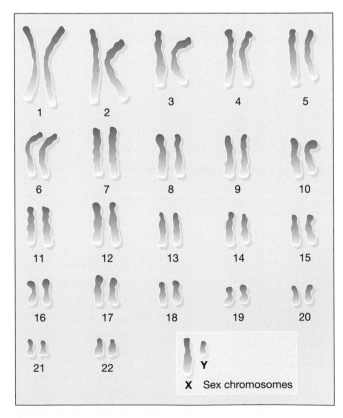

Figure 17.1 Chromosomal complement (karyotype) of a human cell.

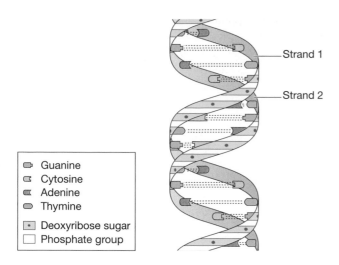

Figure 17.2 Deoxyribonucleic acid (DNA).

DNA

Genes are composed of very long strands of DNA; the total length of DNA in each cell is about a metre. Because this is packaged into chromosomes, which are micro-metres (10^{-6} m) long, this means that the DNA must be tightly wrapped up to condense it into such a small space.

DNA is a double-stranded molecule, made up of two chains of *nucleotides*. Nucleotides consist of three subunits:

- a sugar
- a phosphate group
- a base.

The DNA molecule is sometimes likened to a twisted ladder, with the uprights formed by alternating chains of sugar and phosphate units (Fig. 17.2). In DNA, the sugar is deoxyribose, thus **D**NA. The bases are linked to the sugars, and each base binds to another base on the other sugar/phosphate chain, forming the rungs of the ladder. The two chains are twisted around one another, giving a double helix (twisted ladder) arrangement. The double helix itself is further twisted and wrapped in a highly organised way around structural proteins called *histones*, which are important in maintaining the heavily coiled three-dimensional shape of the DNA. The term given to the DNA – histone material is *chromatin*. The chromatin is supercoiled and packaged into the chromosomes (Fig. 17.3).

The genetic code

The function of DNA is carrying huge amounts of information that determines all biological activities of an organism, and which is transmitted from one generation to the next. The key to how this information is kept is found in the bases within DNA. There are four bases:

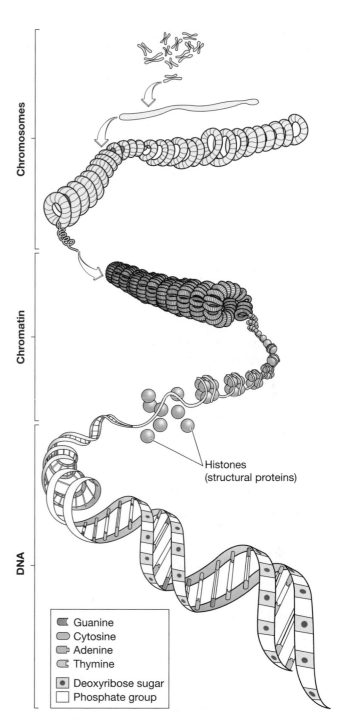

Figure 17.3 The structural relationship between DNA, chromatin and chromosomes.

- adenine (A)
- guanine (G)
- thymine (T)
- cytosine (C).

They are arranged in a precise order along the DNA molecule, making a code that can be read when protein synthesis is required. Each base along one strand of DNA

433

pairs with a base on the other strand in a precise and predictable way. This is known as *complementary base pairing*. Adenine always pairs with thymine (and vice versa), and cytosine and guanine always go together. The bases on opposite strands run down the middle of the helix and bind to one another with hydrogen bonds (Fig. 17.2).

Mutation

Mutation means an alteration in the normal genetic make-up of a cell. Some mutations occur by chance, because of the countless millions of DNA replications and cell divisions that occur normally throughout life. Others may be caused by external factors, such as X-rays, ultraviolet rays or exposure to certain chemicals.

Sometimes the mutation is lethal, because it disrupts some essential cellular function, causing cell death. Often, the mutated cell is detected by immune cells and destroyed because it is abnormal (p. 374). Other mutations do not kill the cell but alter its function in some way that may cause disease, e.g. in cancer (p. 51). Mutations in the genetic material present in the gametes may be passed on to the next generation, e.g. phenylketonuria (p. 439).

434

Protein synthesis

Learning outcomes

After studying this section you should be able to:

- describe the origin and structure of mRNA

- explain the mechanism of transcription

- outline the mechanism of translation.

DNA holds the cell's essential biological information, written within the base code in the centre of the double helix. The products of this information are almost always proteins. Proteins are essential to all aspects of body function, forming the major structural elements of the body as well as the enzymes (p. 25) essential for all biochemical processes within it. The building blocks of human proteins are about 20 different amino acids. The cell's DNA is too big to leave the nucleus, and therefore an intermediary molecule is needed to carry the genetic instructions from the nucleus to the cytoplasm, where proteins are made. This is called *messenger (m)RNA*. Protein synthesis is summarised in Figure 17.4.

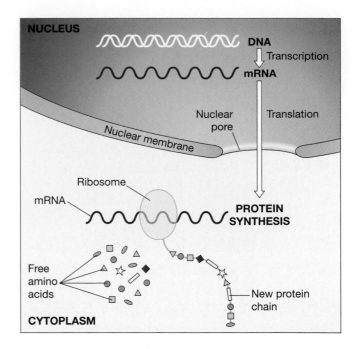

Figure 17.4 The relationship between DNA, RNA and protein synthesis.

Messenger ribonucleic acid (mRNA)

mRNA is a single-stranded chain of nucleotides synthesised in the nucleus from the appropriate gene, whenever the cell requires to make the protein for which that gene codes. There are three main differences between the structures of RNA and DNA:

- it is single instead of double stranded
- it contains ribose as its sugar instead of deoxyribose
- it uses uracil instead of thymine as a base.

Using the DNA as a template, a piece of mRNA is made from the gene to be used. This process is called *transcription*. The message then leaves the nucleus through the nuclear pores and carries its information to the *ribosomes* in the cytoplasm.

Transcription

Because the code is buried within the DNA molecule, the first step is to open up the helix to expose the bases. Only the gene to be transcribed is opened; the remainder of the chromosome remains coiled. Opening up the helix exposes both sets of bases, but the enzyme that makes the mRNA uses only one of them, so the mRNA molecule is single, not double stranded. As the enzyme moves along the opened DNA strand, reading its code, it adds the complementary base to the mRNA. Therefore, if the DNA base is cytosine, guanine is added to the mRNA molecule (and vice versa); if it is thymine, adenine is added; if it is adenine, uracil is added (remember there is no thymine in RNA, but uracil instead) (Fig. 17.5). When the enzyme gets to a 'stop' signal, it terminates synthesis of the mRNA molecule, and the mRNA is released. The DNA is zipped up again by other enzymes, and the mRNA then leaves the nucleus.

Translation

Translation is synthesis of the final protein using the information carried on mRNA. It takes place on ribosomes (p. 31) in the cytoplasm and on rough endoplasmic reticulum. First, the mRNA attaches to the ribosome. The ribosome then 'reads' the base sequence of the mRNA (Fig. 17.5).

Because proteins are built from up to 20 different amino acids, it is not possible to use the four bases individually in a simple one-to-one code. To give enough options, the base code in RNA is read in triplets, giving a possible 64 base combinations, which allows a coded instruction for each amino acid as well as other codes, e.g. stop and start instructions. Each of these specific triplet sequences is called a *codon*; for example, the base sequence ACA (adenine, cytosine, adenine) codes for the amino acid cysteine.

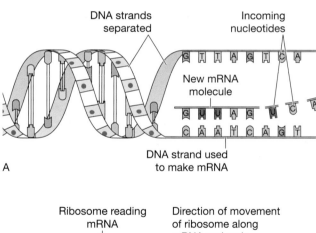

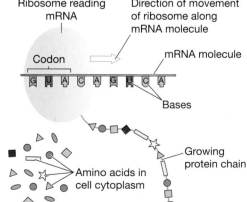

Figure 17.5 Transcription (A) and translation (B).

The first codon is a *start codon*, which initiates protein synthesis. The ribosome slides along the mRNA, reading the codons and adding the appropriate amino acids to the growing protein molecule as it goes. The ribosome continues assembling the new protein molecule until it arrives at a *stop codon*, at which point it terminates synthesis and releases the new protein. Some new proteins are used within the cell itself, and others are exported, e.g. insulin synthesised by pancreatic β-islet cells is released into the bloodstream.

Gene expression

Although all cells (except gametes and red blood cells) have an identical set of genes, each cell type is able to use only those genes related directly to its own particular function. For example, the only cell type containing haemoglobin is the red blood cell, although all body cells carry the haemoglobin gene. This selective gene expression is controlled by various regulatory substances, and the genes not needed by the cell are kept switched off.

Cell division

Learning outcomes

After studying this section, you should be able to:

- explain the mechanism of DNA replication

- compare and contrast the processes of mitosis and meiosis

- describe the basis of genetic diversity from generation to generation.

435

Most body cells are capable of division, even in adulthood. Cell division usually leads to production of two identical diploid daughter cells, *mitosis* (p. 32) and is important in body growth and repair. Production of gametes is different in that the daughter cells have only half the normal chromosome number – 23 instead of 46, i.e. they are haploid. Gametes are produced by a form of cell division called *meiosis*. DNA replication takes place before mitosis and meiosis.

DNA replication

DNA is the only biological molecule capable of self-replication. Mistakes in copying may lead to production of non-functioning or poorly functional cells, or cells that do not respond to normal cell controls (this could lead to the development of a tumour). Accurate copying of DNA is therefore essential.

The initial step in DNA replication is the unfolding of the double helix and the unzipping of the two strands to expose the bases, as happens in transcription. Both strands of the parent DNA molecule are copied. The enzyme responsible for DNA replication moves along the base sequence on each strand, reading the genetic code and adding the complementary base to the newly forming chain. This means that each strand of opened bases becomes a double strand and the end result is two identical DNA molecules (Fig. 17.6). As each new double strand is formed, other enzymes cause it to twist and coil back into its normal highly folded form.

Mitosis

This is described on page 32.

Meiosis

Meiosis produces gametes. On fertilisation, when the male gamete (sperm cell) and the female gamete (ovum)

unite, the resulting *zygote* is diploid, because each gamete was haploid.

Unlike mitosis, meiosis involves two distinct cell divisions rather than one (Fig. 17.7). Additionally, meiosis produces four daughter cells, not two, all different from the parent cells and from each other. This is the basis of genetic diversity and the uniqueness of each human individual.

First meiotic division

This stage (Fig. 17.7) produces two genetically different daughter cells.

DNA replication occurred beforehand, so each pair of chromosomes is now four chromatids, and they gather together into a tight bundle. Because the chromosomes are so tightly associated, it is possible for them to exchange genes. This process is called *crossing over*, and results in the four chromatids having different combinations of genes. Following crossing over, the pairs of chromosomes then separate in preparation for the first meiotic division, and transfer of maternal and paternal chromosomes to either daughter cell is random. This

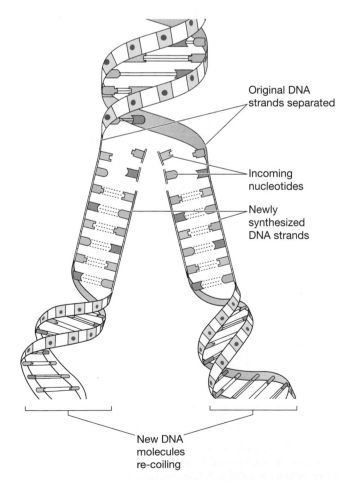

Figure 17.6 **DNA replication.**

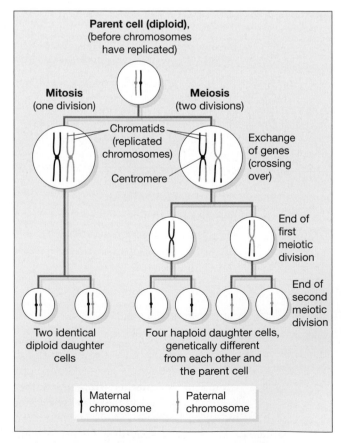

Figure 17.7 **Mitosis and meiosis, showing only one pair of chromosomes**

means that the two daughter cells have an unpredictable assortment of maternal and paternal DNA, giving rise to a huge number of possible combinations of chromosomes in them. This explains why a child inherits a combination of its mother's and father's characteristics.

Each pair of chromosomes separates and one travels to each end of the cell, guided by a spindle as in mitosis, and the cytoplasm divides, producing two genetically unique diploid daughter cells.

Second meiotic division

For a gamete to be produced, the amount of genetic material present in the two daughter cells following the first meiotic division must be halved. This is accomplished by a second division (Fig. 17.7). The centromeres separate and the two sister chromatids travel to opposite ends of the cell, which then divides. Each of the four haploid daughter cells now has only one chromosome from each original pair. Fusion with another gamete creates a diploid cell, which can then go on to grow and develop into a human being by mitosis.

The genetic pattern of inheritance

Learning outcomes

After studying this section, you should be able to:

- describe the basis of autosomal inheritance, including the relevance of recessive and dominant genes

- explain how sex-linked characteristics are passed from one generation to the next.

Mixing up of parental genes during meiosis leads to the huge genetic variety of the human race. It is important to understand how genes interact to produce inherited characteristics.

Autosomal inheritance

Each of a pair of homologous chromosomes contains genes for the same traits. For example, the ability to roll one's tongue is coded for on a single gene. Because one chromosome of each pair is inherited from the father and one from the mother, an individual has two genes controlling the ability to roll the tongue. Such paired genes are called *alleles*. Corresponding alleles contain genes concerned with the same trait, but they need not be identical. An individual may have:

- two identical forms of the gene (*homozygous*)
- two different forms of the gene (*heterozygous*).

One copy of the tongue-rolling gene may code for the ability to roll the tongue, but the corresponding gene on the other chromosome of the pair may be a different form and code for inability to tongue roll. This example involves only two forms of the same gene, but other characteristics are more complex. Eye colour is a diverse trait with a wide range of pigment colours and patterns possible, and is controlled by more than one gene.

Should an individual inherit a tongue-rolling gene from one parent, and the non-rolling gene from the other, he will be able to roll his tongue. This is because the tongue-rolling form of the gene is *dominant*, and takes priority over the non-rolling gene, which is *recessive*. Dominant genes are always *expressed* (active) in preference over recessive genes, and only one copy of a dominant gene is required for that characteristic to be expressed. A recessive gene can only be expressed if it is present on both chromosomes, i.e. individuals unable to tongue-roll have two copies of the recessive, non-rolling gene.

Individuals homozygous for a gene have two identical copies, of either the dominant or the recessive form. Heterozygous individuals have one dominant and one recessive gene.

Punnett squares

The probability of inheriting either form of a gene depends upon parental make-up. Simple autosomal inheritance can be illustrated using a Punnett square. Figure 17.8 shows all the possible combinations of the

437

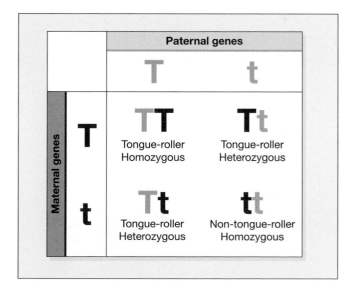

Figure 17.8 Autosomal inheritance. Example shows all possible combinations of tongue-rolling genes in children of parents heterozygous for the trait. T: dominant gene (tongue rolling); t: recessive gene (non-tongue rolling).

tongue-rolling gene in children whose parents are heterozygous for the trait. Using this example, there is a 3 in 4 (75%) chance that the child of these parents will be a tongue roller (TT or Tt), and only a 1 in 4 chance that they would inherit two recessive genes (tt), making them a non-roller.

Prediction of the probability that a baby will be born with an inherited disease e.g. cystic fibrosis, page 266, forms the basis of genetic counselling.

Sex-linked inheritance

The Y chromosome is shorter than, so carries fewer genes than, the X chromosome (Fig. 17.1). Traits coded for on the section of the X chromosome that has no corresponding material on the Y are said to be *sex linked*. The gene that codes for normal colour vision is one example, and is therefore carried on X chromosomes only. It is the dominant form of the gene. There is a rare, recessive form of this gene, which is faulty and codes for red–green colour blindness. If a female inherits a faulty copy of the gene, she is likely to have a normal gene on her other X chromosome, giving normal colour vision. A female carrying the colour blindness gene, even though she is not colour blind, may pass the faulty gene on to her children and is said to be a *carrier*. If the gene is abnormal in a male, he will be colour blind because, having only one X-chromosome, he has only one copy of the gene. Inheritance of colour blindness is shown in Figure 17.9. This illustrates the possible genetic combinations of the children of a carrier mother (one normal gene and one faulty gene) and a normal father (one normal gene).

438

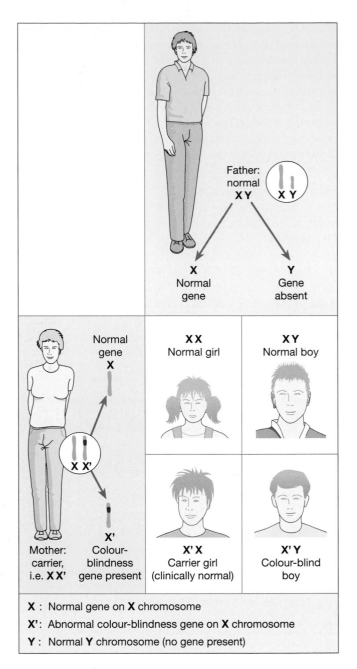

Figure 17.9 Inheritance of the sex-linked red–green colour blindness gene between generations.

Genetic basis of disease

Learning outcomes

After studying this section, you should be able to:

■ outline the link between cancer and cell mutation

■ distinguish between genetic disorders caused by gene mutation and chromosomal abnormalities, giving examples of each.

Cancer

Cancer (malignant growth of new tissue, p. 51) is caused by mutation (p. 434) of cellular DNA, causing its growth pattern to become disorganised and uncontrolled.

Inherited disease

Gene mutation

Many diseases, such as cystic fibrosis (p. 266) and haemophilia (p. 74), are passed directly from parent to child via a faulty gene. Many of these genes have been located by mapping of the human genome, e.g. the gene for cystic fibrosis is carried on chromosome 7. Other diseases, e.g. asthma, some cancers and cardiovascular disease, have a genetic component (run in the family). In these cases, a single faulty gene has not been identified, and inheritance is not as predictable as when a single gene is responsible.

Phenylketonuria

In this disorder, which is an example of an *inborn error of metabolism*, the gene responsible for producing the enzyme phenylalanine hydroxylase is faulty, and the enzyme is absent. This enzyme normally converts phenylalanine to tyrosine in the liver, but in its absence phenylalanine accumulates in the liver and overflows into the blood (Fig. 17.10). In high quantities, phenylalanine is toxic to the central nervous system and, if untreated, results in brain damage and mental retardation within a few months. Because there are low levels of tyrosine, which is needed to make melanin, depigmentation occurs and children are fair skinned and blonde. The incidence of this disease is now low in developed countries because screening of newborn babies detects the condition and treatment is provided.

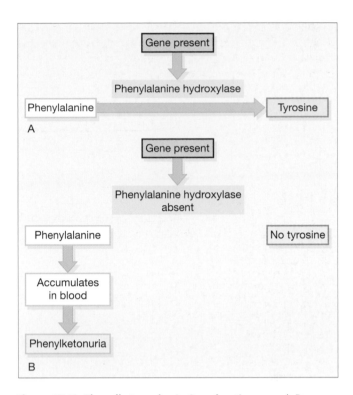

Figure 17.10 Phenylketonuria. A: Gene function normal. **B:** Abnormal gene.

Chromosomal abnormalities

Down syndrome

In this disorder, there are three copies of chromosome 21 (trisomy 21), meaning that an extra chromosome is present, caused by failure of chromosomes to separate normally during meiosis. People with Down syndrome are usually short of stature, with pronounced eyelid folds and flat, round faces. The tongue may be too large for the mouth and habitually protrudes. Learning disability is present, ranging from mild to severe. Life expectancy is shorter than normal, with a higher than average incidence of cardiovascular and respiratory disease. Down syndrome is associated with increasing maternal age, especially over 35 years.

Cri-du-chat syndrome

Cri-du-chat (cat's cry) refers to the characteristic meowing cry of an affected child. This syndrome is caused when part of chromosome 5 is missing, and is associated with learning disabilities and anatomical abnormalities, including gastrointestinal and cardiovascular problems.

439

The reproductive systems

18

The ability to reproduce is one of the properties distinguishing living from non-living matter. The more primitive the animal, the simpler the process of reproduction. In human beings the process is one of sexual reproduction, in which the male and female organs differ anatomically and physiologically.

Both males and females produce specialised reproductive germ cells, called *gametes*. The male gametes are called *spermatozoa* and the female gametes are called *ova*. They contain the genetic material, or *genes*, on *chromosomes*, which pass inherited characteristics on to the next generation. Other body cells possess 46 chromosomes arranged in 23 pairs but the gametes contain only 23, one from each pair. Gametes are formed by *meiosis* (p. 436). At *fertilisation*, the fusion of an ovum and a spermatozoon, the resulting cell is called a *zygote*, and now possesses the full complement of 46 chromosomes.

The zygote embeds itself in the wall of the uterus where it grows and develops during the 40-week *gestation period* before birth.

The functions of the female reproductive system are:

- formation of ova
- reception of spermatozoa
- provision of suitable environments for fertilisation and fetal development
- parturition (childbirth)
- lactation, the production of breast milk, which provides complete nourishment for the baby in its early life.

The functions of the male reproductive system are:

- production of spermatozoa
- transmission of spermatozoa to the female.

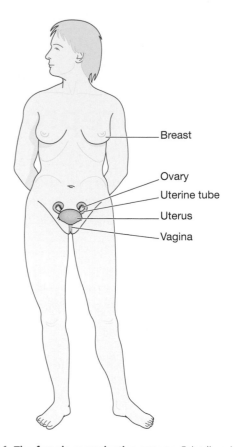

Figure 18.1 The female reproductive organs. Faint lines indicate the positions of the lower ribs and the pelvis.

The female reproductive organs, or genitalia, are divided into external and internal organs (Fig. 18.1).

Female reproductive system

Learning outcomes

After studying this section, you should be able to:

- describe the main structures of the external genitalia
- explain the structure and function of the vagina
- describe the location, structure and function of the uterus and the uterine tubes
- discuss the process of ovulation and the hormones that control it
- outline the changes that occur in the female at puberty, including the physiology of menstruation
- describe the structure and function of the female breast.

External genitalia (vulva)

The external genitalia (Fig. 18.2) are known collectively as the vulva, and consist of the labia majora and labia minora, the clitoris, the vaginal orifice, the vestibule, the hymen and the vestibular glands (Bartholin's glands).

Labia majora

These are the two large folds forming the boundary of the vulva. They are composed of skin, fibrous tissue and fat and contain large numbers of sebaceous glands. Anteriorly the folds join in front of the symphysis pubis, and posteriorly they merge with the skin of the perineum. At puberty, hair grows on the mons pubis and on the lateral surfaces of the labia majora.

Labia minora

These are two smaller folds of skin between the labia majora, containing numerous sebaceous glands.

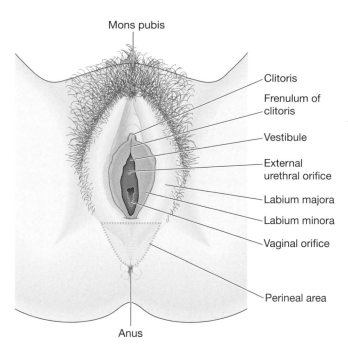

Mons pubis

Clitoris

Frenulum of clitoris

Vestibule

External urethral orifice

Labium majora

Labium minora

Vaginal orifice

Perineal area

Anus

Figure 18.2 The external genitalia of the female.

The cleft between the labia minora is the *vestibule*. The vagina, urethra and ducts of the greater vestibular glands open into the vestibule.

Clitoris
The clitoris corresponds to the penis in the male and contains sensory nerve endings and erectile tissue, but it has no reproductive significance.

Hymen
The hymen is a thin layer of mucous membrane that partially occludes the opening of the vagina. It is normally incomplete to allow for passage of menstrual flow.

Vestibular glands
The vestibular glands (Bartholin's glands) are situated one on each side near the vaginal opening. They are about the size of a small pea and have ducts, opening into the vestibule immediately lateral to the attachment of the hymen. They secrete mucus that keeps the vulva moist.

Blood supply, lymph drainage and nerve supply
Arterial supply. This is by branches from the internal pudendal arteries that branch from the internal iliac arteries and by external pudendal arteries that branch from the femoral arteries.

Venous drainage. This forms a large plexus which eventually drains into the internal iliac veins.

Lymph drainage. This is through the superficial inguinal nodes.

Nerve supply. This is by branches from pudendal nerves.

Perineum
The perineum is the area extending from the base of the labia minora to the anal canal. It is roughly triangular and consists of connective tissue, muscle and fat. It gives attachment to the muscles of the pelvic floor (p. 422).

Internal genitalia

The internal organs of the female reproductive system (Figs 18.3 and 18.4) lie in the pelvic cavity and consist of the vagina, uterus, two uterine tubes and two ovaries.

Vagina

The vagina is a fibromuscular tube lined with stratified squamous epithelium, connecting the external and internal organs of reproduction. It runs obliquely upwards and backwards at an angle of about 45° between the bladder in front and rectum and anus behind. In the adult, the anterior wall is about 7.5 cm long and the posterior wall about 9 cm long. The difference is due to the angle of insertion of the cervix through the anterior wall.

Structure of the vagina

The vagina has three layers: an outer covering of areolar tissue, a middle layer of smooth muscle and an inner lining of stratified squamous epithelium that forms ridges or *rugae*. It has no secretory glands but the surface is kept moist by cervical secretions. Between puberty and the menopause, *Lactobacillus acidophilus* bacteria are normally present, which secrete lactic acid, maintaining the pH between 4.9 and 3.5. The acidity inhibits the growth of most other microbes that may enter the vagina from the perineum.

Blood supply, lymph drainage and nerve supply
Arterial supply. An arterial plexus is formed round the vagina, derived from the uterine and vaginal arteries, which are branches of the internal iliac arteries.

Venous drainage. A venous plexus, situated in the muscular wall, drains into the internal iliac veins.

Lymph drainage. This is through the deep and superficial iliac glands.

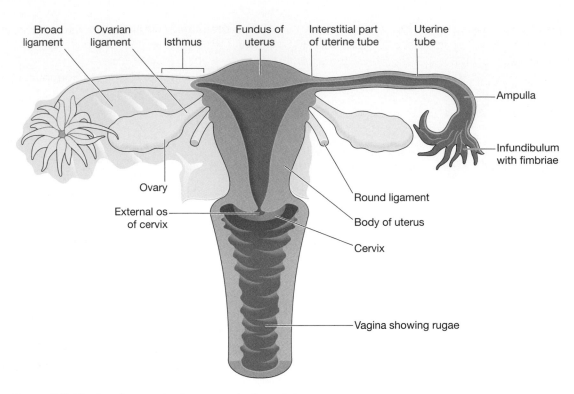

Figure 18.3 The female reproductive organs in the pelvis.

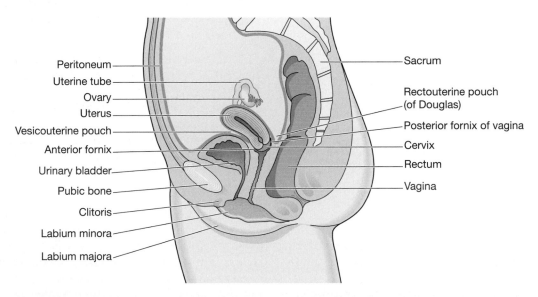

Figure 18.4 Lateral view of the female reproductive organs in the pelvis and their associated structures.

Nerve supply. This consists of parasympathetic fibres from the sacral outflow, sympathetic fibres from the lumbar outflow and somatic sensory fibres from the pudendal nerves.

Functions of the vagina

The vagina acts as the receptacle for the penis during coitus, and provides an elastic passageway through which the baby passes during childbirth.

Uterus

The uterus is a hollow muscular pear-shaped organ, flattened anteroposteriorly. It lies in the pelvic cavity between the urinary bladder and the rectum (Fig. 18.4).

In most women, it leans forward (*anteversion*), and is bent forward (*anteflexion*) almost at right angles to the vagina, so that its anterior wall rests partly against the bladder below, and forming the vesicouterine pouch between the two organs.

When the body is upright, the uterus lies in an almost horizontal position. It is about 7.5 cm long, 5 cm wide and its walls are about 2.5 cm thick. It weighs from 30 to 40 grams. The parts of the uterus are the fundus, body and cervix (Fig. 18.3).

Fundus. This is the dome-shaped part of the uterus above the openings of the uterine tubes.

Body. This is the main part. It is narrowest inferiorly at the *internal os* where it is continuous with the cervix.

Cervix ('neck' of the uterus). This protrudes through the anterior wall of the vagina, opening into it at the *external os.*

Structure

The walls of the uterus are composed of three layers of tissue: perimetrium, myometrium and endometrium (Fig. 18.5).

Perimetrium. This is peritoneum, which is distributed differently on the various surfaces of the uterus (Fig. 18.4).

Anteriorly it extends over the fundus and the body where it is folded on to the upper surface of the urinary bladder. This fold of peritoneum forms the *vesicouterine pouch.*

Posteriorly the peritoneum extends over the fundus, the body and the cervix, then it continues on to the rectum to form the *rectouterine pouch* (of Douglas).

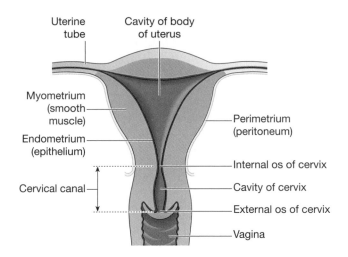

Figure 18.5 A section of the uterus.

Laterally, only the fundus is covered because the peritoneum forms a double fold with the uterine tubes in the upper free border. This double fold is the *broad ligament,* which, at its lateral ends, attaches the uterus to the sides of the pelvis.

Myometrium. This is the thickest layer of tissue in the uterine wall. It is a mass of smooth muscle fibres interlaced with areolar tissue, blood vessels and nerves.

Endometrium. This consists of columnar epithelium containing a large number of mucus-secreting tubular glands. It is divided functionally into two layers.

- The *functional layer* is the upper layer and it thickens and becomes rich in blood vessels in the first half of the menstrual cycle. If the ovum is not fertilised and does not implant, this layer is shed during menstruation.
- The *basal layer* lies next to the myometrium, and is not lost during menstruation. It is the layer from which the fresh functional layer is regenerated during each cycle.

The upper two-thirds of the cervical canal is lined with this mucous membrane. Lower down, however, the mucosa changes, becoming stratified squamous epithelium, which is continuous with the lining of the vagina itself.

Blood supply, lymph drainage and nerve supply
Arterial supply. This is by the uterine arteries, branches of the internal iliac arteries. They pass up the lateral aspects of the uterus between the two layers of the broad ligaments. They supply the uterus and uterine tubes and join with the ovarian arteries to supply the ovaries.

445

Venous drainage. The veins follow the same route as the arteries and eventually drain into the internal iliac veins.

Lymph drainage. Deep and superficial lymph vessels drain lymph from the uterus and the uterine tubes to the aortic lymph nodes and groups of nodes associated with the iliac blood vessels.

Nerve supply. The nerves supplying the uterus and the uterine tubes consist of parasympathetic fibres from the sacral outflow and sympathetic fibres from the lumbar outflow.

Supporting structures

The uterus is supported in the pelvic cavity by surrounding organs, muscles of the pelvic floor and ligaments that suspend it from the walls of the pelvis (Fig. 18.6).

Broad ligaments. These are formed by a double fold of peritoneum, one on each side of the uterus. They hang down from the uterine tubes as though draped over them and at their lateral ends they are attached to the sides of the pelvis. The uterine tubes are enclosed in the upper free border and near the lateral ends they penetrate the posterior wall of the broad ligament and open into the peritoneal cavity. The ovaries are attached to the posterior wall, one on each side. Blood and lymph vessels and nerves pass to the uterus and uterine tubes between the layers of the broad ligaments.

Round ligaments. These are bands of fibrous tissue between the two layers of broad ligament, one on each side of the uterus. They pass to the sides of the pelvis then through the *inguinal canal* to end by fusing with the labia majora.

Uterosacral ligaments. These originate from the posterior walls of the cervix and vagina and extend backwards, one on each side of the rectum, to the sacrum.

Transverse cervical (cardinal) ligaments. These extend one from each side of the cervix and vagina to the side walls of the pelvis.

Pubocervical fascia. This extends forward from the transverse cervical ligaments on each side of the bladder and is attached to the posterior surface of the pubic bones.

Functions of the uterus

After puberty, the endometrium of the uterus goes through a regular monthly cycle of changes, the *menstrual cycle*, under the control of hypothalamic and anterior pituitary hormones (see Ch. 9). The purpose of the cycle is to prepare the uterus to receive, nourish and protect a fertilised ovum. The cycle is usually regular, lasting between 26 and 30 days. If the ovum is not fertilised a new cycle begins with a short period of bleeding (menstruation).

If the ovum is fertilised the zygote embeds itself in the uterine wall. The uterine muscle grows to accommodate the developing baby, which is called an *embryo* during its first 8 weeks, and a *fetus* for the remainder of the pregnancy. Uterine secretions nourish the ovum before it implants in the endometrium, and after implantation the rapidly expanding ball of cells is nourished by the endometrial cells themselves. This is sufficient for only the first few weeks and the *placenta* is the organ that takes over thereafter (see Ch. 5). The placenta, which is attached to the fetus by the umbilical cord, is firmly attached to the wall of the uterus, and provides the route by which the growing baby receives oxygen and nutrients, and gets rid of its wastes. During pregnancy, which normally lasts about 40 weeks, the muscular walls of the uterus are prevented from contracting and expelling the baby early by high levels of the hormone progesterone secreted by the placenta. At the end of pregnancy (at term) the hormone oestrogen, which increases uterine contractility, becomes the predominant sex hormone in the blood. Additionally, oxytocin is released from the posterior pituitary, and also stimulates the uterine muscle. Control of oxytocin release is by positive feedback (see also Fig. 9.5, p. 217). During labour, the uterus forcefully expels the baby by means of powerful rhythmical contractions.

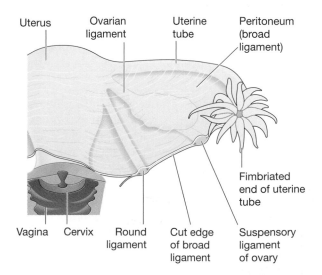

Uterus Ovarian ligament Uterine tube Peritoneum (broad ligament)

Fimbriated end of uterine tube

Vagina Cervix Round ligament Cut edge of broad ligament Suspensory ligament of ovary

Figure 18.6 The main ligaments supporting the uterus. Only one side is shown.

Uterine tubes

The uterine (Fallopian) tubes (Fig. 18.3) are about 10 cm long and extend from the sides of the uterus between the body and the fundus. They lie in the upper free border of the broad ligament and their trumpet-shaped lateral ends penetrate the posterior wall, opening into the peritoneal cavity close to the ovaries. The end of each tube has fingerlike projections called *fimbriae*. The longest of these is the *ovarian fimbria*, which is in close association with the ovary.

Structure

The uterine tubes have an outer covering of peritoneum (broad ligament), a middle layer of smooth muscle and are lined with ciliated epithelium.

Blood supply, lymph drainage and nerve supply

These are as for the uterus.

Functions

The uterine tubes move the ovum from the ovary to the uterus by peristalsis and ciliary movement. The mucus secreted by the mucosa provides ideal conditions for movement of ova and spermatozoa. Fertilisation of the ovum usually takes place in the uterine tube, and the zygote is propelled into the uterus for implantation.

Ovaries

The ovaries (Fig. 18.3) are the female gonads (glands producing sex hormones and the ova), and they lie in a shallow fossa on the lateral walls of the pelvis. They are 2.5 to 3.5 cm long, 2 cm wide and 1 cm thick. Each is attached to the upper part of the uterus by the *ovarian ligament* and to the back of the broad ligament by a broad band of tissue, the *mesovarium*. Blood vessels and nerves pass to the ovary through the mesovarium (Fig. 18.7).

Structure of the ovaries

The ovaries have two layers of tissue.

Medulla. This lies in the centre and consists of fibrous tissue, blood vessels and nerves.

Cortex. This surrounds the medulla. It has a framework of connective tissue, or *stroma*, covered by *germinal epithelium*. It contains *ovarian follicles* in various stages of maturity, each of which contains an ovum. Before puberty the ovaries are inactive but the stroma already contains immature (primordial) follicles, which the female has from birth. During the childbearing years, about every 28 days, one ovarian follicle (Graafian follicle) matures, ruptures and releases its ovum into the peritoneal cavity. This is called *ovulation* and it occurs during most menstrual cycles (Fig. 18.7).

447

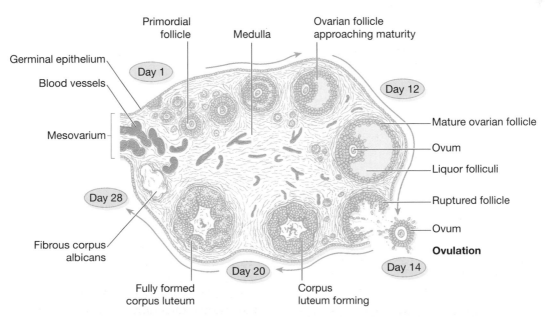

Figure 18.7 A section of an ovary showing the stages of development of one ovarian follicle.

Blood supply, lymph drainage and nerve supply

Arterial supply. This is by the ovarian arteries, which branch from the abdominal aorta just below the renal arteries.

Venous drainage. This is into a plexus of veins behind the uterus from which the ovarian veins arise. The right ovarian vein opens into the inferior vena cava and the left into the left renal vein.

Lymph drainage. This is to the lateral aortic and preaortic lymph nodes. The lymph vessels follow the same route as the arteries.

Nerve supply. The ovaries are supplied by parasympathetic nerves from the sacral outflow and sympathetic nerves from the lumbar outflow.

Functions

Maturation of the follicle is stimulated by follicle stimulating hormone (FSH) from the anterior pituitary, and oestrogen secreted by the follicle lining cells. Ovulation is triggered by a surge of luteinising hormone (LH) from the anterior pituitary, which occurs a few hours before ovulation. After ovulation, the follicle lining cells develop into the *corpus luteum* (yellow body), under the influence of LH from the anterior pituitary. The corpus luteum produces the hormone progesterone and some oestrogen. If the ovum is fertilised it embeds itself in the wall of the uterus where it grows and develops and produces the hormone *human chorionic gonadotrophin* (hCG), which stimulates the corpus luteum to continue secreting progesterone and oestrogen for the first 3 months of the pregnancy (Figs 18.8 and 18.9), after which time this function is continued by the placenta. If the ovum is not fertilised the corpus luteum degenerates and a new cycle begins with menstruation. At the site of the degenerate corpus luteum an inactive mass of fibrous tissue forms, called the *corpus albicans*. Sometimes more than one follicle matures at a time, releasing two or more ova in the same cycle. When this happens and the ova are fertilised the result is a multiple pregnancy.

Puberty in the female

Puberty is the age at which the internal reproductive organs reach maturity. This is called the *menarche*, and marks the beginning of the childbearing period. The ovaries are stimulated by the gonadotrophins from the anterior pituitary: follicle stimulating hormone and luteinising hormone.

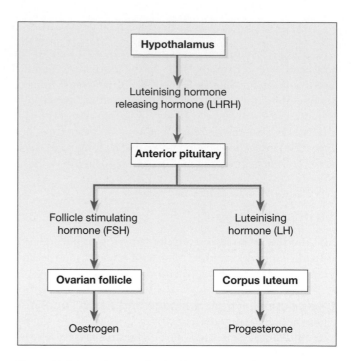

Figure 18.8 Female reproductive hormones and target tissues.

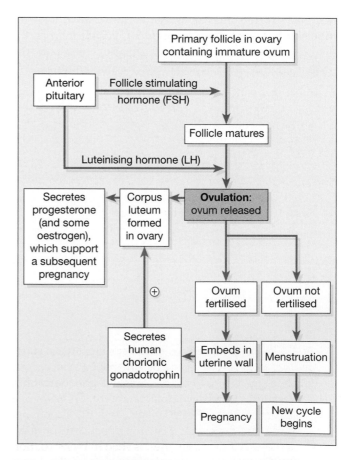

Figure 18.9 Summary of the stages of development of the ovum and the associated hormones.

The age of puberty varies between 10 and 14 years and a number of physical and psychological changes take place at this time:

- the uterus, the uterine tubes and the ovaries reach maturity
- the menstrual cycle and ovulation begin (menarche)
- the breasts develop and enlarge
- pubic and axillary hair begins to grow
- increase in height and widening of the pelvis
- increased fat deposited in the subcutaneous tissue, especially at the hips and breasts.

The menstrual cycle

This is a series of events, occurring regularly in females every 26 to 30 days throughout the childbearing period of about 36 years (Fig. 18.10). The cycle consists of a series of changes taking place concurrently in the ovaries and uterine walls, stimulated by changes in blood concentrations of hormones (Fig. 18.10B and D). Hormones secreted in the cycle are regulated by negative feedback mechanisms.

The hypothalamus secretes luteinising hormone releasing hormone (LHRH), which stimulates the anterior pituitary to secrete (see Table 9.1, p. 212):

- follicle stimulating hormone (FSH), which promotes the maturation of ovarian follicles and the secretion of oestrogen, leading to ovulation
- luteinising hormone (LH), which triggers ovulation, stimulates the development of the corpus luteum and the secretion of progesterone.

The hypothalamus responds to changes in the blood levels of oestrogen and progesterone. It is switched off by high levels and stimulated when they are low.

The average length of the menstrual cycle is about 28 days. By convention the days of the cycle are numbered from the beginning of the *menstrual phase* of the menstrual cycle, which usually lasts about 4 days. This is followed by the *proliferative phase* (about 10 days), then by the *secretory phase* (about 14 days).

Menstrual phase

When the ovum is not fertilised, the corpus luteum starts to degenerate. (In the event of pregnancy, the corpus luteum is supported by human chorionic gonadotrophin (hCG) secreted by the developing embryo). Progesterone and oestrogen levels therefore fall, and the functional layer of the endometrium, which is dependent on high levels of these ovarian hormones, is shed in menstruation (Fig. 18.10C). The menstrual flow consists of the secretions from endometrial glands, endometrial cells, blood

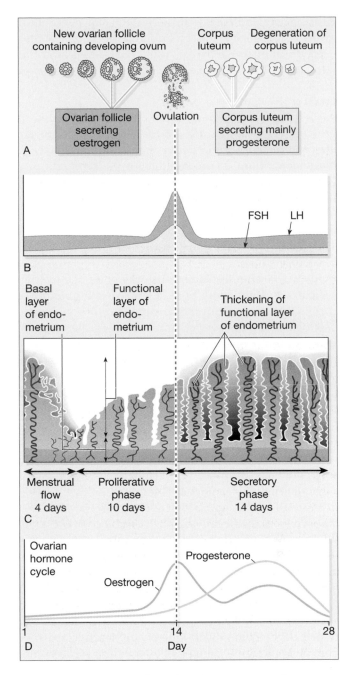

Figure 18.10 Summary of one female menstrual cycle:
A. Ovarian cycle; maturation of follicle and development of corpus luteum. B. Anterior pituitary cycle; LH and FSH levels. C. Uterine cycle; menstrual, proliferative and secretory phases. D. Ovarian hormone cycle; oestrogen and progesterone levels.

from the broken down capillaries and the unfertilised ovum.

High circulating levels of ovarian progesterone and oestrogen inhibit the anterior pituitary, blocking the release of FSH and LH, and should pregnancy occur then rising oestrogen and progesterone levels therefore prevent the maturation and release of another ovum.

449

After degeneration of the corpus luteum, however, falling levels of oestrogen and progesterone lead to resumed anterior pituitary activity, rising FSH levels and the initiation of the next cycle.

Proliferative phase

At this stage an ovarian follicle, stimulated by FSH, is growing towards maturity and is producing oestrogen, which stimulates proliferation of the functional layer of the endometrium in preparation for the reception of a fertilised ovum. The endometrium thickens, becoming very vascular and rich in mucus-secreting glands. This phase ends when ovulation occurs and oestrogen production by the follicle declines.

Secretory phase

Immediately after ovulation, the cells lining the ovarian follicle are stimulated by LH and develop into the corpus luteum, which produces progesterone and some oestrogen. Under the influence of progesterone, the endometrium becomes oedematous and the secretory glands produce increased amounts of watery mucus. This is believed to assist the passage of the spermatozoa through the uterus to the uterine tubes where the ovum is usually fertilised. There is a similar increase in the secretion of watery mucus by the glands of the uterine tubes and by cervical glands that lubricate the vagina.

The ovum may survive in a fertilisable form for a very short time after ovulation, probably as little as 8 hours. The spermatozoa, deposited in the vagina during intercourse, may be capable of fertilising the ovum for only about 24 hours although they can survive for several days. This means that the period in each cycle during which fertilisation can occur is relatively short. Observable changes in the woman's body occur around the time of ovulation. Cervical mucus, normally thick and dry, becomes thin, elastic and watery, and body temperature rises by a small but measurable amount immediately following ovulation. Some women experience abdominal discomfort in the middle of the cycle, thought to correspond to rupture of the follicle and release of its contents into the abdominal cavity.

If the ovum is not fertilised, menstruation occurs and a new cycle begins.

If the ovum is fertilised there is no breakdown of the endometrium and no menstruation. The fertilised ovum (zygote) travels through the uterine tube to the uterus where it becomes embedded in the wall and produces human chorionic gonadotrophin (hCG), which is similar to anterior pituitary luteinising hormone. This hormone keeps the corpus luteum intact, enabling it to continue secreting progesterone and oestrogen for the first 3 to 4 months of the pregnancy, inhibiting the maturation of further ovarian follicles (Fig. 18.9). During that time the placenta develops and produces oestrogen, progesterone and gonadotrophins.

Menopause

The menopause (climacteric) usually occurs between the ages of 45 and 55 years, marking the end of the child-bearing period. It may occur suddenly or over a period of years, sometimes as long as 10 years, and is caused by changes in sex hormone levels. The ovaries gradually become less responsive to FSH and LH, and ovulation and the menstrual cycle become irregular, eventually ceasing. Several other phenomena may occur at the same time, including:

- short-term unpredictable vasodilatation with flushing, sweating and palpitations, causing discomfort and disturbance of the normal sleep pattern
- shrinkage of the breasts
- axillary and pubic hair become sparse
- atrophy of the sex organs
- episodes of uncharacteristic behaviour, e.g. irritability, mood changes
- gradual thinning of the skin
- loss of bone mass predisposing to osteoporosis (p. 426)
- slow increase in blood cholesterol levels that increase the risk of cardiovascular disease in postmenopausal women to that in males of the same age.

Similar changes occur after bilateral irradiation or surgical removal of the ovaries.

Breasts

The breasts or *mammary glands* are accessory glands of the female reproductive system. They exist also in the male, but in only a rudimentary form.

In the female, the breasts are small and immature until puberty. Thereafter they grow and develop under the influence of oestrogen and progesterone. During pregnancy these hormones stimulate further growth. After the baby is born the hormone *prolactin* from the anterior pituitary stimulates the production of milk, and *oxytocin* from the posterior pituitary stimulates the release of milk in response to the stimulation of the nipple by the sucking baby, by a positive feedback mechanism.

Structure

The mammary glands (Fig. 18.11) consist of glandular tissue, fibrous tissue and fatty tissue.

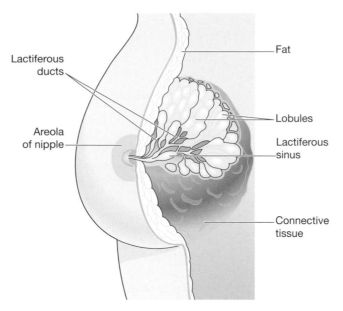

Lactiferous ducts

Fat

Lobules

Areola of nipple

Lactiferous sinus

Connective tissue

Figure 18.11 Structure of the breast.

Each breast consists of about 20 lobes of glandular tissue, each lobe being made up of a number of lobules that radiate around the nipple. The lobules consist of a cluster of alveoli that open into small ducts, and these unite to form large excretory ducts, called *lactiferous ducts*. The lactiferous ducts converge towards the centre of the breast where they form dilatations or reservoirs for milk. Leading from each dilatation, or *lactiferous sinus*, is a narrow duct that opens on to the surface at the nipple. Fibrous tissue supports the glandular tissue and ducts. Fat covers the surface of the gland and is also found between the lobes.

The nipple. This is a small conical eminence at the centre of the breast surrounded by a pigmented area, the *areola*. On the surface of the areola are numerous sebaceous glands (Montgomery's tubercles), which lubricate the nipple during lactation.

Blood supply, lymph drainage and nerve supply
Arterial supply. The breasts are supplied with blood from the thoracic branches of the axillary arteries and from the internal mammary and intercostal arteries.

Venous drainage. This is formed by an anastomotic circle round the base of the nipple from which branches carry the venous blood to the circumference, and end in the axillary and mammary veins.

Lymph drainage (see Fig. 6.1, p. 132). This is mainly into the superficial axillary lymph vessels and nodes. Lymph may drain through the internal mammary nodes if the superficial route is obstructed.

Nerve supply. The breasts are supplied by branches from the 4th, 5th and 6th thoracic nerves, which contain sympathetic fibres. There are numerous somatic sensory nerve endings in the breast, especially around the nipple. When these touch receptors are stimulated by sucking, impulses pass to the hypothalamus and the flow of the hormone oxytocin is increased, promoting the release of milk.

Functions

The mammary glands are only active during late pregnancy and after childbirth, when they produce milk (lactation). Lactation is stimulated by the hormone prolactin (p. 215).

Male reproductive system

Learning outcomes

After studying this section, you should be able to:

- describe the structure and function of the testes
- outline the structure and function of the spermatic cords
- describe the secretions that pass into the spermatic fluid
- explain the process of ejaculation
- list the main changes occurring at puberty in the male.

The male reproductive system is shown in Figure 18.12.

Scrotum

The scrotum is a pouch of deeply pigmented skin, fibrous and connective tissue and smooth muscle. It is divided into two compartments each of which contains one testis, one epididymis and the testicular end of a spermatic cord. It lies below the symphysis pubis, in front of the upper parts of the thighs and behind the penis.

Testes

The testes (Fig. 18.13A and B) are the reproductive glands of the male and are the equivalent of the ovaries in the female. They are about 4.5 cm long, 2.5 cm wide and 3 cm thick and are suspended in the scrotum by the spermatic cords. They are surrounded by three layers of tissue.

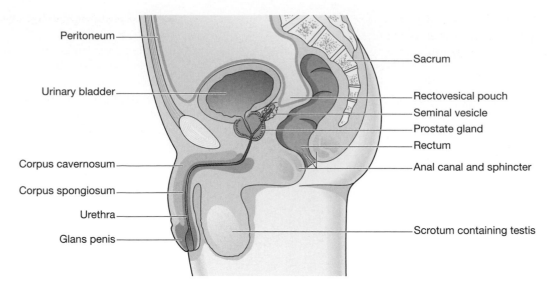

Figure 18.12 The male reproductive organs and their associated structures.

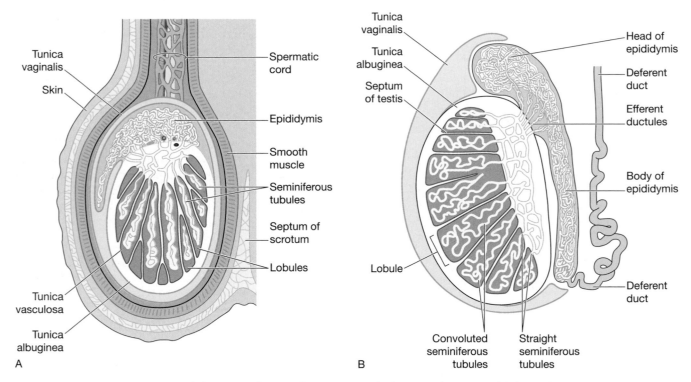

Figure 18.13 The testis: A. Section of the testis and its coverings. B. Longitudinal section of a testis and deferent duct.

Tunica vaginalis. This is a double membrane, forming the outer covering of the testes, and is a downgrowth of the abdominal and pelvic peritoneum. During early fetal life, the testes develop in the lumbar region of the abdominal cavity just below the kidneys. They then descend into the scrotum taking with them coverings of peritoneum, blood and lymph vessels, nerves and the deferent duct. The peritoneum eventually surrounds the testes in the scrotum, and becomes detached from the abdominal peritoneum. Descent of the testes into the scrotum should be complete by the 8th month of fetal life.

Tunica albuginea. This is a fibrous covering beneath the tunica vaginalis that surrounds the testes. Ingrowths form septa, dividing the glandular structure of the testes into *lobules*.

Tunica vasculosa. This consists of a network of capillaries supported by delicate connective tissue.

Structure of the testes

In each testis are 200 to 300 lobules, and within each lobule are 1 to 4 convoluted loops composed of *germinal epithelial cells*, called *seminiferous tubules*. Between the tubules are groups of *interstitial cells (of Leydig)* that secrete the hormone testosterone after puberty. At the upper pole of the testis the tubules combine to form a single tubule. This tubule, about 6 m in its full length, is repeatedly folded and tightly packed into a mass called the epididymis. It leaves the scrotum as the *deferent duct* (vas deferens) in the *spermatic cord*. Blood and lymph vessels pass to the testes in the spermatic cords.

Functions

Spermatozoa (sperm) are produced in the seminiferous tubules of the testes, and mature as they pass through the long and convoluted epididymis, where they are stored. The hormone controlling sperm production is FSH from the anterior pituitary (p. 215). A mature sperm (Fig. 18.14) has a head, a body, and a long whip-like tail used for motility. The head is almost completely filled by the nucleus, containing its DNA. It also contains the enzymes required to penetrate the outer layers of the ovum to reach, and fuse with, its nucleus. The body of the sperm is packed with mitochondria, to fuel the propelling action of the tail that powers the sperm along the female reproductive tract.

Successful spermatogenesis takes place at a temperature about 3 °C below normal body temperature. The testes are cooled by their position outside the abdominal cavity,

and the thin outer covering of the scrotum has very little insulating fat.

Spermatic cords

The spermatic cords suspend the testes in the scrotum. Each cord contains a testicular artery, testicular veins, lymphatics, a deferent duct and testicular nerves, which come together to form the cord from their various origins in the abdomen. The cord, which is covered in a sheath of smooth muscle and connective and fibrous tissues, extends through the inguinal canal (p. 422) and is attached to the testis on the posterior wall.

Blood supply, lymph drainage and nerve supply
Arterial supply. The testicular artery branches from the abdominal aorta, just below the renal arteries.

Venous drainage. The testicular vein passes into the abdominal cavity. The left vein opens into the left renal vein and the right into the inferior vena cava.

Lymph drainage. This is through lymph nodes around the aorta.

Nerve supply. This is provided by branches from the 10th and 11th thoracic nerves.

The deferent duct
This is some 45 cm long. It passes upwards from the testis through the inguinal canal and ascends medially towards the posterior wall of the bladder where it is joined by the duct from the *seminal vesicle* to form the *ejaculatory duct* (Fig. 18.15).

453

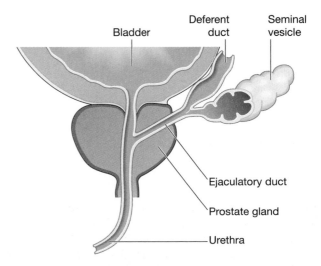

Figure 18.15 Section of the prostate gland and associated reproductive structures on one side.

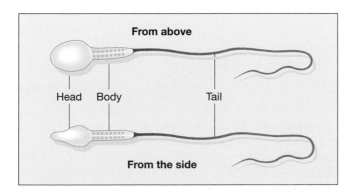

Figure 18.14 A spermatozoon.

Seminal vesicles

The seminal vesicles are two small fibromuscular pouches lined with columnar epithelium, lying on the posterior aspect of the bladder (Fig. 18.15).

At its lower end each seminal vesicle opens into a short duct, which joins with the corresponding deferent duct to form an ejaculatory duct.

Functions

The seminal vesicles contract and expel their stored contents, seminal fluid, during ejaculation. Seminal fluid, which forms 60% of the bulk of the fluid ejaculated at male orgasm, contains nutrients to support the sperm during their journey through the female reproductive tract.

Ejaculatory ducts

The ejaculatory ducts are two tubes about 2 cm long, each formed by the union of the duct from a seminal vesicle and a deferent duct. They pass through the prostate gland and join the prostatic urethra, carrying seminal fluid and spermatozoa to the urethra (Fig. 18.15).

The ejaculatory ducts are composed of the same layers of tissue as the seminal vesicles.

Prostate gland

The prostate gland (Fig. 18.15) lies in the pelvic cavity in front of the rectum and behind the symphysis pubis, surrounding the first part of the urethra. It consists of an outer fibrous covering, a layer of smooth muscle and glandular substance composed of columnar epithelial cells.

Functions

The prostate gland secretes a thin, milky fluid that makes up about 30% of *semen*, and gives it its milky appearance. It contains a clotting enzyme, which thickens the semen in the vagina, increasing the likelihood of semen being retained close to the cervix.

Urethra and penis

Urethra

The male urethra provides a common pathway for the flow of urine and semen, the combined secretions of the male reproductive organs. It is about 19 to 20 cm long and consists of three parts. The *prostatic urethra* originates at the urethral orifice of the bladder and passes through the prostate gland. The *membranous urethra* is the shortest and narrowest part and extends from the prostate gland to the bulb of the penis, after passing through the perineal membrane. The *spongiose* or *penile urethra* lies within the corpus spongiosum of the penis and terminates at the external urethral orifice in the *glans penis*.

There are two urethral sphincters (Fig. 18.16). The *internal sphincter* consists of smooth muscle fibres at the neck of the bladder above the prostate gland. The *external sphincter* consists of skeletal muscle fibres surrounding the membranous part.

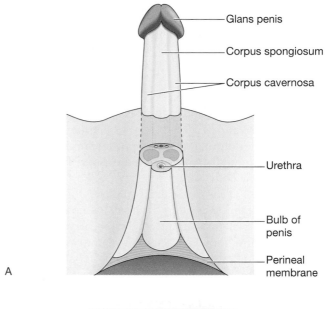

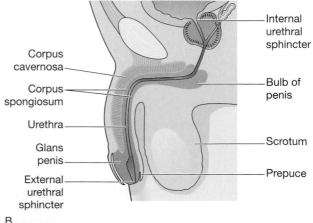

Figure 18.16 The penis: A: Viewed from below. **B:** Viewed from the side.

Penis

The penis (Fig. 18.16) has a *root* and a *body*. The root lies in the perineum and the body surrounds the urethra. It is formed by three cylindrical masses of *erectile tissue* and smooth muscle. The erectile tissue is supported by fibrous tissue and covered with skin and has a rich blood supply.

The two lateral columns are called the *corpora cavernosa* and the column between them, containing the urethra, is the *corpus spongiosum*. At its tip it is expanded into a triangular structure known as the *glans penis*. Just above the glans the skin is folded upon itself and forms a movable double layer, the *foreskin* or *prepuce*. Arterial blood is supplied by deep, dorsal and bulbar arteries of the penis, which are branches from the internal pudendal arteries. A series of veins drain blood to the internal pudendal and internal iliac veins. The penis is supplied by autonomic and somatic nerves. Parasympathetic stimulation leads to filling of the spongy erectile tissue with blood, caused by arteriolar dilatation and venoconstriction, which increases blood flow into the penis and obstructs outflow. The penis therefore becomes engorged and erect, essential for intercourse.

Ejaculation

During ejaculation, which occurs at male orgasm, spermatozoa are expelled from the epididymis and pass through the deferent duct, the ejaculatory duct and the urethra. The semen is propelled by powerful rhythmical contraction of the smooth muscle in the walls of the deferent duct; the muscular contractions are sympathetically mediated. Muscle in the walls of the seminal vesicles and prostate gland also contracts, adding their contents to the fluid passing through the genital ducts. The force generated by these combined processes leads to emission of the semen through the external urethral sphincter (Fig. 18.17).

Sperm comprise only 10% of the final ejaculate, the remainder being made up of seminal and prostatic fluids, which are added to the sperm during male orgasm, as well as mucus produced in the urethra. Semen is slightly

455

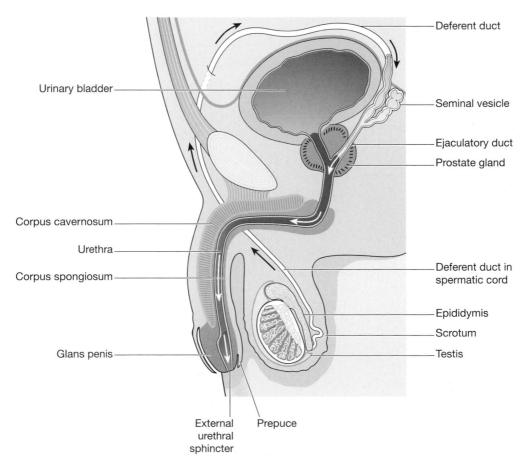

Figure 18.17 **Section of the male reproductive organs.** Arrows show the route taken by spermatozoa during ejaculation.

alkaline, to neutralise the acidity of the vagina. Between 2 and 5 ml of semen are produced in a normal ejaculate, and contain between 40 and 100 million spermatozoa per ml. If not ejaculated, sperm gradually lose their fertility after several months and are reabsorbed by the epididymis.

Puberty in the male

This occurs between the ages of 10 and 14. Luteinising hormone from the anterior lobe of the pituitary gland stimulates the interstitial cells of the testes to increase the production of testosterone. This hormone influences the development of the body to sexual maturity. The changes occurring at puberty are:

- growth of muscle and bone and a marked increase in height and weight
- enlargement of the larynx and deepening of the voice – it 'breaks'
- growth of hair on the face, axillae, chest, abdomen and pubis
- enlargement of the penis, scrotum and prostate gland
- maturation of the seminiferous tubules and production of spermatozoa
- the skin thickens and becomes oilier.

In the male, fertility and sexual ability tend to decline gradually with ageing. The secretion of testosterone gradually declines, usually beginning at about 50 years of age. There is no period comparable to the female menopause.

Sexually transmitted infections

Learning outcomes

After studying this section, you should be able to:

- list the principal causes of sexually transmitted infections

- explain the effects of sexually transmitted infections.

Infection of the reproductive system may be classified as:

- *non-specific*, usually caused by a mixture of microbes, e.g. staphylococci, streptococci, coliform bacteria, *Clostridium perfringens*
- *specific*, caused by sexually transmitted microbes, the most common of which being *Neisseria gonorrhoeae, Trichomonas vaginalis*, chlamydia, herpes viruses, human immunodeficiency virus (HIV) and hepatitis B.

Microbes that cause sexually transmitted infections are unable to survive outside the body for long periods and have no intermediate host.

Chlamydia

The microbe *Chlamydia trachomatis* causes inflammation of the female cervix. Infection may ascend through the reproductive tract and cause pelvic inflammatory disease. In the male, it may cause urethritis, which may also ascend and lead to epididymitis. Chlamydia infection is often present in conjunction with other sexually transmitted diseases. The same organism causes trachoma, an eye infection that is the primary cause of blindness worldwide (p. 208).

Gonorrhoea

This is caused by *Neisseria gonorrhoeae*, which affects the mucosa of the reproductive and urinary tracts. In the male, suppurative urethritis occurs and the infection may spread to the prostate gland, epididymis and testes. In the female the infection may spread from vulvar glands, vagina and cervix to the body of the uterus, uterine tubes, ovaries and peritoneum. Healing by fibrosis in the female may cause obstruction of the uterine tubes, leading to infertility. In the male it may cause urethral stricture.

Non-venereal transmission of gonorrhoea may cause *neonatal ophthalmia* in babies born to infected mothers. The eyes are infected as the baby passes through the vagina.

Syphilis

This disease is caused by *Treponema pallidum*. There are three clearly marked stages although the third is now rarely seen in Britain. After an incubation period of several weeks, the *primary sore* (chancre) appears at the site of infection, e.g. the vulva, vagina, perineum, penis or round the mouth. In the female the primary sore may be undetected if it is internal. After several weeks the chancre subsides spontaneously. *Secondary lesions* appear 3 to 4 months after infection. They consist of skin rashes and raised papules (condylomata lata) on the external genitalia and vaginal walls. These subside after several months and are followed by a latent period of a variable number of years. *Tertiary lesions* (gummas) then develop in many organs, and may involve the nervous system, leading to general paralysis.

Sexual transmission occurs during the primary and secondary stages when discharge from lesions contains microbes. Congenital transmission occurs when microbes from an infected mother cross the placenta to the fetus, often with fatal consequences. Accidental spread of infection may occur by blood transfusion if a donor's blood is taken during the incubation period after microbes have spread to the blood from the site of infection.

Trichomonas vaginalis

These protozoa cause acute vulvovaginitis. It is usually sexually transmitted and is commonly present in women with gonorrhoea.

Candidiasis

The yeast *Candida albicans* (see also p. 316) is frequently a commensal in the normal vagina and causes no problems. It is normally prevented from flourishing by vaginal acidity, but in certain circumstances it proliferates, causing candidiasis (thrush). Common precipitating factors include:

- antibiotic therapy, which kills the bacteria that keep vaginal pH low
- pregnancy
- reduced immune function.

Acquired immune deficiency syndrome (AIDS) and hepatitis B infection

These viral conditions may be sexually transmitted, but there are no local signs of infection. For a description of AIDS and HIV see page 381 and hepatitis B page 330.

457

Diseases of the female reproductive system

Learning outcomes

After studying this section, you should be able to:

- describe the causes and consequences of pelvic inflammatory disease
- discuss the disorders of the vulva
- define the term imperforate hymen
- outline the causes and effects of cervical carcinoma
- discuss the main pathologies of the uterus and uterine tubes
- describe the causes and effects of ovarian disease
- describe the causes of female infertility
- discuss the principal disorders of the female breast.

Pelvic inflammatory disease (PID)

This condition is usually caused by sexually transmitted infections. It usually begins as vulvovaginitis and may spread upwards to the cervix, uterus, uterine tubes and ovaries. Upward spread can also occur when infection is present in the vagina before a surgical procedure, childbirth or miscarriage, especially if some of the products of conception are retained.

Complications of PID include:

- infertility due to obstruction of uterine tubes
- peritonitis
- intestinal obstruction due to adhesions between the bowel and the uterus and/or uterine tubes
- bacteraemia, which may lead to meningitis, endocarditis or suppurative arthritis
- Bartholin's gland abscess or cyst formation if the duct is blocked.

Vulvar dystrophies

Atrophic dystrophy

This is thinning of vulvar epithelium and the formation of fibrous tissue, occurring after the menopause due to oestrogen withdrawal. It predisposes to infection, especially in debilitated women, and to malignant epithelial neoplasia.

Vulvar intraepithelial neoplasia (VIN)

This refers to early neoplastic (cancerous) changes in epithelial cells of the vulva. It is commonest in younger women, often those infected with human papilloma virus, and may proceed to malignancy (see also cervical intraepithelial neoplasia, below).

Imperforate hymen

This congenital abnormality may not be noticed until the onset of menstruation. When complete (imperforate), the hymen forms a barrier in the vagina. Blood accumulates in the vagina, uterus and uterine tubes with each menstrual cycle, and it may enter the peritoneal cavity and cause peritonitis. The uterine tubes may become obstructed by coagulated blood, leading to infertility.

Disorders of the cervix

Cervical carcinoma

Dysplastic changes, referred to as *cervical intraepithelial neoplasia* (CIN) begin in the deepest layer of cervical epithelium, usually at the junction of the stratified squamous epithelium of the lower third of the cervical canal with the secretory epithelium of the upper two-thirds. Dysplasia may progress to involve the full thickness of epithelium. Not all dysplasias develop into malignant disease, but it is not possible to predict how far development will go, and whether it will remain static or regress. Three degrees of dysplasia have been described, although clear distinction between them is not always possible:

- CIN 1 = mild grade
- CIN 2 = moderate grade
- CIN 3 = high grade.

CIN 3 may progress to invasive carcinoma. Early spread is via lymph nodes and local spread is commonly to the uterus, vagina, bladder and rectum. In the late stages spread via the blood to the liver, lungs and bones may occur.

The disease takes 15 to 20 years to develop and it occurs mostly between 35 and 50 years of age. It is likely that a significant proportion of cases are due to the transmission of some sexually transmitted carcinogen. Risk factors include having frequent sexual intercourse with multiple partners from an early age, all of which increase the likelihood of being exposed to a carcinogenic agent. Barrier contraceptives protect against the disease. The human papillomavirus (HPV), which causes genital warts, is strongly associated with this cancer (see also p. 365).

Disorders of the uterine body

Endometritis

This is usually caused by non-specific infection, following childbirth or miscarriage, especially if fragments of membranes or placenta have been retained in the uterus. It may also be caused by an intrauterine contraceptive device (IUD). The inflammation may subside after removal of retained products or the IUD. The infection may spread to surrounding pelvic structures e.g. uterine tubes, or deeper layers of the uterus.

Endometriosis

This is the growth of endometrial tissue outside the uterus, most commonly in the ovaries, uterine tubes and other pelvic structures. The ectopic tissue, like the uterine endometrium, responds to fluctuations in sex hormone levels during the menstrual cycle, causing menstrual-type bleeding into the lower abdomen and, in the ovaries, the formation of coloured cysts, 'chocolate cysts'. There is intermittent pain due to swelling, and recurrent haemorrhage causes fibrous tissue formation. Ovarian endometriosis may lead to pelvic inflammation, infertility and extensive pelvic adhesions, involving the ovaries, uterus, uterine ligaments and the bowel. The cause is not clear but one theory is that menstrual material may have leaked from the uterus through the uterine tubes and into the peritoneum where it established itself.

Adenomyosis

This is the growth of endometrium within the myometrium. The ectopic tissue may cause general or localised uterine enlargement. The lesions may cause dysmenorrhoea and irregular excessive bleeding (menorrhagia), usually beginning between 40 and 50 years of age.

Endometrial hyperplasia

Hyperplasia of the endometrium is associated with high blood oestrogen levels, e.g. in obesity, oestrogen therapy or an ovarian tumour. Sometimes it is associated with increased risk of malignant change.

Leiomyoma (fibroid, myoma)

These are very common, often multiple, benign tumours of myometrium. They are firm masses of smooth muscle encapsulated in compressed muscle fibres and they vary greatly in size. Large tumours may undergo degenerative changes if they outgrow their blood supply, leading to necrosis, fibrosis and calcification. They develop during the reproductive period and may be hormone dependent, enlarging during pregnancy and when oral contraceptives are used. They tend to regress after the menopause. Large tumours may cause pelvic discomfort, frequency of micturition, menorrhagia, irregular bleeding, dysmenorrhoea and reduced fertility. Malignant change is rare.

Endometrial carcinoma

This occurs mainly in nulliparous women (i.e. women who have never been pregnant) between 50 and 60 years of age. The incidence is increased when an oestrogen-secreting tumour is present and in women who are obese, hypertensive or diabetic, because they tend to have a high level of blood oestrogen. The tumour may develop as a diffuse mass, a localised plaque or a polyp and there is often ulceration and bleeding. Endometrium has no lymphatics, so lymph spread is delayed until there is extensive local spread that involves other pelvic structures. Distant metastases, spread in blood or lymph, develop later, most commonly in the liver, lungs and bones. Invasion of the ureters leads to hydronephrosis and uraemia, commonly the cause of death.

Disorders of the uterine tubes and ovaries

Acute salpingitis

Salpingitis is inflammation of the uterine tubes. It is usually due to infection spreading from the uterus, and only occasionally from the peritoneal cavity. The uterine tubes may be left permanently damaged by fibrous scar tissue, which can cause obstruction and infertility. Infection may spread into the peritoneum and involve the ovaries.

Ectopic pregnancy

This is the implantation of a fertilised ovum outside the uterus, most commonly in a uterine tube. As the fetus grows the tube may rupture and its contents enter the peritoneal cavity, causing acute inflammation (peritonitis) and possibly severe intraperitoneal haemorrhage.

Ovarian tumours

The majority of ovarian tumours are benign, usually occurring between 20 and 45 years of age. The rest occur mostly between 45 and 65 years and are divided between borderline malignancy (low-grade cancer) and frank malignancy. There are three main types of cells involved: epithelial cells, germ cells and hormone-secreting cells, called sex-cord stroma cells.

Epithelial cell tumours

Most of these are borderline or malignant tumours. They vary greatly in size from very large to quite small and some are partly cystic. Large tumours may cause pressure, leading to gastrointestinal disturbances, frequency of micturition, dysuria and ascites. Those suspended by a pedicle may twist, causing ischaemia, necrosis, haemorrhage or rupture of a cyst. The principal methods of spread are invasion of local and peritoneal structures. Later lymph- and blood-spread metastases may develop.

They are more common in developed societies and in the higher socioeconomic groups. Pregnancy and suppression of ovulation by the oral contraceptive pill may have a protective effect due to a reduction in the number of ovulatory menstrual cycles.

Germ cell ovarian tumours

These occur mainly in children and young adults and only a few are malignant. Benign *dermoid cysts* are the most common type. These are thick-walled cysts containing a variety of uncharacteristic tissues, e.g. hair, skin, epithelium or teeth. They are usually small and have a tendency to twist on a pedicle, causing ischaemia and necrosis.

Sex-cord stroma cell tumours

These cells are the precursors of the cells lining the ovarian follicles, luteal cells and fibrous supporting cells. Mixed tumours develop, some of which secrete hormones. Oestrogen-secreting tumours cause precocious sexual development in children. In adults the excess oestrogen may cause endometrial hyperplasia, endometrial carcinoma, cystic disease of the breast or breast cancer. Androgen-secreting tumours occasionally develop, causing atrophy of the breast and genitalia and the development of male sex characteristics.

Metastatic ovarian tumours

The ovaries are a common site of metastatic spread from primary tumours in other pelvic organs, the breast, stomach, pancreas and biliary tract.

Female infertility

This may be due to:

- blockage of uterine tubes, often the consequence of pelvic inflammatory disease
- anatomical abnormalities, e.g. retroversion (tilting backwards) of the uterus
- endocrine factors; any abnormalities of the glands and hormones governing the menstrual cycle can interfere with, for example, ovulation or the uterine cycle

- low body weight, e.g. in anorexia nervosa, or severe malnourishment
- endometriosis.

Disorders of the breast

Mastitis (inflammation of the breast)

Acute non-suppurative mastitis

This occurs during lactation and is associated with painful congestion and oedema of the breast. It is of hormonal origin.

Acute suppurative (pyogenic) mastitis

The microbes enter through a nipple abrasion caused by the infant sucking. The most common causative microbes are *Staphylococcus aureus* and *Streptococcus pyogenes* usually acquired by the infant while in hospital. The infection spreads along the mammary ducts of a lobe causing localised swelling and redness. If it does not resolve it can become chronic and an abscess may form.

Tumours of the breast

Benign tumours

Most breast tumours (90%) are benign. Fibroadenomas are the commonest type and occur any time after puberty; incidence peaks in the third decade. Some are cystic and some solid, and they usually occur in women nearing the menopause. They may originate from secretory cells, fibrous tissue or from ducts.

Malignant tumours

The most common types of tumour are usually painless lumps found in the upper outer quadrant of the breast. There is considerable fibrosis around the tumour that may cause retraction of the nipple and necrosis and ulceration of the overlying skin. It is increasingly common between 35 and 70 years.

Early spread beyond the breast is via lymph to the axillary and internal mammary nodes. Local invasion involves the pectoral muscles and the pleura. Blood-spread metastases may occur later in many organs and bones, especially lumbar and thoracic vertebrae. The causes of breast cancer are not known, but an important predisposing factor appears to be high oestrogen exposure. Women with an early menarche, a late menopause, and no pregnancies have a higher than normal risk because they experience more menstrual cycles in their lifetimes, and each monthly cycle brings with it the oestrogen surge seen during the proliferative phase (p. 450). A genetic component is also likely, with close relatives of breast cancer sufferers having a significantly elevated risk of developing the disease. One per cent of all breast cancer occurs in men.

Diseases of the male reproductive system

Infections of the penis

Inflammation of the glans and prepuce may be caused by a specific or non-specific infection. In non-specific infections, or *balanitis*, lack of personal hygiene is an important predisposing factor, especially if *phimosis* is present, i.e. the orifice in the foreskin (prepuce) is too small to allow for its normal retraction. If the infection becomes chronic there may be fibrosis of the foreskin, which increases the phimosis.

Infections of the urethra

Gonococcal urethritis is the most common specific infection. Non-specific infection may be spread from the bladder (cystitis) or be introduced during catheterisation, cystoscopy or surgery. Both types may spread throughout the system to the prostate, seminal vesicles, epididymis and testes. If infection becomes chronic, fibrosis may cause urethral stricture or obstruction, leading to retention of urine.

Epididymis and testes

Infections

Non-specific epididymitis and orchitis are usually due to spread of infection from the urethra, commonly following prostatectomy. The microbes may spread either through the deferent duct (vas deferens) or via lymph.

Specific epididymitis. This is usually caused by gonorrhoea spread from the urethra.

Orchitis (inflammation of the testis). This is commonly caused by mumps virus, blood-borne from the parotid glands. Acute inflammation with oedema occurs about 1 week after the appearance of parotid swelling. The infection is usually unilateral but, if bilateral, severe damage to germinal epithelium of the seminiferous tubules may result in sterility.

Undescended testis (cryptorchidism)

During embryonic life the testes develop within the abdominal cavity, but descend into the scrotum prior to birth. If they fail to do this and the condition is not corrected, infertility is likely to follow and the risk of testicular cancer is increased.

Hydrocele

This is the most common form of scrotal swelling and is accumulation of serous fluid in the tunica vaginalis. The onset may be acute and painful or chronic. It may be congenital or be secondary to another disorder of the testis or epididymis.

Testicular tumours

Most testicular tumours are malignant, the commonest malignancies in young men. They occur in childhood and early adulthood when the affected testis has not descended or has been late in descending into the scrotum. The tumour tends to remain localised for a considerable time but eventually spreads in lymph to pelvic and abdominal lymph nodes, and more widely in the blood. Occasionally, hormone-secreting tumours develop and may cause precocious development in boys.

Prostate gland

Infections

Acute prostatitis is usually caused by non-specific infection, spread from the urethra or bladder, often following catheterisation, cystoscopy, urethral dilatation or prostate surgery. Chronic infection may follow an acute attack. Fibrosis of the gland may occur during healing, causing urethral stricture or obstruction.

Benign prostatic enlargement

Hyperplastic nodules form around the urethra and may obstruct the flow of urine, causing urinary retention.

Urethral stricture may prevent the bladder emptying completely during micturition, predisposing to infection, which may spread upwards, causing pyelonephritis and other complications. Prostatic enlargement is common in men over 50, affecting up to 70% of men aged over 70. The cause is not clear, but it may be an acceleration of the ageing process associated with the decline in androgen secretion, which changes the androgen/oestrogen balance.

Malignant prostatic tumours

These are a relatively common cause of death in men over 50. The carcinogen is not known but changes in the androgen/oestrogen balance may be significant or viruses may be involved. Invasion of local tissues is widespread before lymph-spread metastases develop in pelvic and abdominal lymph nodes. Blood-spread metastases in bone are common and bone formation rather than bone destruction is a common feature. Lumbar vertebrae are common sites, possibly due to retrograde spread along the walls of veins. Bone metastases are often the first indication of malignant prostatic tumours.

Breast

Breast tissue in men consists of ducts and stroma only.

Gynaecomastia

This is proliferation of breast tissue in men. It usually affects only one breast and is benign. It is common in adolescents and older men, and is often associated with:

- endocrine disorders, especially those associated with high oestrogen levels
- cirrhosis of the liver (p. 331)
- malnutrition
- some drugs, e.g. chlorpromazine, spironolactone, digoxin
- Klinefelter's syndrome, a genetic disorder with testicular atrophy and absence of spermatogenesis.

Malignant tumours

These develop in a small number of men, usually in the older age groups.

Male infertility

This may be due to:

- endocrine disorders
- obstruction of the deferent duct
- failure of erection or ejaculation during intercourse
- vasectomy
- suppression of spermatogenesis by e.g. ionising radiation, chemotherapy and other drugs.

Normal values

Note. Some biological measures have been extracted from the text and listed here for easy reference. In some cases slightly different 'normals' may be found in other texts and used by different medical practitioners.

Metric measures, units and SI symbols

Name	SI unit	Symbol
Length	metre	m
Mass	kilogram	kg
Amount of substance	mole	mol
Pressure	pascal	Pa
Energy	joule	J

Decimal multiples and submultiples of the units are formed by the use of standard prefixes.

Multiple	Prefix	Symbol	Submultiple	Prefix	Symbol
10^6	mega	M	10^{-1}	deci	d
10^3	kilo	k	10^{-2}	centi	c
10^2	hecto	h	10^{-3}	milli	m
10^1	deca	da	10^{-6}	micro	μ
			10^{-9}	nano	n
			10^{-12}	pico	p
			10^{-15}	femto	f

Conversion table for kPa/mmHg (for e.g. capillary pressures)

1 mmHg	=	0.13 kPa
1 kPa	=	7.5 mmHg
35 mmHg	=	4.7 kPa
25 mmHg	=	3.3 kPa
15 mmHg	=	2.0 kPa
10 mmHg	=	1.3 kPa

Hydrogen ion concentration (pH)

Neutral = 7   Acid = 0 to 7   Alkaline = 7 to 14

Normal pH of some body fluids	
Blood	7.35 to 7.45
Saliva	5.8 to 7.4
Gastric juice	1.5 to 3.5
Bile	6.0 to 8.5
Urine	4.5 to 8.0

Some normal plasma levels in adults

Calcium	2.12 to 2.62 mmol/l	(8.5 to 10.5 mg/100 ml)
Chloride	97 to 106 mmol/l	(97 to 106 mEq/l)
Cholesterol	3.6 to 6.7 mmol/l	(140 to 260 mg/100 ml)
Glucose	3.5 to 8 mmol/l	(63 to 144 mg/100 ml)
Fasting glucose	3.6 to 5.8 mmol/l	(65 to 105 mg/100 ml)
Potassium	3.3 to 4.7 mmol/l	(3.3 to 4.7 mEq/l)
Sodium	135 to 143 mmol/l	(135 to 143 mEq/l)
Urea	2.5 to 6.6 mmol/l	(15 to 44 mg/100 ml)

Arterial blood gases

PO_2	12 to 15 kPa	(90 to 110 mmHg)
PCO_2	4.5 to 6 kPa	(34 to 46 mmHg)
Bicarbonate	21 to 27.5 mmol/l	
H^+ ions	36 to 44 nmol/l	(7.35 to 7.45 pH units)

Blood pressure
Normal adult 120/80 mmHg.
Blood pressure above 140/90 is generally considered high.

Heart rate
At rest	60 to 80/min
Sinus bradycardia	< 60/min
Sinus tachycardia	> 100/min

Respiration rate
At rest 15 to 18/min
Tidal volume	500 ml
Dead space	150 ml
Alveolar ventilation	15 (500 – 150) = 5.25 l/min

Blood count
Leukocytes	$4 \times 10^9/l$	to	$11 \times 10^9/l$
Neutrophils	$2.5 \times 10^9/l$	to	$7.5 \times 10^9/l$
Eosinophils	$0.04 \times 10^9/l$	to	$0.44 \times 10^9/l$
Basophils	$0.015 \times 10^9/l$	to	$0.1 \times 10^9/l$
Monocytes	$0.2 \times 10^9/l$	to	$0.8 \times 10^9/l$
Lymphocytes	$1.5 \times 10^9/l$	to	$3.5 \times 10^9/l$
Erythrocytes			
female	$3.8 \times 10^{12}/l$	to	$5 \times 10^{12}/l$
male	$4.5 \times 10^{12}/l$	to	$6.5 \times 10^{12}/l$
Thrombocytes	$200 \times 10^9/l$	to	$350 \times 10^9/l$

Diet
Vitamins. Daily requirements see pages 274 to 276.
1 kilocalorie (kcal) = 4.182 kilojoules (kJ)
1 kilojoule   = 0.24 kilocalories

Energy source	Energy released	Recommended proportion in diet
Carbohydrate	1 g = 17 kJ = 4 kcal	55–75%
Protein	1 g = 17 kJ = 4 kcal	10–15%
Fat	1 g = 38 kJ = 9 kcal	15–30%

Urine
Specific gravity	1.020 to 1.030
Volume excreted	1000 to 1500 ml/day

Glucose is normally absent, but appears in urine when blood glucose levels exceed 9 mmol/l

Body temperatures
Normal	36.8°C: axillary
Hypothermia	≤35°C: core temperature
Death when below	25°C

Cerebrospinal fluid pressure
Lying on the side 60–180 mm H_2O

Intraocular pressure
1.3 to 2.6 kPa (10 to 20 mmHg)

Bibliography

Bass P, Carr N, du Boulay C 2004 Master medicine – Pathology, Churchill Livingstone, Edinburgh

Boron W F, Boulpaep E L 2003 Medical Physiology, Saunders, Philadelphia

Bull P D 1996 Diseases of the ear, nose and throat, 8th edn. Blackwell Science, Oxford

Campbell P N, Smith A D 2000 Biochemistry illustrated, 4th edn. Churchill Livingstone, Edinburgh

Department of Health 1991 Dietary reference values of food energy and nutrients for the UK: COMA report. HMSO, London

Drake-Lee A 1996 Clinical otorhinolaryngology, Churchill Livingstone, New York

Garrow J S, James E P T, Ralph A 2000 Human nutrition and dietetics, 10th edn. Churchill Livingstone, Edinburgh

Guyton A C, Hall J E 2000 Textbook of medical physiology, 10th edn. W B Saunders, Philadelphia

Haslett C, Chilvers E R, Boon N A, Colledge N R (eds) 2002 Davidson's principles and practice of medicine, 19th edn. Churchill Livingstone, Edinburgh

Huether S E, McCance K L (eds) 2004 Understanding pathophysiology, 3rd edn Mosby, Missouri

James B, Chew C, Bron A 1997 Ophthalmology, 8th edn. Blackwell Science, Oxford

Kumar P, Clark M (eds) 2002 Clinical medicine, 5th edn. W B Saunders, Edinburgh

Klug W S, Cummings M R 2002 Essentials of genetics, 4th edn. Prentice Hall, New Jersey

Martini F H 2004 Fundamentals of anatomy and physiology, 6th edn. Prentice Hall, New Jersey

Mathews C K, van Holde K E, Ahern K G 2000 Biochemistry, 3rd edn. Benjamin Cummings, San Francisco

Merck manual of diagnosis and therapy 1999 17th edn. Merck Research Laboratories, New Jersey

Mirpuri N, Patel P 1998 Crash course: renal and urinary systems, Mosby, New York

Mueller R F, Young I D 2001 Emery's Elements of medical genetics, 11th edn. Churchill Livingstone, Edinburgh

Roitt I, Brostoff J, Male D 2001 Immunology, 6th edn. Mosby, New York

Selby C 2002 Respiratory Medicine, Churchill Livingstone, Edinburgh

Timbury, M C, McCartney A C, Thakker B, Ward K N 2002 Notes on medical microbiology, Churchill Livingstone, Edinburgh

Thibodeau G A, Patton K T 1999 Anatomy and physiology, 4th edn. Mosby, St Louis

Tortora G J and Grabowski S R 2003 Principles of anatomy and physiology, 10th edn. John Wiley & Sons Inc, New Jersey

Underwood J C E (ed) 2004 General and systematic pathology, 4th edn. Churchill Livingstone, Edinburgh

Vander A J, Sherman J H, Luciano D 1998 Human physiology – the mechanisms of body function, 7th edn. McGraw-Hill, Boston

Van Way C W, Ireton-Jones C 2004 Nutrition secrets, 2nd edn. Hanley & Belfus, Pennsylvania

Williams P L, Bannister L H, Berry M M et al (eds) 1995 Gray's anatomy – the anatomical basis of medicine and surgery, 38th edn. Churchill Livingstone, New York

Young B, Heath J W 2000 Wheater's functional histology – a text and colour atlas, 4th edn. Churchill Livingstone, Edinburgh

Index

Page numbers in **bold** refer to main discussions of anatomy and physiology. Those in ***bold italics*** refer to main discussions of diseases. Page numbers referring to anatomy and physiology are in ordinary type. Those referring to diseases are in *italics*.

A

Abdominal cavity, **47–49**
 arterial supply, 102–104
 contents, 48, 49
 lymph nodes, 135
 regions, 49
 venous return, 104, 105
Abdominal wall
 muscles, 420, **421–422**
 nerves, 167
Abducent nerve (cranial nerve VI), 168, **169**, 202
Abduction, 408, 409
ABO blood group system, 62–63
Abscess, *373*
 deep-seated, *373*
 liver, *331*
 lung, *262*
 pelvic, *322*
 subphrenic, *321, 322*
 superficial, *373*
Absorption, 282–283, **310**
 in large intestine, 303
 by skin, 362
 in small intestine, 300–301
 in stomach, 297
Accessory nerve (cranial nerve XI), 168, **169**
Accommodation, of eyes to light, 200
Acetabular labrum, 412, 413
Acetabulum, 403, 412, 413
Acetylcholine, 146, 147
 in autonomic nervous system, 170
 in neuromuscular transmission, 160, 416–417
Acetyl co-enzyme A, 315
Achalasia, *319*
Achilles (calcanean) tendon, 424, 425
Achondroplasia, *427*
Acid–base balance, 22, 343
Acidosis, 22–23, *351*
Acids, **21–23**
Acne vulgaris, *365–366*
Acoustic meatus, external, 190–191, 392
Acquired disease, *15*
Acquired immune deficiency syndrome (AIDS), *183*, ***381–382***, *457*
Acromegaly, *225, 226*
Acromioclavicular joint, 401
Acromion process, 401
ACTH *see* Adrenocorticotrophic hormone
Actin, 415, 416
Action potential, 143, **144–145**
Acute disease, *15*
Acute disseminating encephalomyelitis, *184*
Acute idiopathic inflammatory polyneuropathy, *187*
Acute lymphoblastic leukaemia (ALL), *73*

Acute myeloblastic leukaemia (AML), *73*
Acute renal failure, *350–351*
Acute tubular necrosis (ATN), *350–351*
Adam's apple, 242
Addisonian crisis, *231*
Addison's disease, ***231***
Adduction, 408, 409
Adductor muscles, hip, 424, 425
Adenocarcinoma, *51*
 oesophagus, *319*
Adenohypophysis *see* Pituitary gland, anterior
Adenoids (pharyngeal tonsils), 241
 enlarged, *257*
Adenoma, *51*
Adenomyosis, uterine, *459*
Adenosine diphosphate (ADP), 24, 25, 66
Adenosine triphosphate *see* ATP
ADH *see* Antidiuretic hormone
Adhesions, *322, 374*
Adipocytes, 36
Adipose tissue, 37
 brown, 37
 subcutaneous, 359
 white, 37
ADP (adenosine diphosphate), 24, 25, 66
Adrenal (suprarenal) arteries, 102, 103, 220
Adrenal cortex, **220–222**
 acute insufficiency, *231*
 chronic insufficiency, ***231***
 disorders, ***229–231***
Adrenal glands, **220–222**
 autonomic control, 173
 response to stress, 222, 223
Adrenaline (epinephrine), 146, 173, **222**, 312
 excess secretion, *128, 231*
 heart rate and, 88
Adrenal medulla, **222**
 disorders, ***231***
 tumours, *231*
Adrenal (suprarenal) veins, 104, 220
Adrenocorticoids, 220–222
Adrenocorticotrophic hormone (ACTH), **215**, 216, 220
 deficiency, *230*
 hypersecretion, *229*
Adult respiratory distress syndrome (ARDS), *266*
Adventitia, **284–285**
Aerobic metabolism, 23, 312–313
Aetiology, *14, 15*
Afferent nerves *see* Sensory nerves
Afterload, 88
Agranulocytes, 63, **65–66**
Agranulocytosis, *72*
AIDS (acquired immune deficiency syndrome), *183*, ***381–382***, *457*
Air, 238

alveolar, 253
 composition, 253
 control of entry into lungs, 249
 expired, 253
 filtering/cleaning, 240, 244, 245
 humidification, 240, 241, 244, 245, 250
 passages, 239–240
 warming, 240, 241, 244, 245, 250
Air sinuses *see* Paranasal sinuses
Airway(s)
 conducting, 247, 248
 fibrosis, in chronic bronchitis, *258*
 obstruction, *265*
 resistance, 252
 upper, 239–240, 241, 244
Albinos, 196
Albumin, 58, *349*
Aldosterone, **221**, 343
 function, 221, 340
 hypersecretion, *230–231*
 hyposecretion, *230, 231*
 regulation of secretion, 341
Aldosteronism *see* Hyperaldosteronism
Alimentary canal, 11–12, 282
 adventitia (serosa), **284–285**
 basic structure, **283–286**
 mucosa, 285–286
 muscle layer, 285
 nerve supply, 286
 submucosa, 285
 see also specific parts
Alkalis, **21–23**
Alkalosis, 22–23
Alleles, 437
Allergen, 65, *379*
Allergic disorders
 asthma, *259*
 conjunctivitis, *208*
 rhinitis, *258*
Allergic reactions, 13, 65, ***379***, *380*
All-or-none law, 417
Alpha$_1$-antitrypsin deficiency, *260*
Altitude, high, 71
Alveolar ducts, 248
Alveolar hypoventilation, *266*
Alveolar ridges, 287, 394
Alveolar ventilation, 253, 464
Alveoli, 11, 248, **249–250**
 air in, 253
 functions, 250
 gas exchange, 253, 254
Alveolitis, extrinsic allergic, *264*
Alzheimer's disease, *181*
Amenorrhoea, *225*
Amino acids, 23–24, **272**
 absorption, 300
 codons, 435
 deamination, 307, 314
 energy release, 314

Main anatomy and physiology: **bold**. Main diseases: ***bold italics***. Anatomy & physiology: ordinary type. Diseases: *italics*.

Main anatomy and physiology: **bold**. Main diseases: ***bold italics***. Anatomy & physiology: ordinary type. Diseases: *italics*.

469

Main anatomy and physiology: **bold**. Main diseases: ***bold italics***. Anatomy & physiology: ordinary type. Diseases: *italics*.

Main anatomy and physiology: **bold**. Main diseases: ***bold italics***. Anatomy & physiology: ordinary type. Diseases: *italics*.

Main anatomy and physiology: **bold**. Main diseases: ***bold italics***. Anatomy & physiology: ordinary type. Diseases: *italics*.

Main anatomy and physiology: **bold**. Main diseases: ***bold italics***. Anatomy & physiology: ordinary type. Diseases: *italics*.

473

Main anatomy and physiology: **bold**. Main diseases: ***bold italics***. Anatomy & physiology: ordinary type. Diseases: *italics*.

474

Main anatomy and physiology: **bold**. Main diseases: ***bold italics***. Anatomy & physiology: ordinary type. Diseases: *italics*.

Main anatomy and physiology: **bold**. Main diseases: ***bold italics***. Anatomy & physiology: ordinary type. Diseases: *italics*.

Main anatomy and physiology: **bold**. Main diseases: ***bold italics***. Anatomy & physiology: ordinary type. Diseases: *italics*.

Main anatomy and physiology: **bold**. Main diseases: ***bold italics***. Anatomy & physiology: ordinary type. Diseases: *italics*.

Main anatomy and physiology: **bold**. Main diseases: ***bold italics***. Anatomy & physiology: ordinary type. Diseases: *italics*.

479

M

Main anatomy and physiology: **bold**. Main diseases: ***bold italics***. Anatomy & physiology: ordinary type. Diseases: *italics*.

Main anatomy and physiology: **bold**. Main diseases: ***bold italics***. Anatomy & physiology: ordinary type. Diseases: *italics*.

481

Main anatomy and physiology: **bold**. Main diseases: ***bold italics***. Anatomy & physiology: ordinary type. Diseases: *italics*.

Main anatomy and physiology: **bold**. Main diseases: ***bold italics***. Anatomy & physiology: ordinary type. Diseases: *italics*.

483

Main anatomy and physiology: **bold**. Main diseases: ***bold italics***. Anatomy & physiology: ordinary type. Diseases: *italics*.

Main anatomy and physiology: **bold**. Main diseases: ***bold italics***. Anatomy & physiology: ordinary type. Diseases: *italics*.

R

S

Main anatomy and physiology: **bold**. Main diseases: ***bold italics***. Anatomy & physiology: ordinary type. Diseases: *italics*.

Main anatomy and physiology: **bold**. Main diseases: ***bold italics***. Anatomy & physiology: ordinary type. Diseases: *italics*.

487

Main anatomy and physiology: **bold**. Main diseases: ***bold italics***. Anatomy & physiology: ordinary type. Diseases: *italics*.

Main anatomy and physiology: **bold**. Main diseases: ***bold italics***. Anatomy & physiology: ordinary type. Diseases: *italics*.

489

Main anatomy and physiology: **bold**. Main diseases: ***bold italics***. Anatomy & physiology: ordinary type. Diseases: *italics*.

Main anatomy and physiology: **bold**. Main diseases: ***bold italics***. Anatomy & physiology: ordinary type. Diseases: *italics*.